# NATIONAL
# OCCUPATIONAL THERAPY ASSISTANT
# CERTIFICATION EXAM
## REVIEW & STUDY GUIDE
## 2ND EDITION

**Rita P. Fleming-Castaldy, PhD, OTL, FAOTA**

University of Scranton
Scranton, PA

**TherapyEd**
Evanston, Illinois
United States of America

**TherapyEd**
500 Davis Street, Suite 512
Evanston, IL  60201
Telephone (847) 328-5361
FAX       (847) 328-5049
www.TherapyEd.com

# CONTRIBUTORS

**Marge E. Moffett Boyd, MPH, OTR/L**
Coordinator of Academic Studies and Fieldwork
Clinical Instructor, Program of Occupational Therapy
Dominican College
Orangeburg, New York

**Ann Burkhardt, OTD, OTR/L, FAOTA**
Director, Post-professional Online Master's Program
in Occupational Therapy
Quinnipiac University
Hamden, Connecticut

**Colleen De Ritis MA, OTR/L**
Senior Occupational Therapist
Meridian Nursing and Rehabilitation
Brick, New Jersey

**Josephine S. Dolera, PT**
Director of Rehabilitation
St. Barnabas Hospital
Bronx, NY 10457

**Jan G. Garbarini, MA, OTR/L**
Research Coordinator
Occupational Therapy Department
Dominican College
Orangeburg, New York

**Glen Gillen, EdD, OTR, FAOTA**
Associate Professor of Clinical Occupational Therapy
Programs in Occupational Therapy
Columbia University
College of Physicians and Surgeons
New York, New York

**Kari Inda, PhD, OTR**
Professional Entry Program Director
Occupational Therapy Department
Mount Mary College
Milwaukee, Wisconsin

**Linda Kahn-D'Angelo, PT, ScD**
Professor
Department of Physical Therapy
College of Health Professions
University of Massachusetts Lowell
Lowell, Massachusetts

**Regina Lehman, MS, OTR/L**
Assistant Vice President
St. Barnabas Hospital
Bronx, New York

**Colleen Maher, MS, OTR, CHT**
Assistant Professor of Occupational Therapy
Mercy College
Dobbs Ferry, New York

**Susan B. O'Sullivan, PT, EdD**
Professor
Department of Physical Therapy
School of Health and Environment
University of Massachusetts Lowell
Lowell, Massachusetts

**Janice Romeo, MA, OTR/L**
Retired, Seattle, WA
Formerly Student Coordinator
Rehabilitation Department
Hagedorn Psychiatric Hospital
Glen Gardner, New Jersey

**Julie Ann Starr, PT, MS, CCS**
Clinical Associate Professor and Chair
Physical Therapy Program
Department of Rehabilitation Sciences
Sargent College of Health and Rehabilitation Sciences
Boston University
Boston, Massachusetts

# ACKNOWLEDGEMENTS

Organizing the depth and breadth of occupational therapy assistant education and practice into a comprehensive review book and study guide can be a daunting task. It can easily become overwhelming if it were not for the capable assistance of others. Annemarie Erdman, Jenna Osborn, and John Patro, University of Scranton graduate assistants, completed essential background research to ensure that this text's content was current. They also provided key production assistance to facilitate the timely completion of this work. Judy Noe of TherapyEd helped obtain and track the copyright permissions which were needed to make sure that this text contained relevant tables and figures to support its content. Past editions of this text benefited from the excellent production and editorial assistance of Kathleen Smyth, personal administrative assistant. I would also like to thank Raymond Siegelman, President of TherapyEd, for his highly competent editorial critique of this work and his ongoing support in bringing this publication to press. A final thanks is due Ruthann Cassidy of Zographix for her expedient and high-quality typography and design of this final product.

# TABLE OF CONTENTS

## Preface

## SECTION I: The NBCOT Examination and Guidelines for Success

## Chapter 1: Certification of the Occupational Therapy Assistant

# Chapter 2: Principles of Effective Examination Preparation

# SECTION II: Foundational Concepts of OT Practice Across the Continuum of Care

# Chapter 3: The Process of Occupational Therapy

# Chapter 4: Professional Standards and Responsibilities

# Chapter 5: Human Development and Aging: Pediatric and Geriatric Practice Considerations for OT Practice

# SECTION III: Clinical Conditions, Disorders, and Diseases

# Chapter 6: Musculoskeletal System Disorders

# Chapter 7: Neurological System Disorders

# Chapter 8: Cardiovascular and Pulmonary System Disorders

# Chapter 9: Gastrointestinal, Renal-Genitourinary, Endocrine, Immunological, and Integumentary Systems Disorders

## Chapter 10: Psychiatric and Cognitive Disorders

# SECTION IV: Evaluation and Intervention Approaches for Occupational Therapy Practice

## Chapter 11: Biomechanical Approaches: Evaluation and Intervention

# Chapter 12: Neurological and Cognitive-Perceptual Approaches: Evaluation and Intervention

# Chapter 13: Psychosocial Approaches: Evaluation and Intervention

# Chapter 14: Evaluation and Intervention for Performance in Areas of Occupation

# Chapter 15: Mastery of the Environment: Evaluation and Intervention

# PREFACE

## PURPOSE OF THIS TEXT

This publication, *National Occupational Therapy Assistant Certification Exam Review & Study Guide,* is primarily designed to assist graduates of accredited occupational therapy assistant (OTA) education programs in their preparation for the certification examination for certified occupational therapy assistants (COTAs). However, since the publication of this text's first edition in 2005, many students have reported that it has served as an invaluable resource for them while they are completing their coursework and clinical affiliations. This *Review and Study Guide* provides a comprehensive overview of current OT practice according to the American Occupational Therapy Association's (AOTA's) *Practice Framework, Guide to Occupational Therapy Practice, and Standards of Practice*; therefore, it can also be helpful to practitioners who are new to the field, changing practice areas, and/or initiating a new role (e.g., fieldwork supervisor). The text chapters include all of the major content areas of the examination as determined by the National Board for Certification in Occupational Therapy (NBCOT). The reader should know that the text contributors did not have access to the actual content of the examination or to specific examination questions. The content of this study guide is based on the most recent OTA examination content outline provided by NBCOT (NBCOT, 2009).

Information that is prerequisite to competent OT practice (i.e., anatomy, physiology, kinesiology and theoretical models) is presented to provide the reader with a solid foundation to clinically reason through practice questions. Essential background material on the foundations of OT, OT tools of practice, clinical conditions, and practice standards is also provided to ensure that the reader acquires the knowledge and skills that NBCOT considers essential to perform professional tasks. Each chapter is presented in an outline format that is easy to read and provides a helpful guide for organizing a study plan.

Specific methods of evaluation and intervention are provided in chapters organized according to clinical approaches, rather than according to diagnosis. This holistic, integrative approach allows for in-depth coverage while eliminating redundancy and reductionism. It also makes this text compatible with a multitude of OTA curriculum designs. For example, the section on cognitive-perceptual approaches includes evaluation and intervention methods for cognitive-perceptual dysfunction that are relevant to many psychiatric and neurological disorders.

The text is not intended to be a substitute for primary resources, such as classroom lectures and course textbooks. However, upon reviewing each chapter's outline, the reader will be able to assess his/her level of comfort with, and mastery of, each content area. The identification of areas of strength can bolster confidence and the identification of weaker areas can help focus studying in an efficient and effective manner. Basically, by first using this text, the reader will not spend time extensively studying information already known; rather, specific areas in which further knowledge is required will be identified, and appropriate study time can be planned.

References are provided at the end of each chapter. These sources served as the foundation for each chapter's content and can supplement this text. Completion of this text's simulated examinations will also help the reader in evaluating his/her preparedness for the certification examination. Overall, the questions are designed to test mastery of basic and fundamental professional knowledge by asking for application of this knowledge to practice situations. Explanations are provided to help the reader understand why one answer is considered the best response and the others are incorrect. The critical analysis of responses to these test questions will provide additional information about areas requiring further study. The critical reasoning skills used to determine the correct responses to the simulated examination questions are also analyzed to provide additional information that can guide successful examination preparation.

# CHAPTER 1

# CERTIFICATION OF THE OCCUPATIONAL THERAPY ASSISTANT

Rita P. Fleming-Castaldy

## I. Credentialing Agencies

### A. National Board for Certification in Occupational Therapy (NBCOT)

1. NBCOT is currently the only national independent credentialing agency for occupational therapy assistants (OTAs) and occupational therapists (OTs).
2. NBCOT develops and implements all policies related to OT professional certification, including the national OTA and OT certification examinations and the certification renewal program.
   a. NBCOT holds the copyright to the designations Certified Occupational Therapy Assistant (COTA) and Occupational Therapist, Registered (OTR). Individuals not certified by NBCOT cannot use these credentials.
   b. NBCOT certification is not equivalent to state certification, licensure, or registration.
   c. NBCOT certification is initially granted for three years. Certification must be renewed every three years according to the procedures of the NBCOT Certification Renewal Program.

### B. State Regulatory Boards (SRBs)

1. SRBs are public bodies created by legislation to define and regulate the qualifications a professional must have to practice within his or her state.
2. State regulation may take the form of certification, registration, or licensure.
   a. Definitions of, and requirements for, state certification, registration or licensure vary from state to state.
   b. OTA practice is not regulated by all states. See text's Appendix 3 for contact information for each state.
3. It is against the law to practice OT without meeting state requirements for certification, registration, or licensure.
4. Most states accept a passing grade on the NBCOT certification examination as one qualifying criterion for initial state licensure, registration and/or certification.
   a. If you want your NBCOT certification examination score to be sent to an SRB you must indicate this on your application and pay a fee in accordance with NBCOT's Handbook guidelines.
   b. Most states do not require ongoing NBCOT certification to maintain licensure, registration and/or certification.
5. States vary in the additional criteria they require to attain and/or maintain licensure, registration and/or certification. A passing NBCOT score does not ensure attainment of licensure.
6. Some states grant temporary licenses to individuals eligible to become licensed in the state.
7. The terms "registration," "licensure" and "certifica-

tion" are often used interchangeably even though they are different types of regulations. Therefore, each state regulation should be carefully reviewed to ensure understanding of its requirements and provisions.

8. SRBs should be contacted directly to obtain their regulations and an application. Most states do not have reciprocal agreements, so one must meet the requirements of every state in which one intends to practice.

# II. Certification Examination Format and Content

## A. Background Information

1. Practice analysis.
   a. To guide the development of items for the examination, NBCOT conducts periodic (every 5-7 years) surveys of occupational therapy practitioners to ensure content validity of the examination.
   b. The analysis of these survey results is used to construct the blueprint of the exam, create test specifications, and guide the writing of test items (NBCOT, 2008).
   c. The exam blueprint implemented in January 2009 was derived from the outcomes of a practice analysis study conducted in 2007 and analyzed in 2008.
      (1) This *Review and Study Guide* presents the most current information available at the time of its publication about the new NBCOT examination content, format, administration, and scoring.
2. Certification Examination Development Committee (CEDC).
   a. The CEDC is composed of experts in the examination content areas who represent a diversity of practice settings, geographic regions, and demographics.
   b. CEDC committee members develop examination items after the completion of an item writing training program.
   c. The CEDC uses the test specifications developed from the practice analysis to guide their item development.
3. Item development.
   a. Test items are developed to differentiate the presence of inadequate from adequate entry-level practice knowledge and skills.
   b. All test items are reviewed for appropriateness

in measuring the knowledge and skills needed for entry-level OTA practice.
   c. All test items are also reviewed to ensure that the language, context, terminology, descriptions and content are unbiased, inoffensive and appropriate to all population groups.

## B. Examination Composition

1. Item bank.
   a. A large item bank is maintained so that each examination will be composed of a unique combination of items drawn from this bank.
   b. Different forms of the examination are offered simultaneously.
   c. Items are selected according to the weightings of examination domains and content areas to ensure each examination contains consistent percentages of each area.
2. Test format.
   a. The examination has 200 items that use a multiple-choice format.
      (1) The 200 items contain a number of items that NBCOT are pre-testing for future examinations.
         (a) The pre-test items are not considered operational and they are not scored.
         (b) The pre-test items are intermixed with the items that are scored. These items have been pre-equated by NBCOT and deemed operational.
         (c) Pre-test items that perform well statistically will become part of the operational pre-equated item bank used for future examinations.
         (d) There are no identifying characteristics to distinguish unscored pre-test items from the scored operational items.
   b. There are four answer options with only one correct response for each item.
   c. No answers are provided in a combination format (e.g., "all" or "none of the above")

## C. Examination Content

1. The NBCOT examination tests three domains of OTA practice with each domain comprising a set percentage of the exam. These domains and percentages are:
   a. Gather information and formulate conclusions regarding the client's needs and priorities to develop a client-centered intervention plan. 33%
   b. Select and implement evidence-based interven-

tions to support participation in areas of occupation throughout the continuum of care - 47%.

   c. Uphold professional standards and responsibilities to promote quality in practice - 20%. (NBCOT, 2009).

2. Specific task and knowledge statements for each domain are provided on NBCOT's website.
3. Examination content reflects language typically used in practice and is not based on any practice framework model.

   a. Certain aspects of a given practice framework (e.g., AOTA's) may be integrated into examination content if they represent test specifications as determined by a NBCOT practice analysis.

## III. Certification Examination Procedures

### A. Eligibility Requirements for the NBCOT Certification Examination

1. General requirements.

   a. Information submitted on the application must be accurate and truthful.

   b. Candidates submitting misleading or inaccurate information will be prohibited from taking the certification examination.

   c. Information related to felonies must be provided by all candidates.

   d. If, after taking the examination, it is determined that a candidate was ineligible to take the examination, (or that eligibility was questionable) NBCOT will either hold or void the examination.

   e. If a candidate was certified and later found to be ineligible for the examination, certification will be revoked. NBCOT's Disciplinary Action Committee will review the case to determine if any disciplinary action is warranted and if the candidate will or will not be permitted to take the examination at a future date.

2. Education requirements.

   a. Must be a graduate of or 'cleared for graduation' from an occupational therapy assistant education program accredited by the Accreditation Council for Occupational Therapy Education (ACOTE).

   b. Must have completed all full-time Level II fieldwork requirements of the education program. Optional additional fieldwork affiliations must be completed before a candidate is eligible to take the examination, if these affiliations are also needed to fulfill degree requirements.

   c. Completion of the above two criteria must be accomplished on or before specific deadlines as set forth in the NBCOT annual Examination Handbook.

   d. Official documentation verifying a candidate's eligibility (i.e., final official transcript or NBCOT Academic Credential Verification Form [ACVF]) must be submitted by the academic institution's registrar to NBCOT, after the candidate has submitted an examination application to NBCOT.

     (1) Transcripts received by NBCOT before an examination application has been filed will not be retained.

     (2) It is the responsibility of the candidate to verify that the final official transcript sent by the registrar contains all of the information required by NBCOT.

     (3) Transcripts using different language from the criteria set forth in the NBCOT Examination Handbook are not accepted, even if the language is similar.

     (4) Transcripts labeled "student copy" are not accepted.

     (5) Candidates who submitted an ACVF in lieu of an official transcript must forward a final official transcript to NBCOT. Certification is withheld until NBCOT receives a final transcript.

3. Examination eligibility limit.

   a. There is no limit to the number of times a candidate is eligible to take the examination.

   b. A candidate can continue to take the examination until he/she successfully passes.

   c. Candidates should consult the SRB of the state in which they seek to obtain a license to determine the state's standards regarding limits on the number of times the examination can be taken to obtain licensure.

### B. Examination Application Process

1. The NBCOT Examination Handbook contains all required forms for the examination application and provides specific instructions for completion of the application.

   a. The Examination Handbook and its corresponding forms are available at http://www.nbcot.org.

     (1) All information from this web site can be printed out.

     (2) The examination application can be completed, submitted, and processed on-line.

(a) NBCOT encourages on-line applications for this process reduces the occurrence of incomplete application submissions.

(b) In addition, it is faster and more efficient to check application status on-line.

2. Application directions and procedures must be adhered to strictly.

a. Applications that are incomplete, inaccurate, or do not follow instructions will be rejected and returned to the applicant.

b. Applications are also returned if there are any problems with the fee payment.

c. Applications returned to candidates can be resubmitted with the fee payment but this reapplication will delay examination administration.

d. Only one application is required. Do not complete an on-line and a paper mailed application.

3. Given the above facts, candidates are wise to submit their application as far in advance of the date on which they intend to take the examination.

4. When the application process is completed, candidates will receive an Authorization to Test (ATT) letter from NBCOT.

a. This ATT letter gives the candidate permission to contact Prometric to schedule an examination administration date.

b. The ATT letter is only valid for 90 days.

(1) If the 90 days expires, the candidate can reactivate the ATT by completing a reactivation form and paying a reactivation fee at any time within one year of the application submission.

(2) If a candidate does not take an examination within one year of the application submission, the ATT cannot be reactivated. A complete application is required.

c. Carefully review your name as it appears on this admission notice.

(1) It must match exactly with the three forms of identification that you will present on the examination day.

(2) To correct any errors on this admissions form (e.g., a missing middle initial) complete the name section on the Change of Address form that is sent with the admissions notice. Forward the correction(s) as per the directions on this form.

d. This admission notice is required for entry into the test administration area.

5. Applications do not "roll-over" from year to year.

## C. Special Accommodations

1. Candidates with disabilities can receive special testing arrangements if the examination application for special testing accommodations is filled out accurately and completely.

a. All documentation must be received by the published deadlines and completed according to the instructions.

b. Incomplete applications, applications with insufficient documentation, or late applications will not be considered by NBCOT and special accommodations will not be made for a candidate.

c. All documentation must establish a current need for accommodation based on candidate's current status.

d. The receipt of accommodations during an OTA education program does not guarantee that accommodations will be provided for the examination.

2. NBCOT uses the definition of disability set forth in the Americans with Disabilities Act (ADA) to determine eligibility for special accommodations.

3. Candidates must have a documented disability, which can include a mental or physical impairment (e.g., learning, cognitive, or psychological disability; hearing, visual, speech or orthopedic impairment) that substantially limits a major life activity.

4. Candidates who have medical or health conditions (e.g. diabetes, a complicated pregnancy) that may require them to have a snack or water and/or take medicine or restroom breaks must also submit requests for special accommodations.

5. Candidates with temporary conditions that do not meet the ADA definition of disability (e.g., fractures) but who may need accommodations (e.g., wheelchair access) should contact NBCOT for information about how to obtain special testing arrangements.

6. NBCOT adheres to ADA's guidelines for accommodations. Accommodations may include:

a. Architecturally accessible test centers or alternative site arrangements.

b. Auxiliary aids and services.

c. Extra time to complete the examination.

d. Other special accommodations based on documented need.

7. Accommodation recommendations made by professionals are considered and reviewed by NBCOT but are not automatically granted.
   a. NBCOT determines if requested accommodations are appropriate, reasonable, and necessary.
   b. NBCOT will not make accommodations that may alter the fundamental nature of the examination.
   c. English as a second language is not considered a disability; therefore, the use of a dictionary and/or extra time to complete the examination due to language difficulty are not permitted for individuals for whom English is not the primary language.
   d. Denials of requests for accommodations can be appealed according to procedures provided in the Examination Handbook.
8. All information about a candidate's disability and request for accommodations is confidential.
   a. NBCOT and its testing agency only communicate with the candidate, the candidate's authorized, verified representative, and/or a professional knowledgeable about the candidate's disability with the candidate's permission.
   b. No information about the candidate's application or request for accommodations is released by NBCOT or its testing agency without the written authorization of the candidate.
9. All accommodations must be approved by NBCOT prior to the test date.
   a. No requests for accommodations will be approved at the test site.
   b. After taking the test, a candidate cannot retroactively declare a disability.
10. There are no additional fees required to request accommodations.
11. NBCOT will not issue an ATT letter until after accommodation decisions have been made.

### D. Examination Administration

1. Test centers.
   a. Prometric Test Centers are the only locations at which the NBCOT examination can be administered.
   b. Candidates must contact a Prometric Center directly to schedule their examination.
      (1) Test center information is located at www.prometric.com.
      (2) Any desired change in location must be

handled directly by the candidate and Prometric staff.

2. Administration schedule.
   a. Examinations are offered on a continuous, on demand basis and can be scheduled by a candidate throughout the year.
   b. Examinations can be scheduled Monday through Saturday for a morning or afternoon administration.
      (1) Some Prometric centers only schedule afternoon sessions after all morning appointments are filled.
      (2) If you are able, try to schedule your examination for the time of day that you are at your best.
   c. Candidates are strongly urged to schedule their examination immediately after receipt of the confirmation of eligibility.
      (1) NBCOT candidates are competing with all other test-takers who use Prometric services.
      (2) A delay in scheduling an examination administration can result in the need to take the examination at a less preferred time and/or site.
      (3) Prometric staff advises that Saturday examinations be scheduled a minimum of 6 weeks in advance; weekday examinations can be scheduled 2-4 weeks in advance.

## IV. The Examination Day

### A. Pre-Preparation Plans

1. Be prepared physically.
   a. Get a good night's sleep.
   b. Eat a well-balanced meal.
   c. Avoid too much caffeine.
   d. Wear clothing that can be comfortable in a warm or cold room and/or be adjustable to room temperature changes (e.g., a long sleeve cotton knit shirt that you can roll the sleeves up and down).
      (1) You can wear a sweater or a jacket into the test area but if you want to remove it you must go into the waiting area.
         (a) Some Prometric sites do not allow the wearing of "hoodies" or jackets with pockets.
      (2) Head coverings worn for religious reasons (e.g., turbans, yarmulkes, scarves,) can be worn into the testing area.
   e. Go to the rest room before checking in.

2. Be prepared emotionally.
   a. Remind yourself of past achievements and adopt the attitude that the examination is one more accomplishment to be added to this list.
   b. Decrease pre-exam stress. If you have never traveled to the test site, do a trial run before your examination date on the same day of the week that you are planning to take the exam.
      (1) Exam day is not the time to discover that mass transportation or traffic patterns are different from those with which you are familiar.
3. If you are late for your exam or need to cancel or reschedule it, you must follow the procedures and pay the fees that are outlined in the Examination Handbook.

**B. Test Center Procedures**
1. The check in period is half an hour before the scheduled examination.
   a. You can call the Prometric Center that you are scheduled to take the examination at to see if earlier arrivals are acceptable.
   b. It is best to arrive as early as possible prior to the scheduled test. This allows sufficient time to calmly check in and complete the computer tutorial.
2. No one is admitted without an ATT letter.
3. Three forms of identification including one primary identification with a photo and signature (e.g., passport, driver's license) and two secondary identifications (e.g., credit card, ATM card) must be presented at the test center.
   a. Copies of identification are not acceptable.
   b. Names on identification must match the name on the examination admission notice exactly.
   c. Both forms of identification must have signatures that match exactly.
   d. No one is admitted without required identification.
4. All candidates are photographed and, at some sites, thumb printed.
5. Upon check in, verify that previously made requests for special accommodations have been met.
6. Only a dry erase board and marker, earplugs, eyeglasses/contacts, and/or medications are allowed into the test administration area.
   a. Earplugs and the dry erase board must be obtained from Prometric personnel.
   b. Some Prometric centers allow tissues, mints, and other small "comfort" items to be brought to the test area. Others do not. All items are carefully checked.
7. A locker is provided to store all other personal possessions (e.g., wallet, purse, watches, cell phones, PDAs).
   a. This locker is not accessible until the conclusion of the examination.
8. Food and/or drink are not allowed in the test area. Food and/or drink can be consumed in the waiting area. Be judicious about your food and drink consumption prior to the exam and during the exam to decrease the need for bathroom breaks.
9. A 10-15 minute tutorial on how to use the computer and complete the examination is available prior to commencement of the examination.
   a. Candidates are strongly advised to take this tutorial.
   b. The time spent on the tutorial before the exam does not count towards its administration time so use it to get physically comfortable (e.g., move the computer screen to decrease glare, adjust the chair, take a bathroom break).
10. Prometric personnel can also provide an orientation to the examination.
    a. They are available prior to the examination's start to answer questions and clarify the examination procedures.
11. If you are assigned an examination location that is dissatisfying for any reason (i.e., poor lighting, computer screen glare, ventilation, noise level), request a change to another computer cubicle before the examination begins.
    a. You cannot change locations once you have begun the examination.
12. There are no scheduled breaks during the examination unless pre-arranged as an accommodation for a disability or medical necessity.
    a. Restroom breaks are allowed during the examination; however, the examination's clock does keep running.
       (1) After taking a break, you will need to re-check in with Prometric staff. This may require waiting while other people check in for their examinations.
13. Prometric centers do not dedicate times just for NBCOT test takers. Many individuals taking a variety of examinations may be coming, going, or receiving orientation during your examination.
    a. Some individuals find the use of earplugs help-

ful in decreasing these auditory distractions.

14. The examination is videotaped and these tapes are reviewed by Prometric personnel.

15. You are not allowed to talk or read aloud during the examination.

16. If you take a break, DO NOT use ANY electronic device (e.g., a cell phone or personal digital assistant). Any candidate who is observed using any electronic device during any part of the exam administration period will have his/her exam terminated.

## C. Examination Time and Time Keeping

1. There are four hours allowed to complete the examination.

2. Additional time is not provided for any reason other than as a pre-approved special accommodation for a disability.

3. A running clock on the computer will indicate the time remaining and a counter will indicate the number of questions left to answer so you can readily see if you are progressing at the needed pace.
   a. Periodically check the clock and/or counter to be sure that you are on track with your timing.
      (1) Avoid spending too much time checking this clock and counter.

4. You should allot an average of one minute to complete each item.
   a. This pace will enable you to complete an average of 50 items in an hour, providing you with a 'bank' of approximately 40 - 50 minutes that you can use to review and answer more challenging MCT items.

5. If you are ahead of schedule, take a brief breather and congratulate yourself; then maintain this pace, for you can use this additional time later during the examination to review more challenging questions.
   a. Some students report feeling listless as the exam progresses and they have found a brief break re-energized them and enabled them to resume the exam with a positive outlook.

6. If you are behind schedule, your pace is too slow and you will need to speed up to complete the exam.
   a. Do not belabor difficult questions. Move on to other questions.

## D. Test Taking Strategies

1. Decrease your anxiety level before you begin by taking the tutorial and asking any and all questions.

2. Don't panic. OTA programs are challenging, but you passed your coursework and fieldwork to get to this point so you must have done something right! Remember this and give yourself credit.

3. Pace yourself. You need to complete 200 questions within a 4 hour period; therefore your goal is to complete at least 50 questions within an hour.
   a. Reading and reasoning skills may deteriorate by hour four so plan to work a bit faster in the first three hours of the examination.
   b. You are permitted to stand and stretch during the examination as long as you do not disturb other test-takers; however, the examination clock does keep running.

4. Select the best answer.
   a. Think logically and eliminate obviously wrong answers.
   b. Jot down notes on the dry erase board that Prometric staff will provide you upon request.
      (1) Often visualizing the remaining options of a familiar list (e.g., Allen's Cognitive Levels) will jog one's memory and make it easier to arrive at a correct answer.
   c. Narrow your choices to the best possible answers and use your knowledge of the clinical condition and OT standards of practice to clinically reason and determine the best answer.
   d. Do not read extra information into the question; just consider what is stated in the question. Decide what the question is basically about by looking for key words.
   e. Avoid thinking "but" and "what if". Often your first instincts are accurate, so decrease second guessing. Do not think about patients you know with this condition or practices you've seen in the clinic; think of the basic OT principles, (i.e., what the book says, not what you saw on fieldwork).
   f. It may help to read the answer choices before you read the question scenario. Then you will be able to focus your reading of the case on issues directly related to the answer choices. It may also help to try to answer the question without reading the answer choices. However, be certain to read all answer choices before making your final choice.
   g. The answer should be grammatically consistent with the question.
      (1) After you have selected your answer, read the question, then your answer. Does it

flow? If not, review other options.

    (2) Save this hint for questions you're not sure of. (Who said APA wouldn't come in handy?!)

    (3) If English is your second language, you must remember to "think" in English when reading and answering questions.

11. Table 1-1 provides general strategies for answering NBCOT examination items.

12. Table 1-2 provides specific strategies for answering multiple choice items.

## TABLE 1-1: GENERAL STRATEGIES FOR ANSWERING NBCOT EXAM ITEMS

- Read the exam item carefully before selecting a response to the question posed.

- Employ relevant clinical experience.
  - Remember trends and consistent cases in your experience.
  - Do not call on unusual cases or atypical presentations.

- Read the exam item for key words that set a priority.

- Apply clinical reasoning skills to determine the relevance of item info. (i.e., diagnosis, setting, intervention, and theoretical principles). See Chapter 2.

- Use your knowledge of medical terminology to decipher unknown terms by applying the meanings of known prefixes, suffixes, and root words. See Appendix 2.

- Select responses that most closely reflect the fundamental tenets of OT; e.g., ethical actions, the use of meaningful occupation.

- Choose client-centered, person-directed actions.

- Identify choices that focus on the emotional well-being of the person.

- Use your clinical judgment to support the best answer.

- Check your answer to see if it is:
  - theoretically consistent with exam item scenario.
  - diagnostically consistent with the exam item scenario.
  - developmentally consistent with the exam item scenario.

- Eliminate choices that contain contraindications as these must be incorrect.

- Consider eliminating options that state "always", "never", "all", or "only" as there are few absolutes in OT practice.

- Eliminate unsafe options.

- Choose answers that reflect entry-level COTA practice.

- Remember the NBCOT exam is *not* a specialty certification exam.

## E. Completion of the Examination

1. Answers can be recorded by using keystrokes or the mouse.

2. Do not skip questions.

    a. Although not every item is scored, there is no way to know which items are operational or not, therefore, you must answer all to the best of your abilities.

3. If you are uncertain of an answer, mark the question by using the mark/unmark button.

    a. You can return to a marked item to review and change the answer, if desired.

        (1) Only change the answer if you have a good reason (e.g., you missed a key word like "initial" or "best").

4. If you remain unsure of an answer, make a logical guess based on the test-taking strategies outlined in Tables 1-1 and 1-2. There is no penalty for guessing but there is for leaving a question unanswered.

5. Do not communicate with anyone other than

## TABLE 1-2: SPECIFIC STRATEGIES FOR ANSWERING MULTIPLE CHOICE (MC) EXAM ITEMS

- Identify the theme of the MC item. Ask yourself, "What is the question posed REALLY asking?"

- Avoid "reading into" the MC item. Read the question asked and nothing but the question.

- Identify choices that seem similar or equally plausible.
  - If two choices basically say the same thing or use synonyms in their answers both cannot be right; therefore, both can be eliminated.

- Carefully consider choices that are opposites of one another. If you cannot eliminate both opposites right away, one may be the correct answer.

- Determine the best answer using strategies identified in Table 1-1.
  - More than one answer may be "correct". Choose the one that is MOST correct.

- Select positive, active choices rather than passive, negative ones.

- Before changing an answer make sure that you have a good reason to eliminate your original choice and a good reason to make your new choice.
  - Good reasons include realizing that you misunderstood the item's theme, missed a key word in the exam item, or you gained a clue from a subsequent exam item.

- Do not let second-guessing talk you out of the correct answer.

Prometric personnel while completing the examination.

   a. An innocent passing remark to another person can be mistaken for an attempt to cheat.

6. Keep your eyes on your own computer screen and do not look at other screens if you take a break.

   a. A fleeting glance at another computer screen can be interpreted as an attempt to cheat.

7. Don't panic if you are stumped by a number of questions.

   a. Focus on what you know, because it is likely you know a lot.

   b. We often tend to remember our "failures" and not our "successes". Be kind to yourself.

8. If you are running out of time and have not completed the test, pick a letter and mark all remaining answers using that one letter choice.

   a. Laws of probability will enable you to get some right.

9. Once you have exited the exam you cannot return to it.

   a. You are able to review the entire examination and make changes, prior to exiting the examination.

      (1) Again, only change an answer if there is a strong reason.

10. Congratulate yourself for what you know and make educated guesses on what you don't know. You do not need to answer 100%, 90% or even 80% of the questions correctly in order to pass the exam.

## V. After the Examination

### A. Examination Administration Complaints

1. Only complaints regarding an administrative or technical problem with the examination are accepted (e.g., the computer screen freezes).

   a. Prometric centers are in the business of providing optimal environments for test-taking, so administrative and technical problems are rare.

2. If you do experience a problem, you must immediately complete an on-site complaint with Prometric staff.

   a. Be very specific about the nature of your complaint, the rationale for the complaint and any actions that were taken to try to deal with the complaint on-site.

   b. Request a 'ticket number' for your complaint.

3. You must email NBCOT *within 24 hours* to provide them with a summary of your complaint and its assigned number.

4. Be certain to adhere to the complaint guidelines in the NBCOT Examination Handbook.

   a. There are no exceptions.

5. Complaints are investigated by NBCOT and the testing agency and written responses are sent to the candidate.

### B. Examination Scoring and Reporting

1. Item analysis.

   a. All examinations use items that have been analyzed as performing well on previous examinations.

   b. All items are pre-equated and determined to have sound statistical attributes.

2. Equating.

   a. The passing score for each examination is statistically adjusted to compensate for differences in the difficulty level of each examination.

   b. This equating aims to ensure that candidates with equivalent abilities will be equally likely to pass the examination.

   c. From NBCOT's and their testing agency's points of view, all examination candidates have a fair and equal chance to pass the examination, regardless of the administration date.

3. Scoring processes.

   a. Only the pre-equated operational items are scored; the pre-operational items that are being field-tested are not scored.

   b. Statistical procedures convert candidates' raw scores (number of correct items) into "scaled scores" which are then comparable for all examinations based upon the equating process.

   c. The examination results are reported on a scale from 300 to 600 points.

   d. A scaled score of at least 450 is needed to pass the examination.

   e. This passing score of 450 remains the same for all examination administration dates. There are no adjustments made after the score is determined by the equating process.

4. Score reporting.

   a. Several steps are followed by the testing agency to produce accurate examination reports in as timely a manner as possible. Early score results are not given.

   b. Exams are scored twice a month. Score dates are available at www.nbcot.org.

      (1) Candidates can typically obtain an unofficial pass/fail score on the next business day

after their exam was scored.

    (a) Candidates must use their user name and password to access this score information.

c. Official score reports are mailed within four to six weeks of the examination administration date.

d. Score reports are held for candidates who submitted an ACVF with their applications.

    (1) Upon receipt of an official transcript, NBCOT will mail the score report.

e. If, after four weeks of taking the exam, you have not received a score, you should submit a Duplicate Score Request form. The form is provided in the Examination Handbook and is available at www.nbcot.org. Do not phone or fax, as you will receive no information.

g. Candidates who pass the examination receive a letter of congratulations, a report with their total score, and a wallet card designating their certification status.

h. Candidates who fail the examination receive a report of their total score and information on their performance on each area of the examination.

i. Score reports are only provided to examination candidates or their legally verified representative.

j. Score reports can be provided to SRBs and other regulatory agencies upon the written authorization of the examination candidate.

**C. Waiting For and Receiving Examination Results**

1. Accept that the exam is done and over with, and move on to other enjoyable activities.

2. Focus on your successes. Congratulate yourself on questions you answered confidently.

3. Avoid focusing on exam difficulties. For example, the exam was not solely about the two obscure diagnoses that you could not recall. Remember, there were 198 other questions.

4. Surround yourself with your "fan club", people who assure you of your competencies.

5. Avoid and ignore individuals who continually question the exam's fairness and perseverate about their ability to pass.

6. Ignore rumors about the examination's pass rate.

    a. No one knows this information until it is received in the mail by the examination takers.

    b. OTA educational programs do not receive this information prior to the students.

    c. OTA educational programs do not receive information identifying the names of students who do not pass the exam.

7. The size of the envelope you receive is not reflective of your score. Thick or thin envelopes do not reflect passing or failing scores, so do not panic! Just open the envelope.

8. If you passed, congratulate yourself and begin your lifelong pursuit of a rewarding career in occupational therapy.

9. If you did not pass, do not denigrate yourself; rather, make a plan to retake the test and succeed.

**D. Implications of Not Passing the Examination**

1. The implications of not passing the examination vary from state to state. You must follow your state regulatory board's (SRB's) procedures for notification of examination failure.

2. If you are currently employed as an OTA or you have specific plans to begin employment, you must notify your employer immediately.

3. Depending on the state, you may be able to continue employment under an extension of a temporary license or have your position reconfigured a rehabilitation aide/associate, with a corresponding decrease in responsibility and salary.

**E. Retaking the Examination**

1. You must wait 45 days after your examination administration date before you can take the examination again.

    a. A new and complete application must be submitted to retake the examination.

2. Obtain support to handle your legitimate disappointment.

3. Review examination results to identify and analyze areas of strength and weakness. Look for patterns in your score report - do not agonize over exact percentages.

4. Reflect on your examination experience to identify behaviors that may have hindered success. Common mistakes include:

    a. Taking too much time to answer difficult questions.

    b. Becoming anxious or upset over a question that seemed to have no good answer (or two good answers).

    c. Becoming distracted by the progress of the other test-takers.

    d. Arriving in a rushed, harried manner just as the examination is about to begin.

5. Be realistic about the obstacles you can change and

those you cannot. For example, if you were stressed due to a traffic jam, you can stay overnight in a nearby hotel. On the other hand, you cannot change the fact that the test is on a computer even though you have technophobic tendencies.

6. Increase your comfort level with taking a computerized examination by using this text's disc.

   a. The disc does not self-destruct after a set number of examination trials; it can be interrupted, returned to, and used repeatedly.

7. If you are eligible for reasonable accommodations, follow NBCOT's guidelines and adhere to the deadline dates to attain needed examination accommodations.

   a. Since the examination requires four hours of computer work, carefully and realistically assess your cognitive, physical, and psychosocial abilities for any potential problems that may warrant accommodations.

8. Develop a plan of action to ensure success.

   a. Review this text's section on examination preparation and critically evaluate what you did to prepare for your first examination.

   b. Take (or re-take) an examination preparatory course; your first-hand examination experience can make this course even more relevant.

   c. Do not rush to take the next scheduled examination, for that may not allow you sufficient time to adequately prepare for the examination. It is better to delay the exam than rush your preparation and risk being under-prepared.

9. Adopt the perspective that your first experience with the exam can be viewed positively, in that you can re-take the examination with a clear idea of what the experience is like.

   a. You are aware of your strong and weak points; therefore, your chances of passing the re-take are greater.

10. Recognize that there are many skilled and competent OTAs who did not pass the certification examination on their first (or even their second) attempt.

   a. You can join their ranks by honestly self-assessing your examination preparedness and taking concrete steps to remediate your difficulties and build upon your strengths.

   b. Being able to practice occupational therapy is well worth the effort.

# References

National Board for Certification in Occupational Therapy (NBCOT). (2010). *The certification exam handbook and application 2010.* Gaithersburg, MD: NBCOT.

Fleming-Castaldy, R. (2010). *Occupational therapy course manual.* Evanston, IL: TherapyED.

National Board for Certification in Occupational Therapy (NBCOT). (2008). *Executive summary for the practice analysis study.*

National Board for Certification in Occupational Therapy (NBCOT). (2008). *The NBCOT official COTA study guide: Certified Occupational Therapy Assistant, certification exam.* Gaithersburg, MD: NBCOT.

Sides, M. & Korcheck, N. (Eds.). (1998). *Successful test-taking: Learning strategies for nurses.* Philadelphia: Lippincott.

# CHAPTER 2

# PRINCIPLES OF EFFECTIVE EXAMINATION PREPARATION

### Rita P. Fleming-Castaldy • Kari Inda

## I. Effective Examination Preparation

### A. Overview and General Guidelines

1. The examination tests general knowledge and fundamentals of OT in an integrated manner.
   a. There are four main levels of objective exam questions.
      (1) Table 2-1 describes each question level and its relevance to the NBCOT exam and provides related examination preparation strategies.
2. Your clinical reasoning skills and critical thinking skills will be vital to use to ensure exam success.
   a. Refer to Section II for a review of the relationship between critical reasoning and the NBCOT exam.

### B. Psychological Outlook

1. When preparing for a professional certification exam, your psychological outlook is a critical aspect of effective exam preparation. See Table 2-2.
   a. Fears, doubts, and negative attitudes must be replaced with a positive "I can" attitude.
   b. Since developing a positive attitude can be difficult to do alone, surround yourself with your "fan club"; people who know that you will be a terrific COTA.
   c. Practice techniques to reduce anxiety during the exam while preparing for the exam.
      (1) Techniques of visual imagery, muscle relaxation, controlled diaphragmatic breathing, cognitive-behavioral strategies, meditation, positive self-talk, and/or exercise can be just as beneficial for you as the individuals you will be working with.
2. Keep your "eye on the prize".
   a. Write down two reasons why you want to be a COTA.
      (1) Keep these statements where you will read them every day so that they help you to stay motivated.
   b. Write down two reasons why you *WILL* pass the exam. For instance, "I will pass the certification exam because I have developed a clear study plan and will implement it." "I passed the hardest class in the world with the most difficult teacher ever".
3. If you have previously failed the exam, *honestly critique* what did not work for you in preparing for and taking this prior exam.
   a. Develop and implement remediation strategies to effectively deal with these difficulties.
   b. Maintain a positive attitude is important but be careful and do not accept false reassurance from others.

## TABLE 2-1 - LEVELS OF EXAM QUESTIONS

| QUESTION LEVEL AND DESCRIPTION | RELEVANCE TO NBCOT EXAM | NBCOT EXAM PREPARATION STRATEGY |
|---|---|---|
| **1. Knowledge**<br>Recall of basic information. For example, DSM-IV-TR diagnoses, spinal cord levels, wheelchair measurements. | A solid knowledge foundation of *ALL* information related to entry-level OTA practice is required to answer NBCOT exam items. It is likely that very few items on the OTA exam will be solely at this level. | A strong commitment to studying is needed to remember all the information acquired during your OTA education. Fortunately, this text provides extensive information in an outline format to ease your review. Memorization of this information is required to be able to readily recall it during the 200 MC items on the OTA exam. |
| **2. Comprehension**<br>Understanding of information to determine significance, consequences, or implications. For example, the impact of a tenodesis grasp on function. | The NBCOT exam is not a matching column type of test; therefore, you cannot only be able to just recall information to succeed on the OTA exam. You must fully understand the content area to be able to understand the nuances of an exam item. All items will require comprehension but only some will be solely at this level. | When studying the text to review basic content and acquire your foundational knowledge, ask yourself how and why this fundamental information is important. Studying with a peer or a study group can provide you with additional insights about the relevance, significance, consequences, and implications of the info. Do not enter the test without strong comprehension of all major areas of OT practice. |
| **3. Application**<br>Use of information and application of rules, procedures, or theories to new situations. For example, the classroom modifications that an OTA would make for a child with autism. | The NBCOT exam requires you to use your knowledge and comprehension as described above, along with the competencies you developed during your clinical fieldworks, in a manner that best fits the specific practice scenario in an exam item. Many OTA exam items will likely be at this level for a main goal of the NBCOT exam is to assess your ability to respond competently to different situations. | Once you have acquired a solid knowledge base and good comprehension skills in all domains of OT as put forth in this text, you should take the computer-based NBCOT simulated practice exams that accompany this text. These exams require you to apply your knowledge in a manner similar to the NBCOT exam. Upon completion of these exams, you receive an analysis of your performance so that you can determine how well you are applying your knowledge. |
| **4. Analysis**<br>Recognition of interrelationships between principles & interpretation or evaluation of data presented. For example, the most appropriate focus for discharge planning sessions for a parent with a traumatic brain injury. | The NBCOT exam assumes that you have mastered and comprehend entry-level knowledge and that you can competently apply this information to diverse situations; therefore it will likely ask you to analyze and respond to ambiguous, not 'straight from the book' situations. Most OTA exam items will likely be at this level for the main objective of the NBCOT exam is to determine your ability to be competent in practice situations. | Use the analyses of text practice exams described above to reflect on your reasoning mistakes. Critically review the extensive rationales provided in the text for the correct exam answers. Reflecting with a peer or a study group can be helpful in determining your gaps in analysis of exam items. Review the chapter's section on critical reasoning skills and reflect on the questions provided in Table 5 to ascertain the actions you need to take to adequately prepare for the complexities of the NBCOT exam. |

## C. Structuring a Review of Professional Education

1. Establish your knowledge and skill level.
   a. The examination tests general knowledge and fundamentals of OT in an integrated manner. Your clinical reasoning skills and critical thinking skills will be vital to use since the NBCOT exam emphasizes the application of knowledge. (See Chapter 3 for a review of the profession's Tools of Practice.)
      (1) Table 2-3 outlines the application of clinical reasoning to multiple choice questions.
   b. Critique your knowledge of the three exam domains listed in Chapter 1 to identify your areas of strength and weakness in order to create a personal study plan.
   c. Review your academic history to help clarify strengths and weaknesses. Honestly appraise which course topics you mastered and which ones you struggled with.
   d. As you proceed through the chapters in this text rate your knowledge of key content according to a scale of know very well, know

## TABLE 2-2: PSYCHOLOGY OF SUCCESSFUL TEST-TAKING

| CONCEPT | PRINCIPLE | ACTIONS |
|---|---|---|
| Control | Only you can determine your future. | • Take charge; determine exactly what is needed to succeed.<br>• Set goals to meet these needs.<br>• Develop and implement concrete plans to succeed. |
| Self-Awareness | Knowing one's innate capabilities enables one to build on strengths and effectively deal with limitations. | • Critically analyze test-taking errors and content knowledge gaps.<br>• Be honest about your test-taking and content knowledge. strengths and limitations.<br>• Avoid self-defeatist behaviors. |
| Self-Confidence | Your past accomplishments provide a solid foundation for future success. | • Review exam content prior to completing practice examinations.<br>• Use a diversity of learning methods to achieve mastery.<br>• Recognize and celebrate your successes and achievements. |
| Self-fulfilling Prophecy | Your self-expectancy will influence the outcomes of your efforts. | • Expect success.<br>• Use positive self-talk throughout exam preparation.<br>• Continue to think positively during the exam administration. |
| Self-esteem | You are a person capable of excellence. | • Remember your personal and academic achievements.<br>• Occupational therapy academic course work and fieldwork are demanding; give yourself well-earned credit for your success. |
| Motivation | Your desire to succeed and a fear of failure can be channeled for success. | • Understand that the early stages of studying will have uncertain results.<br>• Remind yourself of what initially motivated you to enter OT school.<br>• Harness fear and establish a do-able study plan. |
| Courage | Taking responsibility for one's failures is key to success. | • Honestly critique precipitators/reasons for an exam failure.<br>• Do not make excuses.<br>• Do not strive for perfection. |
| Perseverance | You can only succeed if you persevere. | • Re-establish goals.<br>• Seek support for goal attainment.<br>• Utilize multiple resources to stay on track. |
| Freedom | You can freely choose your attitude. | • View test-taking as an opportunity.<br>• Keep your "eye on the prize".<br>• Exam success equates to achievement of your goal to become an OT practitioner. |

Reference: Sides, M. (1998). Forming the psychology of test-taking success. In M. Sides and N. Korcheck. (Eds). Successful test-taking: Learning strategies for nurses (pp. 49-61). Philadelphia: Lippincott.

adequately, know very little, know nothing.
  (1) Based on this critical self assessment, make a personal "Knowledge Continuum" listing topics from strongest to weakest.
    (a) Your aim is to enter the examination with solid knowledge in all critical content areas.
2. Develop an individualized study plan.
  a. Content areas that are rated as 'know nothing' or 'know very little' will become your *"Must Study"* list.
  b. Content areas that are rated as 'know very well'

or 'know adequately' will become your *"Review"* list.
  c. Organize both your *"Must Study"* list and *"Review"* list into a logical schedule. For example, if you are weak in your knowledge about biomechanical evaluation and intervention approaches but have a good recall of clinical conditions, study the biomechanical chapter and then review the chapter on musculoskeletal conditions. Studying these two chapters together will provide an integrative learning experience since diagnoses will be includ-

ed in examination items testing your knowledge about evaluation and intervention approaches.

  d. Allocate study time according to your "Knowledge Continuum", *"Must Study"* list, and *"Review"* list; begin with your weakest area first,

    (1) After you master a weak content area, reward yourself by reviewing a content area of strength.

    (2) Continue studying to progress along your knowledge continuum, alternating between your *"Must Study"* list and *"Review"* list. This will help prevent examination preparation fatigue and burnout.

  e. Plan to spend more time studying areas that compose a greater percent of the examination content, especially if these areas are on the low end of your "Knowledge Continuum" and on your *"Must Study"* list.

  f. Allow yourself sufficient time to study over a period of time, and set aside enough time to master your weakest areas and to review all areas in general.

    (1) Be realistic about your inherent capabilities (e.g., being a poor memorizer) and your external constraints (e.g. being a single parent who must rely on childcare) when planning the amount of study time needed to ensure success.

    (2) Studying in cram sessions can increase anxiety and result in burnout.

  d. Critically assess the study habits you used throughout your OTA education to identify routines that worked most effectively for you.

  e. Establish a study schedule and routine and adhere to it strictly.

    (1) Study one major content area per study session.

    (2) Limit interruptions (lock the cell phone in your car's glove compartment, turn on voice mail and/or the answering machine, and arrange for childcare). *DO NOT* study by a computer; the latest TravelZoo ad will be far more interesting than supervisory guidelines.

    (3) If an unexpected event results in a loss of planned study time, immediately schedule time to make up for this loss.

3. *DO NOT* take the practice examinations in this text until after you have implemented your study plan and gained mastery of your *"Must Study"* list.

  a. Completing a practice exam before you have attained mastery of essential content will only reinforce that you have key gaps in your foundational knowledge.

    (1) This can diminish confidence, lower self-esteem, and make the prospect of studying more overwhelming.

  b. Completing a practice examination after the implementation of your study plan will provide you the opportunity to demonstrate your acquired knowledge.

    (1) This can increase confidence, boost self-esteem, and enable your subsequent studying to be more targeted on areas that you had initially not focused on in depth.

4. Complete the first practice examination in this text

---

## TABLE 2-3 – CLINICAL REASONING APPLIED TO MULTIPLE-CHOICE QUESTIONS

**PROCEDURAL REASONING**

What does the question tell/ask you about:
- diagnosis?
- symptoms?
- etiology?
- prognosis?
- occupational therapy assessment?
- occupational therapy treatment?
- potential discharge settings?
- occupational therapy philosophy?
- theory to support procedures?

**CONDITIONAL REASONING**

What does the question tell/ask you about:
- the individual's unique roles, values, goals?
- impact of illness on this person's function?
- how the course of the disease will influence person's future?
- where the person will be able to live after discharge?

**INTERACTIVE REASONING**

What does the question tell/ask you about:
- rapport building?
- family/caregiver involvement?
- therapeutic use of self?
- teaching/learning styles?
- ways to successfully collaborate?

**PRAGMATIC REASONING**

What does the question tell/ask you about:
- length of stay?
- practice setting characteristics?
- reimbursement concerns and legal responsibilities?
- referral options?
- person's socioeconomic status?

using the test taking strategies provided in Chapter 1.

   a. Revise your study plan based on the provided analysis of your examination performance.

     (1) Implement this revised study plan to address identified knowledge gaps.

5. Complete the second practice examination in this text using the test taking strategies provided in Chapter 1.

6. Answering examination questions can further assist in identifying content areas of strength and weakness and in identifying your test-taking personality.

   a. Table 2-4 outlines typical test-taking personalities and their corresponding behavior management strategies.

7. Be certain to complete each practice examination in its entirety during a continuous 4 hour period to increase comfort with the cognitive, visual and

## TABLE 2-4: PERSONALITIES OF TEST-TAKERS

| PERSONALITY TYPE | CHARACTERISTICS | STRATEGIES |
|---|---|---|
| The Rusher | • Impatient.<br>• Jumps to conclusions.<br>• Skips key words.<br>• Inadequate consideration of questions. | • Take practice exams in a timed manner to establish a non-desperate pace.<br>• Recognize that the time allotted for the test is sufficient.<br>• Use positive self-talk and relaxation techniques during exam. |
| The Turtle | • Overly slow and methodical.<br>• Over attention to extraneous detail.<br>• Reads and re-reads test item's details.<br>• Misses theme of question. | • Take practice exams in a timed manner to establish a pace of completing 50 questions per hour.<br>• Study in bullet format. |
| Squisher/ Procrastinator | • Puts things off.<br>• Does not reschedule missed study time. | • Focus on developing a step-by step study plan.<br>• Dig in and get started.<br>• Adopt a "no excuses" attitude. |
| Philosopher | • Is a thoughtful, talented, intelligent, and disciplined student.<br>• Excels in essay questions.<br>• Over-analyzes and reads into questions.<br>• Wants to know everything and answer everything about the topic.<br>• Over-applies clinical knowledge. | • Focus only on the test question.<br>• Study in bullet, not paragraph form.<br>• Look for simple, straightforward answers. |
| Lawyer | • Is a thoughtful, talented, intelligent and disciplined student.<br>• Picks out some bit of information and builds a case on that.<br>• Reads information into a test item to make a case for the preferred answer instead of determining what the question is asking. | • Focus on what the question is asking and only what the question is asking.<br>• Remember you can train to be an NBCOT exam item writer and write "better" questions after you pass the exam. |
| Second-Guesser | • Looks at the question from every angle.<br>• Keeps changing answers, increasing anxiety, thinking less clearly and then changing answers more rapidly. | • Focus on only using the 'light bulb' strategy to change answers.<br>• Identify a good reason to reject an old answer and a good reason to select a new answer before changing answer. |

Reference: Korchek, N. (1998). Personalities of test-takers. In M. Sides and N. Korcheck (Eds). Successful test-taking: Learning strategies for nurses (77-89). Philadelphia: Lippincott.

drawn based on facts, laws, rules, or accepted principles.
2. The reverse thinking process of inductive reasoning.
3. Starts with information about larger circumstances, broader principles, and general theories and applies this knowledge to specific situations.
   a. For example, an OTA applies the OT ethical principle of veracity to conclude that a fellow therapist who falsely documents a treatment procedure to fraudulently bill Medicare is behaving in an unethical manner.
4. Provides important guidelines for OT practice by putting forth protocols (e.g., diagnostic-specific clinical pathways), procedures (e.g., correlation data analysis), rules (e.g., OT code of ethics), and laws (e.g., IDEA, ADA) that can be applied to a specific practice scenario without necessitating independent judgment for the situation.
5. Deductive reasoning must be used cautiously when answering NBCOT exam items because erroneous assumptions about the premises of a theory can be made and then mistakenly applied to a specific circumstance.
   a. For example, an OTA who staunchly adheres to the belief that all persons with disabilities want to be independent in all ADL would be wrong to apply this viewpoint to a person from a cultural background that views family-provided assistance as a sign of loving care. This OTA would be deducing from a flawed premise which would lead to a faulty conclusion.
   b. Recognizing the limitations of deductive reasoning is an important part of successful exam performance; the soundness and trustworthiness of the applied procedures, theories, principles, and concepts must be thoughtfully critiqued before they are applied to a specific situation.
6. To help you identify NBCOT exam items that require their correct answer to be based on facts, laws, rules, or accepted principles, the analysis of your performance on this text's two practice examinations will have a picture of a microscope next to deductive reasoning items.

E. Analytical Reasoning or Analysis
1. The process of interpreting the meaning of information, determining relationships within the information presented, and then making assumptions or judgments about that information.
   a. Helps to examine ideas and concepts and the relationships between them.
2. Information presented in the form of graphs, charts, tables, and pictures encourage analytical reasoning skills because one must interpret the information that is depicted and determine what it precisely means.
   a. Information can also be presented in a narrative manner that requires one to make a "mental chart" of the information presented.
3. Used in OT practice to interpret test results (e.g., ECG), categorize information (e.g., define a symptom based on a behavioral description, or determine a diagnosis based on a cluster of reported symptoms).
   a. Important in OT practice, because it helps the OTA determine the potential impact of a clinical condition on occupational performance.
4. Analysis is required to correctly answer many NBCOT exam questions.
   a. Analytical reasoning is used when some descriptors are included in an item stem (e.g., member characteristics of a mature-level group), but some key descriptors needed to answer the question are not provided (e.g., the leader's role in a mature group) leaving the test taker to make assumptions about what the best answer would be (e.g., type of activity used in the group) based on the partial information provided.
5. Analysis questions are often frustrating since limited information upon which an answer must be selected is provided; however, they accurately reflect the practice reality that OT practitioners rarely have complete information about a person or group.
6. To help you identify NBCOT exam items that require the examination of ideas and concepts and the relationships between them, the analysis of your performance on this text's two practice examinations will have a picture of a beaker next to analytical reasoning items.

F. Inferential Reasoning or Inference
1. The process of drawing conclusions or making logical judgments based on facts, concepts, and evidence rather than direct observations.
2. Used in practice situations when an OTA infers the symptoms to expect based on a diagnosis (e.g., a person with a left CVA will exhibit right hemiplegia and aphasia) or the likely progression of a disease or disorder (e.g., Amyotrophic Lateral

Sclerosis will steadily progress until death while the course of Multiple Sclerosis is characterized by exacerbations and remissions).

    a. Inferences about the nature of a disease, all of its possible symptoms and its sequelae are not guaranteed to be 100% accurate; therefore, skilled inference must be based on the OT practitioner's knowledge and experience.

3. Inferential reasoning is also utilized in practice situations when OTAs have to decide on a best course of action.

    a. Inferences about clinical courses of action are not guaranteed to be 100% accurate. For example, when treating an individual with a rotator cuff tear, an OTA cannot be 100% certain that the chosen intervention will result in the successful therapeutic outcome of improved occupational performance. Therefore, skilled inference must be based on the OT practitioner's knowledge and experience.

4. Inferential reasoning is regularly used by OT practitioners in their decision making process and this reality is precisely why the skill is important for successful NBCOT exam performance.

5. Inference is required to correctly answer many NBCOT exam questions.

    a. Questions that ask the test taker to determine what is best, most important, or most likely to occur often require inferential reasoning.

    b. Questions of this nature can be difficult because they ask the test-taker to determine what is believed to be true even though there is no 100% assurance that the selected answer is correct; however, they accurately reflect the realistic uncertainties of OT practice.

6. Inferential reasoning must be used cautiously when answering NBCOT exam questions because inadequate consideration of the information presented in an exam item or the use of faulty or hasty logic to determine what may occur in certain situations can lead to the selection of an incorrect answer.

    a. For example, an OTA determines that it is most appropriate for a person with T12 paraplegia to focus on the upper trapezius and levator scapulae muscles in preparation for functional mobility with crutches, rather than the triceps and lower trapezius muscles. This decision is erroneous because it does not consider the nature of the task at hand (i.e., ambulation with crutches) or tie the muscle functions with the use of crutches for functional mobility.

7. Since quick decisions can lead to suboptimal intervention, the NBCOT exam requires judicious use of inferential reasoning.

8. To help you identify NBCOT exam items that require you to draw conclusions or make logical judgments based on facts, concepts, and evidence rather than direct observations, the analysis of your performance on this text's two practice examinations will have a picture of a light bulb next to inferential reasoning items.

## G. Evaluative Reasoning or Evaluation

1. The process by which the merits of an argument are weighed for their validity and the inherent value of the argument itself is critiqued.

    a. The determination that an argument "holds any water" or not.

    b. If there is value found in the argument itself, the assignment of a value to it.

2. People make judgments about the merits and value of the information they receive all the time and are often unconscious of the thought process that is involved.

3. In OT practice, evaluative reasoning must be conscious.

    a. A good evaluative thinker listens with a skeptical ear to determine the trustworthiness of information before assigning a value to it.

    b. Accepting information at face value can be a reasoning pitfall since there can be additional information needed to complete an accurate assessment of a situation.

4. Evaluative reasoning helps guide thinking about a correct course of action.

5. Evaluation is often used in OT practice when difficult decisions must be made in areas that have no clear cut answers.

    a. Practice situations can be ambiguous and require the OTA to evaluate the situation, weigh the information presented, and determine a correct course of action, given his/her knowledge and experience.

    b. These dilemmas pose a challenge to practitioners since the correct course of action must be determined.

    c. For example, during an intervention session, an OTA observes bruises on an elder resident in a skilled nursing facility and must determine if the correct course of action is immediately notifying the charge nurse, the physician, adult protective services, and/or the family; or asking the resident to explain the source of the bruises; or documenting the observation and continuing with the session as planned.

6. Pitfalls in evaluative reasoning lie in assigning great value to information that has little value to the situation, not assigning enough value to highly valuable information, and finally not utilizing principles and guidelines that are put into place to help guide one's thinking (e.g., OT Code of Ethics, treatment protocols).

   a. For example, an OTA working in home care with a patient who becomes short of breath must determine if he/she should immediately call 911, notify the occupational therapist, notify the physician, or continue with the treatment session.

      (1) It would help the OTA to know if the shortness of breath is an expected symptom given the patient's diagnosis, medical history, and past response to treatment. This information would guide the OTA's thinking about a correct course of action.

      (2) Evaluative reasoning is important in this clinical situation because the OTA could overreact to the situation and call 911 for expected shortness of breath that often accompanies chronic obstructive pulmonary disease or under-react and fail to call 911 when a person is also complaining of co-occurring severe unremitting substernal pain which can be indicative of a myocardial infarction.

7. Evaluative reasoning is often required during the NBCOT exam to correctly answer questions about ethical dilemmas.

8. To help you identify exam items that pose challenging practice situations and ethical dilemmas, the analysis of your performance on this text's two practice examinations will have a picture of a cogwheel next to evaluative reasoning items.

## H. Developing Critical Reasoning Skills for NBCOT Exam Success

1. Since critical reasoning is not learned during a quick lesson or improved upon by simply reading the above basic descriptions of them, practice with items that test reasoning skills and provide feedback on your performance is essential.

   a. The good news is that this *Review and Study Guide* provides 400 opportunities to develop your reasoning skills.

(1) Each MCT item in this text's two simulated practice exams has an accompanying rationale for the correct and incorrect answer choices and an explanation of its corresponding critical reasoning sub-skill and the knowledge or skill required to select the correct answer.

2. When reviewing the analysis of your examination performance on this text's two simulated practice examinations, pay particular attention to the five types of critical reasoning that are listed with each MCT item.

   a. The five symbols assigned to designate the different types of critical reasoning are:

 Binoculars = Inductive Reasoning.

 Microscope = Deductive Reasoning.

 Beaker = Analytical Reasoning.

 Light bulb = Inferential Reasoning.

 Cogwheels = Evaluative Reasoning.

3. Carefully review this feedback to identify any performance patterns that emerge.

   a. Is your exam performance weaker in a certain area of reasoning?

      (1) Since critical reasoning skills are based on knowledge and day-to-day experiences, it is not uncommon to be stronger in certain areas of reasoning than others.

4. If you have a weakness in a certain area(s) of reasoning, do not despair.

   a. Being aware of your gaps in reasoning is the first essential step in the development of a corrective plan of action.

5. As you review the rationales provided for the practice exam items in this *Review and Study Guide,* refer back to your incorrect responses and see if there is a pattern to the types of questions you are answering incorrectly related to a sub-skill of critical reasoning.

a. Do you notice that you have difficulty with certain types of questions?

6. Once you have identified a weakness in critical reasoning, take some time to reflect on why this is so.

a. Ask yourself the questions identified in Table 2-5 and determine if they are reflective of your exam performance.

(1) Questions answered affirmatively can help you identify critical reasoning skills that can be improved.

(2) Implement the corresponding suggested examination preparation strategies to develop needed critical reasoning skills.

7. An honest appraisal of your performance patterns will help build your knowledge of and experience with the application of critical reasoning skills and prepare you to successfully meet the challenges of the NBCOT exam.

## TABLE 2-5: CRITICAL REASONING SELF-ASSESSMENT QUESTIONS

| OBSERVED EXAM DIFFICULTY | REASONING CHALLENGE | NBCOT EXAM PREPARATION STRATEGY |
| --- | --- | --- |
| **Do you:**<br>- have difficulty with taking specific information and applying it to larger populations?<br>- select incorrect answers because you can not generalize your knowledge? | Inductive | When studying a specific content area, think about how the discrete information that you are reviewing can be applied to a diversity of situations. Use a reflective "what if" stance to think how this information may be generalized to a broader context. This can be a fun and effective study group activity. |
| **Do you:**<br>- prefer to follow your instincts rather than the guidelines that a protocol may provide?<br>- select incorrect answers because you are unfamiliar with established practice standards or major theoretical approaches? | Deductive | Be sure when you study that you master all major facts, laws, rules, and accepted principles that guide OT practice. Carefully review all of the frames of reference, practice models, and intervention protocols and procedures provided in Chapters 11 - 15 and the AOTA Code of Ethics and legislation information provided in Chapter 4. |
| **Do you:**<br>- tend to misinterpret information provided and make poor judgments and apply inadequately conceived assumptions about it?<br>- select incorrect answers because you misjudged the effects of a clinical condition on occupational performance? | Analytical | Be sure to obtain a solid knowledge of all major clinical conditions, their symptoms, diagnostic testing and criteria, anticipated sequelae, and expected outcomes. This information is extensively reviewed in Chapters 6 - 10 to help you make accurate judgments and correct assumptions about the potential impact of a clinical condition on occupational performance. |
| **Do you:**<br>- have difficulty with thinking about how clinical conditions and practice situations may evolve over time?<br>- assume information is valid when in fact it is not true?<br>- select incorrect answers because you have difficulty deciding the best course of action in a practice scenario? | Inferential | When studying the clinical conditions in the Chapters identified above, be sure to think about how the presentation of these conditions may sometimes vary from textbook descriptions. Use the knowledge and experience you acquired during your clinical fieldworks to assess the trustworthiness of your assumptions. Study the frames of reference and practice models presented in Chapters 11 - 13 to develop a solid foundation on how to decide the best course of action based on facts, concepts, and evidence. |
| **Do you:**<br>- feel anxious when you have questions that are ambiguous and you cannot find answers to them in a textbook?<br>- rely on protocols and guidelines more than gut instinct?<br>- select incorrect answers because you become overwhelmed by questions that present ethical dilemmas? | Evaluative | When reviewing specific content, think about the practice ambiguities and ethical dilemmas you observed during your fieldworks related to these areas. Be sure to study the guidelines for ethical decision making that are provided in Chapter 4. to help you evaluate NBCOT item scenarios, weigh the information presented, and determine a correct course action. |

This table was adapted with permission from Kari Inda's research on critical reasoning and the OT certification examination.

# References

Facione, P. (2006). *Critical thinking: What it is and why it counts.* Millbrae, CA: California Academic Press.

Facione, P. (1990a). *Critical thinking: A statement of expert consensus for purposes of educational assessment and instruction. Research findings and recommendations.* Newark, DE: American Psychological Association.

Facione, P. (1990b). *Critical thinking: A statement of expert consensus for purposes of educational assessment and instruction ("Executive summary: The Delphi report").* Millbrae, CA: California Academic Press.

Facione, N. C., & Facione, P. A. (2006). *The health sciences reasoning test HSRT: Test manual 2006 edition.* Millbrae, CA: California Academic Press.

Fleming-Castaldy, R. (2010). *Occupational therapy course manual.* Evanston, IL: TherapyED.

Sides, M. & Korcheck, N. (Eds.). (1998). *Successful test-taking: Learning strategies for nurses.* Philadelphia: Lippincott.

Sladyk, K. Gilmore, S. Tufano, R. (2005). *OT exam review manual,* (4th ed.) Thorofare, NJ: Slack.

# CHAPTER 3

# THE PROCESS OF OCCUPATIONAL THERAPY

Rita P. Fleming-Castaldy

## I. The Process of Occupational Therapy

### A. Overview

1. The OT process is comprised of three main aspects of service delivery: evaluation, intervention, and outcomes.
2. This process is client-centered, interactive, and dynamic.
3. The NBCOT examination places a heavy emphasis on the OT process with 80% of the examination focused on service delivery to individuals and populations.

## II. Referral, Screening, and Evaluation

### A. Referral

1. The basic request for occupational therapy services. This may also be termed an order or a consultation.
2. Sources include the individual, family or caregivers, physicians, social workers, physical therapists, nurse practitioners, allied health professionals, teachers, administrators, insurance companies, employers, state and local/public and private agencies.
3. The content and form of a referral/order varies among program types and practice areas and can range from the highly specific (e.g., a resting hand splint) to the very general (e.g., evaluate for developmental delay).

4. While anyone can refer themselves or others to occupational therapy services, the ability of the OT practitioner to act upon the referral is determined by state licensure laws and/or third party reimbursers.
5. If an OTA receives a referral, the OTA must give the referral to the OT supervisor who is responsible for responding to the referral.

### B. Screening

1. The acquisition of information to determine the need for an in depth evaluation and to obtain a preliminary understanding of the individual's needs, limitations, assets, and resources.
2. Screening procedures are usually brief and easy to administer since they must be applied to a large number of individuals (i.e., all persons who receive an OT referral need to be screened to determine the appropriateness of the referral).
3. The OTA contributes to the screening process,
   a. The OTA can collect screening data and report information with OT supervision.
   b. The amount of supervision required will depend upon the OTA's experience and the establishment of service competency.
4. Screening tools measure broad performance abilities and include chart/medical record review, checklists, structured observations, and/or brief interviews with the individual, family, and/or caregivers.

5. Data collected during screening will be analyzed by the OT to determine the areas of performance, performance components, and/or performance contexts that require further evaluation.

**C. Evaluation**

1. The comprehensive process of obtaining and interpreting the data necessary to understand the individual, system, or situation." (Hinojosa, Kramer, & Crist, 2005, p. 2).

2. The OTA contributes to the evaluation process.
   a. The OTA can assist with the collection of evaluation data once service competency is established with OT supervision.
   b. The level of supervision required depends upon the OTA's experience and established service competency.

3. If the individual and the OT practitioner do not share a common language, an interpreter must be used to ensure the validity of the information obtained.

4. The OT supervisor determines which assessment will attain information essential for setting goals and planning intervention.
   a. The OTA contributes to this determination process.
   b. Considerations in determining appropriate assessments.
      (1) Individual's baseline functional level, major concerns, and pressing needs as determined through the screening process.
      (2) The environmental context in which the assessment will be conducted.
         (a) The length of stay of the setting influences comprehensiveness of evaluation.
         (b) The primary focus of the setting, (e.g., prevocational versus self management).
         (c) Legislative guidelines and restrictions (e.g., in a school setting, assessments must focus on areas related to the child's educational needs).
         (d) The facility's resources of space, equipment, and supplies.
      (3) The environmental context of the individual's current and expected environment.
         (a) Sociocultural aspects including roles, values, norms, supports. (For example, in some cultures home management is only considered a valued role for females, so there is no need to do a home management evaluation for a male of this cultural background.)
         (b) Physical environment characteristics. (For example, it would be essential to measure functional mobility endurance for a person who lives in a third floor walk-up apartment.)
      (4) The temporal context of the individual and his/her disability.
         (a) Person's chronological and developmental age.
         (b) Anticipated duration of disability (e.g., short-term, long-term, permanent).
         (c) Recent occurrence of illness or exacerbation of a long-standing, chronic condition.
         (d) Stage of illness (e.g., acute stage versus terminal stage).
      (5) The evaluation tool's compatibility with frame of reference selected to guide intervention planning.
      (6) The existing evidence to support evaluation's use.
      (7) Consider ethical concerns and potential ethical conflicts. (Table 3-1).

5. If service competency is established, the OTA administers the assessment according to recommended guidelines, administration protocols, and/or standardized procedures with OT supervision.
   a. Standard precautions are observed. (Tables 3-2 and 3-3).

6. The OTA and/or occupational therapist scores or rates assessment results according to published guidelines or standardized procedures.

7. The occupational therapist interprets the assessment results in relation to uniform terminology, the practice framework, and/or a specific frame of reference. The OTA collaborates with the occupational therapist to:
   a. Integrate referral, screening, and diagnostic information and data gathered from assessment.
   b. Relate all information to functional abilities and disabilities relevant to person's roles, occupational performance areas, and environmental contexts relevant to the individual.
   c. In school/educational settings, assessment information must be related to the multiple aspects of educational performance.
      (1) Academic.
      (2) Mobility.

## TABLE 3-1 - QUESTIONNAIRE FOR IDENTIFYING POTENTIAL CONFLICTS

### OCCUPATIONAL THERAPIST

- Am I competent to do this assessment? Do I have the necessary knowledge, skills, and attitudes to select, administer, and interpret the results of each evaluation?
- Am I competent to supervise other occupational therapy personnel in the collection of data for this assessment? Am I sure that all delegated tasks are being carried out properly by competent individuals?
- Have I accurately documented the services provided? Is the summary assessment an accurate reflection of the separate evaluations?

### OCCUPATIONAL THERAPY ASSISTANT

- Am I competent to carry out the data collection that I am responsible to perform?
- Am I receiving adequate training and supervision to carry out the assigned portions of the assessment process?
- Have I accurately reported the data and contributed to the overall assessment process?

### INDIVIDUAL WHO IS BEING ASSESSED (FAMILY, SIGNIFICANT OTHERS, GUARDIAN)

- Has the consumer been informed about the purpose of the assessment, how it will be administered, and by whom? Does this person understand how the results of the assessment will be used?
- Has the individual been informed about how this service will be billed?
- Has the person been given the opportunity to decide if the assessment should be done?
- Are the individual's goals the basis for developing and carrying out the assessment process?

### EMPLOYER (FACILITY, AGENCY, COMPANY)

- Is the assessment consistent with the mission of the facility?
- Will there be an accurate billing for services?
- How will the interpretation and recommendations of the therapist be used?

### PAYER

- Is the assessment a necessary and billable service?
- If there is not coverage by third-party reimbursement, does the client know this? Has this individual given consent before the initiation of the evaluations?
- Will the therapist and the billing office request fair compensation for the services and request payment only for the services provided?

### PROFESSIONAL COLLEAGUES

- Is the referral consistent with the client's goals and needs?
- Is this assessment necessary?
- Are you communicating the results of the assessment clearly so that other members of the service delivery team have useful information?
- Have copyrighted evaluation materials been used according to the laws regulating their use?
- Is it necessary to pay fees to use the evaluation tool? Have they been paid?
- Must the practitioner obtain permission to use the materials?
- Is there specific training and supervision required to conduct the evaluation?
- Does the person carrying out the evaluation hold the appropriate credentials to do so?
- Have you used the correct forms and procedures in conducting the evaluation and reporting the results?
- If it is a standardized evaluation, have you followed the procedures exactly?

### COMMUNITY AND SOCIETY

- Is this assessment consistent with the concepts of due process, reparation for wrongs that have been done (physical or emotional), and the fair and equitable distribution of occupational therapy services to individuals needing those services?

From Lesson 10: Ethical considerations. In C.B. Royeen (ed.), *AOTA self-study series. Assessing functions*, (p.9) by Hansen, R.A. Copyright 1990 by the American Occupational Therapy Association. Reprinted with permission.

## TABLE 3-2 - STANDARD PRECAUTIONS

### AIRBORNE PRECAUTIONS

Standard Precautions combine the major features of Universal Precautions (UP) and Body Substance Isolation (BSI) and are based on the principle that all blood, body fluids, secretions, excretions except sweat, nonintact skin, and mucous membranes may contain transmissible infectious agents. Standard Precautions include a group of infection prevention practices that apply to all patients, regardless of suspected or confirmed infection status, in any setting in which health care is delivered. These include hand hygiene; use of gloves, gown, mask, eye protection, or face shield, depending on the anticipated exposure; and safe injection practices. Also, equipment or items in the patient environment likely to have been contaminated with infectious body fluids must be handled in a manner to prevent transmission of infectious agents (e.g., wear gloves for direct contact, contain heavily soiled equipment, properly clean and disinfect or sterilize reusable equipment before use on another patient). The application of Standard Precautions during patient care is determined by the nature of the health care worker (HCW)–patient interaction and the extent of anticipated blood, body fluid, or pathogen exposure. Standard Precautions are also intended to protect patients by ensuring that health-care personnel do not carry infectious agents to patients on their hands or via equipment used during patient care.

Assume that every person is potentially infected or colonized with an organism that could be transmitted in the health-care setting and apply the following infection control practices during the delivery of health care.

### HAND HYGIENE

1. During the delivery of health care, avoid unnecessary touching of surfaces in close proximity to the patient to prevent both contamination of clean hand from environmental surfaces and transmission of pathogens from contaminated hands to surfaces.
2. When hands are visibly dirty, contaminated with proteinaceous material, or visibly soiled with blood or body fluids, wash hands with either a nonantimicrobial soap and water or an antimicrobial soap and water.
3. If hands are not visibly soiled, or after removing visible material with nonantimicrobial soap and water decontaminate hands in the clinical situations described in a-f below. The preferred method of hand decontamination is with an alcohol-based hand rub. Alternatively, hands may be washed with an antimicrobial soap and water. Frequent use of an alcohol-based hand rub immediately following hand washing with nonantimicrobial soap may increase the frequency of dermatitis. Perform hand hygiene:
   a. Before having direct contact with patients.
   b. After contact with blood, body fluids or excretions, mucous membranes, nonintact skin, or wound dressings.
   c. After contact with a patient's intact skin (e.g., when taking a pulse or blood pressure or lifting a patient).
   d. If hands will be moving from a contaminated body site to a clean body site during patient care.
   e. After contact with inanimate objects (including medical equipment) in the immediate vicinity of the patient.
   f. After removing gloves.
4. Wash hands with nonantimicrobial soap and water or with antimicrobial soap and water if in contact with spores (e.g., Clostridium difficile or Bacillus anthracis) is likely to have occurred. The physical action of washing and rinsing hands under such circumstances is recommended because alcohols, chlorhexidine, iodophors, and other antiseptic agents have poor activity against spores.
5. Do not wear artificial fingernails or extenders if duties include direct contact with patients at high risk for infection and associated adverse outcomes (e.g., those in intensive care units [ICUs] or operating rooms).
   a. Develop an organizational policy on the wearing of non-natural nails by health-care personnel who have direct contact with patients outside of the groups specified above.

### PERSONAL PROTECTIVE EQUIPMENT (PPE)

1. Observe the following principles of use:
   a. Wear PPE, as described in 2–4 below, when the nature of the anticipated patient interaction indicates that contact with blood or body fluids may occur.
   b. Prevent contamination of clothing and skin during the process of removing PPE.
   c. Before leaving the patient's room or cubicle, remove and discard PPE.
2. Gloves
   a. Wear gloves when it can be reasonably anticipated that contact with blood or other potentially infectious materials, mucous membranes, nonintact skin, or potentially contaminated intact skin (e.g., of a patient incontinent of stool or urine) could occur.
   b. Wear gloves with fit and durability appropriate to the task.
      (1) Wear disposable medical examination gloves for providing direct patient care.

      (2) Wear disposable medical examination gloves or reusable utility gloves for cleaning the environment or medical equipment.
   c. Remove gloves after contact with a patient and/or the surrounding environment (including medical equipment) using proper technique to prevent hand contamination.
      (1) Do not wear the same pair of gloves for the care of more than one patient. Do not wash gloves for the purpose of reuse since this practice has been associated with transmission of pathogens.
   d. Change gloves during patient care if the hands will move from a contaminated body site (e.g., perineal area) to a clean body site (e.g., face).
3. Gowns
   a. Wear a gown that is appropriate to the task to protect skin and prevent soiling or contamination of clothing during procedures and patient-care activities when contact with blood, body fluids, secretions, or excretions is anticipated.
      (1) Wear a gown for direct patient contact if the patient has uncontained secretions or excretions.
      (2) Remove gown and perform hand hygiene before leaving the patient's environment.
   b. Do not reuse gowns, even for repeated contacts with the same patient.
   c. Routine donning of gowns upon entrance into a high-risk unit (e.g., ICU, neonatal intensive care unit [NICU], hematopoietic stem cell transplantation [HSCT] unit) is not indicated.
4. Mouth, nose, eye protection.
   a. Use PPE to protect the mucous membranes of the eyes, nose, and mouth during procedures and patient-care activities that are likely to generate splashes or sprays of blood, body fluids, secretions, and excretions. Select masks, goggles, face shields, and combinations of each according to the need anticipated by the task performed.
5. During aerosol-generating procedures (e.g., bronchoscopy, suctioning of the respiratory tract [if not using in-line suction catheters], endotracheal intubation) in patients who are not suspected of being infected with an agent for which respiratory protection is otherwise recommended (e.g., M. tuberculosis, SARS, orhemorrhagic fever viruses), wear one of the following: a face shield that fully covers the front and sides of the face, a mask with attached shield, or a mask and goggles (in addition to gloves and gown).

### RESPIRATORY HYGIENE/COUGH ETIQUETTE

1. Educate healthcare personnel on the importance of source control measures to contain respiratory secretions to prevent droplet and fomite transmission of respiratory pathogens, especially during seasonal outbreaks of viral respiratory tract infections (e.g., influenza, respiratory syncytial virus [RSV], adenovirus, parainfluenza virus) in communities.
2. Implement the following measures to contain respiratory secretions in patients and accompanying individuals who have signs and symptoms of a respiratory infection, beginning at the point of initial encounter in a health-care setting (e.g., triage, reception and waiting areas in emergency departments, outpatient clinics, and physician offices).

## TABLE 3-2 - STANDARD PRECAUTIONS CONTINUED

a. Post signs at entrances and in strategic places (e.g., elevators, cafeterias) within ambulatory and inpatient settings with instructions to patients and other persons with symptoms of a respiratory infection to cover their mouths/noses when coughing or sneezing, use and dispose of tissues, and perform hand hygiene after hands have been in contact with respiratory secretions.

b. Provide tissues and no-touch receptacles (e.g., foot pedal–operated lid or open, plastic-lined waste basket) for disposal of tissues.

c. Provide resources and instructions for performing hand hygiene in or near waiting areas in ambulatory and inpatient settings; provide conveniently located dispensers of alcohol-based hand rubs and, where sinks are available, supplies for hand washing.

d. During periods of increased prevalence of respiratory infections in the community (e.g., as indicated by increased school absenteeism, increased number of patients seeking care for a respiratory infection), offer masks to coughing patients and other symptomatic persons (e.g., persons who accompany ill patients) upon entry into the facility or medical office and encourage them to maintain special separation, ideally a distance of at least 3 feet, from others in common waiting areas.
   (1) Some facilities may find it logistically easier to institute this recommendation year-round as a standard of practice.

### PATIENT PLACEMENT

1. Include the potential for transmission of infectious agents in patient placement decisions.
   a. Place patients who pose a risk for transmission to others (e.g., uncontained secretions, excretions or wound drainage, infants with suspected viral respiratory or gasrointestinal infections) in a single-patient room when available.
2. Determine patient placement based on the following principles:
   a. Route(s) of transmission of the known or suspected infectious agent.
   b. Risk factors for transmission in the infected patient.
   c. Risk factors for adverse outcomes resulting from a hospital-acquired infection (HAI) in other patients in the area or room being considered for patient placement.
   d. Availability of single-patient rooms.
   e. Patient options for room sharing (e.g., cohorting patients with the same infection).

### PATIENT-CARE EQUIPMENT AND INSTRUMENTS/DEVICES

1. Establish policies and procedures for containing, transporting, and handling patient-care equipment and instruments/devices that may be contaminated with blood or body fluids.
2. Remove organic material from critical and semicritical instrument/devices, using recommended cleaning agents before high-level disinfection and sterilization to enable effective disinfection and sterilization processes.
3. Wear PPE (e.g., gloves, gown), according to the level of anticipated contamination, when handling patient-care equipment and instruments/devices that are visibly soiled or may have been in contact with blood or body fluids.

### CARE OF THE ENVIRONMENT

1. Establish policies and procedures for routine and targeted cleaning of environmental surfaces as indicated by the level of patient contact and degree of soiling.
2. Clean and disinfect surfaces that are likely to be contaminated with pathogens, including those that are in close proximity to the patient (e.g., bed rails, over bed tables) and frequently touched surfaces in the patient-care environment (e.g., door knobs, surfaces in and surrounding toilets in patients' rooms) on a more frequent schedule compared to that for other surfaces (e.g., horizontal surfaces in waiting rooms).
3. Use Environmental Protection Agency (EPA)–registered disinfectants that have microbiocidal (i.e., killing) activity against the pathogens most likely to contaminate the patient-care environment. Use in accordance with manufacturer's instructions.
   a. Review the efficacy of in-use disinfectants when evidence of continuing transmission of an infectious agent (e.g., rotavirus, C. difficile, norovirus) may indicate resistance to the in-use product and change to a more effective disinfectant as indicated.
4. In facilities that provide health care to pediatric patients or have waiting areas with child play toys (e.g., obstetric/gynecology offices and clinics), establish policies and procedures for cleaning and disinfecting toys at regular intervals.
   a. Use the following principles in developing this policy and procedures:
      (1) Select play toys that can be easily cleaned and disinfected.
      (2) Do not permit use of stuffed furry toys if they will be shared.
      (3) Clean and disinfect large stationary toys (e.g., climbing equipment) at least weekly and whenever visibly soiled.
      (4) If toys are likely to be mouthed, rinse with water after disinfection; alternatively wash in a dishwasher.
      (5) When a toy requires cleaning and disinfection, do so immediately or store in a designated labeled container separate from toys that are clean and ready for use.
5. Include multiuse electronic equipment in policies and procedures for preventing contamination and for cleaning and disinfection, especially those items that are used by patients, those used during delivery of patient care, and mobile devices that are moved in and out of patient rooms frequently (e.g., daily).
   a. No recommendations are provided for use of removable protective covers or washable keyboards. This is an unresolved issue.

### TEXTILES AND LAUNDRY

1. Handle used textiles and fabrics with minimum agitation to avoid contamination of air, surfaces, and persons.
2. If laundry are used, ensure that they are properly designed, maintained, and used in a manner to minimize dispersion of aerosols from contaminated laundry.

### SAFE INJECTION PRACTICES

These are not included here since OT practitioners do not give injections. See CDC website.

### WORKER SAFETY

Adhere to federal and state requirements for protection of health-care personnel from exposure to bloodborne pathogens.

Reference: Centers for Disease Control and Prevention. (2007). Guideline for isolation precautions: Preventing transmission of infectious agents in healthcare settings. Retrieved March 9, 2010 from http://www.cdc.gov/ncidod/dhqp/gl_isolation_standard.html

      (3) Psychosocial.
      (4) Behavioral.
      (5) Self care.
8. The occupational therapist and OTA collaborate with the individual, family, caregivers, and other team members to obtain a broader picture of the person's situation and to put the OT assessment results into a larger context.
   a. In school/educational settings, medically necessary OT must be separated from educationally relevant OT.
   b. Referrals to after school, home care, and/or community-based OT services are indicated for non-educational OT.

## TABLE 3-3 - TRANSMISSION-BASED PRECAUTIONS

There are three categories of Transmission-Based Precautions: Contact Precautions, Droplet Precautions, and Airborne Precautions. Transmission-Based Precautions are used when the route(s) of transmission is (are) not completely interrupted using Standard Precautions alone. For some diseases that have multiple routes of transmission (e.g., SARS), more than one Transmission-Based Precautions category may be used. When used either singly or in combination, they are always used in addition to Standard Precautions. When Transmission-Based Precautions are indicated, efforts must be made to counteract possible adverse effects on patients (i.e., anxiety, depression and other mood disturbances, perceptions of stigma, reduced contact with clinical staff, and increases in preventable adverse events in order to improve acceptance by the patients and adherence by health care workers.

### AIRBORNE PRECAUTIONS

In addition to Standard Precautions, use Airborne Precautions, or the equivalent, for patients known or suspected to be infected with serious illness transmitted by airborne droplet nuclei (small-particle residue) that remain suspended in the air and that can be dispersed widely by air currents within a room or over a long distance (for example, Mycobacterium tuberculosis, measles virus, chickenpox virus).

1. Respiratory isolation room.
2. Wear respiratory protection (mask) when entering room.
3. Limit movement and transport of patient to essential purposes only. Mask patient when transporting out of area.

### DROPLET PRECAUTIONS

In addition to Standard Precautions, use Droplet Precautions, or the equivalent, for patients known or suspected to be infected with serious illness microorganisms transmitted by large particle droplets that can be generated by the patient during coughing, sneezing, talking, or the performance of procedures (for example, mumps, rubella, pertussis, influenza).

1. Isolation room.
2. Wear respiratory protection (mask) when entering room.
3. Limit movement and transport of patient to essential purposes only. Mask patient when transporting out of area.

### CONTACT PRECAUTIONS

In addition to Standard Precautions, use Contact Precautions, or the equivalent, for specified patients known or suspected to be infected or colonized with serious illness transmitted by direct patient contact (hand or skin-to-skin contact) or contact with items in patient environment.

1. Isolation room.
2. Wear gloves when entering room; change gloves after having contact with infective material; remove gloves before leaving patient's room; wash hands immediately with an antimicrobial agent or waterless antiseptic agent. After glove removal and handwashing, ensure that hands do not touch contaminated environmental items.
3. Wear a gown when entering room if you anticipate your clothing will have substantial contact with the patient, environmental surfaces, or items in the patient's room, or if the patient is incontinent or has diarrhea, ileostomy, colostomy, or wound drainage not contained by dressing. Remove gown before leaving patient's room; after gown removal, ensure that clothing does not contact potentially contaminated environmental surfaces.
4. Single-patient-use equipment.
5. Limit movement and transport of patient to essential purposes only. Use precautions when transporting patient to minimize risk of transmission of microorganisms to other patients and contamination of environmental surfaces or equipment.

Reference: Centers for Disease Control and Prevention. (2007). *Guideline for isolation precautions: Preventing transmission of infectious agents in healthcare settings.* Retrieved March 9, 2010 from http://www.cdc.gov/ncidod/dhqp/gl_isolation_standard.html

9. The OT supervisor prioritizes identified problems in collaboration with the OTA and the individual to develop intervention plan.

### D. Assessment Tools

1. The OTA can utilize a diversity of assessment tools with OT supervision and the establishment of service competency.
2. Observation involves visual assessment of an individual, his/her behavior, and environmental contexts. (See Section E for an overview of the skills needed for accurate observations).
3. Interviews involve the practitioner asking the individual specific questions. (See Section F for an overview of interviewing techniques).
4. Self report requires the individual to disclose personal information in an organized manner, e.g., through the completion of a questionnaire.

5. Checklists require the use of a predetermined listing of items against which a person's performance is checked to determine the presence or absence of these items.
6. Rating scales require the individual or occupational therapist /OTA to rate reactions, performance, or set criteria according to an established scale.
7. Performance tests involve structured guidelines and/or standardized procedures for engaging the individual in performing an activity and for scoring this activity.
8. Norm-referenced assessments produce scores that compare the individual's performance to a set population's performance.
9. Criterion-referenced assessments provide scores that compare the individual's performance to a pre-established criterion.

10. The OTA can utilize assessment tools upon the establishment of service competency with OT supervision.
    a. State licensure laws, regulations, and statutes may limit the OTA's role in assessment but this variability will not be tested on the NBCOT examination.

**E. Observation Skills**
1. Observation of a person during actual occupational performance is critical.
2. Observation of performance must be done in different contexts and in structured and unstructured situations.
3. Observation of environmental contexts is also important to assess physical and sociocultural supports or barriers.
4. Use of a structured tool to note observations can increase reliability.
5. Observations must be ongoing to assess the nuances of performance and subtle changes in function.
6. The OTA must be aware of his/her own sociocultural background, as this is the lens through which he/she observes and it can influence the interpretation of observations (e.g., appropriateness of the individual's non-verbal behavior).
7. The OTA shares his/her observations with the OT supervisor.
    a. Interpretation of these observations is made by the OT supervisor in collaboration with the OTA.
    b. Interpretations must be validated by the individual and/or caregiver.

**F. Interviewing Guidelines**
1. Establish the purpose of the interview.
    a. Questions asked and information sought should be consistent with stated purpose.
    b. Interviewee should feel each question is relevant and significant.
    c. Irrelevant, spurious, and/or extraneous questions should not be asked.
2. Establish rapport with interviewee.
    a. Initial interview is often the beginning of a long-term therapeutic relationship.
    b. Set an atmosphere of trust by maintaining confidentiality.
    c. Set an atmosphere of respect by being on time, asking pertinent questions, and actively listening.
3. Ask questions in an organized, formalized manner.
    a. Interviews are not casual conversations.
    b. A haphazard approach will not obtain information needed to achieve the purpose of the interview.
    c. Numerous assessment tools are available to guide the interview.
        (1) The OTA can use these tools with OT supervision upon establishment of service competence.
4. Observe interviewee's non-verbal communications during the interview.
    a. What is not said during an interview can be as important as what is said.
        (1) Gaps in information presented.
        (2) Affect and mood.
        (3) Physical mannerisms.
        (4) Speech patterns and inflections.
    b. Interpret with OT supervision the congruence or incongruence of non-verbal behaviors with actual verbalizations.
5. Listen before talking.
    a. Counteracts preconceived views of interviewee.
    b. Prevents premature recommendations.
6. Question and re-question, as needed, to obtain essential information.
    a. Follow up questions should be specific.
    b. Open-ended, leading questions facilitate discussion.
    c. Questions that can be answered by yes or no should be avoided.
7. Comment in a limited manner and only when directly related to the stated purpose of the interview.
    a. Reassuring comments are used to facilitate interviewee's participation.
    b. Specific suggestions or advice should only be given if intervention is part of interview's purpose.
8. Answer personal questions directed to interviewer by interviewee in a direct and honest manner.
    a. Purposes of personal questions asked by interviewee.
        (1) To show a general polite interest in interviewer.
        (2) To move the therapeutic relationship to a closer level.
        (3) To indirectly introduce a personal concern of his/her own.
    b. Interviewer should immediately re-direct interviewee to purpose of interview and to him/herself after providing a brief, truthful answer.
9. Lead and direct interview to achieve stated purpose.

10. Maintain confidentiality at all times.
11. The OTA shares interview results with the OT supervisor.
    a. The OT supervisor interprets verbalizations and nonverbal communications to formulate hypotheses about interviewee's situation.
12. The OT supervisor develops a plan in collaboration with the OTA based on the information obtained from the interview and the hypotheses formulated about the person's situation.
    a. Plan can include the need for further evaluation and more information.
    b. The use of an interview to formulate a plan can prevent interviewing just for the sake of interviewing.
    c. Plans for intervention should be developed collaboratively with the individual using a client-centered approach.

## III. Intervention

### A. Types of Intervention
1. Prevention: interventions designed to promote wellness, prevent disabilities and illnesses, and maintain health.
    a. Primary prevention: the reduction of the incidence or occurrence of a disease or disorder within a population that is currently well or considered to be potentially at risk (e.g., parenting skills classes for teen parents to prevent child neglect or abuse).
        (1) In the AOTA practice framework, primary prevention is termed 'create/promote' and 'health promotion'.
            (a) Interventions focus on providing enrichment experiences to enhance person's occupational performance in their natural contexts.
    b. Secondary prevention: the early detection of problems in a population at risk to reduce the duration of a disorder/disease and/or minimize its effects through early detection/diagnosis, early appropriate referral and early/effective intervention (e.g., the screening of infants born prematurely for developmental delays and the immediate implementation of intervention for identified delays).
    c. Tertiary prevention: the elimination or reduction of the impact of dysfunction on an individual (e.g., the provision of rehabilitation services to maximize community integration).
    d. In the AOTA practice framework, the term 'dis-ability prevention' is used to designate interventions that address the needs of persons with or without disabilities who are considered at risk for problems with their occupational performance.
        (1) Interventions focus on preventing the occurrence or minimizing the effects of barriers to occupational performance.
2. Meeting health needs: interventions designed to satisfy inherent, universal human needs. These needs are not automatically met and they include:
    a. Psychophysical: the need for adequate shelter, food, material goods, sensory stimulation, physical activity and rest (e.g., institutionalized orphans confined to cribs require sensorimotor interventions to counter environmental deprivation).
    b. Temporal balance and regularity: the need for a satisfying balance between work/productive activities, leisure/play, and rest (e.g., forced leisure due to involuntary unemployment requires intervention to achieve temporal balance).
    c. Safety: the need to be in an environment free from hazards or threats (e.g., living in a chaotic, abusive home does not meet this need and interventions are needed to ensure safety).
    d. Love and acceptance: the need to be accepted and loved for one's personal attributes and uniqueness, not for one's accomplishments (e.g., the barriers caused by aphasia and ataxia can hinder meeting this need; therefore, supportive interventions are indicated).
    e. Group association: the need to feel a connection to others who share similar interests and goals (e.g., the stigma and symptoms of mental illness can prevent regular interactions with a group; therefore, interventions to develop social interaction skills and provide community supports are indicated).
    f. Mastery: the need to successfully complete an activity or meet a goal because it is interesting and challenging (e.g., deficits in performance components can hinder successful performance and block mastery, therefore interventions to develop performance skills and/or adapt activities are needed).
    g. Esteem: the need to be recognized for one's accomplishments (e.g., a lack of opportunity to do activities perceived as worthwhile by others requires interventions to facilitate recognized contributions).
    h. Sexual: the need for recognition of one's sexu-

ality and the satisfaction of sexual drives (e.g., institutional rules against adult consensual sex prohibit meeting this need and require review and revision). Also, physical impediments to sexuality may require activity adaptations and environmental modifications.

    i. Pleasure: the need to do things just for fun (e.g., the child on an intensive school and home physical rehabilitation program needs an intervention plan supportive of spontaneous play).

    j. Self actualization: the need to engage in activities just for one's self and for personal satisfaction (e.g., the person who writes poetry through an augmentative communication device for the joy of free expression).

3. The change process: interventions designed to achieve behavioral changes and functional outcomes.

    a. This type of intervention is the most commonly used in OT practice and is the most reimbursable.

    b. This process is often the only form of intervention discussed or documented.

    c. Guidelines for intervention planning and intervention implementation relate directly to this process.

    d. In the AOTA practice framework, the terms 'establish/restore/remediation/restoration' are used to distinguish interventions that change a person in some manner.

       (1) Interventions focus on establishing a skill or ability that a person had never developed and/or restoring a skill or ability that the person had lost due to impairment.

4. Management: interventions designed to reduce or minimize disruptive or undesirable behavior that interfere with therapeutic activities or procedures needed to change areas of dysfunction that are the main focus of intervention (e.g., an individual becomes excessively anxious during his/her first use of a wheelchair in an environment outside of the hospital. Supportive interventions are needed to decrease anxiety, thereby enabling the person to work on essential community mobility skills).

    a. In the AOTA practice framework, the terms 'modify/compensation/adaptation' are used to distinguish interventions that alter the context or demands of an activity to reduce distracting features.

       (1) Compensation and adaptation techniques are also used to alter the context or demands of an activity to support the person's ability to engage in areas of occupation (e.g., the provision of cues).

5. Maintenance: interventions designed to support and preserve the individual's current functional level (e.g., a reminiscence group to maintain the cognitive and social skills of individuals with early to mid-stage Alzheimer's disease).

    a. No improvement in function is planned due to the chronicity of the disorder or the progression of the disease.

    b. A decline in function is prevented, as much and for as long as possible.

    c. Maintenance programs include familial, environmental, and social supports and consistent and regularly scheduled follow-ups.

    d. While maintenance is not often reimbursed by third-party payers, it is a major type of OT intervention due to the chronic and progressive nature of many disorders with which we work.

    e. In the AOTA practice framework, the term 'maintain' is used to designate these interventions.

## B. Intervention Planning

1. The formulation of the plan for intervention based upon an analysis of evaluation results according to selected frame(s) of reference.

2. The OT supervisor is responsible for the intervention plan.

    a. The OTA contributes to this plan in a collaborative process.

3. Collaboration with the individual, family, significant others, and/or caregivers is essential to establish a relevant, meaningful plan that will be followed.

4. Prioritization of problem areas to be addressed in intervention.

    a. Values, interests, and needs of the individual, family, significant others, and caregivers.

    b. Individual's current and expected roles and environmental contexts.

    c. The treatment setting's characteristics, resources, and limitations (e.g., length of stay).

    d. The likelihood that the problem will respond to intervention within the given setting.

       (1) Concrete and specific problems are more likely to be effectively resolved than abstract global ones.

       (2) Services must be available within the setting to effectively address the problem; otherwise a referral is indicated.

5. Formats of written intervention plans can vary from setting to setting.
6. Intervention plan content.
   a. Long term goals (LTGs): the change in activity limitations and participation restriction that will occur, prior to the termination of intervention, in order to achieve the desired functional occupational performance outcome.
   b. Short term goals (STGs) or objectives: the component subskills which are to be achieved over shorter time frames, leading to the attainment of the long term goal.
      (1) STGs must be directly related to the LTG.
      (2) Due to the reality of very brief lengths of stay (LOS) in some settings, only STGs may be accomplished prior to the termination of intervention.
      (3) Referrals to other settings with longer LOS or home care services may be required for intervention to attain LTGs.
   c. Intervention methods.
      (1) The meaningful occupations and purposeful activities and their associated tasks, techniques, procedures, and modalities that are used to achieve goals.
      (2) Methods of intervention must be clearly related to, and theoretically consistent with, the established goals.
      (3) Home programs and/or family caregiver training may be included.
      (4) Adaptive/assistive equipment, orthotics, prosthetics, and/or environmental modifications to meet individual's needs are specified.
   d. Duration, frequency, and number and type of intervention sessions planned to attain goals are specified (e.g., 10 community mobility groups, meeting for 1 hour, 3 times per week).
   e. Recommendations for additional OT services and referrals, if needed, to other professionals are provided.
   f. Clinical reasoning must be used when designing intervention plans to ensure that each plan's primary focus is on the individual's engagement in occupation and participation in his/her chosen contexts.
   g. The existing evidence to support potential interventions must be reviewed and used to guide the intervention plan.

## C. Intervention Implementation
1. Fundamental OT principles are used to guide OT interventions. See Table 3-4, "Principles of Occupations".
2. The OTA is responsible for intervention implementation with OT supervision.
   a. Clinical reasoning is used to guide the implementation of intervention. See this chapter's Section V G.
   b. State licensure laws, regulations, and statutes may limit the OTA's role in the implementation of intervention but this variability will not be tested on the NBCOT examination.
3. Overview of OT intervention methods.
   a. Purposeful activities and meaningful occupations are used therapeutically.
      (1) See this chapter's sections on tools of practice, occupation, purposeful activities, and activity analysis and synthesis. (Section V).
   b. Environmental modifications and adaptations are provided to enhance function.
   c. Promotion of engagement in valued occupations is used to foster health and wellness.
   d. Adaptive equipment, assistive technology, and orthotic devices are designed, fabricated, and applied to facilitate function.
   e. Adaptive equipment, assistive technology, orthotics, and prosthetic use training are provided to promote independence.
   f. Physical agent modalities are used to prepare for, or as an adjunct to, engagement in therapeutic functional activities.
   g. Ergonomic principles are applied to the performance of meaningful occupations.
   h. Standard precautions are observed.
      (1) Standard precautions are the primary strategy for control of nosocomial infection and are used in the care of all persons (Table 3-2).
   i. Transmission-based precautions are used for persons with known or suspected infections of highly transmissible or epidemiologically important pathogens.
      (1) Includes airborne precautions, droplet precautions and contact precautions (Table 3-3).
3. Individual, group or population interventions may be used.
   a. Refer to Table 3-5 for a comparison of indications for "Individual vs. Group interventions".
   b. See this chapter's sections on the teaching-learning process, therapeutic use of self, and group process.

## TABLE 3-4 - PRINCIPLES OF OCCUPATIONS THAT SUPPORT THEIR VALUE AND USE IN INTERVENTION

| PRINCIPLE | EXPLANATION | EXAMPLE |
|---|---|---|
| Occupations and activities act as a therapeutic change agent to *remediate* or *restore*. | People have the potential to improve performance skills, patterns (habits, routines, and rituals), and body functions. | A homemaker who has impairments and problems in motor skills resulting from a stroke benefits more from working in the actual occupation of preparing meals in conjunction with exercises to increase her ROM, muscle strength, and coordination as opposed to solely using exercise equipment and objects stimulating the motor actions of the activity (Gasser-Wieland &Rice, 2002). |
| The use of new occupations as interventions provides the means for *establishing* performance skills and for developing habits. | The features of the context and environment may have changed and thus may demand the use of new performance skills and habits for the client to perform successfully. | Women with developmental delays and psychiatric conditions had a reduced rate of inappropriate behaviors and increased rate of socially appropriate behaviors in a new community living arrangement when given positive reinforcement in perusing everyday occupations (Holm, Santangelo, Fromuth, Brown, & Walter, 2000). |
| Valued occupations are *inherently motivating*. | Chosen occupations often are a reflection of what people value and enjoy and thus are more likely to be satisfying | Older adults were motivated to resume engagement in occupations because of opportunities to reestablish relationships with others during engagement in valued occupations (Chan & Spencer, 2004). |
| Occupations promote the identification of *values and interests*. | Values influence occupational choice. When active in occupations, one experiences pleasure and satisfaction, thus generating interests (Kielhofner, 2002). | Older adults living within their communities related the three most important activities required for them to remain in their communities as using the telephone, using transportation, and reading; health professionals' list consisted of using the telephone, managing medications and preparing snacks (Fricke & Unsworth, 2001). |
| Occupations create opportunities to *practice* performance skills and to *reinforce* performance. | The client must have the opportunity to develop patterns that include the remediated skill in routine daily tasks (Holm, Rogers, & Stone, 2003, p.477). | Elementary students with learning disabilities and handwriting problems who practiced keyboarding in a training program improved written communication skills for performance at school (Handley-More, Deitz, Billingsley, & Coggins, 2003). |
| Active engagement in occupations produces *feedback*. | Corrective feedback regarding performance helps the client modify behavior. | A computer system was modified for a person with a head injury to provide an auditory prompt to mark the commencement of each planned activity. "I was just sitting there on the sofa doing something like reading a newspaper, and had completely forgotten the swimming bath, the computer started to bleep; oh, what had I forgotten now?" (Erikson, Karlsson, Soderstrom, & Tham, 2004, p. 267). |
| Engagement in occupations facilitates *mastery or competence* in performing daily activities. | Successes motivate further change and continued use and practice of newly learned performance skills during engagement in occupations. | People with severe mental illness developed skills and competence in work and social activities while participating in a supported work setting (Gahnstrom-Strandqvist, Liukko, & Tham, 2003). |
| Selected occupations promote *participation* with individuals or groups. | Interventions designed to eliminate physical and social barriers increase opportunities for social interaction, leading to increased interaction and sense of control in context and environment. | Children with impaired performance skills used an adapted powered-mobility riding toy, which increased opportunities for participation with other children and adults during the occupation of play (Deitz, Swinth, & White, 2002). |

## TABLE 3-4 - PRINCIPLES OF OCCUPATIONS THAT SUPPORT THEIR VALUE AND USE IN INTERVENTION CONTINUED

| PRINCIPLE | EXPLANATION | EXAMPLE |
|---|---|---|
| Through engagement in occupations, people learn to *assume responsibility for their own health and wellness.* | Interventions that focus on improving a client's ability to self-direct change in lifestyle choices can lead to a sense of control . | People with chronic disorders who participated in community-based group services developed responsibility for their own health by empowerment of the group members (Taylor, Braveman, & Hammel, 2004). |
| Occupations exert a positive influence on *health* and *well-being* (Law, 2002b). | Regardless of the presence of impairments, a person may remain active and engaged in healthy occupations. | People with fibromyalgia who successfully used activity modification strategies to complete daily activities reported positive quality of life and health (Lindberg & Schkade, 2001). |
| Occupations provide the means for people to *adapt* to changing needs and conditions. | A person's capacity for performance is affected by the status of body structures and functions. Permanent loss of capacity necessitates modification of the context and environment and of activity demands. | Patients who had hip fractures demonstrated more efficiency and greater satisfaction in recovering performance skills in daily occupations when modified activity procedures were emphasized (Jackson & Schkade, 2001). |
| Occupations contribute to the creation and maintenance *of identity* (AOTA, 2002; Christainsen, 1999). | Discovering identity is related to what a person does and to those people with whom they come in contact during daily occupations and activities. | People with injuries to the hand resumed occupations that facilitated resumption of their identity (Chan & Spencer, 2004). |
| Successful performance in occupation can positively affect *psychological* functioning. | A person's evaluation of performance in occupations and activities influences perceptions about himself or herself. | People recovering from a stroke demonstrated positive views and acceptance of the need for a wheelchair, described opportunities for continuity of previous life activities, maintenance of mobility, and decreased burden on the caregiver (Barker, Reid, & Cott, 2004). |
| Occupations have unique *meaning* and *purpose* for each person, which influences the quality of performance (AOTA, 2002). | The meaning of occupations refers to the subjective experience one has when engaging in activities. | People recovering from a stroke stood longer when performing personally meaningful tasks (Dolecheck & Schkade, 1999). |
| Engagement in occupations gives a sense of *satisfaction* and *fulfillment* (AOTA, 2002). | Performance of valued occupations provides for achievement of personal goals in a variety of roles. | Satisfaction through occupations was found when older adults maintained daily routines and engaged in fulfilling occupations (Bontje, Kinebanian, Josephsson, & Tamura, 2004). Goldberg, Brintell, and Golberg (2002) found a correlation between engagement in meaningful activites and life satisfaction. |
| Occupations influence how people spend time and *make decisions* (AOTA, 2002). | People occupy time through engagement in activity. | In a study of time use, older people spent most of their time completing activities that were meaningful for them and not necessarily the activities that were necessary for them to remain in the community (Fricke & Unsworth, 2001). |

## TABLE 3-5 - INDIVIDUAL VS. GROUP INTERVENTION

| | |
|---|---|
| Individual | Learning capacity of the person |
| | Amount of attention and skill required from the occupational therapy practitioner owing to body structure and function impairments |
| | Need for privacy |
| | Need for greater control over the context and environment |
| | Difficulty or complexity of occupation and activity demands, performance skills and performance patterns |
| | Inappropriate or dangerous behavior of the person |
| Group | Developing interpersonal skills |
| | Engaging in socialization |
| | Receiving feedback from people experiencing similar conditions |
| | Being motivated by peer role models |
| | Learning from other people |
| | Placing one's own condition into perspective |
| | Developing group normative behavior for successful performance in shared occupations (e.g., work, study, and leisure groups |

From Moyers, P.A. & Dale, L (2007). *The guide to occupational therapy practice*, 2nd edition, p. 47. Copyright 2007 by the American Occupational Therapy Association. Reprinted with permission.

## IV. Reevaluation/Intervention Review

### A. Overview

1. The process of determining whether the individual's occupational performance has improved, declined, or remained the same after intervention.
2. Frequent monitoring of an individual's response to intervention is an integral part of all OT interventions.
3. Effective interventions resulting in the individual's progress require intervention plan modification and an upgrading of goals, as long as there is a reasonable expectation that the individual can improve functional performance.
4. If the individual is not progressing according to plan, different intervention methods, referral(s) to experts in the field or other professions or to another level of care, and/or discharge from intervention may be indicated.

### B. The Role of the OTA

1. The OT supervisor is responsible for the review of intervention and reevaluation process.
   a. The OTA contributes to this process in a collaborative manner.
2. The OTA shares all observations regarding an individual's response to intervention and any other information that may affect intervention and intervention plans.
   a. The OT supervisor is responsible for intervention plan modification.
   b. The OTA contributes to this process.

### C. Discharge Planning

1. The process for planning for discontinuation of services.
2. The OT supervisor is responsible for this process.
   a. The OTA contributes to this process in a collaborative manner.
3. Reasons for discharge.
   a. The individual's goals have been met.
   b. The individual has reached a functional plateau.
   c. The individual does not require skilled services, for maximum benefit has been achieved.
   d. An exacerbation of an illness or a medical crisis requires discharge to a higher level of care.
   e. The person's allotted length of stay in the setting has expired and extension of LOS is not possible.
4. General principles.
   a. Discharge planning begins with the initial evaluation and is an inherent part of the intervention planning process. All interventions should be planned with consideration of the expected, planned discharge environment.
   b. Collaboration with the individual, family, significant others, caregivers, other professionals on the team, employers, and reimbursers is required for an effective and realistic discharge plan.
   c. Discharge may include transfer to a long-term care setting (e.g., a skilled nursing or assistive living facility), to an intermediate care facility (e.g., a halfway house), or to a home setting.
      (1) A pre-discharge home evaluation must be completed to ensure the individual will be safe and to identify needed home adaptations or supports (e.g., bathroom modifications, home health aide).
   d. A well planned discharge facilitates community integration and maintenance of functional gains.

5. Follow-up referrals for further OT intervention and/or other supportive services must be made.
   a. Home programs.
      (1) Recommendations to the individual, family, significant others, and caregivers on techniques and procedures to maintain and/or improve functional status.
      (2) Training should be provided prior to discharge.
      (3) Information on additional supports should be provided.
   b. Community resources.
      (1) Recommendations and referrals to specific services in the community that can support function (e.g., AA, day treatment).

## V. OT Tools of Practice

### A. Definition
1. The established, legitimate means by which the practitioners of a profession achieve the profession's goals and meet society's needs.

### B. Relevance to Examination
1. While it is unlikely that the NBCOT examination will ask direct questions about the following tools of practice, the use and application of these tools of practice will be needed to decide the best possible answer to a question about practice.

### C. Occupation
1. Definition: Goal-directed pursuits which typically extend over time.
   a. They have purpose, value, and meaning to the performer, and involve multiple tasks.
   b. They are the ordinary and familiar things that people do every day.
2. Basic concepts of occupation.
   a. Every individual has multiple occupations that are meaningful (e.g., self-care, home management, work and leisure) and needed to function in roles (e.g., parent, worker, student, hobbyist).
   b. Humans are innately occupational beings and are driven by an inherent need for mastery, self-actualization, self-identity, competence, and social acceptance.
   c. Occupations have social, cultural, physical, and temporal contextual dimensions because they involve activities within specific settings and extend over time.
   d. Occupations have symbolic and spiritual dimensions, as individuals infuse individualized meanings into occupations.

   e. Occupations are interdependent (e.g., one must work to pay for leisure; one must have leisure to sustain and renew oneself for work).
   f. Health is attained when the dynamic balance between occupations and rest is appropriate and meets the needs of the individual.
   g. Occupation can be viewed and used as a "means" or a method to change an individual's performance (e.g., playing a board game to increase motor skills).
   h. Occupation can also be viewed and used as an "end" or desired outcome (e.g., playing a board game to improve the ability to engage in age-appropriate social play).
   i. Engagement in occupation to support the individual's participation in environment(s) of choice is the overriding desired outcome of OT.
3. Areas of occupation.
   a. Activities of daily living: activities that involve care of self; often called personal activities of daily living (PADL) or basic activities of daily living (BADL).
   b. Instrumental activities of daily living: activities that involve environmental interaction; they are more complex than self-care and can be optional (e.g., home maintenance, care of others and community mobility activities).
   c. Work: all productive activities that contribute services, goods, or commodities to society, whether financially compensated or not (i.e., a student or a volunteer is working).
   d. Education: activities that involve the student role and participation in an educational environment.
   e. Play/leisure: all activities engaged in for pleasure, relaxation, amusement, and/or self-fulfillment.
   f. Social participation: activities involving interaction with community, family, and peers/friends.

### D. Purposeful Activities
1. Definition.
   a. Doing processes that are directed toward a desired and intended outcome and require energy and thought to engage in and complete.
   b. The goal-directed tasks and/or behaviors that make up occupations.
2. Characteristics of purposeful activities.
   a. Universally, people participate in purposeful activities, although there are personal and soci-

ocultural differences in the manner in which activities are performed (e.g., dressing).

b. Fundamental to the development and acquisition of performance component skills is active participation in purposeful activities (e.g., the development of eye-hand coordination through play).

c. Fundamental to occupational performance areas is the performance of purposeful activities (e.g., to work involves completion of multiple tasks).

d. Purposeful activities are composed of identifiable parts that can be analyzed.

e. Purposeful activities are holistic.

f. Purposeful activities can be manipulated and adapted to be appropriate to, and/or therapeutic for, the individual.

g. Purposeful activities can be graded along many dimensions to meet the needs of an individual.

h. Determination of the individual's differential responses to purposeful activities can provide information for the selection of appropriate activities for use in evaluation and intervention.

i. Verbal and nonverbal communication is facilitated through engagement in purposeful activities.

j. Organization and ability to focus are enhanced, because purposeful activities provide concrete structure.

k. Doing is emphasized.

l. Involvement in, and with, the nonhuman environment is enhanced.

m. Purposeful activities can vary on a continuum from conscious to not conscious/unconscious.

n. Purposeful activities vary on a continuum from real to symbolic.

o. Purposeful activities vary on a continuum from simulated in a clinical setting to real in the individual's natural environment.

**E. Activity/Task Analysis and Synthesis**

1. Activity/task analysis
   a. The breaking down and identification of the component parts of an activity/task.
   b. Determination of the abilities needed to effectively perform and successfully complete the activity/task.
   c. Determination if the activity/task has therapeutic value.
   d. Methods of activity/task analysis.
      (1) Specify the exact activity/task to be analyzed (i.e., not just "dressing" but "donning a sweatshirt").
      (2) Identify and know the procedures, materials, and tools needed to complete the specific activity/ task.
      (3) Analyze the activity/task as it is typically performed under ordinary circumstances.
      4) Use AOTA's practice framework to be certain that all client factors, performance skills, and activity/task performance components and contexts are considered.
      (5) Select a frame of reference to determine which aspects of the activity/task are to be emphasized in the analysis.

2. Activity synthesis.
   a. The process of designing an activity for OT evaluation or intervention.
   b. Combines information obtained from the activity analysis with assessment information about the individual to ensure that a suitable match is made between the activity requirements and the person's needs and abilities.
   c. Effective activity synthesis often requires the adaptation and/or gradation of the selected activity.

3. Purposes and methods of activity analysis and synthesis.
   a. Teaching an activity.
      (1) Analyze the nature and sequence of the subtasks within the activity.
      (2) Synthesize to determine the best way to present the activity as a learning experience.
   b. Determining whether an individual can perform an activity.
      (1) Analyze the performance component requirements of the activity.
      (2) Synthesize by comparing the activity requirements with the individual's functional level.
   c. Adapting an activity.
      (1) Evaluate the individual's functional capabilities.
      (2) Analyze what parts of the activity can be changed.
      (3) Identify what functional aids can be used to allow the individual to successfully perform the activity.
   c. Grading an activity.
      (1) Determine what aspects can be changed along a continuum of performance.
      (2) Identify the individual's performance

deficit(s) and/or client factors requiring intervention.

(3) Synthesize to upgrade or downgrade complexity or difficulty level of the activity to meet the needs of the individual.

## F. The Teaching-Learning Process

1. Definition: The process by which the OT practitioner designs experiences to facilitate the individual's acquisition of the knowledge and skills needed for living.

2. Principles of learning.
   a. Learning is influenced by the individual's interests, age, sex, sociocultural factors, and current assets and limitations.
   b. Attention to the learning experience and perception of the situation influence learning.
   c. The learner's sources of motivation must be identified and used for engagement in learning experiences.
   d. Learning goals made by the individual are more likely to be met than goals determined by others.
   e. Learning is enhanced when the individual understands the reason for and purpose of the learning activity.
   f. Learning is increased when it recognizes the individual's current functional level, and is initiated within the person's capabilities (i.e., not too high or too low).
   g. Learning is enhanced when activities and experiences proceed at a rate that is comfortable for the individual.
   h. Individuals who actively participate in the learning process learn more, for experiential learning is more effective than didactic learning.
   i. Reinforcement and feedback on the individual's behavior and/or task performance are important parts of the learning experience and can be used to support desired behaviors and extinguish undesirable behaviors.
   j. Learning can be enhanced through trial and error, shaping, and imitation of models.
   k. Frequent repetition and practice in different situations facilitates learning and encourages generalization.
   l. Planned movement from simplified wholes to more complex wholes facilitates integration of what is to be learned.
   m. Inventive solutions to problems (as well as more useful or typical solutions) should be encouraged.

n. The environment of the learning experience can strongly influence the success of that experience.

o. Individual differences in the way anxiety affects the individual's learning must be considered.

p. Conflicts and frustrations, inevitably present in the learning situation, must be recognized and provisions made for their resolution or accommodation.

q. Continuity between the planned therapeutic learning experiences and the real-life situations for which the individual needs to be prepared facilitates the effective transfer of learning and the generalization of knowledge and skills.

3. Teaching methods.
   a. Definition: ways to present information and/or a task to an individual on a one-to-one basis or in a group.
   b. Demonstration and performance.
      (1) The OT practitioner performs the task and the individual imitates the OT practitioner's performance.
      (2) For example, the OT practitioner demonstrates one-handed cooking techniques, and the use of adaptive equipment, and the individual with a unilateral upper extremity amputation imitates therapist's task performance.
   c. Exploration and discovery.
      (1) A diversity of activities is made available and the individual is permitted to choose any activity and try it without specific instructions or directions.
      (2) For example, in an expressive arts group, members can select from a diversity of media and create individual works.
   d. Explanation and discussion.
      (1) A verbal explanation of the task and a discussion of the activity components to either plan an activity or to review what occurred during the activity are provided by the therapist.
      (2 For example, in a vocational group, the steps for applying for a job are explained and what happened during a job interview is reviewed.
   e. Role play.
      (1) The OT practitioner and/or individual(s) assume roles and act out scenarios to practice behaviors prior to doing the behavior in

a real situation.

    (2) For example, the OT practitioner plays the interviewer and the individual plays the job applicant.

  f. Simulation.

    (1) The individual acts out an activity performance using simulated tasks and/or objects.

    (2) For example, using a driving simulator prior to driving in a car on a roadway.

  g. Problem solving.

    (1) The process of teaching a person to analyze a situation, define the problem, outline potential solutions, select the solution that appears to be most viable, implement the solution, evaluate the outcome to determine if problem is resolved, and re-try a new solution, if needed.

    (2) For example, an individual living in a supportive apartment is having a problem getting his/her roommate to share household tasks.

  h. Audiovisual aids.

    (1) The use of slides, videos, and/or audio cassettes to teach material with or without the presence of a therapist.

    (2) For example, an individual with anxiety is provided with relaxation tapes to use at home.

  i. Repetition and practice.

    (1) The repetitious engagement in a task to increase accuracy and speed.

    (2) For example, repeatedly closing the fasteners on clothing to decrease the time needed to get ready for work in the morning.

  j. Behavioral management.

    (1) The identification of behaviors that require development (e.g., appropriate social skills) and/or require extinction (e.g., hitting people).

    (2) The implementation of a structured program to facilitate the desired behavioral change.

    (3) For example, appropriate social skills are rewarded with praise, whereas aggressive acts lead to a solitary "time out" period.

  k. Consumer/family/caregiver education.

    (1) An organized, systematic approach to formally present information to increase knowledge.

    (2) The nature of the illness or disease, including etiology, signs and symptoms, func-

tional implications, prognosis, and intervention are explained.

    (3) The maintenance of roles and occupational performance is emphasized.

    (4) Methods for the prevention of secondary problems (e.g, decubiti), are provided.

    (5) Community resources and supportive services are explored with appropriate referrals made.

## G. Clinical Reasoning

  1. Definition: The complex mental processes the therapist uses when thinking about the individual, the disability and the personal, social, and cultural meanings the individual gives to the disability, the uniqueness of the situation, and him/herself.

  2. Value for OTAs in practice.

    a. Improves clinical decision-making by giving OTAs tools for self-conscious reflection on their decisions.

    b. Improves ability to explain the rationales behind OTAs' decisions to consumers, family members, team members, and medical finance agencies (e.g., insurers).

    c. Improves job satisfaction by making OTAs more aware of the complexity of their work, the value of their practice.

  3. Types of clinical reasoning.

    a. Procedural reasoning/scientific reasoning.

      (1) Involves identifying OT problems, goal setting, and treatment planning.

      (2) Involves implementing treatment strategies via systematic gathering and interpreting of client data.

      (3) The actual technical "doing" of practice.

      (4) The reasoning that is documented the most for reimbursement purposes.

    b. Interactive reasoning.

      (1) Deals with how the disability or disease affects the person; focuses on the client as a person.

      (2) Involves the therapeutic relationship between the OTA, the individual, and caregivers.

      (3) Facilitates effective treatment, as it focuses on the personal meaning of illness and disability which can influence how a person engages in treatment (i.e., how motivational issues affect client's performance).

      (4) Congruent with the profession's philosophy and heritage of caring.

c. Narrative reasoning.
   (1) Deals with the individual's occupational story and focuses on the process of change needed to reach an imagined future.
   (2) Identifies what activities and roles were important to the person prior to illness/injury.
   (3) Analyzes what valued activities and roles the individual can perform now.
   (4) Explores what valued activities and roles are possible in the future, given the person's disability.
   (5) Asks what valued activities and roles the individual would choose as priorities for the future.
   (6) Neglects larger practice area issues in which the client/practitioner interaction is occurring (e.g., pragmatic constraints imposed by reimbursement, equipment, and/or organizational culture).
d. Pragmatic reasoning.
   (1) Considers the context in which the OT practitioner's thinking occurs.
   (2) States that mental activities are shaped by the situation (i.e., is setting long term or acute?).
   (3) Considers the treatment environment and OT practitioner's values, knowledge, abilities, and experiences.
   (4) Focuses on the treatment possibilities within a given treatment setting.
   (5) Reframes understanding of the influence of personal and practical constraints on OT practice.
   (6) The most effective OT practitioners are able to negotiate pragmatic contextual issues in favor of quality care.
e. Conditional reasoning.
   (1) Involves an ongoing revision of treatment.
   (2) Focuses on current and possible future social contexts.
   (3) Represents an integration of interactive, procedural, and pragmatic reasoning in the context of the client's narrative.
   (4) Requires multidimensional thinking.

## H. Therapeutic Use of Self

1. Definition: The practitioner's conscious, planned interaction with the individual, family members, significant others, and/or caregivers.
   a. The conscious, planned use of one's personali-

ty, unique characteristics, perceptions and insights during the therapeutic process.
2. Purposes of therapeutic use of self.
   a. Provide reassurance and/or information.
   b. Give advice.
   c. Alleviate anxiety and/or fear.
   d. Obtain needed information.
   e. Improve and maintain function.
   f. Promote growth and development.
   g. Increase coping skills.
3. Essential characteristics of therapeutic use of self.
   a. Perception of the individuality and uniqueness of each person.
   b. Respect for the dignity and rights of each individual regardless of past or present situation or possible future potential.
   c. Empathy to enter and share the experiences of an individual while maintaining one's own sense of self.
   d. Compassion to be kind and want to alleviate pain and suffering.
   e. Humility to recognize one's own limitations.
   f. Unconditional positive regard to be non-judgmental and accept, respect, and show concern and liking for each individual as a human being, regardless of presenting behaviors.
   g. Honesty to be truthful and straightforward.
   h. A relaxed manner to leave other concerns aside and schedule sufficient time to be with the person so that external issues do not impede on the relationship.
   i. Flexibility to modify behavior to meet the needs of each individual and deal with circumstances as they arise or change.
   j. Self-awareness to accurately know one's assets and limitations and to be able to make changes as needed to interact more effectively in therapeutic relationships.
   k. Humor to appropriately recognize and/or use what is amusing and comical.
4. Common issues and responses that can affect therapeutic relationships.
   a. Negative attitudes, fear or hostility towards individuals who are different and/or towards the unknown.
   b. Resistance to establishing a rapport due to past rejections and/or fear of future rejection.
   c. Communication difficulties.
      (1) Incongruence between verbal and non-verbal communications, (when spoken words

do not match a person's facial expression, tone of voice, gestures, or postures), resulting in confusion.

 (2) Language difficulties.

  (a) Psychiatric symptoms such as blocking, circumstantiality, flight of ideas, confabulation, grandiosity, articulated delusions, loosening of association, and/or poverty of content can hinder effective communication.

  (b) Cultural, class, educational, and/or regional differences can result in misunderstandings or lack of comprehension between individuals.

  (c) Misinterpretations can occur due to differences in primary language.

 d. Dependency that is excessive, and hinders the individual's growth towards interdependence and/or independence.

 e. Transference and countertransference.

  (1) Transference is an unconscious response to an individual that is similar to the way one has responded to a significant person (e.g., the practitioner is responded to as a parent).

  (2) Countertransference is an unconscious response to transference in which the individual responds in a manner that is expected and desired by the person who has transference towards him/her (e.g., the practitioner assumes a parental role towards a client).

 f. Difficulty in expressing feelings due to personal reticence or cultural background.

 g. Over involvement that results in a loss of objectivity or a fear of involvement that leads to detachment.

 h. Difficulty with developing an individual therapeutic style that is a comfortable "fit" so that being a therapist becomes a natural part of one's self.

5. Supervision and support.

 a. Develops the ability to use oneself therapeutically.

 b. Assists with the common issues and responses noted in Section 4.

 c. Increases effectiveness in applying therapeutic principles in daily practice.

## I. Group Process, Therapeutic Groups, and Activity Groups

1. Overview of group dynamics.

 a. Group dynamics are the forces which influence the nature of small groups, the interrelationships of their members, the events that typically occur in small groups and ultimately, the outcome(s) of these groups.

 b. Group dynamics can be examined according to the group's structure, content, and process.

2. Group development: the stages groups typically go through from their initial beginnings to their termination.

 a. Origin phase involves the leader composing the group protocol and planning for the group (e.g., size of the group, member characteristics, location of meetings).

 b. Orientation phase involves members learning what the group is about, making a preliminary commitment to the group, and developing initial connections with other members.

 c. Intermediate phase involves members developing interpersonal bonds, group norms, and specialized member roles through involvement in goal-directed activities and clarification of group's purpose.

 d. Conflict phase involves members challenging the group's structure, purposes, and/or processes, and is characterized by dissension and disagreements among members.

  (1). Unsuccessful resolution of this phase results in dissolution of the group.

  (2). Successful resolution of this phase results in modifications to the group that are acceptable to members, enabling the group to proceed to the next phase of development.

 e. Cohesion phase involves members regrouping after the conflict with a clearer sense of purpose and a reaffirmation of group norms and values, leading to group stability.

 f. Maturation phase involves members using their energies and skills to be productive and to achieve group's goals.

 g. Termination phase involves dissolution of the group due to lack of engagement of members, inability to resolve conflict, administrative constraints (e.g., only 4 sessions allotted for a discharge planning group), goal attainment, or task accomplishment.

3. Group roles: describe the patterns of behavior that are typical within groups.

 a. Instrumental roles are functional and assumed to help the group select, plan, and complete the group's task (e.g., initiator, organizer).

 b. Expressive roles are functional and are

assumed to support and maintain the overall group and to meet members' needs (e.g., encourager, compromiser).

   c. Individual roles are dysfunctional and contrary to group roles, for they serve an individual purpose and interfere with successful group functioning (e.g., aggressor, blocker).

4. Group norms: the standards of behavior and attitudes that are considered appropriate and acceptable to the group.

   a. Behavior that falls outside of the group's range of acceptable behavior is considered deviant and is often negatively sanctioned.

   b. Norms can be explicit and clearly verbalized (e.g., confidentiality is maintained by all group members, aggression is not tolerated).

   c. Norms can be non-explicit and not verbalized (e.g., discussion topics that are taboo).

   d. Norms can vary in different groups and can change as a group develops and/or membership changes.

   e. Therapeutic norms.

     (1) Encourage self-reflection, self-disclosure, and interaction among members.

     (2) Reinforce the value and importance of the group by being on time and well-prepared.

     (3) Establish an atmosphere of support and safety.

     (4) Maintain confidentiality and respect.

     (5) Regard group members as effective agents of change by not placing the group leader in the expert role.

5. Group goals: the desired outcomes of the group that are shared by a sufficient number of the group's members.

   a. The group's effort is mostly aimed at attaining these goals.

   b. Group goals provide focus for the group and guidelines for group activities and interactions.

   c. Group goals are not a compilation of individual member goals. Members may have diverse goals but attainment of the group goal will facilitate personal goal achievement.

   d. Benefits of member participation in group goal setting.

     (1) A match between members' goals and group's goal(s).

     (2) Increased understanding of the requirements for achievement of the goal(s).

     (3) Increased appreciation of each member's

contribution to achieving group's desired outcomes.

6. Group communication: the process of giving, receiving, and interpreting information through verbal and non-verbal expression.

   a. Effective group communication is a prerequisite to, and a requirement for, all group functioning.

   b. Effective communication occurs in a group when a member sends a message and the message is interpreted by the other group members receiving the message in the manner that the sender intended.

   c. Sending and receiving messages often takes place simultaneously due to the dynamic process of verbal and non-verbal communication.

   d. Communication can take many forms, including monologue, criticism, orders, questions and answers, and open give-and-take.

   e. Group communication that is adaptive may include clarifying goals and the sharing of ideas, experiences, and feelings.

   f. Group communication that is maladaptive may include seeking to control the group by controlling the channels of communication, and avoidance of specific issues or persons.

7. Group cohesiveness: the degree to which members are committed to a group and the extent of members' liking for the group (i.e., the sense of "we-ness").

   a. Factors that contribute to cohesiveness.

     (1) Extensive interaction between members.

     (2) Similarity or complementariness in member characteristics.

     (3) Perception of relevance of group to individual needs.

     (4) Members' expectation of goal attainment and successful group outcome.

     (5) Democratic leadership and member cooperation.

8. Group decision making: The process of agreeing on a resolution to a problem. The solution may be obtained through different processes.

   a. Unanimous decision in which all group members agree.

   b. Consensus in which members agree to the majority's decision but retain the right to reconsider their decision.

   c. Majority rule in which the majority's decision is accepted with no reevaluation of the decision by members.

d. Compromise in which a combination of different points of view results in a decision that is different from each distinct point of view.

9. Group leadership styles and membership roles.
    a. Directive leadership takes place when the OT practitioner is responsible for the planning and structuring of much of what takes place in the group.
        (1) This is style needed when the members' cognitive, social, and verbal skills, as well as engagement, are limited (e.g., parallel or project level groups).
        (2) Directive leaders select the activities to be used in the group.
        (3) They provide clear verbal and demonstrated instruction to complete tasks.
        (4) Group maintenance roles and feedback is predominately provided by the directive leader.
        (5) The directive leader's goal is task accomplishment.
    b. Facilitative leadership occurs when the OT practitioner shares responsibility for the group and for group process with the members.
        (1) This style is advised when members' skill levels and engagement are moderate (e.g., ego-centric cooperative, or cooperative).
        (2) Facilitative leaders collaborate with group members to select the activities to be used in a group.
        (3) Members and leaders share instruction throughout the group's process.
        (4) Group maintenance roles and feedback are provided by members with the leader facilitating the process.
        (5) The facilitative leader's goal is to have members acquire skills through experience.
    c. Advisory leadership takes place when the OT practitioner functions as a resource to the members, who set the agenda and structure the group's functioning.
        (1) This style is assumed when members' skills and engagement are high (e.g., mature groups).
        (2) Members select and complete the group's activity with leader's advice, if needed.
        (3) Group maintenance roles are independently assumed by group members.
        (4) Feedback occurs as a natural part of the group's self-directed process.
        (5) The advisory leader's goal is to have members understand and self-direct the process.
    d. Refer to Table 3-6 for Medicare guidelines for group therapy member selection and Table 3-7 for Medicare guidelines for group leadership responsibility.
        (1) These guidelines are relevant and helpful standards to apply to all settings that use group interventions.

10. Co-leadership: Occurs when there is sharing of group leadership between two or more therapists and/or OTAs.
    a. Advantages.
        (1) Each leader can assume different leadership roles, tasks and styles.
        (2) Both leaders can provide and obtain mutual support.

## TABLE 3-6 - MEDICARE INDICATORS FOR GROUP MEMBERSHIP

**THE INDIVIDUAL IS ABLE TO:**

- engage willingly in group
- attend to group guidelines/procedures
- actively participate in group process
- benefit from group leadership input
- benefit from group membership/peer input
- respond appropriately throughout group process
- incorporate feedback
- complete activities toward goal attainment
- attain greater benefit from the group intervention than from 1:1 intervention

Reference: Adapted from United States Government Printing Office Code of Federal Regulations, Title 42, Volume 3. Retrieved from http://www.cms.gov. December 21, 2003.

## TABLE 3-7 - MEDICARE CRITERIA FOR GROUP LEADERSHIP

**THE LEADER:**

- provides active leadership
- instructs members as a group
- monitors and documents individual's participation and response to intervention
- provides individualized guidance and feedback
- documents person's progress toward goals defined in the individual intervention plan in objective, measurable, functional terms

Reference: Adapted from United States Government Printing Office Code of Federal Regulations, Title 42, Volume 3. Retrieved from http://www.cms.gov. December 21, 2003.

(3) Observations and objectivity can increase.

(4) Co-leaders can share knowledge and skills.

(5) Co-leaders can model effective behaviors.

b. Disadvantages may arise and must be dealt with for effective co-leadership.

  (1) Splitting by group member(s) of one leader against the other.

  (2) Excessive competition among co-leaders.

  (3) Unequal responsibilities resulting in an unbalanced work load among co-leaders.

11. Curative factors of groups as defined by Yalom.

a. Altruism is the giving of oneself to help others.

b. Catharsis is the relieving of emotions by expressing one's feelings.

c. Universality comes from recognizing shared feelings and that one's problems are not unique.

d. Existential factors address accepting the fact that the responsibility for change comes from within oneself.

e. Self-understanding (insight) involves discovering and accepting the unknown parts of oneself.

f. Family reenactment leads to understanding what it was like growing up in one's family through the group experience.

g. Guidance comes from accepting advice from other group members.

h. Identification involves benefiting from imitation of the positive behaviors of other group members.

i. Instillation of hope is experiencing optimism through observing the improvement of others in the group.

j. Interpersonal learning occurs when receiving feedback from group members regarding one's behavior (input).

k. Interpersonal learning also occurs by learning successful ways of relating to group members (output).

l. The conscious understanding and facilitation of these curative factors enhances the therapeutic value of a group.

12. Taxonomy of activity groups:

a. Mosey (1996) provided a standard classification to identify major types of activity groups.

b. Evaluation group.

  (1) Purpose/focus: to enable client and OT practitioner to assess client's skills, assets, and limitations regarding group interaction.

  (2) Assumption: to accurately evaluate an individual's functional abilities, one must observe the person in a setting where the skills can be demonstrated.

  (3) Type of client: all individuals who will be involved in groups or who lack group interaction skills.

  (4) Role of the OTA group leader.

    (a) Orients clients to group's purpose.

    (b) Provides needed supplies for activities that were selected by the OT for their collaborative and interactive aspects.

    (c) Does not participate or intervene in group (except to maintain safety, if needed), but observes and reports members' interaction and functional skill level to the OT supervisor.

    (d) Closes group by sharing general observations with members.

    (e) Asks for clients' input and reports feedback to the OT supervisor.

  (5) Suitable activities: tasks that can be completed in one session and require interaction to complete.

c. Thematic group.

  (1) Purpose/focus: to assist members in acquiring the knowledge, skills, and/or attitudes needed to perform a specific activity.

  (2) Assumptions.

    (a) Improvement of ability to engage in activities outside of group can result from teaching of these activities within group.

    (b) Learning is facilitated by practicing and experiencing needed behaviors, with reinforcement of appropriate behaviors given.

  (3) Type of client.

    (a) Determined by the specific goals of the group.

    (b) Members' needs, concerns, and goals must match the objectives of the group.

    (c) Members must have a minimal group interaction skill level equal to a parallel group skill level.

  (4) Role of the OTA group leader.

    (a) Contributes to the selection, structuring, and gradation of suitable activities to teach needed skills.

    (b) Interventions vary according to group's

level, needs, and goals.

    (c) May range on a continuum from a highly structured, supportive director to a resource advisor.

    (d) Reinforces skill development.

    (e) Attention is not paid to intra- and interpersonal conflicts unless they interfere with or are directly related to the activity.

  (5) Suitable activities.

    (a) Simulated, clearly defined, structured activities which enable members to practice and learn needed skills, attitudes, and knowledge within the group.

    (b) Activities selected are directly related to the skills needed to perform the activity outside of the group (e.g., a cooking group to learn how to cook).

d. Topical group.

  (1) Purpose/focus: to discuss specific activities that members are engaged in outside of group to enable them to engage in the activities in a more effective, need-satisfying manner.

    (a) Concurrent topical groups are concerned with activities already engaged in outside of group (e.g., a parenting skills group for parents of children with developmental disabilities).

    (b) Anticipatory topical groups are concerned with activities that are expected to be done in the future (e.g., a discharge planning group for persons completing short-term rehabilitation).

  (2) Assumptions.

    (a) Improvement of ability to engage in specific activities outside of group results from discussion of these activities.

    (b) Discussion of problem areas and potential solutions, reinforcement of appropriate behaviors, and experiential learning facilitate skill acquisition.

  (3) Type of client.

    (a) Individuals who share similar current or anticipatory problems in functioning.

    (b) Members must be at an ego-centric-cooperative group skill level.

    (c) Sufficient verbal and cognitive skills to engage in discussion and to problem-solve are present.

  (4) Role of the OTA group leader.

    (a) Facilitates group discussion while maintaining focus on the circumscribed activity.

    (b) Helps members problem-solve, gives feedback and support, reinforces skill acquisition.

    (c) Shares leadership with members; acts as a role model.

  (5) Suitable activities.

    (a) Group activity is a verbal discussion on a circumscribed activity that members are engaged in (concurrent) or will be engaged in (anticipatory) outside of group (e.g., parenting, home maintenance, discharge from hospital, work, and leisure).

    (b) Discussion may include members' current or anticipated fears and problems, potential solutions, and coping mechanisms.

    (c) Role play and "homework" may be utilized.

e. Task-oriented group.

  (1) Purpose/focus.

    (a) To increase clients' awareness of their needs, values, ideas, feelings, and behaviors as they engage in a group task.

    (b) To improve intra- and interpsychic functioning by focusing on problems which emerge in the process of choosing, planning and implementing a group activity.

  (2) Assumptions.

    (a) Activities elicit feelings, thoughts, and behaviors.

    (b) Activities are the means by which members can explore and experience these thoughts, feelings, and actions.

    (c) Through activities members can increase their self-awareness and practice new behaviors.

  (3) Type of client.

    (a) Individuals whose primary dysfunction is in the cognitive and socioemotional areas due to psychological or physical trauma.

    (b) Clients with fair verbal skills who can interact with others.

(4) Role of the OTA group leader.
  (a) Initially, very active, defines group goals and structure.
  (b) Assists with activity selection, offers guidelines and suggestions.
  (c) Facilitates discussion among members.
  (d) Gives feedback and support.
  (e) Assists members in exploring relationships between thoughts, feelings, and actions.
  (f) Encourages members to experiment with new behavior patterns.
  (g) As the group develops, the leader is less active, helps members give more feedback and input; however, the OT practitioner remains the leader and ensures that the task is a means to the end, not the end itself.
(5) Suitable activities.
  (a) Activities that are chosen by members and will create an end product or demonstrable service for the group itself or for persons outside the group.
  (b) Activities are selected, planned, and carried out by members with the understanding that the task is a means to study, understand, and practice behavior.
f. Developmental group.
  (1) A continuum of groups consisting of parallel, project, egocentric-cooperative, cooperative, and mature groups.
  (2) Purpose/focus is to teach and develop members' group interaction skills.
    (a). Parallel.
      • To enable members to perform individual tasks in the presence of others.
      • To minimally interact verbally and non-verbally with others even though task does not require interaction for successful completion.
      • To develop a basic level of awareness, trust, and comfort with others in group.
    (b) Project.
      • To develop the ability to perform a shared, short-term activity with another member in a comfortable, cooperative manner.
      • To develop interactions beyond those that the activity requires.

• To enable members to give and seek assistance.
  (c) Egocentric-cooperative.
    • To enable members to select and implement a long-range activity which requires group interaction to complete.
    • To enable members to identify and meet the needs of themselves and others (e.g., safety, esteem).
  (d) Cooperative.
    • To enable members to engage in a group activity which facilitates free expression of ideas and feelings.
    • To develop sense of trust, love and belonging, and cohesion.
    • To enable members to identify and meet socio-emotional needs.
  (e) Mature group.
    • To enable members to assume all functional socio-emotional and task roles within a group.
    • To enable members to reinforce behaviors which result in need satisfaction and task completion.
(3) Assumptions.
  (a) Learning principles are the basis. They are utilized throughout the five developmental levels.
  (b) Members are made aware of and helped to engage in appropriate group behavior.
  (c) Feedback and reinforcement are utilized. Learning of needed behaviors occurs when adaptive behaviors are reinforced and when maladaptive behaviors are not.
  (d) Maladaptive behaviors result from deviations, lags, or insufficiencies in development. These developmental deficiencies can be treated by participating in groups that are similar to the ones in which the skills would have been developed.
  (e) Subskills fundamental to mature group function must be acquired in a sequential manner.
(4) Type of clients: individuals with decreased group interaction skills.
(5) Role of the OTA group leader.

(a) Contributes to the assessment process and the placement of individuals in the appropriate group, with OT supervision in the appropriate group.

(b) Orients all members to group's goals, structure, and norms.

(c) The OTA provides group leadership with OT supervision.
  • Lower level groups require more active, direct leadership.
  • As group matures and attains a higher level of group interaction, leadership is shared among members.

(6) Parallel group leadership role.

(a) Provide unconditional positive regard to develop trust.

(b) Actively fill all leadership functions and meets all members' needs.

(c) Reinforce all behaviors appropriate to group, no matter how small.

(d) Provide structure.

(e) Facilitate interaction.

(7) Project group leadership role.

(a) Select and structure activities that can be shared by two or more members.

(b) Fulfill all of members' needs while encouraging members to give and seek assistance and interact beyond activity requirements.

(c) Reinforce cooperation, mild competition, sharing, and interactions.

(8) Egocentric-cooperative group leadership role.

(a) Less of an active, direct leader.

(b) Facilitate and allow members to fulfill functional leadership roles to function independently.

(c) Provide guidelines and assistance as needed.

(d) Reinforce members' meeting needs of self and others.

(e) Serve as a role model.

(9) Cooperative group leadership role.

(a) Act as an advisor, not as a direct leader.

(b) Leader and members are mutually responsible for giving feedback, identifying and meeting needs, and reinforcing behavior.

(10) Mature group leadership role.

(a) Acts as a peer, an equal, a group member.

(b) Members assume all roles with the OT group leader filling in only if and when needed to maintain group.

(c) All members satisfy needs and reinforce behavior while maintaining a balance between need satisfaction and task completion.

(11) Suitable activities.

(a) Parallel.
  • Members perform activities independently of others but in the presence of others.
  • Interactions are not required to successfully complete activity.
  • Activities should be similar or utilize common tools or materials to facilitate interaction and sharing.
  • Activities should be relevant to a person's ability, age, gender, and interest so he/she is more able to interact with and about it.

(b) Project.
  • Task is short-term and requires the participation of two or more people.
  • Task is shareable and requires interaction to successfully complete.
  • Group interaction, not project completion, is emphasized.

(c) Egocentric-cooperative.
  • Activity allows 5-10 people to work together.
  • It is selected and implemented by members.
  • It is longer-term, requiring more than two meetings to complete.

(d) Cooperative.
  • Activities facilitate and allow for free expression of ideas and feelings.
  • Activity is secondary to need fulfillment and may not produce an end product.

(e) Mature.
  • Activity requires a number of people to work together.
  • It requires an end product or has an inherent time limit for completion.
  • During group, activity may be stopped for members to explore what is going on within the group.

g. Instrumental group.
   (1) Purpose/focus.
       (a) To help members function at their highest possible level for as long as possible.
       (b) To meet mental health needs.
   (2) Assumption.
       (a) Individuals are functioning at their highest possible level and cannot change or progress.
       (b) A supportive, structured environment which provides appropriate activities can prevent regression, maintain function, and meet mental health needs.
   (3) Type of client.
       (a) Individuals who have demonstrated in treatment an inability to change or progress.
       (b) Individuals who can't independently meet their mental health needs and/or need assistance to maintain function due to cognitive, psychological, perceptual-motor, and/or social deficits.
   (4) Role of OTA group leader.
       (a) Provide unconditional positive regard, support, and structure to create a comfortable, safe environment for patients.
       (b) Select and design activities that will meet member's health needs and maintain highest possible level of function.
       (c) Assist members with activity as needed.
       (d) Make no attempt to change client.
   (5) Suitable activities.
       (a) Members can successfully complete activities with structure and assistance of therapist as needed.
       (b) Non-threatening and non-demanding.
       (c) Interesting, enjoyable and attractive to members.
       (d) Meet mental health needs of patient by enabling him/her to experience pleasure, have fun, socialize with others, etc.
       (e) Maintain function by providing sensory, cognitive, perceptual-motor, and social input.
h. Role of the OTA in group work.
   (1) The OTA is active in all aspects of group work.
   (2) Refer to Chapter 13 for additional group information

# References

American Occupational Therapy Association. (2006). *Reference manual of the official documents of the American Occupational Therapy Association* (11th ed.). Bethesda, MD: Author.

American Occupational Therapy Association. (2005). Standards of practice for occupational therapy. *American Journal of Occupational Therapy, 59*, 663-665.

Case-Smith, J. (Ed.). (2005). *Occupational therapy for children (5th ed.).* St. Louis, MO: Elsevier Mosby.

Cole, M.B. (1998). *Group dynamics in occupational therapy; the theoretical basis and practice application of group treatment* (2nd ed.). Thorofare, NJ: Slack.

Fleming, M.H. (1996). The therapist with the three-track mind. In R.P. Cottrell (Ed.), *Perspectives on purposeful activity: Foundation and future of occupational therapy* (pp. 341-349). Bethesda, MD: American Occupational Therapy Association.

Hansen, R.A. (1990). Lesson 10: *Ethical considerations.* In C.B. Royeen (Ed.), AOTA self study series. Assessing function. Bethesda, MD: American Occupational Therapy Association.

Hinojosa, J., & Kramer, P., & Crist, P. (Eds.) (2005). *Evaluation: Obtaining and interpreting data* (2nd ed.). Bethesda, MD: American Occupational Therapy Association.

Hopkins, H. & Smith, H. (Eds.). (2003). *Willard and Spackman's occupational therapy (10th ed.).* Philadelphia: J.B. Lippincott.

Jacobs, K., & Logigian, M.K. (1999). *Functions of a manager in occupational therapy.* Thorofare, NJ: Slack.

Law, M., Baum, C., & Dunn, W. (2005). *Measuring occupational performance: Supporting best practice in occupational therapy.* Thorofare, NJ: Slack.

Leary, D.A. & Mardirossian, J. (2000, Sept 11), *Ethical knowledge = Collaborative power OT Practice,* 19-22.

Mattingly, C. (1996). The narrative nature of clinical reasoning. In R.P. Cottrell (Ed.), *Perspectives on purposeful activity: Foundation and future of occupational therapy* (pp. 351-359). Bethesda, MD: American Occupational Therapy Association.

50

McCormack, G.; Jaffe, E.; Goodman-Lavey, M. (Eds.). (2003). *The occupational therapy manager, (4th ed.).* Bethesda, MD: American Occupational Therapy Association.

*Mosey, A.C. (1996). Psychosocial components of occupational therapy.* New York: Raven Press.

Moyers, P. & Dale, L. (2007). *The guide to occupational therapy practice.* Bethesda, MD: American Occupational Therapy Association.

United States *Government Printing Office Code of Federal Regulations, Title 42, Volume 3.* Retrieved from http://www.cms.gov. December 21, 2003.

# CHAPTER 4

# PROFESSIONAL STANDARDS AND RESPONSIBILITIES

Rita P. Fleming-Castaldy

## I. Professional Ethics

### A. Code of Ethics Overview

1. Developed by AOTA as a statement to the public to identify the values and principles used to promote and maintain high standards for the behavior of occupational therapy practitioners.
2. A set of principles that apply to all levels of occupational therapy personnel.
3. Actions that are in violation of the purpose and spirit of AOTA's Code of Ethics are considered unethical by AOTA.
4. All OT practitioners are obligated to uphold these standards for themselves and their colleagues.

### B. Occupational Therapy Code of Ethics

1. "Principle 1. Occupational therapy personnel shall demonstrate a concern for the safety and well-being of the recipients of their services (beneficence). Occupational therapy personnel shall:
   a. Provide services in a fair and equitable manner. They shall recognize and appreciate the cultural components of economics, geography, race, ethnicity, religious and political factors, marital status, sexual orientation, gender identity, and disability of all recipients of their services.
   b. Strive to ensure that fees are fair and reasonable and commensurate with services performed. When occupational therapy practitioners set fees, they shall set fees considering institutional, local, state, and federal requirements, and with due regard for the service recipient's ability to pay.
   c. Make every effort to advocate for recipients to obtain needed services through available means.
   d. Recognize the responsibility to promote public health and the safety and well-being of individuals, groups, and/or communities.
2. Principle 2. Occupational therapy personnel shall take reasonable precautions to avoid imposing or inflicting harm upon the recipient of services or to his or her property (nonmaleficence). Occupational therapy personnel shall:
   a. Maintain relationships that do not exploit the recipient of services sexually, physically, emotionally, financially, socially, or in any other manner.
   b. Avoid relationships or activities that interfere with professional judgment and objectivity.
   c. Refrain from any influences that may compromise provision of service.
   d. Exercise professional judgment and critically analyze directives that could result in potential harm before implementation.
   e. Identify and address personal problems that may adversely impact professional judgment and duties.

f. Bring concerns regarding impairment of professional skills of a colleague to the attention of the appropriate authority when or if attempts to address concerns are unsuccessful.

3. Principle 3. Occupational therapy personnel shall respect the recipient and/or their surrogate(s) as well as the recipient's rights (autonomy, privacy, confidentiality).

   a. Occupational therapy practitioners shall collaborate with service recipients and if they desire, families, significant others, and/or caregivers in setting goals and priorities throughout the intervention process including full disclosure of the nature, risks, and potential outcomes of any interventions.

   b. Occupational therapy practitioners shall obtain informed consent from participants involved in research activities and ensure that they understand potential risks and outcomes.

   d. Occupational therapy personnel shall respect the individual's right to refuse professional services or involvement in research or educational activities.

   e. Occupational therapy personnel shall protect all privileged confidential forms of written, verbal, and electronic communication gained from educational, practice, research, and investigational activities unless otherwise mandated by local, state, or federal regulations.

4. Principle 4. Occupational therapy personnel shall achieve and continually maintain high standards of competence (duty).

   a. Occupational therapy practitioners shall hold the appropriate national and state credentials for the services they provide.

   b. Occupational therapy practitioners shall use procedures that conform to AOTA standards of practice and official documents.

   c. Occupational therapy practitioners shall take responsibility for maintaining and documenting competence in practice, education, and research by participating in professional development and educational activities.

   d. Occupational therapy practitioners shall be competent in all topic areas in which they provide instruction to consumers, peers, and/or students.

   e. Occupational therapy practitioners shall critically examine and keep current with emerging knowledge relevant to their practice so they may perform their duties on the basis of accurate information.

   f. Occupational therapy practitioners shall protect service recipients by ensuring that duties assumed by or assigned to other occupational therapy personnel match credentials, qualifications, experience, and scope of practice. (This ethical standard can be tested in NBCOT question scenarios that involve an OT supervisor assigning responsibilities to an OTA).

   g. Occupational therapy practitioners shall provide appropriate supervision to individuals for whom the practitioners have supervisory responsibility in accordance with Association official documents; local, state, and federal or national laws and regulations; and institutional policies and procedures. (This ethical standard can be tested in question scenarios regarding OT supervision of an OTA).

   h. Occupational therapy practitioners shall refer to or consult with other service providers whenever such a referral or consultation would be helpful to the care of the recipient of service. The referral or consultation process should be done in collaboration with the recipient of service.

5. Principle 5. Occupational therapy personnel shall comply with laws and Association policies guiding the profession of occupational therapy (justice).

   a. Occupational therapy personnel shall familiarize themselves with and seek to understand and abide by applicable Association policies; local, state, and federal/national/international laws.

   b. Occupational therapy practitioners shall be familiar with revisions in those laws and Association policies that apply to the profession of occupational therapy and shall inform employers, employees, and colleagues of those changes.

   c. Occupational therapy practitioners shall encourage those they supervise in occupational therapy-related activities to adhere to the Code of Ethics. (This ethical standard is often tested in scenarios regarding practices involving questionable ethics).

   d. Occupational therapy practitioners shall take reasonable steps to ensure employers are aware of occupational therapy's ethical obligations, as set forth in this Code of Ethics, and of the implications of those obligations for occupational therapy practice, education, and research. (This standard can be tested in question scenarios in which employers request that the OT supervisor and OTA perform tasks that are not consistent with occupational therapist/OTA supervisory standards).

    e. Occupational therapy practitioners shall record and report in an accurate and timely manner all information related to professional activities.

6. Principle 6. Occupational therapy personnel shall provide accurate information when representing the profession (veracity).

    a. Occupational therapy personnel shall represent their credentials, qualifications, education, experience, training, and competence accurately. This is of particular importance for those to whom occupational therapy personnel provide their services or with whom occupational therapy practitioners have a professional relationship.

    b. Occupational therapy personnel shall disclose any professional, personal, financial, business, or volunteer affiliations that may pose a conflict of interest to those with whom they may establish a professional, contractual, or other working relationship.

    c. Occupational therapy personnel shall refrain from using or participating in the use of any form of communication that contains false, fraudulent, deceptive, or unfair statements or claims.

    d. Occupational therapy practitioners shall identify and fully disclose to all appropriate persons errors that compromise recipients' safety.

    e. Occupational therapy practitioners shall accept the responsibility for their professional actions which reduce the public's trust in occupational therapy services and those that perform those services.

7. Principle 7. Occupational therapy personnel shall treat colleagues and other professionals with fairness, discretion, and integrity (fidelity).

    a. Occupational therapy personnel shall preserve, respect, and safeguard confidential information about colleagues and staff, unless otherwise mandated by national, state, or local laws.

    b. Occupational therapy practitioners shall accurately represent the qualifications, views, contributions, and findings of colleagues.

    c. Occupational therapy personnel shall take adequate measures to discourage, prevent, expose,

and correct any breaches of the Code of Ethics and report any breaches of the Code of Ethics to the appropriate authority.

    d. Occupational therapy personnel shall use conflict resolution and/or alternative dispute resolution resources to resolve organizational and interpersonal conflicts.

    e. Occupational therapy personnel shall familiarize themselves with established policies and procedures for handling concerns about this Code of Ethics, including familiarity with national, state, local, district, and territorial procedures for handling ethics complaints. These include policies and procedures created by the AOTA, licensing and regulatory bodies, employers, agencies, certification boards, and other organizations who have jurisdiction over occupational therapy practice (AOTA, 2005).

**C. Ethics in Practice**

1. Ethics guide the behavior and decision making of occupational therapy practitioners to help them determine the morally right course of action

    a. OTAs often are faced with issues and events that challenge their values and beliefs.

    b. Decisions about what is the right or wrong course of action are based on our profession's code of ethics.

2. These ethical standards are often the guide by which other bodies judge professional behaviors to determine if malpractice has occurred.

3. NBCOT examination questions may include practice scenarios that reflect ethical distress or ethical dilemmas.

    a. Ethical distress.

        (1) When a practitioner knows the correct action to take but an existing barrier prevents the practitioner from taking this course of action.

        (2) For example, when an admissions policy to a day treatment program excludes persons with substance abuse histories, yet this program would provide appropriate intervention for a client who is mentally ill and chemically addicted (MICA).

    b. Ethical dilemmas.

        (1) When there are two or more potentially morally correct ways to solve a problem. However, these solutions are exclusive; therefore, choosing one course of action prohibits acting on the other choices.

(2) For example, a group of OT private practitioners has the opportunity to bid on a lucrative contract for the provision of OT services in a school system. However, none of the OTAs have pediatric experience and the practice relies on OTAs to implement treatment. The options in this case may include not bidding on the contract or bidding on the contract and if the contract is won, incurring the expense of hiring pediatric-trained OTAs to implement treatment.

**D. Patient/Client Abuse[1]**

1. Ethical responsibility of occupational therapy practitioners.
   a. In accordance with Principle 1 of the AOTA code of ethics occupational therapy personnel must act to ensure "the safety and well-being of the recipients of their services" (AOTA, 2005).
   b. As a result, practitioners are obligated to report any observed or suspected incidents of patient/client abuse or neglect.
      (1) The party to whom reporting is required varies from state to state, as does the penalties for not reporting.
      (2) Minimum reporting standards require reporting to one's immediate supervisor.
   c. Occupational therapy practitioners should also provide interventions to victims of abuse and/or neglect. These can include:
      (1) Treatment for physical and emotional injuries.
      (2) Development of a trusting relationship.
      (3) Provision of support to family and loved ones.
      (4) Referral to appropriate disciplines and agencies.
      (5) Contributor to staff training programs to prevent abuse.
2. Facts and figures.
   a. All ages are at risk for abuse.
      (1) Refer to Chapter 5 for specific information on child and elder and vulnerable adult abuse.
   b. Facts and figures for patient/client abuse are subsumed into institutional elder abuse and abuse of the mentally ill.
3. Definition of abuse.
   a. Abuse is defined as deliberately hurting a patient physically, mentally or emotionally.
   b. Neglect is defined as deliberately withholding

services that are necessary to maintain an individual's physical, mental, and emotional health.
   c. Legal definitions may vary from state to state.
4. Signs of patient/client abuse.
   a. Individual's report of abuse and/or neglect.
   b. Frequent unexplained injuries or complaints of pain without obvious injury.
   c. Burns or bruises suggesting the use of instruments, cigarettes, etc.
   d. Passive, withdrawn, and emotionless behavior.
   e. Lack of reaction to pain.
   f. Sexually transmitted diseases or injury to the genital area.
   g. Unexplained difficulty in sitting or walking.
   h. Fear of being alone with caretakers.
   i. Obvious malnutrition.
   j. Lack of personal cleanliness.
   k. Habitually dressed in torn or dirty clothes.
   l. Obvious fatigue and listlessness.
   m. Begs for food, water, or assistance (especially in regard to toileting).
   n. In need of medical or dental care.
   o. Left unattended for long periods.
   p. Bedsores and skin lesions.

**E. Ethical Decision Making**

1. Identify the ethical issues and potential dilemmas.
2. Gather relevant information.
   a. Identify all individuals affected by the issue.
   b. Determine prior history of the issue.
   c. Analyze the dynamics and culture of the setting(s).
   d. Ask open ended questions to obtain descriptive data.
3. Determine conflicting values and areas of agreement.
   a. A commitment to patient autonomy versus the principles of beneficence and nonmaleficence may need to be considered.
4. Consult and collaborate with the OT supervisor to:
   a. Identify as many relevant alternative courses of action as possible.
      (1) Consider who would take these actions and when these actions would need to occur.
   b. Determine all possible positive and negative outcomes for each possible action.
      (1) Include outcomes for all participants in the dilemma. An ethical dilemma never involves just one person.
      (2) It can take time and thought to identify all

---

[1]Janice Romeo contributed this section on patient/client abuse.

those who may possibly have a "stake" or will be touched by a specific decision.

c. Weigh, with care, the consequences of each outcome.

(1) This step includes the process of reordering or rearranging parts of different decisions to arrive at a new alternative which may be the best possible course of action.

d. Seek input from others (i.e., rehabilitation director, OT supervisor).

(1) Provide information in an anonymous fashion which enables the individual to give advice in a more objective manner and to provide recommendations that cannot be construed to be biased or prejudicial.

e. Apply best professional judgment to choose the action(s) to recommend.

f. Contact any and all agencies that have jurisdiction over a practitioner if there are questions about potential ethical violations that could cause harm or have the potential to cause harm to a person.

g. Determine desired and/or potential outcome of filing an ethical complaint.

## II. Ethical Jurisdiction of Occupational Therapy

### A. American Occupational Therapy Association (AOTA)

1. The profession's official membership organization which develops, publishes, and disseminates the field's ethical code.

a. Represents and promotes the interest of those individuals who choose to become members.

b. Since membership is voluntary, the AOTA has no direct authority over practitioners (occupational therapists and OTAs) who are not members, and no direct legal mechanism for preventing non-members who are incompetent, unethical, or unqualified from practicing.

2. Actions that are in violation of the purpose and spirit of AOTA's Code of Ethics are considered unethical by AOTA.

a. These ethical standards are often the guide by which other bodies judge professional behaviors to determine if malpractice has occurred.

3. Ethics Commission.

a. The component of the AOTA that is responsible for the Code of Ethics, and the Standards of Practice of the profession.

b. The Ethics Commission is responsible for informing and educating members about current ethical issues, upholding the practice and education standards of the profession, monitoring the behavior of members, and reviewing allegations of unethical conduct.

(1) Ethical complaints filed with the Ethics Commission initiate an extensive, confidential review process according to the AOTA's established enforcement procedures for occupational therapy Code of Ethics.

### B. National Board for Certification in Occupational Therapy (NBCOT)

1. The national credentialing agency.

a. Certifies qualified persons as COTA®s and OTR®s through a written examination for entry-level practitioners.

b. NBCOT also maintains COTA® and OTR® certification through a voluntary certification renewal program.

c. Jurisdiction is over all NBCOT certified occupational therapy practitioners as well as those eligible for NBCOT certification.

2. As a voluntary credentialing agency, NBCOT has no direct authority over practitioners (occupational therapists and OTAs) who are not certified by NBCOT, and no direct legal mechanism for preventing uncertified practitioners who are incompetent, unethical, or unqualified from practicing.

3. NBCOT has developed investigatory and disciplinary action procedures for NBCOT certified practitioners whose practices raise concern due to incompetence, unethical behavior, and/or impairment.

### C. State Regulatory Boards (SRBs)

1. Public bodies created by state legislatures to assure the health and safety of the citizens of that state.

a. Their specific responsibility is to protect the public from potential harm that might be caused by incompetent or unqualified practitioners.

b. State regulation may be in the form of licensure, registration or certification. Refer to Appendix 3.

(1) Not all states regulate OTAs.

c. Each state has legal guidelines that usually specify the scope of practice of the profession, and the qualifications that must be met to practice in that state.

2. Ethical jurisdiction.
   a. SRBs usually provide a description of ethical behavior. In many instances, SRBs have adopted AOTA's Code of Ethics for this purpose.
   b. By the very nature of their limited jurisdiction (i.e., only over therapists and assistants practicing in their state), SRBs can monitor a profession closely.
   c. SRBs have the authority by law to discipline members of a profession if the public is determined to be at risk due to malpractice.
   d. SRBs also intervene in situations where the individual has been convicted of an illegal act that is directly connected with professional practice (i.e., fraud or misappropriation of funds through false billing practices).
   e. Since SRBs are primarily concerned with the protection of the public from harm, they will limit their review of complaints to those involving such a threat.

**D. Disciplinary Actions for Ethical Violations & Professional Misconduct**
1. When the AOTA, NBCOT, and/or a SRB determine that a person has violated their standards for ethical practice, different actions can be used as a disciplinary measure.
   a. These actions are based on agency internal investigations to determine the severity of an infraction and can include:
   (1) Reprimand: the private communication of the respective agency's disapproval of a practitioner's conduct.
   (2) Censure: a public statement of the respective agency's disapproval of a practitioner's conduct.
   (3) Ineligibility: the removal of eligibility for membership, certification, or licensure by the respective agency for an indefinite or specific time period.
   (4) Probation: the requirement that a practitioner meet certain conditions (e.g., further education, extensive supervision, individual counseling, participation in a substance abuse rehabilitation program) to retain membership, certification, or licensure by the respective agency.
   (5) Suspension: the loss of membership, certification, or licensure for a specific time period.
   (6) Revocation: the permanent loss of membership, certification, or licensure.

2. All of the above actions (except for reprimand) are made public by the respective agencies.
   a. Disciplinary actions that are made public by one agency (e.g., NBCOT) can trigger an investigation into a practitioner's professional conduct by other practice jurisdictions (e.g., SRBs).

**E. Common Law Related to Ethical Violations/ Malpractice**
1. Common law evolves from legal decisions and can impact occupational therapists and OTAs.
   a. Malpractice suits can be filed by individuals and/or their caregivers if the OTA is viewed to be personally responsible for negligence or other acts that resulted in harm to a client.
   (1) Negligence.
       (a) Failure to do what other reasonable practitioners would have done under similar circumstances.
       (b) Doing what other reasonable practitioners would not have done under similar circumstances.
       (c) The end result was harm to the individual.
       (d) Every individual (OTA, occupational therapist, student OTA, or student occupational therapist) is liable for their own negligence.
   b. Supervisors or superiors may also assume the liability of their workers if they provided faulty supervision or inappropriately delegated responsibilities.
   c. The institution usually assumes liability if an individual was harmed as a result of an environmental problem.
   (1) Falls resulting from slippery floors, poorly lit areas, lack of grab bars.
   d. The institution is also liable if an employee was incompetent or not properly licensed.
   e. Personal malpractice insurance is advisable for all levels of OT practitioners.

# III. OT Practitioner Roles

## A. General Information
1. OT practitioners include occupational therapy assistants (OTAs) and occupational therapists.
2. OT aides have an important role but are not considered OT practitioners. See Section C below.
3. OT practitioners can assume a variety of roles including entry to advanced level practitioner, peer and/or consumer educator, fieldwork educator, supervisor, administrator, consultant, fieldwork

coordinator, faculty member, academic program director, researcher/scholar, and/or entrepreneur.

4. Role development and advancement depends on practitioner's experience, education, practice skills, and professional development activities (i.e., self study, continuing education, advanced degrees).

**B. OT Assistant (OTA) Information**

1. OTAs are graduates of ACOTE accredited technical educational programs which are generally 2 years in duration, resulting in an Associate's degree or a Certificate.

2. An OTA can expand their role by establishing service competency.

   a. Service competency is the ability to use the specified intervention in a safe, effective, and reliable manner, (i.e., the OTA and occupational therapist can perform the same or equivalent procedure and obtain the same results).

      (1) Frequently performed procedures are easier to establish service competency.

      (2) Procedures performed infrequently require more supervision.

   b. OTAs who establish service competency do not become independent; they continue to work under the occupational therapist's supervision.

3. OTA's primary role is to implement treatment.

   a. OTAs can contribute to the evaluation process but they cannot independently evaluate or initiate treatment prior to the occupational therapist's evaluation.

   b. OTAs can contribute to development and implementation of the intervention plan and the monitoring and documenting of the individual's response to intervention under the occupational therapist's supervision. See Section IV.

4. OTAs can be activities directors in skilled nursing facilities (SNFs) and can supervise OT aides.

5. AOTA supports the independent practice of OTAs with advanced level skills who work for independent living centers.

   a. State licensure laws and scope of practice legislation may supersede this recommendation.

**C. OT Aide Roles**

1. Occupational therapy aides are not considered OT practitioners, according to the AOTA Standards of Practice.

   a. OT aides cannot perform OT practice tasks or be delegated skilled tasks that are performed by OTAs or occupational therapists.

2. The use of OT aides has increased in response to changes in the health care system (i.e., pressures to control costs have resulted in the delegation of non-skilled tasks to aides).

   a. Medicare Part A only provides guidelines for the use of therapy aides in skilled nursing facilities.

      (1) According to Medicare, therapy aides in skilled nursing facilities can only perform services within 'line of sight' supervision of an occupational therapist.

         (a) Therapy aides cannot perform any services outside of the occupational therapist's vision at any time.

   b. Despite the Medicare ruling, most state occupational therapy licensure laws, regulations, and statutes do not allow the use of therapy aides to provide OT services.

3. OT aides can be delegated supportive, non-skilled tasks by OTAs or occupational therapists.

   a. Non-skilled tasks aides may perform include routine maintenance and clerical activities, preparation of clinic area for intervention, and/or specified, supervised aspects of a treatment session (e.g., contact guarding a client while an OTA teaches transfers).

## IV. Supervisory Guidelines for OT Personnel

**A. General Supervision Information**

1. Supervision is the process in which two or more individuals collaborate to establish, maintain, promote, or enhance a level of performance and quality of service.

2. It is a mutually respectful joint effort between supervisor and supervisee.

3. It promotes professional growth and development and facilitates mentoring.

4. It ensures appropriate training, education, and use of resources for safe and effective service provision.

5. Supervision facilitates innovation, supports creativity, and provides encouragement, guidance, and support while working toward attainment of a shared goal.

6. Only OT practitioners can supervise OT practice, OT aides cannot supervise OT practice.

**B. Methods of Supervision**

1. Direct: face-to-face contact between supervisor and supervisee.

   a. Includes co-treatment, observation, instruction, modeling, and discussion.

2. Indirect, non face-to-face contact between supervisor and supervisee.
   a. Includes electronic, written and telephone communications.

**C. The Supervision Continuum**

1. Supervision occurs along a continuum that includes close, routine, general, and minimum.
   a. Close: daily, direct contact at the site of work.
   b. Routine: direct contact at least every 2 weeks at the site of work, with interim supervision occurring by other methods such as telephone or written communication.
   c. General: at least monthly direct contact with supervision available as needed by other methods.
   d. Minimal: provided only on a needed basis, and may be less than monthly.

2. Formal supervision can be supplemented by functional supervision, which is the provision of information and feedback to coworkers (a sharing of expertise).

3. The degree, amount, and pattern of supervision required can vary depending on the practitioner's competence, service demands, state laws and licensure requirements, facilities procedures, and case characteristics (i.e., an acutely ill person with rapidly changing status on an acute inpatient unit will require a closer occupational therapist/OTA partnership than a more stable client in a long-term care residential facility).
   a. For example, a novice OTA requires frequent and direct supervision while an OTA with 15 years experience may require monthly minimal supervision.

4. The supervising occupational therapist determines the type of supervision that is most appropriate.

5. Ethically, the OT supervisor must ensure that the type, amount, and pattern of supervision match the supervisee's level of role performance. (Table 4-1)

6. OT aide supervision may be intermittent or continuous depending on the task being performed.
   a. Intermittent supervision is sufficient for non-patient related tasks. It requires periodic discussion, demonstration, or contact between the supervisor and aide on at least a monthly basis.
   b. Continuous supervision is required for patient-related tasks. A supervisory OTA or occupational therapist must be within auditory and/or visual contact in the immediate area of the aide during the aide's task performance.

**D. Specific OT Roles and Supervisory Guidelines**

1. Practitioner: Occupational therapist.
   a. Functions to provide quality OT services (assessment, intervention, program planning and implementation, discharge planning, related documentation and communication).
   b. Can be direct, indirect, or consultative in nature, and can range from entry level to advanced level depending on experience, education, and practice skills.
   c. The occupational therapist has ultimate responsibility for service provision.
   d. Occupational therapists that do not have access to formal supervision are advised to seek mentoring to facilitate professional growth and develop best practice skills.

2. Practitioner: Occupational therapy assistant (OTA).
   a. Functions to provide quality OT services to assigned individuals under supervision of an occupational therapist.
   b. Can range from entry level to advanced level depending on experience, education, and practice skills.
   c. Development from entry level to advanced level is dependent upon development of service competency.

3. Educator.
   a. Functions to develop and provide training or educational offerings related to OT's domain of concern to consumer, peer, and community groups or individuals.
   b. Can be an occupational therapist or an OTA with appropriate supervision.

4. Fieldwork educator.
   a. Functions as the manager of Level I and/or II fieldwork in a practice setting, providing students with opportunities to practice and implement practitioner competence.
      (1) Entry level OTAs and occupational therapists may supervise Level I fieldwork students.
      (2) Occupational therapists with one year practice-based experience may supervise OT Level II students.
      (3) OTAs with 1 year of practice experience may supervise OTA Level II fieldwork students.
      (4) Three years of experience are recommended for individuals supervising programs with multiple students and multiple supervisors.

## TABLE 4-1  GUIDE FOR SUPERVISION OF OCCUPATIONAL THERAPY PERSONNEL

| OCCUPATIONAL THERAPY PERSONNEL | SUPERVISION | SUPERVISES |
|---|---|---|
| Entry-level OT* (working on initial skill development or entering new practice) (AOTA, 1993a, p.1088) | Not required. Close supervision by an intermediate-level or an advanced-level OT recommended. | Aides, technicians, all levels of OTAs, volunteers, Level I fieldwork students |
| Intermediate-level OT* (working on increased skill development and mastery of basic role functions, and demonstrates ability to respond to situations based on previous experience) (AOTA,1993a, p.1088) | Not required. Routine or general supervision by an advanced-level OT recommended. | Aides, technicians, all levels of OTAs, Level I and Level II fieldwork students, entry-level OTs |
| Advanced-level OT* (refining specialized skills with the ability to understand complex issues affecting role functions) (AOTA, 1993a, p.1088) | Not required. Minimal supervision by an advanced-level OT is recommended. | Aides, technicians, all levels of OTAs, Level I and Level II fieldwork students entry-level and intermediate-level OTs. |
| Entry-level OTA* (working on initial skill development or entering new practice) (AOTA, 1993a, p.1088) | Close supervision by all levels of OTs, or an intermediate or an advanced-level OTA who is under the supervision of an OT. | Aides, technicians, volunteers. |
| Intermediate-level OTA* (working on increased skill development and mastery of basic role functions, and demonstrates ability to respond to situations based on previous experience) (AOTA, 1993a, p.1088) | Routine or general supervision by all levels of OTs, or an advanced-level OTA, who is under the supervision of an OT. | Aides, technicians, entry-level OTAs, volunteers, Level I OT fieldwork students, Level I and II OTA fieldwork students. |
| Advanced-level OTA** (refining specialized skills with the ability to understand complex issues affecting role functions) (AOTA, 1993a, p.1088) | General supervision by all levels of OTs, or an advanced-level OTA, who is under the supervision of an OT. | Aides, technicians, entry-level and intermediate-level OTAs, volunteers, Level I OT fieldwork students, Level I and Level II OTA fieldwork students. |
| Personnel other than occupational therapy practitioners assisting in occupational therapy service (aides, paraprofessionals, technicians, volunteers)*** (AOTA, 1993a, p1088) | For non-client related tasks, supervision is determined by the supervising practitioner. For client-related tasks, continuous supervision is provided by all levels of practitioners. | No supervisory capacity. |

* Refer to the *Occupational Therapy Roles* document for descriptions of entry-level, intermediate-level, and advanced-level OTs and OTAs (AOTA, 1993a).

** Although specific state regulations may dictate the parameters of certified occupational therapy assistant practice, the American Occupational Therapy Association supports the autonomous practice of the certified occupational therapy assistant practitioner in the independent living setting (AOTA, 1993b, p.1079). (*Note.* Removed from active files and placed in archives April 1999).

*** Students are not addressed in this category. The student role as a supervisor is addressed in the Essentials and Guidelines for an Accredited Educational Program for the Occupational Therapist (AOTA, 1991a) and Essentials and Guidelines for an Accredited Educational Program for the Occupational Therapy Assistant (AOTA, 1991b).

From Guide for supervision of occupational therapy. *American Journal of Occupational Therapy, 53* (p. 594) by the American Occupational Therapy Association Commission on Practice. Copyright 1999 by the American Occupational Therapy Association. Reprinted with permission.

5. Supervisor.
   a. Functions as the manager of the overall daily operation of OT services in a defined practice area(s).
   b. Can be an OTA or an occupational therapist.
   c. Experienced OTAs may supervise other OTAs administratively as long as service protocols and documentation are supervised by an occupational therapist.
6. Administrator.
   a. Functions to manage department, program, services, or agency providing OT services.

b. Can be an occupational therapist with a graduate degree or continuing education relevant to management and experience appropriate to the size and scope of department and program(s), (i.e., a minimum of 3-5 years of experience).

7. Consultant.
   a. Functions to provide OT consultation to individuals, groups, or organizations.
   b. Can be an OTA or an occupational therapist at the intermediate or advanced practice level.
   c. The OTA and occupational therapist are responsible for obtaining the appropriate level of supervision to meet regulatory and professional standards.

8. Academic setting fieldwork coordinator.
   a. Functions to manage fieldwork within the OT academic setting.
   b. Can be an OTA or an occupational therapist with a recommended three years of practice experience and experience in supervising fieldwork students.
   c. General supervision by the OT academic program director is recommended.
   d. Close to routine supervision is recommended for new faculty.

9. Faculty.
   a. Functions to provide formal academic education to OT students.
   b. Can be an OTA or an occupational therapist with an appropriate advanced professional degree and intermediate to advanced skills in teaching.
   c. General supervision is recommended by academic program director.
   d. Close to routine supervision for new, adjunct, and part-time faculty by program director.

10. Program director (academic setting).
    a. Functions to manage the OT education program with an appropriate advanced professional degree, experience as a faculty member, and experience or continuing education in academic management.
    b. General to minimal administrative supervision from designated administrative officer (e.g., Academic Dean).

11. Researcher/scholar.
    a. Functions to perform scholarly work of the profession, i.e., examining, developing, refining, and/or evaluating the profession's theoretical base, philosophical foundations, and body of knowledge.

b. Can be an occupational therapist or an OTA o with additional self study, continuing education, experience and formal education related to research and scholarly activities.
c. Additional academic qualifications are needed for OTAs to be principal investigators.
d. OTAs without additional education can contribute to research process.
e. Supervision needs range from close to minimal depending on skills of researcher/scholar and scope of the project.

12. Entrepreneur.
    a. Functions as a partially or fully self-employed individual who provides OT services.
    b. Can be an OTA or an occupational therapist who meets state regulatory requirements.
    c. OTAs who provide direct service have the responsibility to obtain appropriate supervision from an occupational therapist.

# V. Team Roles and Principles of Collaboration

## A. Overview

1. A team is a group of equally important individuals with common interests collaborating to develop shared goals and build trusting relationships to achieve these shared goals.
2. Members of the team include the patient/client/consumer; his/her family, significant others, and/or caregivers; healthcare professionals; and the reimburser's gatekeepers.
3. Professional members on team will vary according to practice setting.
4. The consumer, family, significant other, and/or caregiver role on the team has become increasingly important. Collaboration with these individuals is even mandated by law (e.g., OBRA, IDEA; see this chapter's section on legislation).

## B. Principles of Collaboration

1. Factors that influence effective team functioning.
   a. Member skill and knowledge.
   b. Membership stability.
   c. Commitment to team goals.
   d. Good communication.
   e. Membership composition.
   f. A common language.
   g. Effective leadership.
2. Recognize that all members of the team are equally important.
   a. No one's opinion or area of competence takes

precedence over the other.

   (1) Facility chain of command guidelines will determine who is ultimately responsible for the team's decision.

3. Understand principles of team collaboration and that correct exam answers will adhere to these principles.

4. Know the different types of teams and their respective limits and benefits for team efficacy.

5. Know all potential team members and their respective role responsibilities. NBCOT exam items can ask questions that require an answer that includes a referral to another team member.

6. Recognize that OT practitioners are competent in many domains of concern but our scope of practice does have its limits.

   a. Be prepared to recognize these limits. For example, a parent distraught over his/her child's traumatic brain injury angrily questions the meaning of life and the relevance of his/her faith. A correct answer would include active listening and a referral to pastoral care.

**C. Lay Team Members and Role Responsibilities**

1. Consumer.

   a. The most important and primary member of the treatment team.

   b. The consumer's occupations, values, interests, and goals must be determined and used in all treatment planning.

      (1) If the consumer and the therapist do not share a common language, an interpreter must be used.

2. Family/primary caregiver.

   a. Family's sociocultural background, socioeconomic status, and caregiving tasks, needs, and skills must be considered as they can impact on the outcome of intervention.

      (1) If the family and the therapist do not share a common language, an interpreter must be used.

**D. Para-professional Team Members and Role Responsibilities**

1. Home health aides (HHAs)/Personal care assistants (PCAs).

   a. Individuals who provide primary care to enable a person with a disability to remain in his or her own home.

   b. Most states require some minimum training and certification as an HHA/PCA. Standards and educational requirements can vary greatly from state to state.

   c. Responsibilities.

      (1) Personal care such as bathing, grooming, dressing, and feeding.

      (2) Home management such as shopping, cleaning, and cooking.

      (3) Supervision of home programs as directed by a health care practitioner (e.g., nurse, therapist).

   d. Due to the tremendous importance this role has in maintaining a person with a disability in his or her own home, OT practitioner collaboration with HHAs/PCAs is critical.

   e. OT practitioners can also educate and train consumers on the hiring, training, and supervision of HHAs/PCAs.

**E. Professional Team Members and Role Responsibilities**

1. Primary care physician (PCP).

   a. A physician who serves as the "gatekeeper" of services for consumers in managed health care systems.

   b. Provides primary health care services and manages routine medical care.

   c. Makes referrals, as needed, to other health care providers and services including specialty tests and examinations, rehabilitation services, and occupational therapy.

2. Physiatrist.

   a. A physician who specializes in physical medicine and rehabilitation and is certified by the American Board of Physical Medicine and Rehabilitation.

   b. Leads the rehabilitation team and works directly with occupational, speech, and physical therapists and others to maximize rehabilitation outcome for persons with physical disorders.

   c. Diagnoses and medically treats individuals with musculoskeletal, neurological, cardiovascular, pulmonary, and/or other body systems disorders.

3. Psychiatrist.

   a. A physician who specializes in mental health and psychiatric rehabilitation.

   b. Leads the rehabilitation team and works directly with occupational therapists, psychologists, social workers, and others to maximize rehabilitation outcomes for persons with psychiatric disorders.

   c. Diagnoses and medically treats individuals with psychiatric disorders.

   d. Responsible for ordering transfers to long term

care settings and for determining competence and the need for involuntary treatment.

4. Psychologist.
   a. A professional with a Ph.D. in psychology.
   b. Evaluates psychological and cognitive status with standardized and non-standardized assessments including intelligence/IQ (Stanford-Binet, Wechsler), Projective (Rorschach), Personality (Minnesota Multiphasic Personality Inventory), Neuropsychological and Interest Inventories (Strong-Campbell).
   c. Provides individual, couple, family, and group supportive therapy, cognitive retraining, and behavior modification.
5. Physician's assistant (PA).
   a. A professional who is a graduate of an accredited physician's assistant educational program and who has passed a national certification examination.
   b. Performs routine diagnostic, therapeutic, preventative, and health maintenance services.
   c. Specializations can include family medicine, geriatrics, pediatrics, obstetrics, emergency care, and orthopedics.
   d. Must work under the direction of and be supervised by a physician.
6. Registered nurse (RN).
   a. A licensed professional who is a graduate of an accredited nursing education program.
   b. Serves as the primary liaison between the individual and physician. Also, often serves as the primary case manager.
   c. Monitors vital signs, symptoms, and behaviors.
   d. Dispenses medications and assists the physician with the titration of medications.
   e. Performs or supervises bedside care and assists with ADL.
   f. Conducts group and individual interventions related to wellness and prevention and disease and symptom management (e.g., medication education).
   g. Performs patient, family, and caregiver education to facilitate recovery and maximize quality of life.
   h. Supervises and is assisted by licensed practical nurses (LPNs), certified nursing assistants (CNAs), and aides.
      (1) Due to the major role LPNs and CNAs have in providing direct care to individuals. OT collaboration with these team members is

essential.

7. Dietician/Clinical Nutritionist.
   a. A licensed professional who is a graduate of an accredited educational program and who passed a national registration examination.
      (1) Practitioners who pass this registration examination are credentialed as Registered Dietician (RD) or Dietician Technician, Registered (DTR), depending on level of education.
   b. Evaluates individuals' nutritional status and dietary needs.
   c. Provides nutrition therapy for diseases such as diabetes and preventive counseling for issues such as obesity.
8. Respiratory therapy technician certified (CRT).
   a. A technically trained professional with an Associate's Degree who has passed a national certification examination.
   b. Administers respiratory therapy as prescribed and supervised by a physician.
   c. Performs pulmonary function tests and intervenes through oxygen delivery, aerosols, and nebulizers.
9. Physical therapist (PT).
   a. A licensed professional who is a graduate of an accredited physical therapy education program currently at a graduate level.
   b. Evaluates clients' physical motor skills.
   c. Develops plan of care, and administers or supervises treatment to develop, improve and/or maintain client's physical motor skills, to alleviate pain, and to correct or minimize physical deformity.
   d. Delegates portions of treatment program to supportive personnel, e.g., physical therapist assistant (PTA).
   e. Supervises and directs supportive staff (PTA, PT aide) in designated tasks.
   f. Re-evaluates and adjusts plan of care as appropriate.
   g. Performs and documents final evaluation and establishes discharge and follow-up plans.
10. Physical therapist assistant (PTA).
    a. A skilled allied health care technologist, usually with a two year associate's degree.
    b. Must work under the supervision of a physical therapist.
       (1) If the supervisor is off-site, delegated responsibilities must be safe and legal prac-

tice with ready access to the supervisor.

    (2) In home health, required periodic joint on-site visits or treatments with physical therapist.

  c. Able to adjust treatment procedure in accordance with the patient's status.

  d. May not evaluate, develop, or change plan of care or write discharge plan or summary.

11. Athletic trainer.

  a. An allied health professional.

  b. Assesses athletes' risk for injury, conducts injury prevention programs, and provides treatment and rehabilitation under the supervision of a physician when athletic trauma occurs.

12. Chiropractor (DC).

  a. A professional who is a graduate of an educational program in chiropractory who is usually licensed by state boards.

  b. Assesses the individual's spinal column and intervenes to restore and maintain health, and decrease and eliminate pain.

13. Certified orthotist (CO).

  a. Evaluates the need for orthotic equipment (splints, braces).

  b. Designs, fabricates, and fits orthoses for individuals to prevent or correct deformities and/or support body parts weakened by injury, disease, or congenital deformity.

  c. Educates the client on purpose of orthoses, recommended care, and wearing schedule.

  d. May be an OT, a PT, or an individual with specialized training.

14. Certified prosthetist (CP).

  a. Evaluates the need for a prosthesis.

  b. Designs, fabricates, and fits prosthesis for an individual to ensure proper fit and to promote functional abilities.

  c. Educates client and/or caregiver(s) about the use and care of the prosthesis.

  d. Works directly with OTs, PTs, and physicians.

15. Biomedical engineer.

  a A graduate of an engineering program who specializes in the biomedical application of engineering theory and technology.

  b. Serves as a technical expert to recommend commercial products, adapt available devices, and/or modify existing environments.

  c. Develops, designs, and fabricates customized equipment, devices, and techniques.

16. Speech-language pathologist (SLP) or speech therapist (ST).

  a. A professional who is a graduate of an accredited educational program in speech-language pathology.

  b. Assesses language and speech abilities and impairments.

  c. Develops and conducts intervention programs to restore, improve, or augment the communication of persons with speech and/or language impairments.

  d. May receive advanced training and specialize in oral-motor functioning (e.g., the evaluation and treatment of dysphagia).

17. Audiologist.

  a. A professional who is a graduate of an educational program in audiology.

  b. Administers assessments to determine an individual's auditory acuity, level of hearing impairment, and damage site(s) in the auditory system.

  c. Provides recommendations for assistive devices (e.g., hearing aids) and/or special training to enhance residual hearing and/or adapt to hearing loss.

18. Optometrist/vision specialist.

  a. A professional who is a graduate of an educational program in optometry.

  b. Examines the eye to determine visual acuity, level of visual impairments, and damage to or disease in the visual system.

  c. Prescribes assistive devices (e.g., corrective lenses) and recommends other appropriate treatment (e.g., visual-motor training).

  d. Optometrists can refer individuals to outpatient OT.

19. Special educator/teacher.

  a. A professional teacher certified to provide education to children with special needs.

    (1) Visual and/or hearing impairments.

    (2) Emotional and psychosocial disabilities.

    (3) Physical and sensorimotor disabilities.

    (4) Developmental disabilities.

    (5) Learning and cognitive disabilities.

  b. Assesses and monitors student learning, plans and implements instructional activities, and addresses the special developmental and educational needs of each student.

  c. Advanced training in instructional methods for teaching children with special needs to develop to their fullest educational potential is required.

  d. Additional training in teaching children with

multiple disabilities is often needed.

  e. May be assisted by teacher aides who provide direct care and "hands-on" support to students in the classroom.

    (1) Collaboration with aides is required for effective follow-through of OT programming in school settings.

20. Vocational rehabilitation counselor.

  a. A professional who is a graduate of an educational program in vocational rehabilitation.

  b. If certified, the counselor is able to use the credential of Certified Rehabilitation Counselor (CRC).

  c. Evaluates prevocational skills and vocational interests and abilities via standardized and non-standardized assessments to determine an individual's employability.

  d. Provides counseling to maximize the individual's vocational potential.

  e. Refers individual to appropriate vocational programming and/or job placement.

  f. Serves as liaison between the individual and state educational and vocational departments for persons with disabilities to obtain funding for needed services.

21. Social worker.

  a. A licensed/registered professional who is a graduate of an accredited educational social work program at a baccalaureate level (BSW) or at a graduate level (MSW).

  b. Upon passing a national certification examination, a social worker is eligible to use the credentials Certified Social Worker (CSW).

  c. Assesses client's social history and psychosocial functioning via clinical interviews and structured assessments.

  d. Assists clients, families and caregivers with accessing social support services (e.g., home care, support groups) and obtaining needed reimbursement/funding (e.g., Medicaid, food stamps) through the completion of required application processes and through active advocacy.

  e. Provides individual, couple, and family counseling.

  f. Serves as a primary care manager, enabling individual to function optimally and maintain quality of life.

  g. Provides crisis intervention and recommendations for additional services.

  h. Contributes to discharge plan and completes tasks needed for implementation of discharge orders (e.g., application to a SNF).

  i. Supervises and is assisted by social work assistants (SWAs) and mental health technicians (MHTs).

22. Substance abuse counselor.

  a. A professional who may come from a diversity of educational backgrounds (psychology, social work, occupational therapy) who has completed a specialized training program.

  b. Provides individual and/or group intervention.

  c. Certified Alcohol Counselor (CAC) and Certified Alcohol and Drug Counselor (CADC) are the two main credentials designating this specialized role.

23. Recreational therapist/therapeutic recreation specialist.

  a. A professional who is a graduate of a recreation therapy education program.

  b. Conducts individual and/or group interventions to develop leisure interests and skills; to facilitate community, social, and recreational integration; to manage stress and symptoms; and to adjust to disability.

  c. May be called an Activities Therapist but the two positions are not synonymous. Activities Therapists may only have on-the-job training.

24. Expressive/creative arts therapist.

  a. Professionals who are graduates of specialized education programs.

  b. Depending on the state, they may or may not be licensed or registered.

  c. Includes art, dance/movement, music, horticulture, and poetry therapists.

  d. Conducts individual and/or group interventions which use select expressive modalities to facilitate self-expression, self-awareness, social skills, symptom reduction and management.

25. Pastoral care.

  a. Serves as the spiritual advisor to the individual, his/her family, caregivers, and the team.

  b. Provides individual, couple, and family counseling in a non-denominational manner.

26. Alternative practitioners.

  a. May include massage therapists, acupuncturists, Reiki practitioners, and others.

  b. Training and licensure requirements vary greatly.

  c. The roles and tasks of alternative practitioners will be determined by state practice regulations and reimburser's guidelines.

# VI. The United States Health Care System

## A. Overview

1. A group of decentralized subsystems serving different populations.
2. Overwhelmingly private ownership of health care delivery.
3. Relatively small federal and state governmental programs work in conjunction with a large private sector; however, the government pays for a large portion of these private sector services through Medicare and Medicaid reimbursement.
4. Decentralization results in overlap in some areas and competition in others; therefore, health care is primarily a business that is market-driven.
   a. Patients are viewed as consumers due to this economic focus.
   b. Cost containment while maintaining quality of service is a delicate balancing act that is not always achieved.
5. Primary care physicians have increased significance as the first line for evaluation and intervention, and the referral source for specialized and/or ancillary services.

## B. Health Care Regulations

1. Health care is a highly regulated industry with most regulations mandated by law.
2. Legally mandated regulations are set forth by the Centers for Medicare and Medicaid Services (CMS), a division of U.S. Department of Health and Human Services (HHS).
   a. CMS is the federal agency which develops rules and regulations pertaining to federal laws, in particular the Medicare and Medicaid programs.
   b. Facilities that participate in Medicare and/or Medicaid programs are monitored regularly for compliance with CMS guidelines by federal and state surveyors.
   c. Facilities that repeatedly fail to meet CMS guidelines lose their Medicare and/or Medicaid certification(s).
   d. Long-term settings, i.e., skilled nursing facilities (SNFs), are strongly influenced by CMS regulations since Medicare and/or Medicaid pays for all or most of the expense of long-term care.
   e. CMS is divided into three centers.
      (1) The Center for Beneficiary Choices which focuses on Medicare Choice and Medigap.
      (2) The Center for Medicare Management which focuses on traditional fee-for-service Medicare.
      (3) The Center for Medicaid and State Operations which focuses on state administered programs like Medicaid and State Children's Health Insurance Program (SCHIP).
3. Standards related to safety are set forth and enforced by the Occupational Safety and Health Administration (OSHA), a division of the U.S. Department of Labor.
   a. Structural standards and building codes are established and enforced by OSHA to ensure the safety of structures.
   b. The safety of employees and consumers is regulated by OSHA standards for handling infectious materials and blood products, controlling blood borne pathogens, operating machinery, and handling hazardous substances.
4. State accreditation to obtain licensure for a health care facility is mandatory. Individual states develop their own requirements, with state agencies enforcing these regulations.
5. Local or county entities also develop regulations pertaining to health care institutions (e.g., physical plant safety features such as fire, elevator and boiler regulations).

## C. Voluntary Accreditation

1. Voluntary accreditation and self-imposed compliance with established standards is sought by most health care organizations; e.g., hospitals, skilled nursing facilities (SNFs), home health agencies, preferred provider organizations (PPOs), rehabilitation centers, health maintenance organizations (HMOs), behavioral health including mental health and chemical dependency facilities, physicians' networks, hospice care, long term care facilities, and others.
2. Accreditation is a status awarded for compliance with established standards.
3. Accreditation ensures the public that a health care facility is adequately equipped and meets high standards for patient care, and employs qualified professionals and competent staff.
4. Accreditation affirms the competence of practitioners and the quality of health care facilities and organizations.
5. Accreditation through an accrediting agency is voluntary; however, it is mandatory to receive third party reimbursement and to be eligible for

federal government grants and contracts.

6. CMS and many states accept certain national accreditations as meeting their respective requirements for participation in the Medicare and Medicaid programs and for a license to operate.

7. Voluntary accrediting agencies include the Joint Commission (JCAHO), Commission on Accreditation of Rehabilitation Facilities (CARF), and the Accreditation Council for Services for Mentally Retarded and Other Developmentally Disabled Persons (AC-MRDD) and others.

**D. The Accreditation Process**

1. Accreditation is initiated by the organization submitting an application for review or survey by the accrediting agency.

2. A self-study or self-assessment is conducted to examine the organization based on the accrediting agency's standards.

3. An on-site review is conducted by an individual reviewer or surveyor or a team visiting the organization.

4. The accreditation and the reaccreditation process involve all staff. Tasks include document preparation, hosting the site visit team, and interviews with accreditors.

5. Once accredited, the organization undergoes periodic review, typically every three years.

**E. Value of Accreditation to Occupational Therapy**

1. Self-study and self-assessment can be an opportunity to identify areas of strength, validate competence, and promote excellence.

2. Areas needing improvement can be identified (i.e., procedures can be streamlined and additional resources can be obtained, team communication can be enhanced).

3. Program goals are clarified.

4. Practice is defined and documented.

5. Accreditors can share information regarding "best practice".

6. An increased recognition of the OT practitioners' contributions to the agency and identification of functional outcomes can result in increased visibility for OT and increased referrals.

# VII. Payment for Occupational Therapy Services

**A. Key Terms**

1. Beneficiary: a person receiving services. In skilled nursing facilities (SNFs), the term "resident" is used.

2. Capitation.

   a. Payment system under which the provider is paid prospectively (i.e., on a monthly basis) a set fee for each member of a specific population (i.e., health plan members) regardless if no covered health care is delivered or if extensive care is delivered.

   b. Payment is typically determined in terms of "per member per month" (PMPM).

   c. The healthier the enrollees (and the fewer services used), the more the provider retains of the total PMPM payment.

3. Co-insurance: the monetary amount to be paid by a patient, usually expressed as a percentage of total charge.

4. Clinical/critical pathway: a standardized recommended intervention protocol for a specific diagnosis.

5. Deductible: the amount a patient must pay to a provider before the insurance benefits will pay. Usually expressed as an annual dollar amount.

6. Denial: the refusal by a payer to reimburse a provider for services rendered. Reasons for denial include benefits exhausted, duplication of services, and services not indicated.

7. Diagnosis code: a code that describes a patient's medical reason or condition that requires health service.

8. Diagnostic related groups (DRGs): the descriptive categories established by CMS that determine the level of payment at a per case rate.

9. Fee for service: the payment system under which the provider is paid the same type of rate per unit of service. Traditionally, payer pays 80% and patient or provider is responsible for the remaining 20%.

10. Health maintenance organization (HMO): a common form of managed care. Maintains control over services by requiring enrollees to see only doctors within the HMO network and to obtain referrals before seeking specialty or ancillary care.

11. Managed care: a method of maintaining some control over costs and utilization of services while providing quality health care. Typically refers to HMOs and PPOs.

12. Per diem: a negotiated, per day fee for service. Typically used for inpatient hospital stays and skilled nursing facilities.

13. Preferred provider organization (PPO): a form of managed care that is similar to an HMO but usual-

ly offers a greater choice of providers. However, as choices increase, percentage of payment decreases.

14. Private payment: the individual receiving services is responsible for payment.

15. Procedure codes: codes that describe specific services performed by health professionals.

16. Prospective payment system (PPS): the nationwide payment schedule that determines the Medicare payment for each inpatient stay of a Medicare beneficiary based on DRGs.

17. Provider: the entity responsible for the delivery and quality of services. Providers bill Medicare, HMOs and PPOs for services rendered.

18. Third party payers: agencies and companies who are the primary reimbursers for health care in the U.S. (e.g., Blue Cross). HMOs and PPOs are also third party payers.

19. Usual and customary rate (UCR): the average cost of specific health care procedures in a geographic area. This is the maximum amount the insurer will pay for a service and covered expense.

20. Vendor/supplier: the entity which supplies services.

**B. Private Insurance and Managed Care Plans**
1. Largest source of insurance payment in U.S.
   a. There are broad variations among plans and plan options.
   b. They can be for profit or not for profit.
2. Many private insurers contract with Medicare to handle the day to day operations of Medicare. They are called intermediaries.
3. Insurers (e.g., Blue Cross/Blue Shield, Aetna, MetLife, and Prudential), offer many insurance products including PPOs, HMOs, and managed care.
4. Coverage cannot be assumed based on the name of plan alone.
   a. Coinsurance, deductibles and copayments are common.
   b. Most plans cover for OT in hospitals.
   c. Outpatient coverage varies greatly.
   d. Total number of visits and/or type and amount of services per diagnosis are limited.
5. Insurers are not federally regulated. Each state determines its own requirements and regulations for insurers who operate within their borders.
6. Cost controlling payment strategies such as case management, precertification or preauthorization, mandatory second opinions, and preferred provider networks are often implemented.
7. OT practitioners can join health care provider pan-

els and/or a preferred provider network.

8. Due to the great variability in private insurance coverage, the NBCOT examination will not ask specific questions about private insurance. However, knowledge of industry trends such as those identified above will be helpful in answering service management questions.

**C. Medicare Overview**
1. General information.
   a. Largest single payer for OT services.
   b. Administered by CMS.
   c. Intermediaries determine if services provided are within Medicare guidelines.
   d. Persons eligible for Medicare medical coverage for health care services.
      (1) Persons 65 years or older.
      (2) Individuals with permanent kidney failure, black lung disease, and/or other long-term disability specified in the law.
      (3) Persons who have been on some social security program for 24 months.
      (4) Medicare does not cover chronic illness (except for black lung disease and renal failure as noted above), long term supportive care, or all medical expenses incurred when ill.
2. Part A: pays for services provided by hospitals, inpatient SNFs, home health agencies, rehabilitation facilities, and hospices.
   a. Part A is automatically provided to all who are covered by the Social Security System that meet the above coverage criteria.
   b. Services provided in acute care hospitals, long-term hospitals, rehabilitation facilities, home health, hospice, and SNFs receive a prospective, predetermined rate per inpatient based on the expected amount of resources a patient will use.
      (1) The prospective payment system (PPS) per case rate covers all services including OT.
      (2) In inpatient acute care hospitals, PPS is based on a patient classification system called diagnosis related groups (DRGs).
         (a) It is a fixed dollar amount for patient care for each diagnosis regardless of length of stay (LOS) or number of services provided.
         (b) Treatment supplies (i.e., adaptive equipment, splints) are included in this per case rate.
         (c) Individual hospitals determine the

combination of services a patient will receive.

(3) In inpatient rehabilitation facilities (IRFs), the PPS is based on the Inpatient Rehabilitation Facility Patient Assessment Instrument (IRF PAI).

(4) In inpatient psychiatric facilities and long-term care hospitals, the PPS is based on diagnosis and other factors.

(5) In home care, the PPS is based on a classification system called Home Health Resource Groups (HHRGs) to determine an episode payment rate.

    (a) This rate per episode of care reimbursement system applies to all home health services including all forms of therapy and medical supplies.

    (b) Durable medical equipment is excluded from home health PPS.

    (c) An episode is defined as a 60 day period beginning with the first billable visit and ending 60 days after the start of care.

(6) In skilled nursing facilities, reimbursement is based upon resource utilization groups (RUGs).

(7) In hospice, payment rates are based on four categories: routine home care, continuous home care, inpatient respite, and general inpatient care.

c. Part A covered services have specific time limits and also require deductible and coinsurance payments by the beneficiary.

(1) Annual deductible fees must be paid by patient.

(2) Twenty percent of home health care must be paid by patient.

3. Part B: pays for physician services, hospital outpatient, durable medical equipment, orthotics, prosthetics, supplies, and other professional services including OT services provided by independent practitioners.

a. Part B is considered a Supplemental Medical Insurance Program and therefore must be purchased by the beneficiary, usually as a monthly premium.

b. Part B services have no specific time limit and require 20% copayment.

4. The primary difference between Part A and Part B is the frequency in which the individual receives services. Inpatient Part A coverage requires services for a minimum of 5 days per week services. Part B typically covers 3 days per week outpatient services.

5. Part C is called Medicare Advantage.

a. It is private insurance alternative to the federal government's Part A and B

6. Part D is an optional buy-in coverage plan for prescription drugs.

**D. Medicare Coverage of Occupational Therapy Services**

1. Criteria for coverage of OT services.

a. Person must be under the care of a physician.

b. OT services must be prescribed by a physician or furnished according to a physician-approved/certified plan of care.

c. Performed by a qualified occupational therapist or an OTA under the general supervision of an occupational therapist.

d. Service is reasonable and necessary for treatment of individual's injury or illness.

e. Diagnosis can be physical, psychiatric, or both. There are no diagnostic restrictions for coverage.

f. OT must result in a significant, practical improvement in the person's level of functioning within a reasonable period of time.

2. OT in skilled nursing facilities (SNFs) is covered if the patient requires skilled nursing or skilled rehabilitation (i.e., OT, PT, ST) on a daily basis (i.e., minimum 5 days/week).

a. Reimbursement for OT services is also provided for the designing of a maintenance plan and for the occasional reevaluation of this plan's effectiveness.

b. Reimbursement is not provided for a therapist or OTA to carry out the maintenance plan.

c. Evaluation and training of caregivers is considered part of the design and reevaluation of a maintenance plan.

d. The competence of caregivers to carry out the maintenance plan must be documented prior to discharge from OT.

3. OT in home care is covered if the individual is homebound and needed intermittent skilled nursing care, PT, or ST before OT began. OT services can continue after need for skilled nursing, PT, or ST has ended.

a. Homebound status criteria.

(1) The person is typically not able to leave the

home; i.e., is 'confined' to the home.

    (a) "Confinement" may be due to the need for the aid of ambulatory devices, the assistance of others, or special transportation.

    (b) It considers medical, physical, cognitive, and psychiatric conditions.

  (2) If the person leaves the home it requires "considerable and taxing effort" (CMS 2009, Ch., para. 30.1.1).

  (3) A person may leave his/her home for medical appointments (e.g., kidney dialysis) and non-medical short-term and infrequent appointments /events (e.g., a trip to a hairdresser, attendance at religious services).

  (4) The need for adult day care does not preclude a person from receiving home health services.

b. An initial assessment visit and a comprehensive assessment using the Outcome and Assessment Information Set (OASIS) must be completed to verify the person's eligibility for Medicare home health benefits, the continuing need for home care, and to plan for the person's nursing, medical, social, rehabilitative, and discharge needs.

  (1) OT practitioners can complete the initial OASIS if the need for OT establishes program eligibility.

  (2) The initial assessment must be completed within 48 hours of referral or within 48 hours of the person's return home.

  (3) OT practitioners can conduct follow-up, transfer, and discharge evaluations.

c. AOTA is actively working to change federal legislation to have OT identified as an initial qualifying service for home health care, so barriers to OT home health services may be removed in the future.

4. OT in hospice care is provided to persons who are certified as terminally ill (medical prognosis of fewer than 6 months to live). OT services are provided to enable a patient to maintain functional skills and ADL performance and/or to control symptoms.

5. OT is covered as an outpatient service when provided by or under arrangements with any Medicare Certified provider (i.e., hospital, SNF, home health agency, rehabilitation agency, a clinic) or when provided as part of comprehensive rehabilitation facility services (CORF).

6. OT services can also be covered if provided by a Medicare certified OT in independent practice (OTIP) when services are provided by the OT in the OT's office or in the patient's home.

a. Payment is according to the fee schedule entitled the Resource Based Relative Value Scale (RBRVS).

7. Criteria for coverage of OT services rendered in a physician's office or in a physician-directed clinic.

a. The OTA or OT is employed by the physician or clinic.

b. The service is furnished under physician's direct supervision and the services are directly related to the condition for which the physician is treating the patient.

c. OT service fees are included on the physician's bill to Medicare.

8. Criteria for coverage of partial hospitalization services in a hospital-affiliated or community mental health psychiatric day program.

a. The beneficiary would otherwise have required inpatient psychiatric care.

b. OT services are covered under general Medicare guidelines (i.e., MD's prescription, reasonable and necessary, function expected to improve).

c. Active treatment incorporating an individualized multi-disciplinary intervention plan to attain measureable, time-limited, medically necessary, functional goals directly related to the reason for admission must be provided.

  (1) Psychosocial programs that provide structured diversional, social, and or recreational, services or vocational rehabilitation do not meet the criteria for active treatment in a PHP and are not reimbursable under Medicare.

9. All of the above standards can change when and if new federal legislative guidelines are passed for Medicare.

**E. Medicare Coverage of Durable Medical Equipment, Prostheses, and Orthoses**

1. Rental or purchase expenses for durable medical equipment (DME) are covered if used in beneficiary's home and if necessary and reasonable to treat an illness or injury or to improve functioning.

2. A physician's prescription is needed and must include diagnosis, prognosis, and reason for DME need.

3. Criteria for durable medical equipment.
   a. Repeated use can be withstood.
   b. Primarily and customarily used for a medical purpose (e.g., a wheelchair or walker).
   c. Generally not useful to a person in the absence of injury or illness.
4. Self help items, bathtub grab bars, and raised toilet seats are not reimbursable because other people can use them and they are not considered medically necessary.

F. **Medicaid**
1. General information.
   a. A state/federal health insurance program for persons who have an income that is below an established threshold and/or have a disability.
   b. States administer the program but receive at least 50% of their funding from the federal government.
   c. Includes federally mandated services and state optional services.
   d. Mandated services must be provided if a state receives federal funds.
2. Coverage of optional services varies greatly from state to state.
   (1) As a result, questions about state specific Medicaid coverage cannot be on the NBCOT examination.
3. Mandated Medicaid services.
   a. Inpatient and hospital services.
   b. Outpatient (e.g., laboratory work, x-rays, skilled nursing) and physicians' services.
   c. Home health (level and amount of care can vary).
   d. Early periodic screening diagnosis, and treatment services (EPSDT) for persons 21 years-old and younger.
   e. Services identified as needed to treat a condition during EPSDT (including OT) must be provided.
   f. SNFs receiving Medicaid must provide skilled rehabilitation services (including OT) to residents who require them.
4. Optional Medicaid services.
   a. Occupational therapy, physical therapy, speech language therapy.
   b. Durable medical equipment.
   c. Services provided by independently practicing licensed professionals including psychologists, psychiatric social workers, and other mental health professionals.
   d. Targeted case management.
   e. Prescription medication.
   f. Dental care, eyeglasses.
   g. Crisis response services.
   h. Transportation.
   i. Psychiatric inpatient services for persons aged under 21 or over 65.
   j. Related services (including OT) provided by school systems to children with disabilities. (Note: This provision overlaps IDEA legislation and has led to questioning as to whether services to individual children should be funded as an educational or a health care service.)
5. Medicaid reform.
   a. Due to rapidly rising costs there is an increased press for cost containment.
   b. States are examining ways to reformulate Medicaid benefits.
   c. Reform options may include placing caps or other limitations on types and length of therapy, reducing or eliminating optional benefits, and/or developing and implementing managed care approaches.
   d. Individual states can apply to the federal government for a waiver which gives the state flexibility in the types of services and delivery systems they provide under Medicaid.

G. **Worker's Compensation**
1. General information.
   a. Designed to compensate employees who have job-related illness or injuries.
   b. Funded jointly by individual employers or groups of employers and state governments.
   c. Each state has a workers' compensation commission board which determines regulations for employer participation, benefit provision, employee coverage, and insurance administration.
   d. Administration can be through contract with private insurance companies or through individual employers or groups of employers who administer their own programs. This is known as self-insuring.
   e. Coverage varies from state to state, with many states initiating cost-containment measures including limits on choice of providers, use of set fee schedules, utilization review, and managed care.
   f. Workers compensation programs include cash benefits and medical benefits. OT may be included.

g. Rehabilitation and disability management to return the person to gainful employment is a primary focus. See Chapter 14 for information on work evaluation and intervention.

### H. Personal Payment and "Pro Bono" Care

1. Individuals whose health insurance has discontinued coverage of OT services may elect to pay for these services personally, providing that benefit can be derived from continued services.
2. Individuals without health insurance or with no coverage for rehabilitative services may also pay for OT personally.
3. OT services provided in non-medical settings, (e.g., wellness and prevention programs) are generally not covered by insurers so their clients must private pay.
4. "Pro Bono" or free or reduced rate care may be supported by the individual practitioner's personal donation of services or through philanthropic donations.

### I. Documentation for Reimbursement

1. See Section F in the following section on documentation for guidelines for documenting effectively in order to receive payment for services.

## VIII. Occupational Therapy Documentation Guidelines

### A. Purpose of Documentation

1. Provides a legal, serial record of client's condition, evaluation and re-evaluation results, course of therapeutic intervention and response to intervention from referral to discharge.
2. Serves as an information resource for client care, can be used by a covering occupational therapist/OTA in absence of primary occupational therapist/OTA.
3. Enhances communication among healthcare or educational team members.
4. Provides data for use in intervention, program evaluation, research, education and reimbursement.

### B. OTA Documentation Guidelines

1. OTAs are qualified to write notes in medical charts.
2. AOTA does not require OTA notes to be cosigned by an occupational therapist, but state and federal governments may consider cosigning a tangible way to demonstrate compliance with laws and regulations governing OTAs.
3. Cosignature of OTA documentation by an occupational therapist is viewed as tangible evidence that supervision has been provided.
   a. Cosignature can also support that occupational therapist/OTA collaboration occurred.
4. AOTA does recommend OTA notes for inclusion in medical charts and Individualized Education Plans (IEPs) be cosigned by an occupational therapist, since these are official documents and are subject to subpoena.

### C. General Documentation Standards

1. Use legible handwriting.
   a. Illegible notes may result in denial of reimbursement.
2. Be correct in grammar and spelling.
   a. Errors detract from a professional presentation.
3. Be concise but complete.
   a. If it is not written down it does not exist and never happened.
   b. Non-important, extraneous details (i.e., color of clothing) should be left out.
4. Be objective, with clear distinctions between facts and behavioral data and opinions and interpretations.
5. Be current and accurate.
   a. Occupational therapy notes/records are legal documents.
6. Follow institution and/or program guidelines, as well as reimbursers'/third party payers' guidelines.
   a. Non-compliance can result in services and/or payment being denied.
7. Only use standard, well recognized abbreviations (i.e., ROM).
   a. Avoid alphabet soup.
   b. Write in functional terms using uniform terminology consistent with AOTA's Standards of Practice and state practice acts.
8. Use person first language at all times (e.g., "a mother with schizophrenia", or "the student with developmental delays", not "the schizophrenic", "the retarded").
9. Client's name and ID number should be on every page.
10. No whiting out or blocking out of information is accepted.
    a. Errors must be crossed out with one line, initialed, and dated. Black or blue ink is used at all times.
11. Include the date, including month, day and year.
12. Identify the type of documentation (i.e., initial note, progress note, discharge plan).

13. Comply with confidentiality standards (i.e., do not put other clients' names in a note).
14. Informed consent for treatment can only be given by a competent adult.
    a. Minors or adults determined to be incompetent must have written consent provided by a parent, legal guardian, person with power of attorney, or proxy.
15. Sign with a full signature (first and last name with professional designations) directly following content with no space left between content and signature.
16. Countersignature by an occupational therapist on documentation written by an OTA or a student if required by law or the facility.
17. All documentation may be subject to subpoena; therefore, documentation standards must be adhered to.

**D. Content of Documentation**
1. Identification and background information.
    a. Name, age, sex, date of admission, treatment diagnosis, and case number if one exists.
    b. Referral source, reason for referral, chief complaint relevant to OT's domain of concern.
    c. Pertinent history that indicates prior levels of function and support systems, including applicable developmental, educational, vocational, socioeconomic, and medical history. This can be brief.
    d. Secondary problems or preexisting conditions that may affect function or treatment outcomes.
    e. Precautions, risk factors and contraindications, medications, surgery dates.
2. Evaluation and reevaluation documentation.
    a. Assessments administered and the results.
    b. Summary and analysis of assessment findings in measurable, functional terms.
        (1) Sufficient baseline objective data.
        (2) In reevaluation, compare findings to initial findings.
            (a) Indicate change, if any.
    c. References to other pertinent reports and information including relevant psychological, social, and environmental data.
    d. Occupational therapy problem list, specific and sufficient to develop intervention plan.
    e. Recommendations for occupational therapy services (can include recommendation that no OT services are indicated).
    f. Client's understanding of current status and problems, his or her subjective complaints.
    g. Client's interest and desire to participate in therapy.
3. Intervention plan documentation.
    a. A prioritized problem list.
    b. Goals related to problem list and indicating potential for function and improvement.
    c. The structure of a goal statement.
        (1) The person who will exhibit the skill, almost always written as "the patient/client will". However, the caregiver, family member, and/or teacher may be the focus of the goal.
        (2) The desired functional behavior that is to be demonstrated or increased as the outcome of intervention.
        (3) The underlying factors (e.g., performance skill deficits, client factors) that must be remediated to achieve functional outcome.
        (4) The circumstances under which the behavior must be performed or the conditions necessary for the behavior (e.g., independent, with cueing, with assistance).
        (5) The degree at which the behavior is exhibited (e.g., 3 out of 4 times, minimum number of repetitions).
    d. Short and long term goals written in a SMART manner.
        (1) Specific. For example, not "increase self-care skills"; rather, "develop ability to button shirt using non-dominant hand."
        (2) Measurable, as to number of times or a percent.
        (3) Attainable, as to what can be realistically achieved. For example, one hundred percent return is unlikely.
        (4) Relevant, to roles and expected environment.
        (5) Time-limited, anticipated time to achieve goals.
            (a) Time allotted for goal attainment must be relevant to setting's LOS (e.g., in acute care, goals are measured in days whereas in long term care, weekly or monthly goals are acceptable).
    e. Long term goals must indicate the final desired functional outcome before discharge, regardless of LOS.
        (1) A clear reason for skilled therapeutic intervention.

(2) Statement of potential functional outcome that is clearly related to goal.

f. Activities and/or treatment procedures and methods related to stated goals and problems.

g. Type, amount, frequency of treatment needed to accomplish goals (how many times/week/day? how long are sessions?).

h. Explanation of treatment plan to client and a provision of statement of goals in client's words.

4. Intervention implementation documentation.

a. Activities, procedures, and modalities used.

b. Client's response to treatment and the progress toward goal attainment as related to problem list.

c. Goal modification when indicated by the response to treatment. Rationale for changes in goals needed.

d. Change in anticipated time to achieve goals with rationale for change and new time frame specified.

e. Attendance and participation with treatment plan (attendance can be a check format).

f. Statement of reason for individual missing treatment.

g. Assistive/adaptive equipment, orthoses, and prostheses if issued or fabricated, and specific instructions for the application and/or use of the item, including wearing schedule and care.

h. Patient-related conferences and communication with physicians, third party payers, case manager, team members, etc.

i. Home programs developed and taught to client and/or caregiver(s).

j. Client's and/or caregiver's compliance with home program.

5. Discharge plan documentation.

a. Summary of evaluation and intervention.

b. Compare initial and discharge status.

c. Specify number of sessions, goals achieved, and functional outcome.

d. Reason for discharge.

(1) Goals attained.

(2) Client no longer making functional gains.

(3) Client refuses or is noncompliant with intervention.

(4) Client moves to another location.

(5) Setting not appropriate to individual's needs.

e. Home programs to be followed after discharge.

f. Client and family education.

g. Equipment provided and/or ordered.

h. Follow-up plans/recommendations with rationales.

i. Referral(s) to other health care providers and community agencies.

E. **Specific Documentation Formats**

1. Problem Oriented Medical Record (POMR): a system of providing structure for progress note writing that is based on a list of problems based on assessment.

a. SOAP notes.

(1) Subjective: information reported by the client, family, or significant other.

(2) Objective: diagnosis, medical information and history, and measurable, observable data obtained through formal assessments.

(3) Assessment: therapist's interpretation and clinical reasoning based on objective data includes analysis of client's status and goals and a prioritized problem list.

(4) Plan: the therapist's specific plan of intervention to resolve identified problems and meet stated goals.

2. Consultation reports: meetings and/or phone conversations with team members, other professionals, the individual, and his/her caregivers.

3. Critical incident reports: significant, out of the norm events that may occur during OT evaluation or intervention (e.g., the individual slips during a transfer).

4. All of the above must comply with general documentation standards and contain all fundamental components of documentation.

F. **Documentation for Reimbursement**

1. Coding and billing for services.

a. To be reimbursed, OT services must be properly coded and billed, as required by reimbursers.

b. Practitioners must represent their services in terms of diagnosis and procedure codes.

c. Diagnosis codes describe person's condition or medical reason for requiring services.

d. Procedure codes describe the specific services provided by health care professionals.

(1) Codes are updated annually. Due to these annual updates, the NBCOT examination would not include specific codes.

e. Specific billing forms are used by institutional providers (i.e., hospitals and home health agencies) and by physicians and OT practitioners in independent practice for Medicare, Medicaid, and most states' workers' compensation programs. Form numbers may change, so NBCOT should not ask questions about specific forms.

f. OTAs are generally not eligible for direct payment because they require supervision and do not practice independently.

2. Documentation "red flags".

a. The use of certain words, terms, and/or physician's errors can result in delay, denial, and/or discharge from services.

b. Avoid these in all documentation, unless they are true and accurate representations of a client's status.

c. If a client has met his/her goals and/or is no longer making significant functional gains, this must be documented and the client must be discharged from services.

d. Words to avoid, for they do not reflect progress.

(1) Chronic.

(2) Status quo, no change in status.

(3) Maintaining.

(4) Little change.

(5) Plateau.

(6) Making slow progress.

(7) Stable or stabilizing.

e. Words to avoid, for they do not reflect potential for improvement.

(1) Same as.

(2) Uncooperative, noncompliant.

(3) Dislikes therapy.

(4) Confused/disoriented.

(5) Inability to follow directions.

(6) Patient refused to participate.

(7) Custodial care needed.

(8) Treatment repeated.

(9) Repeated instruction.

(10) Unmotivated.

(11) Extreme depression.

(12) Fair to poor potential.

(13) Chronic/long-term condition.

(14) General weakness.

## G. Documentation for Medicare Reimbursement

1. Overview.

a. Many private reimbursers and state Medicaid programs follow federal Medicare guidelines, so if documentation meets Medicare standards it will generally be acceptable to other insurers.

b. It is advisable to get copies of state and individual insurers' guidelines for OT services, as adherence to these guidelines will be critical for reimbursement. Due to the potential wide variance in these guidelines, the NBCOT examination should not test information beyond the established federal Medicare guidelines.

c. Previously stated standards and guidelines for documentation apply to reimbursement for Medicare.

2. Intervention documentation.

a. Content must indicate that the treatment shows a level of complexity and sophistication, or the condition of the patient must be of a nature that requires the judgment, knowledge, and skills of a qualified practitioner. This statement is as per Medicare.

b. Skilled rehabilitation intervention is mandatory.

(1) Delineate the specific skilled care rendered. This is the biggest cause for retroactive denial.

(2) Notes must show therapeutic intervention. Example: dressing itself does not indicate therapeutic concerns. Decreasing extensor tone to accomplish dressing meets these criteria.

c. Skilled care rendered must match the diagnosis and the physician's order.

d. Services must be unique to OT and not sound like PT or SLP. Medicare does not pay for duplication of services.

e. In home care, homebound status due to functional limitations must be clearly delineated.

(1) If the diagnosis may not render the individual homebound, explain why this particular person is homebound.

(2) Do not give a reviewer any doubt that this person does not meet Medicare homebound criteria (e.g., do not state client not at home when you arrive. Rather state there was no answer to a locked door.)

f. Document honestly, but not over optimistically. Medicare reviewers are interested in determining the need for continued intervention.

(1) Write the note in such a way that the patient has remaining limitations and needs further care instead of the patient improving rapidly.

(2) Provide behavioral observations that substantiate need for further care.

g. Practical improvement is noted with functional change.

(1) If improvements are not made, the client should be discharged in a timely fashion.

(2) If there is a reason for the lack of progress, it should be noted.

h. Documentation must also demonstrate that the patient is making significant functional improvement in a reasonable and generally predictable period of time.

(1) Some improvement must be made at least on a weekly basis; otherwise treatment will be considered maintenance.

(2) If progress is slower than expected, document extenuating circumstances and/or limiting factors (e.g., a secondary diagnosis).

(3) Medicare does not reimburse for maintenance treatment.

(4) Payment for designing a maintenance program and making periodic but infrequent evaluations of the program's effectiveness is provided.

i. The service must be reasonable and necessary.

(1) Was the service effective and completed in a timely fashion?

(2) In long term care, if the treatment does not lessen the amount of care needed by staff, what made the service worthwhile?

# IX. Federal Legislation Related to Occupational Therapy

## A. Overview

1. Historically, the opportunities available to and the roles afforded to persons with disabilities have been influenced by federal legislation.

2. Federal laws establish numerous standards and provide funding for health benefits, medical services, rehabilitation, early intervention, education, vocational programming, professional training, and research.

3. These laws directly affect the profession of occupational therapy by establishing practice guidelines and reimbursement standards.

4. Major social movements that have precipitated federal legislation and/or have resulted from federal legislation include deinstitutionalization, early intervention, mainstreaming, and full inclusion.

5. State laws also influence OT practice but, due to their variability, would not be included in a national examination.

6. To ensure best practice, OTAs have an ethical responsibility to know federal and state laws and regulations.

## B. Health Insurance and Portability Accountability Act (HIPAA)

1. Sets standards and safeguards to assure the individual's right to continuity in healthcare coverage and to ensure privacy and security of health care records.

2. All persons must be informed of the setting's privacy policies and a good faith effort must be made to obtain written acknowledgement from each person about his/her attainment of this knowledge.

a. If the person refuses to sign, the provider should document the efforts made; failure to obtain written acknowledgement is not a violation of the rule.

b. Written consent must be obtained from a person before any personal health information is used or disclosed in the provision of treatment, obtainment of payment, or the carrying out of any healthcare related operations.

(1) Exemptions to the written notification/acknowledgement are allowed if the attainment of this will prevent or delay timely care (i.e., emergency care). Written acknowledgement must be obtained as soon as possible.

(2) If language barriers preclude signed acknowledgement, treatment can occur if the physician believes consent is implied.

3. Prior to discussing a person's status with a family member/significant other or other provider, the provider must obtain the person's permission or give the person the opportunity to object.

a. Providers can use their clinical judgment to determine whether to discuss the person's case with others if the person cannot give permission or objects.

(1) Documentation for this decision is essential (e.g., person is at risk of harming self due to lack of judgment; consultation with a specialist is essential to ensure quality of care).

b. All information used or disclosed about a person's status must be limited to the minimum needed for the immediate purpose.

4. The HIPAA Privacy Rule requires that all providers protect patient confidentiality in all forms (i.e., oral, written, and electronic) and implement appropriate physical, technical, and administrative safeguards to assure this privacy.

a. Settings must reduce the physical identifiability of patient information; i.e., door tags and white boards can only list last names, no diagnoses or treatment procedures may be listed, sign-in sheets with names only are allowed.

b. Charts and any documentation with patients' names or other identifiers must be stored out of public view and in secure locations.

c. Opaque covers should be used for clipboards that contain paperwork with patient information.

d. All computers that are used to record, document, or transmit patient information should be equipped with monitor privacy screens.

e. All faxes must contain cover sheets noting confidentiality of accompanying information and be sent only to dedicated fax machines in secure locations.

f. All e-mails must use password protection and encryption if going over the Internet.

g. All faxes and computer printouts must be immediately destroyed or placed in the person's chart, as most appropriate.

h. All conversations regarding a person's health status must be done in private areas, in low tones, and with minimal disclosure.

5. An individual has the right to access all of his/her records.

a. Providers can charge reasonable copying costs and have 30-60 days to respond.

b. Individuals have the right to request that information in their record be amended.

(1) The provider can refuse the request, providing his/her rationale.

(2) The provider can comply with the request by documenting the request and the reason for compliance. The original documentation should not be removed/excised.

6. HIPAA does not exclude treatment from occurring in group settings or open clinics.

a. Discussion regarding treatment should be done quietly and, if possible, behind a screen/room divider.

7. HIPAA does not require a guarantee of 100% confidentiality; it does require reasonable and vigilant safeguards.

8. HIPAA guidelines for research are complex but they are congruent with the established guidelines for human subject research and Institutional Review Board (IRB) standards.

a. A "limited data set" that does not include any identifiable patient information can be used in research without patient approval (e.g., diagnosis, age, length of stay).

9. The Administrative Simplification rules also provide standardization of codes and formats for medical data.

10. HIPAA does not override state laws that further restrict privacy and it defers to state laws governing minors.

C. **Key Legislation Related to Overall Disability Rights**

1. Medicare Title 18-PL 89-97.

a. Established Medicare and Supplemental Security Income (SSI).

b. SSI enables persons with disabilities to receive a monthly income enabling them to live in the community. This was a major contributor to the deinstitutionalization movement.

2. Rehabilitation Act of 1973.

a. Prohibits discrimination on the basis of disability in any program or activity that receives federal assistance.

b. Required all federal agencies to develop action plans for the hiring, placement, and advancement of persons with disabilities.

c. Required contractors who received federal contracts over a pre-set amount to take affirmative action to employ persons with disabilities.

3. Fair Housing Act.

a. Prohibits discrimination on the bases of disability, religion, sex, color, race, national origin, and familial status.

b. Required owners of housing to make reasonable exceptions to their standard tenant policies to allow individuals with disabilities equal housing opportunities (e.g., allowing a seeing eye or service dog in a "no-pets" apartment).

c. Required that tenants with disabilities be allowed to make reasonable modifications to common use areas and to their private living space to enable access.

(1) The housing owner is not required to fund these modifications.

e. Required that newly constructed multifamily residences (4 or more apartments) be built to meet established accessibility standards.

4. Omnibus Budget Reconciliation Act (OBRA) (PL 97-35).

a. Affirmed application of Section 504 of the

Rehabilitation Act of 1973, which prohibits discrimination in federally funded programs to a diversity of services (i.e., Head Start programs, block grant programs, community development programs).

b. Provided Medicaid financing for community-based services for people with developmental disabilities when services were demonstrated to be less expensive than institutional care. This, combined with the availability of SSI, resulted in a tremendous growth in community residential programs and an emptying of institutions for persons with developmental disabilities.

5. Americans with Disabilities Act (ADA).

a. Prohibits discrimination against qualified persons with disabilities in employment, transportation, accommodations, telecommunications, and public services.

b. Criteria for classifying an individual as disabled.

(1) A person with a physical or mental impairment that substantially limits one or more major life activities.

(2) A person having a record of such an impairment.

(3) A person regarded as having such an impairment.

c. Individuals who are actively abusing substances or compulsively gambling or persons who have kleptomania, pyromania, or sexual behavior disorders are not protected by ADA.

d. Title I - Employment

(1) Prohibits employers from discriminating against persons with disabilities in any aspect or phase of employment including recruitment, hiring, working conditions, hours, promotion, training opportunities, termination, social activities, and other privileges of employment.

(2) Allows questions about one's ability to perform a job but prohibits inquiries as to whether one has a disability.

(3) Prohibits employment tests that tend to screen out people with disabilities.

(4) A "qualified individual with a disability" means a person with a disability who is able to perform the "essential functions" of a job (that is, the tasks fundamental to the position) with or without reasonable accommodations.

(5) "Reasonable accommodations" must be provided by businesses with 15 or more employees to persons with disabilities to enable them to perform essential job functions unless such accommodations would impose an "undue" hardship on the business.

(a) Types of reasonable accommodations.
- Acquisition or modification of equipment or devices.
- Modifications or adjustments to examinations, training materials, or publications.
- Provision of ancillary aids or services.
- Modified or part time work schedules, job restructuring, or reassignment to a vacant position.
- Improvement of existing facilities used by employee so they are usable by and accessible to persons with disabilities and/or other similar accommodations.

(b) Types of auxiliary aids and services.
- Taped texts, qualified readers, or other methods that can effectively make visually delivered materials accessible to persons with visual impairments.
- Qualified interpreters or other methods that can effectively make aurally delivered materials accessible to persons with hearing impairments.
- Modification or acquisition of devices or equipment.
- Similar actions or services that increase accessibility.

(c) Undue hardship is defined as action that would be significantly difficult or overly expensive given the financial resources of the employer, its size, and major functions.

(6) The United States Government, Indian Tribes, and/or private tax-exempt membership clubs are exempt from ADA employer guidelines.

e. Title II Public Services.

(1) Mandates that state and local governments and their departments, agencies, and/or component parts may not discriminate

against, exclude, or deny persons with disabilities participation in or benefit from the services, programs, or activities of these public entities.

  (a) This includes transportation, public education, employment, recreation, social services, health care, courts, town meetings, and voting.

f. Title III Public Accommodations and Services operated by Public Entities.

  (1) Mandates that places of public accommodation (i.e., hospitals, health care providers' offices, schools, day care centers, and other places of accommodation) may not discriminate against persons with disabilities with respect to their participation in or ability to benefit from the service, goods, facility, use, or other programming aspects.

  (2) All new construction of public accommodations must be accessible.

  (3) Public transportation systems must be accessible.

  (4) Physical barriers in existing facilities must be removed if removal is able to be carried out without much difficulty or expense.

  (5) Private services that serve the public (e.g., restaurants, stores, and theaters) cannot discriminate in the provision of services.

  (6) Private transportation systems must be accessible and non-discriminatory (e.g., livery services, taxis, tour bus companies).

g. Title IV Telecommunications

  (1) All televisions manufactured after 1993 must include closed captioning.

  (2) Telephone companies must provide telecommunications relay services (TRS) to persons with hearing or speech impairments 24 hours per day, 7 days per week.

6. Ticket to Work and Work Incentives Improvement Act (TWIIA).

  a. Strives to make it more realistic and easier for a person with a disability to work.

  b. Removes a major disincentive to work by allowing individuals with disabilities to maintain their Medicare or Medicaid health care benefits.

    (1) Allows an individual with a disability to keep Medicare benefits for an additional 54 months after starting work.

    (2) Eliminates limits on Medicaid "buy in" options.

  c. Enables consumers to have a choice in their service provider beyond public assistance programs.

  d. Establishes community-based vocational planning and assistance programs.

  e. Increases consumer choices for accessing employment support services.

  f. All states can design their own program.

7. Work Investment Act (WIA).

  a. Established a federally sponsored national employment and vocational training system entitled "America's Workforce Network" and local boards entitled "Local Workforce Investment Boards (LWIBs)".

  b. Established a "One-Stop" delivery system for all adults aged 18 or older seeking access to employment and training services. This means traditionally separate "unemployment" offices and "vocational rehabilitation services" are now available at a "One-Stop Center".

    (1) Availability of all employment and training services at a One Stop Center is aimed to allow for "universal access" for person with disabilities - a core principle of WIA.

    (2) Categories of One-Stop services.

      (a) Core services, which include outreach, intake and orientation; initial assessment; eligibility determination for services; assistance with job search and placement; job market information and career counseling.

      (b) Intensive services for individuals who do not attain successful employment after receipt of core services. Services can include comprehensive assessments of service needs and skill level, development of individualized plans for employment, case management, and counseling.

      (c) Training services for individuals who do not attain successful employment after receipt of core and intensive services. These services are typically provided off-site from the One-Stop Center and can include adult education and literacy training, on-the-job training, and individualized vocational training.

(3) The One Stop system of services is provided through a network in each state. The names of these systems can vary from state to state.

c. Persons determined to be eligible for WIA services receive an Individual Training Account (ITA) which is used to obtain services from any approved provider. Specific ITA procedures can vary from state to state.

d. Services for youth (aged 14-21) with disabilities are also provided for in the WIA to assist in a successful transition from school to work.

## D. Select Legislation Specific to Technology

1. Technology Related Assistance for Individuals with Disabilities Act.
   a. Funded the development of technology and technologic aids for persons with disabilities to improve communication, mobility, self-care, transportation, and education.
2. Telecommunications Act of 1996.
   a. Required providers of telecommunications systems and manufacturers of telecommunications equipment to make services and equipment useable by and accessible to individuals with disabilities, if at all possible.
   b. Examples of services and equipment covered by this act are cell phones, pagers, call waiting, caller ID, and operator assistance.
3. Title IV Telecommunications of the ADA. See Section C.5.g.

## E. Legislation Specific to Pediatric Practice

1. Child Abuse Prevention and Treatment Act.
   a. Defines child abuse and neglect as mental or physical injury, negligent treatment, maltreatment, or sexual abuse of a child less than 18 years of age by a person responsible for the child's welfare under circumstances that indicate that a child's welfare or health is being threatened or harmed.
   b. Mandates for professionals to report abuse and neglect to law enforcement officials were established.
   c. OT practitioners were included in this list of mandated reporters.
   d. OTAs and occupational therapists can also serve as child welfare advocates.
   e. Direct OT intervention may be needed to remediate the emotional or physical disorders that result from abuse.
2. Early Intervention and Education Acts.

a. Multiple acts have provided the foundation for current early intervention and education services. These include:
   (1) Mandates for free and appropriate education (FAPE) for all children regardless of ability or disability, (aged 3-21) in the least restrictive environment.
       (a) Mainstreaming (i.e., integrating children with disabilities into classrooms) was the means to ensure education is provided in the least restrictive environment
   (2) Requirements that public schools provide OT to special education students if OT is needed for the student to benefit from the special education.
   (3) The designation of occupational therapy as a primary early intervention service.
   (4) Funding for family support services and programs to train professionals in early intervention.
   (5) Recommendations for states to develop infant and toddler programs (birth to 3 years).
       (a) Programs are voluntary and vary from state to state but all states participate to some degree.
       (b) OT is considered a primary developmental service.

3. Reauthorization and Amendment of Individuals with Disabilities Education Act (IDEA)
   a. Emphasizes that the purpose of the Individualized Education Plan (IEP) is to address the child's unique needs as related to his/her disability and decide how these needs can be served so the child has full access to the general education curriculum and can participate in the general education classroom.
   b. Clarifies that the individual education plan (IEP) can include consideration of assistive technology and behavioral interventions, strategies, and supports (an area in which OT can offer a great deal).
   c. States that IEP planning team is open to related personnel at the request of the parent or school, in addition to the regular education teacher, if the student is in a regular education class.
   d. States that the education the student receives should prepare him/her for independent living and employment in adult life.

(1) Transitional planning begins at the age of 14 (or younger if indicated) to help the student plan a course of study that will lead to post-school goals.

(2) Transition services begin at the age of 16 (or younger if indicated) to provide student with a coordinated set of services to attain post-school goals.

    (a) These services can include community experience, specific instruction, and/or ADL and vocational assessment and intervention.

(3) The student must be invited to attend IEP meetings that discuss his/her transition planning and services to allow for self-advocacy and self determination.

(4) This transition plan must be updated annually with appropriate service revision provided.

e. Maintains the established definition of related services (including OT).

f. Expands orientation and mobility services by broadly interpreting them to include all children with disabilities.

g. Students with disabilities may be punished in the same manner as other students for serious offenses (i.e., carrying illicit drugs or a weapon). However, disciplinary prevention measures are stressed.

h. Educational and related services still must be received by the child even if he/she is removed to an alternative placement.

i. Clarifies early intervention services and systems.

(1) Mandates an Individual Family Service Plan (IFSP) for children 0-2 years of age.

(2) OT is identified as a primary early intervention service.

4. Individuals with Disabilities Education Improvement Act (IDEA 2004).

a. Directly addresses the student's functional performance along with academic performance.

(1) Requires that evaluations for IDEA eligibility include relevant functional and developmental information, not just academic achievement data.

(2) Expands the IEP's annual goals to include academic and functional goals.

(3) Specifies that accommodations must be provided as needed to measure the functional performance and academic achievement of all students with disabilities.

b. Provides for the piloting of a multi-year (not to exceed 3 years) IEP to allow for long-term planning and to coincide with a child's 'natural' transitions (e.g., pre-school to elementary school, middle school to high school).

(1) Plan is optional for parents.

c. Provides for increased flexibility in IEP meetings.

(1) Allows IEP team members to be excused from IEP meetings if their area of concern is not being addressed or modified at the meeting or if a written report is submitted prior to the meeting.

    (a) District and parental approval for a team member's absence is required.

    (b) Parental approval must be in writing.

(2) Allows IEP revisions and/or amendments to be made by parents and districts after an annual IEP meeting.

    (a) Parents must be provided with a written copy of the revised/amended IEP.

(3) Allows the use of technological alternatives to face-to-face IEP meetings (i.e., video-conferences conference calls).

d. Requires that recommendations for early intervention, special education, related, and supplementary services and aids be made based on peer-reviewed research to the extent that this is practical.

(1) This requirement raises concern that established intervention methods may be questioned due to a real or perceived lack of evidence supporting their efficacy.

(2) This requirement may spur research on early intervention and school-based OT to support evidence-based practice.

e. Clarifies that a screening done by a specialist is not equivalent to an evaluation for eligibility for IDEA services.

(1) OT practitioners can conduct informal classroom-based screenings and provide consultations for classroom modifications and other teaching strategies without completing a formal evaluation according to IDEA procedures.

f. Requires that all students with disabilities be assessed in compliance with the No Child Left Behind Act.

(1) The IEP team determines if the student should take an alternative assessment or the standard assessment with or without accommodations.

g. Provides for early coordinated intervening services for general education students from kindergarten through 12th grade who do not require special education services but who do need additional supports to succeed in school.

h. Clarifies that the purpose of the IDEA is to prepare children with disabilities for further education, employment, and independent living.

i. Allows school personnel to individually consider each case of a student with a disability who violates the school's code of conduct.

   (1) Students with disabilities who are disciplined must:
      (a) Be provided with services to continue to progress towards achieving their IEP goals.
      (b) Receive appropriate functional behavioral assessments and interventions and service modifications as needed to address their conduct violation(s).

j. Allows each state to define developmental delay criteria to determine if an infant or toddler is eligible for early intervention in that state.

   (1) Typically, states define developmental delays quantitatively (e.g. a percentage of delay according to a standardized developmental assessment).

k. Requires that an IFSP be completed to include:
   (1) The infant's or toddler's developmental level.
   (2) Family priorities, concerns, and resources,
   (3) The infant's or toddler's natural environments
   (4) Measureable outcomes.
   (5) Projected, length, frequency and duration of research-based services.
   (6) Transition plans to pre-school or other services, as appropriate.

l. Clarifies the role of the parent and IFSP team in determining the site for service provision.
   (1) Requires states to maximize the provision of early intervention services in the infant's or toddler's natural environments, as appropriate.

m. Requires states to establish procedures for the referral of infants and toddlers who are victims of abuse and/or neglect to early intervention services.
   (1) This provision was also included in the Keeping Children and Families Safe Act.

5. No Child Left Behind Act (NCLB).
   a. A general education law which emphasizes standards-based education.
   b. Considers occupational therapists to be pupil services personnel and sets no requirements for OT services.
   c. Requires schools to provide accommodations, if needed by students, for mandated tests.
      (1) OT practitioners can recommend testing alternatives and/or classroom accommodations.

F. **Legislation Specific to Gerontic Practice**
   1. Age Discrimination in Employment Act.
      a. Prohibits employment practices that discriminate or unfairly affect workers 40 years and older.
      b. Prohibits mandatory retirement of older workers. Employers cannot fix a retirement age.
   2. Freedom to Work Act.
      a. Amended the Social Security Act to enable Americans receiving retirement Social Security (SS) benefits (currently 65 years old) to be able to work without affecting their SS income.
         (1) There are no income restrictions in this amendment.
   3. Omnibus Budget Reconciliation Act (OBRA) of 1990.
      a. Applied to all nursing homes that receive federal money for Medicare or Medicaid patients.
      b. Emphasized attending to resident rights, autonomy, and self determination; providing quality of care; and enhancing quality of life within nursing homes.
      c. Mandated a comprehensive resident assessment system, the Minimal Data Set (MDS), which is administered upon admission and thereafter on an annual basis, unless there is a significant change in the resident's condition.
         (1) MDS is coordinated by an RN. OTs can contribute information.
      d. Psychosocial wellbeing and activity pursuit patterns must be considered along with the resident's physical condition and cognitive abilities.
         (1) This has broadened OT's role in nursing

homes.

e. Mandated that the evaluation and treatment of conditions found during the MDS follow specific guidelines called the Resident Assessment Protocols (RAPS).

   (1) The structured approach to assessment is called the Resident Assessment Instrument (RAI).

   (2) Individualized care plans must be established within specific time frames.

f. The enhancement of quality of life through restraint reduction and the provision of restraint-free environments are strongly emphasized.

   (1) Nursing homes must show evidence of consultation by an OT or PT for consideration of interventions that are less restrictive than restraints.

   (2) OT practitioners are frequently consulted for ADL treatment, seating adaptations, positioning ideas, environmental modifications, psychosocial interventions, and activity programming.

g. Aims to guarantee that residents have the right to choose how they want to receive care and live their lives.

   (1) Residents should have a choice in determining their ADL, including community activities.

   (2) Residents should be able to function as independently as possible.

h. Post discharge plans must meet specific criteria including client or caregiver education.

# X. Service Delivery Models and Practice Settings

## A. Overview

1. A working knowledge of service delivery models and practice settings ensures that OT practitioners make educated decisions about their employment and competent referrals for their clients.

2. As a result of legislative initiatives and health care system changes, service delivery models and practice settings are evolving from medical-based models and settings to more community-based models and settings, (e.g., IDEA has solidified schools as a practice setting).

3. Implications for OT practice.

   a. Fewer practitioners are working in hospitals and long term care facilities.

   b. More practitioners are working in community based settings (e.g., day treatment, home care, school settings).

## B. Models of Practice

1. Criteria for determining a model of practice.

   a. The type of setting.

   b. Philosophy and mission of the particular setting and department.

   c. The role the practitioner plays as a team member within that particular setting.

2. Medical model.

   a. Views the individual with a disability as a person who has incurred a physiological insult that has resulted in reduced functional capacity.

   b. Focus is placed on identifying the disease or dysfunction.

   c. Treatment addresses the disease or dysfunction (performance skills) contributing to decreased functional skills.

   d. OT frames of reference address the pathological process of the disease or dysfunctions (e.g., biomechanical, neurodevelopmental).

3. Education model.

   a. Views the individual with a disability as lacking knowledge or skills.

   b. Focus is placed on learning and making the behavioral changes needed to interact successfully in the environment.

   c. An individual's skill deficits are determined, and related goals are established, to promote learning to adequately perform within a particular environment.

   d. Behaviors are measured in terms of obtaining skills, knowledge, and competency to successfully meet the demands of the environment.

   e. OT frames of reference are based on learning theories to facilitate adaptation in the environment (e.g., role acquisition, cognitive remediation).

4. Community model.

   a. Views the individual with a disability as lacking skills, resources, and supports for community integration.

   b. Focus is placed on identifying and developing the skills needed for one's expected environment.

   c. If skills cannot be developed, community resources and supports are identified and developed to enable functioning within one's chosen environment.

d. OT frames of reference promote development of performance skills and/or areas of occupation within the individual's performance contexts (e.g., life-style performance, occupation adaptation).

**C. Institutional Practice Settings**

1. Acute care hospitals.
   a. Admission is for a medical or psychiatric diagnosis that cannot be treated on an outpatient basis.
      (1) Initial onset of a new illness or major health problem.
      (2) Acute exacerbation of a chronic illness.
      (3) In psychiatry, a person may be involuntarily admitted to an acute unit if he/she is considered to be a danger to self or others, or as having a grave disability.
   b. Length of stay (LOS) is determined by diagnosis and presenting symptoms.
      (1) LOS can be limited to 1-7 days.
      (2) Longer LOS requires significant documentation to justify need for further hospitalization.
      (3) Ongoing need for care frequently results in discharge to another setting.
   c. OT evaluation process focuses on quick and accurate screening of major difficulties impeding function (e.g., cognitive status, home safety skills).
   d. OT intervention focus.
      (1) Stabilization of client's status.
      (2) Engagement of the client in the therapeutic relationship and purposeful activities/ meaningful occupations so that he/she can see that change is possible, thereby increasing motivation to pursue follow-up.
      (3) Discharge planning and after-care referrals.
      (4) Family, caregiver, and consumer education.
   e. The role of an acute care OT practitioner can be a generalist or a specialist (e.g., neonatology, burns).
      (1) Specialized practice roles require advanced knowledge and skills and therefore would not be evaluated on the NBCOT examination.

2. Sub-acute care/intermediate care facilities (ICFs).
   a. Admission is for a medical or psychiatric diagnosis that has progressed from an acute stage but has not stabilized sufficiently to be treated on an outpatient basis.
   b. Length of stay (LOS) is determined by diagnosis and presenting symptoms.
      (1) LOS can range from 5-30 days.
      (2) Longer LOS requires significant documentation to justify need for further hospitalization.
      (3) Ongoing need for intervention or long-term care frequently results in discharge to another setting.
   c. OT evaluation can include more in-depth assessments and more thorough observations of client's functional performance.
   d. OT intervention focus.
      (1) Functional improvements in performance components and performance areas.
      (2) Active engagement of the client in the treatment planning, implementation, and re-evaluation process.
      (3) Discharge planning to expected environment.
   f. Sub-acute care and ICFs can be housed in hospitals or skilled nursing facilities (SNFs).

3. Long-term acute care hospital (LTAC).
   a. Admission is for chronic or catastrophic illnesses or disabilities that require extensive medical care and/or dependency on life support or ventilators.
      (1) Patients often have multiple diagnoses with major complications.
   b. The average length of stay is greater than 25 days to maintain Medicare certification.
   c. OT evaluation and intervention is often limited by the population's severe and complex medical needs.
      (1) For all clients, evaluation and intervention is concerned with palliative care and the prevention and treatment of complications (e.g., positioning to prevent decubiti and contractures).
      (2) For individuals who are cognitively intact, the focus of evaluation and intervention is mastery of the environment and the attainment of client-centered goals.

4. Rehabilitation hospitals.
   a. Admission is for a disability that is medically stable but which has residual functional deficits requiring skilled rehabilitation services.
   b. Length of stay (LOS) is determined by presenting deficits and rehabilitation potential.
      (1) LOS can range from a week to months.

(2) Documentation requirements supporting the need for an extended LOS are dependent upon institutional, state, and third party payer guidelines.

(3) LOS ends when coverage is expended. The client is then discharged to the appropriate environment.

(a) A skilled nursing facility.

(b) A supportive community residence.

(c) Home/independent living.

c. OT evaluation can be extensive and focus on all areas of occupation, performance skills, and occupational roles that will be required in the expected environment.

(1) Environmental assessments of planned discharge environment must be completed.

d. OT intervention focus.

(1) Functional improvement in performance areas, performance skills, and occupational roles.

(2) Development of compensatory strategies for residual deficits.

(3) Provision of adaptive equipment and training in use of the equipment to promote independent function.

(4) Modification of the discharge environment, as needed, to enhance function.

(5) Education of the individual, family, and caregivers on abilities, limitations, compensatory techniques, and advocacy skills.

5. Long-term hospitals.

a. Admission is for a medical or psychiatric diagnosis that is chronic with the presence of symptoms that cannot be treated on an outpatient basis.

b. Length of stay (LOS) is determined by diagnosis and presenting symptoms.

(1) LOS can range from a month to years.

(2) Documentation requirements supporting need for increased LOS are dependent upon institutional, third-party payer, and/or state guidelines.

(3) LOS in private long-term hospitals is determined by insurance coverage. When coverage is expended, an alternative discharge environment is needed for the client.

(a) A state run long-term hospital.

(b) A skilled nursing facility.

(c) Home or supportive residence.

c. OT evaluation can be extensive due to increased LOS.

d. OT intervention focus.

(1) Functional improvements in performance skills and performance areas.

(2) Development of compensatory strategies for residual deficits.

(3) Maintenance of quality of life.

(4) Development of skills for discharge to the least restrictive environment.

6. Skilled nursing facilities (SNFs)/Extended care facilities (ECFs).

a. Admission is for a medical or psychiatric diagnosis that is chronic and requires skilled care, but the individual's illness is stable with no acute symptoms.

b. Due to managed care constraints on acute hospital stays, many individuals are being admitted to SNFs for medical care and rehabilitation.

c. Length of stay (LOS) can range from 1 month to the individual's lifetime. Several factors influence LOS.

(1) The progression of the illness.

(2) Availability of family or community supports.

(3) Insurance coverage.

d. OT evaluation and intervention is guided by Medicare standards.

(1) For individuals with rehabilitation potential, the focus of evaluation and intervention is the same as identified under Rehabilitation Hospitals.

(2) For individuals without rehabilitation potential, evaluation and intervention is more concerned with palliative care and the maintenance of quality of life.

7. Forensic settings.

a. Admission is due to engagement in criminal activity by a person. The person can be remanded to a variety of settings depending on the nature of the crime and if he/she has a psychiatric diagnosis.

(1) Jail: a city or county facility which is the individual's first entry into the criminal justice system and the placement for those convicted of crimes with sentences of less than a year.

(2) Prison: a state or federal facility for individuals found guilty of crimes with sentences greater than a year.

(3) Forensic psychiatric hospital or unit: a spe-

cialized hospital or unit within a hospital which provides inpatient psychiatric care for individuals convicted of a crime and found guilty but mentally ill or not guilty by reason of insanity.

b. Length of stay is determined by court-ordered directives and criminal sentences.

c. The availability and quality of services varies greatly from none in most jails to extensive in some forensic hospitals.

d. Due to serious gaps in mental health services, the incarceration rate of persons with mental illness has increased significantly (e.g., a homeless person with schizophrenia steals food due to hunger).

e. OT evaluation and intervention focus.
   (1) Determination of individual's competency to stand trial, in forensic psychiatry settings.
   (2) Areas similar to those described under Rehabilitation Hospitals to develop community living skills needed for successful community reintegration upon release.
   (3) Facilitation of skills and provision of structured programs to enable the person to function at his/her highest level within their current environment since discharge may be delayed or not possible, depending on the nature of the crime.
   (4) Restoration of competency to stand trial in forensic psychiatry settings.

8. Outpatient/ambulatory care.
   a. An individual who does not require hospitalization but has functional deficits requiring evaluation and intervention may receive OT services on an outpatient basis in private clinics, medical offices, and/or hospital satellite centers.
   b. Focus of outpatient care is diagnostic evaluations, interventions to increase functional performance, consumer education, and prevention.

**D. Community-Based Practice Settings**

1. Early intervention programs.
   a. Acceptance criteria for an early intervention evaluation are based on "at risk" status of the infant/child.
      (1) Birth complications.
      (2) Suspected delays in development.
      (3) Failure to thrive.
      (4) Maternal substance abuse during pregnancy.
      (5) Birth to an adolescent/teen mother.
      (6) Established disability/diagnosis.
   b. Acceptance criteria for early intervention services are based on the following criteria.
      (1) The extent of the delay (typically a 33% delay in one area of development or a 25% delay in two areas).
      (2) An established diagnosis/disability.
   c. Length of service provision.
      (1) If the infant/child qualifies for services, an infant family service plan is completed by the service coordinator after a review of all assessments and in collaboration with the family and early intervention team.
      (2) Six month reviews are submitted by all professionals to determine if services should continue.
   d. Occupational therapy evaluation.
      (1) Assessment of five developmental areas.
         (a) Cognitive.
         (b) Physical.
         (c) Communication.
         (d) Social-emotional.
         (e) Adaptive.
      (2) Determination of the effects of performance skills on the areas of occupation of play and self care.
      (3) Evaluations need to be written in a strength-oriented manner.
      (4) Functional goals must be written in family friendly terms and include levels of functioning, unique needs, and recommended services.
   e. Occupational therapy intervention process.
      (1) Development of cognitive, psychosocial, and sensorimotor components.
      (2) Development of play, self-care, and developmental skills.
      (3) Provision of family education.
      (4) Provision of advocacy and advocacy training.
      (5) Transition planning from early intervention to preschool is essential.

2. Schools.
   a. Acceptance criteria for OT services as a related service in an educational setting.
      (1) The child requires special education services, and OT will enable the child to benefit from special education.
      (2) OT will facilitate the child's participation in educational activities.

(3) Referrals are received from the previous agency that provided early intervention services, the child's teacher, and/or school's child study team.

(4) The school reviews the referral and, if indicated, recommends an OT evaluation.

    (a) If an OT evaluation has already been completed, the need for OT intervention services is discussed.

    (b) The frequency, length of sessions, and duration of the intervention are also determined.

b. Length of services is dependent upon the impact of OT services on the child's abilities and prevention of loss of abilities.

(1) If OT services can improve the child's ability to participate in education-related activities and allow full access to the general education curriculum, services can be continued.

(2) A review of services and progress made towards the child's individualized education plan (IEP) is conducted annually.

c. OT evaluation.

(1) Assess client factors, performance skills and patterns and areas of occupation that impact on the educational performance of the child within the school.

    (a) Findings are used to contribute to the IEP, in which goals and objectives are formulated to address the overall educational needs of the student.

(2) Assess the child's functional and developmental level to contribute to the Functional Behavioral Analysis.

d. OT intervention focus.

(1) Based on an educational model versus a medical model.

(2) Addresses the student's functional performance along with academic performance.

(3) Activities are utilized to address the goals and objectives documented in the IEP using both corrective and compensatory methods.

(4) Assistive technology and transition services, in accordance with the regulations of IDEA, are provided.

(5) Client factors and performance skill deficits (i.e., sensorimotor, cognitive, and psychosocial) are treated to improve the child's ability to participate in and perform education-related activities within a school setting.

(6) Skills in the occupational performance areas of ADL, school, and play are developed to improve the child's ability to participate in and perform education-related activities within a school setting.

(7) Skills for adult life post-school are developed in accordance with the student's transition plan.

e. The OT practitioner needs to know the school district's and state's funding sources, and regulations and interpretations of the federal laws regarding education (see this chapter's section on legislation).

f. The role of OT practitioners in school-based practice has expanded beyond IDEA related services to include programs that address students' psychosocial needs and prevent school violence.

(1) Behavioral Intervention Plans which include Response to Intervention (RtI), Early Intervening Services (EIS), and Positive Behavioral Supports (PBS) may be a component of school-based OT service provision

    (a) Response to Intervention (RtI) is an evidence-based, structured intervention approach that uses Early Intervening Services (EIS) to address academic difficulties and Positive Behavioral Supports (PBS) to address behavioral problems early in a child's education.

3. Supported education programs.

a. Participant criteria include adolescents or adults who require intervention to develop skills that are needed to succeed in secondary and/or post-secondary education.

(1) The person may have never developed these skills or lost them due to a psychiatric disability or mental health problems.

b. Length of stay is determined by agency's funding and person's attainment of goals.

(1) Discharge is upon entry into, or completion of, an educational program or the attainment of a graduate equivalency degree (GED).

c. OT evaluation is focused on the individual's client factors, performance skills and patterns that impact on the occupational role of student.

d. OT intervention focus.

(1) Improvement in performance skills and patterns that are needed for the occupational role of student (e.g., time management and task prioritization)

(2) Education and training in compensatory strategies to support academic performance (e.g., studying in a quiet room).

(3) Exploration of participant's educational interests and aptitudes to ensure self-determined engagement in a school, college, technical training program, or community-based adult-education class(es).

4. Prevocational programs.

a. Participant criteria include adolescents or adults who require intervention to develop skills that are prerequisite to work.

(1) The person may have never developed these skills due to developmental delays, environmental insufficiencies, illness, or disability.

(2) Person may have lost these skills due to illness or disability.

b. Length of stay is determined by agency's funding and person's attainment of goals.

(1) Discharge is usually to a vocational program.

(2) Discharge to a work setting can occur if sufficient abilities are developed.

c. OT evaluation is focused on the individual's task skills, social interaction skills, work habits, interests, and aptitudes.

d. OT intervention focus.

(1) Improvement in task skills and social skills that are prerequisite to vocational training or work.

(2) Development of work habits and abilities.

(3) Exploration of work interests and aptitudes to ensure discharge to a relevant vocational training program, school, or work setting.

5. Vocational programs.

a. Acceptance is for development of specific vocational skills.

(1) Person has the prerequisite abilities to work (e.g., good task skills and work habits) but requires training for a specific job and/or ongoing structure, support and/or supervision to maintain employment.

(2) Person has to develop his/her work capaci-

ties to a level acceptable for competitive employment (e.g., strength and endurance).

b. Length of stay is determined by agency's funding and attainment of goals.

(1) In vocational rehabilitation workshops (formerly called sheltered workshops) and supportive employment programs, discharge is not always a goal. Maintenance of the person in these specific work environments can be the desired objective for some individuals while others will be discharged to other programs or to work.

(2) Transitional employment programs (TEPs) are generally time limited (3-6 months) with discharge to competitive employment, supportive employment, or rehabilitation workshops.

(3) Employee Assistance Programs (EAPs) provide ongoing support, intervention, and referrals as needed to a company's employees to enable these individuals to maintain this employment.

c. OT evaluation is focused on the individual's functional skills and deficits related to work in his/her current and expected vocational environment.

d. OT intervention focus.

(1) Remediation of underlying performance component deficits that affect the work performance area.

(2) Development of general work abilities and specific job skills.

(3) Consultation to and/or supervision of vocational direct care staff.

(4) Identification and implementation of reasonable accommodations in accordance with ADA.

(5) Referral to state offices of vocational and educational services for persons with disabilities for further evaluation, education and training. (According to the TWIIA, these offices are entitled "One Stop Centers").

6. Residential programs.

a. Admission is for a developmental, medical or psychiatric condition that has resulted in functional deficits that impede independent living but are not severe enough to require hospitalization.

(1) Residential programs are on a continuum from 24 hour supervised quarterway houses,

halfway houses, or group homes, to supportive apartments with weekly or biweekly "check-in" supervision.

    (2) The degree of functional impairment determines the residential level of care needed.

b. Length of stay for transitional living programs (e.g., quarterway and halfway house programs) is determined by agency's funding. Long-term and permanent housing options (i.e., group homes and supportive apartments) are available and are funded through the individual's social service benefits.

c. OT evaluation is focused on assessment of the individual's skills for living in the community and determination of the social and environmental resources and supports needed to maintain the individual in his/her current and expected living environment.

d. OT intervention focus.

    (1) Consultation to and/or supervision of residential program staff.

    (2) Remediation of underlying client factors and performance skill deficits that affect independent living skills.

    (3) ADL training, activity adaptation, and environmental modifications to facilitate community living skills.

    (4) Referral to appropriate residential services along the continuum of care as individual's functional level improves.

    (5) Education about ADA, the Fair Housing Act, and Section 8 Housing.

7. Partial hospitalization/day hospital programs.

a. Admission is for a medical or psychiatric condition that has been sufficiently stabilized to enable an individual to be discharged home or to a community residence (e.g., a halfway house or supported apartment); however, the individual still has symptoms remaining which require active treatment.

b. Treatment is up to 5 days per week with multiple interventions scheduled each day.

c. Length of stay (LOS) is determined by diagnosis, presenting symptoms, and response to treatment.

    (1) LOS can vary from 1 week to 6 months.

    (2) Documentation requirements supporting the need for an extended LOS are dependent upon institutional, state, and/or third party payer guidelines.

    (3) Once LOS is expended, discharge is usually to a less intensive community day program and/or clubhouse.

d. OT evaluation is focused on the individual's functional skills and deficits in his/her performance areas and the occupational roles that are required in his/her current and expected environment(s).

e. OT intervention focus.

    (1) Functional improvement in performance areas and occupational role functioning.

    (2) Remediation of underlying performance skill deficits that affect functional performance.

    (3) Development of skills for community living and identification of community supports for community integration.

8. Clubhouse programs.

a. Membership is open to adults and elders with a current mental illness or a history of mental illness.

    (1) All members have equal access to all clubhouse functions and opportunities regardless of functional level or diagnosis.

    (2) Individuals who pose a significant and direct threat to the safety of the clubhouse community are the only persons excluded.

b. Services are provided by staff and members with the responsibilities of operating the clubhouse shared equally by staff and members under the oversight of a director.

    (1) Due to this role equality, it can be difficult to distinguish between members and paid staff.

    (2) Staff's main role is to engage membership and provide needed support and structure.

c. Individual schedules will vary to meet each person's unique needs and interests.

    (1) Clubhouses are typically open at least 5 days per week. Many are open 7 days per week.

    (2) The daily schedule is organized around the "work-ordered" day, which parallels typical working hours to engage members and staff in the running of the clubhouse.

    (3) Evening and weekend schedules are focused on avocational interests and recreational pursuits.

    (4) Additional services that can be provided include literacy and education programs, transitional employment placements, inde-

pendent employment assistance, community support and outreach services, housing programs, and legal and financial advisement.

d. Length of stay is indefinite and members can exit and re-enter a clubhouse community at will.

e. OT evaluation and intervention are not provided in a formalized manner.

   (1) The role of the OT is integrated into the clubhouse model which has staff acting as generalists who contribute to the development and enrichment of members' abilities and the attainment of recovery.

9. Adult day care.

a. Admission is for adults and elders with chronic physical and/or psychosocial impairments, and/or for individuals who are frail but semi-independent.

b. Services are provided in a congregate or group setting.

c. Individual schedules will vary.

   (1) Flexibility in scheduling is provided to address daily caregiver needs and allow for planned respite.

   (2) Schedules can range from one afternoon per week to 5 full days.

d. Length of stay is indefinite.

   (1) Ongoing services are provided to individuals with chronic conditions who might otherwise be institutionalized or to individuals who are frail and need ongoing support (e.g., cooked meals, socialization opportunities).

e. OT evaluation is focused on the individual's client factors, functional skills and deficits in the performance areas, his/her home environment, and the adult day center's environment.

f. OT intervention focus.

   (1) Maintenance of the healthy, functional aspects of the individual and facilitation of adaptation to impairments.

   (2) Engagement in purposeful activities that provide appropriate stimulation, reflect lifelong interests, develop new interests, and foster a sense of community with other participants.

   (3) Caregiver education, support groups, home visits, consultations, and referrals to community resources.

   (4) Modifications to the day care center's environment and the individual's home envi-

ronment to maximize the person's comfort in, and mastery and control of, these environments.

10. Outpatient/ambulatory care.

a. Admission is for a medical or psychiatric condition that is not serious enough to warrant hospitalization or for a condition that has sufficiently stabilized to enable the individual to be discharged from a hospital but remaining symptoms require active treatment.

b. Treatment is usually provided in short 30-60 minute sessions once a day for up to 5 days a week.

c. Length of stay is determined by diagnosis, presenting symptoms, response to treatment, and insurance coverage or ability to pay a fee for service.

d. OT evaluation focused on the individual's functional assets and deficits in his/her performance skills, his/her areas of occupation, and his/her home, work, leisure, and social participation environments.

e. OT intervention focus.

   (1) Active engagement of the client in the treatment planning, implementation, re-evaluation, and discharge process.

   (2) Remediation of underlying performance skill deficits that affect functional performance.

   (3) Functional improvements in occupational performance areas and occupational roles.

   (4) Compensatory strategies for remaining deficits.

   (5) Consumer, family, and caregiver education.

11. Home health care.

a. Acceptance criteria for home health services.

   (1) Presence of a medical or psychiatric condition that is not serious enough to warrant hospitalization or for a condition that has sufficiently stabilized to enable the individual to be discharged from a hospital but that still has remaining symptoms requiring active treatment.

   (2) Reimbursers can have strict and variable criteria for qualifying for home health care. See earlier section on Medicare and third-party reimbursers.

b. Treatment is usually provided in 60 minute sessions, once a day for up to 5 days a week, as determined by insurance coverage.

c. Length of stay is determined by diagnosis, pre-senting symptoms, response to treatment, insurance coverage, or ability to pay a fee for service.

d. OT evaluation is focused on the individual's functional assets and deficits in his/her perform-ance skills, his/her areas of occupation, and the occupational roles that are required in the per-son's current and expected environment(s).

e. OT intervention focus.

(1) Active engagement of the client, family, and caregivers in the treatment planning, implementation, and re-evaluation process.

(2) Functional improvement in areas of occu-pation and occupational role functioning within the home.

(3) Remediation of underlying performance skill deficits that affect functional perform-ance within the home.

(4) Education of the family, caregivers, and/or home health aides to provide appropriate care and/or assistance as needed.

(5) Environmental modifications and activity adaptations that maintain optimal function-ing and improve quality of life.

(6) Increasing ability to resume occupational roles outside of the home.

(7) Prevention of hospitalization and avoid-ance or delay of residential institutional placement.

12. Hospice.

a. Acceptance criteria for hospice services.

(1) Terminal illness that has a life expectancy of 6 months or less.

b. Services are most often provided in the home with the type and quantity of services deter-mined by the needs of the individual, his/her family, significant others, and caregivers.

(1) Hospice services may also be provided in an independent facility or in a special unit of a SNF or a hospital.

c. Length of stay is determined by the person's terminal outcome.

d. OT evaluation is focused on determining the individual's occupational functioning and his/her physical, psychosocial, spiritual, and environmental needs that are most important to him/her.

e. OT intervention focus.

(1) Maintenance of the individual's control over his/her life.

(2) Facilitation of engagement in meaningful occupations and purposeful activities that are consistent with the individual's roles, values, choices, interests, aspirations, abili-ties, and hopes and that contribute to a sat-isfactory quality of life.

(3) Reduction or removal of distressing symp-toms and pain.

(4) Environmental modifications and activity adaptations that maintain optimal function-ing and improve quality of life.

(5) Caregiver and family education and sup-port to maintain optimal functioning and improve quality of life for all.

13. Case management programs.

a. There are two different focuses to case man-agement programs: one is clinical, one is administrative.

(1) Clinical case management provides indi-vidualized support and intervention to a client with a serious illness which signifi-cantly limits his/her ability to access and/or engage in existing community services and/or therapeutic programs, ensuring that the person is able to remain in the commu-nity and not be re-hospitalized.

(2) Administrative case management connects a person with a serious illness to the appropri-ate and needed community services and/or therapeutic programs, overseeing this serv-ice provision to ensure that quality of care in a cost-effective manner is achieved.

b. Services can be provided in an office and/or in the individual's home and community.

c. Length of stay is determined by the individ-ual's ability to independently access needed services and by funding availability.

d. OT evaluation is focused on the individual's functional assets and deficits in his/her perform-ance skills, areas of occupation, and the occupa-tional roles that are required in his/her current expected environment.

(1) Assessment of the individual's supports and barriers for community integration is critical.

e. Case management interventions can be purely referral-based in the administrative model or encompass the full range of interventions in the clinical model, (e.g., one-on-one counseling, family education, ADL training, community re-entry, etc.).

    (1) Both models aim to prevent regression and re-hospitalization and promote optimal functioning and quality of life.

    (2) Both models actively engage the individual and family in treatment planning, implementation, and the reevaluation process.

    (3) Both models plan discharge, if appropriate, to an environment that will best serve an individual's needs.

14. Wellness and prevention programs.
    a. Acceptance is most often by individual's self-referral to meet a personal need or by an institution's provision of a program to its members or employees (e.g., a parenting skills class for pregnant teens in a school).
    b. Programs have been developed to serve populations considered at risk and are held in offices or individual's residences and/or at community sites.
    c. Length of stay is determined by the individual. It is usually influenced by program's planned length (e.g., a six-week joint protection program) or by individual's achievement of a desired outcome (e.g., smoking cessation).
    d. OT evaluation focuses on risk factors for illnesses and disabilities and the individual's functional skills and deficits in the occupational roles that are required in his/her current and expected environment.
    e. OT intervention focus.
        (1) Disease prevention and health promotion.
        (2) Interventions can range from the traditional domain of OT (e.g., home safety and environmental modifications), to contemporary areas of concern (e.g., stress management, life coaching).
        (3) Refer to Chapter 3 for definitions of and specific interventions for primary, secondary, and tertiary prevention.

### E. Private/Independent Practice

1. In any and all of the above community and institutional settings, the OT practitioner can work in an entrepreneurial manner by negotiating a fee for service agreement and/or a long term contract.
2. OTAs in private independent practice must receive supervision from an occupational therapist and abide by all state and federal regulations for OT practice.

## XI. Service Management

### A. Management Principles, Functions, and Strategies

1. Management that has a positive attitude about change and innovation fosters best practice.
2. Successful management supports open communication, team building, decentralization of resources, and the sharing of power.
3. Management that utilizes strategic thinking in a systems model can respond proactively to market demands and changes.
4. The use of different management styles (i.e., the manager's characteristic way of performing management tasks) has a significant impact on productivity, change and growth. See text's section on leadership styles in Chapter 3.
5. Management's understanding and application of theories of motivation and behavior facilitates appropriate and effective responses to situations, fosters program efficacy, and promotes employee satisfaction.
6. Administrative functions of management include program development, fiscal and personnel management, and program evaluation. See separate sections for specifics on each major function.

### B. Program Development

1. Purposes of developing specific programs.
    a. To directly meet the needs of a specific population(s) or group(s).
    b. To clearly focus evaluation and intervention efforts and activities.
    c. To increase visibility and use of available services (e.g., offering an outpatient cardiac rehabilitation program is more visible than individual referrals, resulting in increased recognition and utilization of this service).
    d. To convert an idea into a practice reality.
2. Role of the OTA.
    a. Collaborate with occupational therapist to assess needs, develop program plan, and implement evaluation program.
    b. Perform specific tasks with OT supervision.
    c. If employed as an activities director, an OTA may be primarily responsible for all program development steps.
3. Four basic steps of program development.
    a. Needs assessment.
        (1) Describe the community; its physical, social, cultural and economic factors; and populations at risk.

(2) Describe the target population's demographics, disorder(s), functional level(s), and presenting problem(s).

(3) Identify specific needs of target population.

(4) Establish unmet needs according to priority.

(5) Identify resources available for program implementation.

   (a) Formal or institutional resources such as staff, supplies, money, space.

   (b) Informal resources such as family, friends, cultural or religious figures, self-help/consumer groups.

(6) Needs assessment methods.

   (a) Survey, interview, or self report of target population. A representative sample is required.

   (b) Key informant, which involves the surveying of specific individuals who are knowledgeable about the target population needs.

   (c) Community forums to obtain information through public meetings or panels.

   (d) Service utilization review of records and reports.

   (e) Analysis of social indicators to identify social, cultural, environmental, and/or economic factors that can predict problems.

b. Program planning.

(1) Define a focus for the program based on the needs assessment results.

   (a) Problem areas, functional limitations, and unmet needs that are relevant to the majority of the target population are the priority focus.

   (b) Program level of difficulty as determined by the range of population's functional levels and the level required by the current and expected environment.

(2) Adopt a frame or frames of reference that are most likely to successfully address and meet the needs that are program's focus.

(3) Establish objectives and goals of the program specifically related to primary focus.

   (a) Individual goals which will be met by the program are set.

   (b) Programmatic goals which establish standards for program evaluation are determined.

(4) Describe integration of program into existing system of care.

   (a) Establish realistic timetable for program implementation.

   (b) Define staff roles, responsibilities, and assignments.

   (c) Identify methods for professional collaboration.

   (d) Determine the physical setting and space requirements.

   (e) Consider potential barriers to program implementation.

   (f) Develop methods to effectively deal with identified obstacles before program implementation.

(5) Develop a system of referral for entry into, completion of, and discharge from the program.

   (a) Evaluation protocols to standardize information to be obtained from each person referred to the program and to assess the type of program services needed.

   (b) Criteria for acceptance into the program and for movement through program levels.

   (c) Discharge criteria to determine when an individual has achieved maximum gain from the program, usually defined as the achievement of program goals.

(6) Describe the fiscal implications of program plan.

   (a) Determine projected volume or service demand to estimate revenue.

   (b) Identify resource utilization and projected expenses to estimate costs.

   (c) Directly compare estimated revenue and estimated expenses to determine financial viability of program.

c. Program implementation.

(1) Initiate program according to timetable and steps set forth in the program plan.

(2) Document program activities, procedures, and use.

(3) Communicate and coordinate with other programs within the system.

(4) Promote program to ensure it reaches target population.

d. Program evaluation. See this chapter's section on program evaluation and quality improvement.

## C. Personnel Management

1.  The oversight of OT practitioners and support personnel and the services they provide.
2.  Role of the OTA.
    a.  Collaborate with the OT and perform specific management tasks as delegated by an occupational therapist and with OT supervision.
    b.  If employed as an activities director, an OTA may be primarily responsible for all aspects of personnel management for the activities department.
3.  Purposes of personnel management.
    a.  To serve as the link between the individuals working for an organization and the larger organizational structure.
    b.  To attain best practice from personnel.
4.  Major personnel management tasks.
    a.  Design work roles and write job descriptions.
    b.  Recruit, select, and orient personnel to perform the roles.
    c.  Supervise and evaluate personnel to ensure adequate role performance and the attainment of organizational goals.
    d.  Support personnel's ongoing professional development.
    e.  Deal with difficult personnel issues as they arise.

## D. Program Evaluation and Quality Improvement

1.  The systematic review and analysis of care provided to determine if this care is at an acceptable level of quality.
2.  Role of the OTA
    a.  Collaborate with the occupational therapist and contribute to the process by performing specific tasks with OT supervision (e.g., the collection of outcome data).
    b.  An OTA may assume primary responsibility for this process if an OTA is directly responsible for program outcome (e.g., as the director of an activities program in a SNF).
3.  Purposes of program evaluation.
    a.  To measure the effectiveness of a program; that is, were program goals accomplished?
    b.  To use information obtained in the evaluation to improve services and assure quality.
    c.  To meet external accreditation standards (see this chapter's section on voluntary accreditation).
    d.  To identify program problems/limitations and to resolve them.
4.  Major types and terms.
    a.  Continuous quality improvement (CQI): a sys-

tem-oriented approach that views limitations and problems proactively as opportunities to increase quality.
    (1)  Prevention is emphasized.
    (2)  Blame is not attributed to persons; problems are related to organizational improvement needs.
    b.  Total quality management (TQM): the creation of an organizational culture that enables all employees to contribute to an environment of continuous improvement to meet or exceed consumer needs.
    c.  Performance assessment and improvement (PAI): a systematic method to evaluate the appropriateness and quality of services.
    (1)  Utilization of an interdisciplinary systems focus.
    (2)  A client-centered approach which focuses on the rights, assessment, care, and education of the person.
    (3)  Organizational ethics, improved organizational performance, leadership and management are emphasized.
    d.  Utilization review: a plan to review the use of resources within a facility.
    (1)  Determination of medical necessity and cost efficiency.
    (2)  Often a component of a CQI or PAI system.
    e.  Statistical utilization review: reimbursement claims data are analyzed to determine the most efficient and cost-effective care.
    f.  Peer review: a system in which the quality of work of a group of health professionals is reviewed by their peers.
    g.  Professional review organization (PRO): groups of peers who evaluate the appropriateness of services and quality of care under reimbursement and/or state licensure requirements.
    h.  Prospective review.
    (1)  Evaluation of proposed intervention plan that specifies how and why care will be provided.
    (2)  Used by third party payers to approve proposed occupational therapy intervention program.
    i.  Concurrent review.
    (1)  Evaluation of ongoing intervention program during hospitalization, outpatient, or home care treatment.
    (2)  Method to ensure appropriate care is being

delivered.

(3) Often a component of a CQI or PAI system.

j. Retrospective review.

(1) Audits of medical records after intervention were rendered.

(2) Method to ensure appropriate care was given.

(3) A UR tool for third party payers that can be time consuming and costly.

k. Risk management: a process that identifies, evaluates, and takes corrective action against risk and plans, organizes and controls the activities and resources of OT services to decrease actual or potential losses.

(1) Potential risks are client or employee injury and property loss or damage with resulting liability and financial loss.

(2) OT practitioners are responsible to ensure proper maintenance of equipment and a safe treatment environment.

(3) Staff education and training (e.g., annual certification/recertification in CPR) is required.

(4) Effective communication with consumers (e.g., informed consent) and with team members is required.

(5) Risk management is an integral part of program evaluation.

(6) If risk management fails and an incident occurs, completion of an incident report according to setting's standards is required.

**E. Fieldwork Education**

1. A key service management function is to develop, implement, and support clinical fieldwork education for OTA and OT students.

a. ACOTE guidelines for Level I and Level II fieldwork education are to be followed.

b. Supervisory qualifications and guidelines for fieldwork educators are provided in this chapter's section on OT practitioner roles and supervision.

2. Fieldwork education managerial tasks.

a. Collaboration with the academic education program to develop specific fieldwork learning objectives and activities consistent with facility's and school's philosophies and missions.

b. Development of professional development plans and activities for the students' clinical supervisors to ensure adequate fieldwork supervision.

c. Establishment of departmental policies and procedures for a student program and its supervision.

d. Assurance of quality care provided by student(s) according to established program standards and professional ethics.

e. Evaluation and supervision of students' performance and completion of ACOTE's evaluation tool.

f. Completion of cost-benefit analysis to collect data for institutional support of clinical education.

---

# References

Alexander, T.C. (October 20, 2003). Capital briefing: Members want to know. *OT Practice, 7.*

American Dietetic Association. (2005). *Scope of dietetics practice framework.* Chicago: American Dietetic Association.

American Occupational Therapy Association. (2007). Enforcement procedures for occupational therapy code of ethics (edited 2007). *American Journal of Occupational Therapy, 61,* 679-685.

American Occupational Therapy Association. (2006). *The new IDEA: Summary of the Individuals with Disabilities Education Improvement Act of 2004* (P.L. 108-446). Bethesda, MD: Author.

American Occupational Therapy Association. (2006). *Reference manual of the official documents of the American Occupational Therapy Association* (11th ed.). Bethesda, MD: Author.

American Occupational Therapy Association. (2005). Occupational therapy code of ethics. *American Journal of Occupational Therapy, 59,* 639-642.

American Occupational Therapy Association. (2005). Enforcement procedures for occupational therapy code of ethics. *American Journal of Occupational Therapy, 59,* 643-652.

American Occupational Therapy Association. (2005). Standards of practice for occupational therapy. *American Journal of Occupational Therapy, 59,* 663-665.

American Occupational Therapy Association. (2004). Guidelines for supervision, roles, and responsibilities. *American Journal of Occupational Therapy, 58,* 663-667.

Case-Smith, J. (Ed.). (2005). *Occupational therapy for children* (5th ed.). St. Louis, MO: Elsevier Mosby.

Centers for Medicare and Medicaid Services (CMS). (2009). *Medicaid benefit policy manual.* Washington DC: Author.

Chandler, B. (2008, January 21). School System Special Interest Section. *OT Practice, 25.*

Clark, G. (2008). The infants and toddlers with disabilities program (Part C of IDEA). *OT Practice, 131*(1), CE-1 – CE-8.

Clifton, D. (2004, December). Workers' Comp: A plethora of opportunities. *Rehab Management, 32,* 34-36.

Department of Training, *Training manual* (2001). Department of Health and Human Services, Trenton New Jersey.

Diffendal, J. (2001, April 30). Coming out of retirement: Do working retirees need your services? *OT Advance, 33,* 36.

Grossman, J., & Bortone, J. (2000). Program development. In R.P. Cottrell (Ed.), *Proactive approaches in psychosocial occupational therapy.* (pp 39-45) Thorofare, NJ: Slack..

Hopkins, H. & Smith, H. (Eds.). (2003). *Willard and Spackman's occupational therapy* (10th ed.). Philadelphia: J.B. Lippincott.

Hussey, S.; Sabonis-Chafee, B.; & O'Brien, J. (2007). *Introduction to occupational therapy,* (3rd ed.). St. Louis, MO: Elsevier Mosby.

International Center for Clubhouse Development. (1994). *Standards for clubhouse programs.* New York, Author.

Jacobs, K. (2000). Innovation to action: Marketing occupational therapy. In R.P. Cottrell (Ed.), *Proactive approaches in psychosocial occupational therapy.* (pp 505-507) Thorofare, NJ: Slack.

Jacobs, K., & Logigan, M.K. (1999). *Functions of a manager in occupational therapy.* Thorofare, NJ: Slack.

Job Accommodation Network (2009). *Accommodation and compliance series: The ADA Amendments Act of 2008.* Morgantown, WV: Author.

Johnson, K.V. (2000, September). Home health PPS: The new payment system. *OT Practice.* CE1-CE8.

Kornblau, B. & Starling, S. (2000). *Ethics in rehabilitation.* Thorofare, NJ: Slack.

Kyler, P. (Ed.). (2005). *Reference guide to the occupational therapy code of ethics.* Bethesda, MD: American Occupational Therapy Association.

Leary, D., & Mardirossian, J. (2000, Sept. 11) Ethical knowledge = collaborative power. *OT Practice,* 19-22.

McCormack, G.; Jaffe, E.; Goodman-Lavey, M. (Eds.). (2003). *The occupational therapy manager,* (4th ed.). Bethesda, MD: American Occupational Therapy Association.

Medcom. (2003). HIPAA: *A guide for health care workers.* Cypress, CA: Author.

Moyers, P. & Dale, L. (2007). *The guide to occupational therapy practice.* Bethesda, MD: American Occupational Therapy Association.

Murer. C. (2007, October). Psychiatric partial hospitalization: An overview. *Rehabilitation Management,* 48 -49.

National Board for Certification of Occupational Therapy. (2008). *NBCOT 2008 candidate handbook.* Gaithersburg, MD: Author.

National Board for Certification in Occupational Therapy (NBCOT). (2008). *Qualifications and compliance review information.* Gaithersburg, MD: Author

National Board for Certification in Occupational Therapy. (NBCOT). (2007, Fall/Winter). *Report to the profession.* Gaithersburg, MD: Author.

National Council on Disability and National Urban League. (2000). A *guide to disability rights laws.* Washington, DC: Author.

Opp, A. (2007, September 27). Reauthorizing No Child Left Behind: Opportunities for OT. *OT Practice,* 9-13.

*Patient and elder abuse* (2001). Tennessee Bureau of Investigation, "Tennessee Anytime", Available: www.tbi.state.tn.us/PATIENTABUSE

Scaffa, M. (2001). *Occupational therapy in community-based practice settings.* Philadelphia, PA: F.A. Davis.

Schindler, V.P. (2000). Occupational therapy in forensic psychiatry. In R.P. Cottrell (Ed.), *Proactive approaches in psychosocial occupational therapy* (pp 319-325). Thorofare, NJ: Slack.

Sladyk, K., & Ryan. S. E. (2001) *Ryan's occupational therapy assistant: Principles, Practice issues and techniques.* (3rd ed.). Thorofare, NJ: Slack.

Vance, K., McGuire, M. J., & Nanof, T. (2009). Medicare coverage of occupational therapy in the home and community. *OT Practice, 14*(13), CE-1 –CE-8.

Wilmarth, C. (2009, November 9). Using aides to provide therapy. *OT Practice,* 8.

# CHAPTER 5

# HUMAN DEVELOPMENT AND AGING: PEDIATRIC AND GERIATRIC PRACTICE CONSIDERATIONS FOR OT PRACTICE

Marge E. Moffett Boyd • Jan G. Garbarini • Linda Kahn D'Angelo • Susan B. O'Sullivan

## I. Development

### A. Definition

1. Sequential changes in the function of the individual.
   a. Qualitative or quantitative.
   b. Influenced by biologic determinants and biopsychosocial environmental experiences.

## II. Sensorimotor Development

### A. Fetal Sensorimotor Development

1. Gestational age: age of the fetus or newborn, in weeks, from first day of mother's last normal menstrual period.
   a. Normal gestational period 38-42 weeks.
   b. Gestational period divided into three trimesters.
2. Conceptual age: age of a fetus or newborn in weeks since conception.

### B. Development of Sensorimotor Integration

1. Prenatal period.
   a. Responds first to tactile stimuli.
   b. Reflex development.
   c. Innate tactile, proprioceptive, and vestibular reactions.
2. Neonatal period.
   a. Tactile, proprioceptive and vestibular input are critical from birth onward for the eventual development of body scheme.
   b. Vestibular system, although fully developed at birth, continues to be refined and impacts on the infant's arousal level.
      (1) Helps the infant to feel more organized and content.
   c. Visual system develops as infant responds to human faces and items of high contrast placed approximately 10 inches from face.
   d. Auditory system is immature at birth and develops as the infant orients to voices and other sounds.
3. First six months.
   a. Vestibular, proprioceptive, and visual systems become more integrated and lay the foundation for postural control, which facilitates a steady visual field.
   b. Tactile and proprioceptive systems continue to be refined, laying the foundation for development of somatosensory skills.
   c. Visual and tactile systems become more integrated as the child reaches out and grasps objects, laying the foundation for eye-hand coordination.
   d. Infant movement patterns progress from reflexive to voluntary and goal-directed.
4. Six to twelve months.
   a. Vestibular, visual, and somatosensory responses increase in quantity and quality as the infant becomes more mobile.

b. Tactile and proprioceptive perception becomes more refined, allowing for development of fine motor and motor planning skills.

c. Tactile and proprioceptive responses also lead to midline skills and eventual crossing of midline.

d. Auditory, tactile, and proprioceptive perception is heightened allowing for development of sounds for the purpose of communication.

e. Tactile, proprioceptive, gustatory, and olfactory perception is integrated, allowing for primitive self-feeding.

5. Thirteen to twenty-four months.

a. Tactile perception becomes more precise allowing for discrimination and localization to further refine fine motor skills.

b. Further integration of all systems promotes complexity of motor planning as the child expands his/her repertoire of movement patterns.

c. Symbolic gesturing and vocalization promotes ideation, indicating the ability to conceptualize.

d. Motor planning abilities contribute to self concept as the child begins to master the environment.

6. Two to three years.

a. This is a period of refinement as the vestibular, proprioceptive, and visual systems further develop, leading to improved balance and postural control.

b. Further development of tactile discrimination and localization lead to improved fine motor skills.

c. Motor planning and praxis ideation also progress during this period.

7. Three to seven years.

a. Child is driven to challenge his/her sensorimotor competencies through roughhouse play, playground activities, games, sports, music, dancing, arts and crafts, household chores, and school tasks.

(1) These provide opportunities to promote social development and self-esteem.

## C. Reflex Development and Integration

1. Predictable motor response elicited by tactile, proprioceptive, or vestibular stimulation.

2. Primitive reflexes are present at or just after birth and typically integrate throughout the first year.

3. The persistence or reemergence of these primitive reflexes are indicative of central nervous system (CNS) dysfunction that may interfere with motor milestone attainment, patterns of movement, musculoskeletal alignment, and function.

4. Refer to Table 5-1 for reflex timetables, stimulus, response, and functional relevance.

5. Refer to Figures 5-1 through 5-10 for pictures of some key reflexes.

## D. Motor Development

1. Performance of occupational roles can be enhanced or inhibited based on the reflex development and integration noted above and in additional areas noted below.

a. Crossing the midline: as the child becomes more mobile, movement against gravity and weight-shift increase, leading to eventual

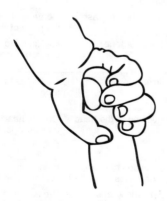

**Figure 5-1** Palmar Grasp Reflex
Groenweghe, Marisa with permission.

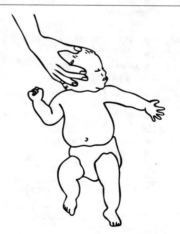

**Figure 5-2** Asymmetric Tonic Neck Reflex (ATNR)
Groenweghe, Marisa with permission.

crossing of the midline, often in an attempt to reach for a toy, while weight bearing on the opposing upper extremity for balance (begins at 9 - 12 months).

b. Laterality: hemispheric specialization for specific tasks varies with different individuals (handedness is considered to be stable by age 5; however, strong preferences can be seen much earlier).

c. Bilateral integration: as the child experiments with movement, his/her nervous system is stimulated, and these sensations help the child to coordinate the two sides of the body (begins at 9 - 12 months).

d. Fine coordination and dexterity. See section on development of hand skills.

e. Visual-motor integration is dependent upon the lower level skills of visual attention, visual memory, visual discrimination, kinesthesia, position in space, figure-ground, form constancy, and spatial relations.

f. Oral-motor control, which is developed in the area of feeding, provides the foundation for early oral communication and later language development.

## TABLE 5-I - OVERVIEW OF THE MOST IMPORTANT REFLEXES

| REFLEX | ONSET AGE | INTEGRATION AGE | STIMULUS | RESPONSE | RELEVANCE |
|---|---|---|---|---|---|
| Rooting | 28 wks gestation | 3 months | Stroke the corner of the mouth, upper lip, and lower lip | Movement of the tongue, mouth, and/or head toward the stimulus | Allows searching for and locating feeding source |
| Suck-swallow | 28 wks gestation | 2-5 months | Place examiner's index finger inside infant's mouth with head in midline | Strong, rhythmical sucking | Allows ingestion of nourishment |
| Traction | 28 wks gestation | 2-5 months | Grasp infant's forearms and pull-to-sit | Complete flexion of upper extremities | Enhances momentary reflexive grasp |
| Moro | 28 wks gestation | 4-6 months | Rapidly drop infant's head backward | First phase: arm extension/abduction, hand opening Second phase: arm flexion and adduction | Facilitates ability to depart from dominant flexor posture: protective response |
| Plantar grasp | 28 wks gestation | 9 months | Apply pressure with thumb on the infant's ball of the foot | Toe flexion | Increases tactile input to sole of foot |
| Galant | 32 wks gestation | 2 months | Hold infant in prone suspension, gently scratch or tap alongside the spine with finger, from shoulders to buttocks | Lateral trunk flexion and wrinkling of the skin on the stimulated side | Facilitates lateral trunk movements necessary for trunk stabilization |
| Asymmetric tonic neck | 37 wks gestation | 4-6 months | Fully rotate infant's head and hold for 5 seconds | Extension of extremities on the face side, flexion of extremities on the skull side | Promotes visual hand regard |
| Palmar grasp | 37 wks gestation | 4-6 months | Place examiner's finger in infant's palm | Finger flexion; reflexive grasp | Increases tactile input on the palm of the hand |
| Tonic labyrinthine - Supine | > 37 wks gestation | 6 months | Place infant in supine | Increased extensor tone | Facilitates total-body extensor tone |
| Tonic labyrinthine - Prone | > 37 wks gestation | 6 months | Place infant in prone | Increased flexor tone | Facilitates total-body flexor tone |
| Labyrinthine/optical (head) righting | birth - 2 months | persists | Hold infant suspended vertically and tilt slowly (about 45°) to the side, forward, or backward | Upright positioning of the head | Orients head in space; maintains face vertical |
| Landau | 3-4 months | 12-24 months | Hold infant in horizontal prone suspension | Complete extension of head, trunk, and extremities | Breaks up flexor dominance; facilitates prone extension |
| Symmetric tonic neck | 4-6 months | 8-12 months | Place infant in the crawling position and extend the head | Flexion of hips and knees | Breaks up total extensor posture; facilitates static quadruped position |

From *Foundations for practice in the neonatal intensive care unit and early intervention*, (Volume 2, p. 34) by Vergara, E. Copyright 1993 by the American Occupational Therapy Association, Bethesda, MD. Reprinted with permission.

## TABLE 5-1 - OVERVIEW OF THE MOST IMPORTANT REFLEXES CONTINUED

| REFLEX | ONSET AGE | INTEGRATION AGE | STIMULUS | RESPONSE | RELEVANCE |
|---|---|---|---|---|---|
| Neck righting (NOB) | 4-6 months | 5 years | Place infant in supine and fully turn head to one side | Log rolling of the entire body to maintain alignment with the head | Maintains head/body alignment; initiates rolling (first ambulation effort) |
| Body righting (on body) (BOB) | 4-6 months | 5 years | Place infant in supine, flex one hip and knee toward the chest and hold briefly | Segmental rolling of the upper trunk to maintain alignment | Facilitates trunk/spinal rotation |
| Downward parachute (protective extension downward) | 4 months | Persists | Rapidly lower infant toward supporting surface while suspended vertically | Extension of the lower extremities | Allows accurate placement of lower extremities in anticipation of a surface |
| Forward parachute (protective extension forward) | 6-9 months | Persists | Suddenly tip infant forward toward supporting surface while vertically suspended | Sudden extension of the upper extremities, hand opening, and neck extension | Allows accurate placement of upper extremities in anticipation of supporting surface to prevent a fall |
| Sideward parachute (protective extension sideward) | 7 months | Persists | Quickly but firmly tip infant off-balance to the side while in the sitting position | Arm extension and abduction to the side | Protects body to prevent a fall; supports body for unilateral use of opposite arm |
| Backward parachute (protective extension backward) | 9-10 months | Persists | Quickly but firmly tip infant off-balance backward | Backward arm extension or arm extension to one side | Protects body to prevent a fall; unilaterally facilitates spinal rotation |
| Prone tilting | 5 months | Persists | After positioning infant in prone, slowly raise one side of the supporting surface | Curving of the spine toward the raised side (opposite to the pull of gravity); abduction/extension of arms and legs | Maintain equilibrium without arm support; facilitate postural adjustments in all positions |
| Supine tilting and Sitting tilting | 7-8 months | Persists | After positioning infant in supine or sitting, slowly raise one side of the supporting surface | Curving of the spine toward the raised side (opposite to the pull of gravity); abduction/extension of arms and legs | Maintain equilibrium without arm support; facilitate postural adjustments in all positions |
| Quadruped tilting | 9-12 months | Persists | After positioning infant on all fours, slowly raise one side of the supporting surface | Curving of the spine toward the raised side (opposite to the pull of gravity); abduction/extension of arms and legs | Maintain equilibrium without arm support; facilitate postural adjustments in all positions |
| Standing tilting | 12-21 months | Persists | After positioning infant in standing, slowly raise one side of the supporting surface | Curving of the spine toward the raised side (opposite to the pull of gravity); abduction/extension of arms and legs | Maintain equilibrium without arm support; facilitate postural adjustments in all positions |

From *Foundations for practice in the neonatal intensive care unit and early intervention,* (Volume 2, p. 35) by Vergara, E. Copyright 1993 by the American Occupational Therapy Association, Bethesda, MD. Reprinted with permission.

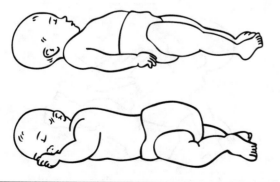

**Figure 5-3** Tonic Labyrinthine Reflex (TLR)
Groenweghe, Marisa with permission.

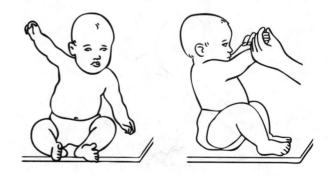

**Figure 5-4** Optical Righting Reaction
Groenweghe, Marisa with permission.

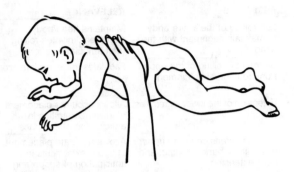

**Figure 5-5** Landau Reaction
Groenweghe, Marisa with permission.

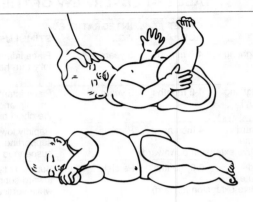

**Figure 5-6** Neck on Body (NOB)
Groenweghe, Marisa with permission.

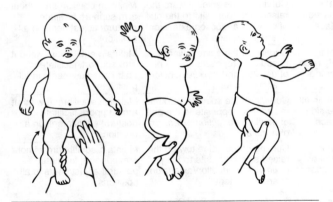

**Figure 5-7** Body Righting Reaction on Body (BOB)
Groenweghe, Marisa with permission.

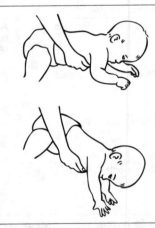

**Figure 5-8** Protective Extension Reaction Forward
Groenweghe, Marisa with permission.

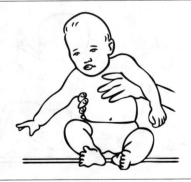

**Figure 5-9** Protective Extension Reaction Sideward
Groenweghe, Marisa with permission.

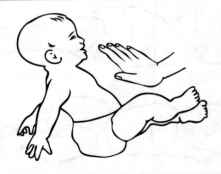

**Figure 5-10** Protective Extension Reaction Backward
Groenweghe, Marisa with permission.

2. General principles of motor development.
   a. Occurs in a cephalocaudal/proximal to distal direction.
   b. Progresses from gross to fine movement.
   c. Progresses from stability to controlled mobility.
   d. Occurs in a spiraling manner, with periods of equilibrium and disequilibrium.
   e. Sensitive periods occur when the infant/child is affected by environmental input.
3. Normal sensorimotor development in key positions. See Tables 5-2 and 5-3.
4. Important aspects in the development of upper extremity function.
   a. Head and trunk control.
   b. Eye/hand interaction/sensory-perceptual interaction.
   c. Shoulder (scapular) stability/mobility.
   d. Humeral control.
   e. Elbow control.
   f. Forearm control.
   g. Wrist control.
   h. Thumb opposition and stability.
   i. Palmar arches of hand.
   j. Isolated finger control.
5. Important components in the development of hand skills.
   a. Reaching skills.
      (1) Visual regard accompanied by swiping/batting, with closed hand and abducted shoulder (newborn).
      (2) Hands come together at midline for bilateral reaching with shoulders abducted with partial internal rotation, forearm pronation, and full finger extension (four months).
      (3) Increased dissociation of body sides, allows for unilateral reaching with less abduction and internal rotation of the shoulder, and the hand is more open (six months).
      (4) As trunk stability improves, shoulder flexion with slight external rotation, elbow extension, forearm supination, and slight wrist extension begin to emerge (nine months).
   b. Grasping skills according to Erhardt Prehension Developmental Levels.
      (1) Grasp of the pellet (prone or sitting).
         (a) No voluntary grasp or visual attention to the object (natal).
         (b) No attempt to grasp, but visually attends to the object (three months).
         (c) Raking and contacting object (six months).
         (d) Inferior-scissors grasp: raking object into palm with adducted totally flexed thumb and all flexed fingers, or two partially extended fingers (seven months).
         (e) Scissors grasp: between thumb and side of curled index finger, distal thumb joint slightly flexed, proximal thumb joint extended (eight months).
         (f) Inferior pincer grasp: between ventral surfaces of thumb and index finger, distal thumb joint extended, beginning of thumb opposition (nine months).
         (g) Pincer grasp: between distal pads of thumb and index finger, distal thumb joint slightly flexed, thumb opposed (ten months).
         (h) Fine pincer grasp: between fingertips or fingernails, distal thumb joint flexed (twelve months).
         (i) Refer to Figure 5-11.
      (2) Grasp of the cube.
         (a) Neonate visually attends to object, grasp is reflexive.
         (b) Visually attends to object and may swipe. Sustained voluntary grasp possible only upon contact, ulnar side used, no thumb involvement, wrist flexed (three months).
         (c) Primitive squeeze grasp: visually attends to object, approaches if within 1 inch, contact results in hand pulling object back to squeeze precariously against the other hand or body, no thumb involvement (four months).
         (d) Palmar grasp: fingers on top surface of object press it into center of palm with thumb adducted (five months).[1]
         (e) Radial-palmar grasp: fingers on far side of object press it against opposed thumb and radial side of palm (six months), with wrist straight (seven months).
         (f) Radial-digital grasp: object held with the opposed thumb and fingertips, space visible between (eight months) with wrist extended (nine months).
         (g) Refer to Figure 5-12.

---

[1] Although Erhardt did not specifically name or describe ulnar palmar grasp in her developmental stages, this term is often used in practice. This grasp occurs before the palmar grasp and has been placed within a 3.5 to 4.5 month stage of development. In the ulnar-palmar grasp, the infant presses small objects against the palm using digits 3, 4, and 5, with flexed wrist and no thumb involvement.

## TABLE 5-2 - SENSORIMOTOR DEVELOPMENT MOBILITY AND STABILITY

| AGE | GROSS MOTOR SKILL |
|---|---|
| **Prone Position** | |
| 0-2 mo | Turns head side to side |
| | Lifts head momentarily |
| | Bends hips with bottom in air |
| | Lifts head and sustains in midline |
| | Rotates head freely when up |
| | Able to bear weight on forearms |
| | Able to tuck chin and gaze at hands in forearm prop |
| | Attempts to shift weight on forearms, resulting in shoulder collapse |
| 5-6 mo | Shifts weight on forearms and reaches forward |
| | Bears weight and shifts weight on extended arms |
| | Legs are closer together and thighs roll inward toward natural alignment |
| | Hips are flat on surface |
| | Equilibrium reactions are present |
| 5-8 mo | Airplane posturing in prone position; chest and thighs lift off surface |
| 7-8 mo | Pivots in prone position |
| | Moves to prone position to sit |
| 9 mo | Begins to dislike prone position |
| **Supine Position** | |
| 0-3 mo | Head held to one side |
| | Able to turn head side to side |
| 3-4 mo | Holds head in midline |
| | Chin is tucked and neck lengthens in back |
| | Legs come together |
| | Lower back flattens against the floor |
| 4-5 mo | Head lag is gone when pulled to a sitting position |
| | Hands are together in space |
| 5-6 mo | Lifts head independently |
| | Brings feet to mouth |
| | Brings hands to feet |
| | Able to reach for toy with one or both hands |
| | Hands are predominantly open |
| 7-8 mo | Equilibrium reactions are present |
| **Rolling** | |
| 3-4 mo | Rolls from prone position to side accidentally because of poor control of weight shift |
| | Rolls from supine position to side |
| 5-6 mo | Rolls from prone to supine position |
| | Rolls from supine position to side with right and left leg performing independent movements |
| | Rolls from supine to prone position with right and left leg performing independent movements |
| 6-14 mo | Rolls segmentally with roll initiated by the head, shoulder, or hips |
| **Creeping** | |
| 7 mo | Crawls forward on belly |
| 7-10 mo | Reciprocal creep |
| 10-11 mo | Creeps on hands and feet |
| 11-12 mo | Creeps well |

## TABLE 5-2 - SENSORIMOTOR DEVELOPMENT MOBILITY AND STABILITY (CONT.)

| AGE | GROSS MOTOR SKILL |
|---|---|
| **Sitting** | |
| 0-3 mo (held in sitting) | Head bobs in sitting |
| | Back is rounded |
| | Hips are apart, turned out, and bent |
| | Head is steady |
| | Chin tucks; able to gaze at floor |
| | Sits with less support |
| | Hips are bent and shoulders are in front of hips |
| 5-6 mo (supports self in sitting) | Sits alone momentarily |
| | Increased extension in back |
| | Sits by propping forward on arms |
| | Wide base, legs are bent |
| | Periodic use of "high guard" position |
| | Protective responses present when falling to the front |
| 5-10 mo (sits alone) | Sits alone steadily, initially with wide base of support |
| | Able to play with toys in sitting position |
| 6-11 mo | Gets to sitting position from prone position |
| 7-8 mo | Equilibrium reactions are present |
| | Able to rotate upper body while lower body remains stationary |
| | Protective responses are present when falling to the side |
| 8-10 mo | Sits well without support |
| | Legs are closer; full upright position, knees straight |
| | Increased variety of sitting positions, including "w" sit and side sit |
| | Difficult fine motor tasks may prompt return to wide base of support |
| 9-18 mo | Rises from supine position by first rolling over to stomach then pushing up into four-point position |
| 10-12 mo | Protective extension backwards, first with bent elbows then straight elbows |
| | Able to move in and out of sitting position into other positions |
| 11-12 mo | Trunk control and equilibrium responses are fully developed in sitting position |
| | Further increase in variety of positions possible |
| 11-24 mo + | Rises from supine by first rolling to side then pushing up into sitting position |
| **Standing** | |
| 0-3 mo | When held in standing position, takes some weight on legs |
| 2-3 mo | When held in standing position, legs may give way |
| 3-4 mo | Bears some weight on legs, but must be held proximally |
| | Head is up in midline, no chin tuck |
| | Pelvis and hips are behind shoulders |
| | Legs are apart and turned outward |
| 5-10 mo | Stands while holding onto furniture |
| 5-6 mo | Increased capability to bear weight |
| | Decreased support needed; may be held by arms or hands |
| | Legs are still spread apart and turned outward |
| | Bounces in standing position |

## TABLE 5-2 - SENSORIMOTOR DEVELOPMENT MOBILITY AND STABILITY (CONT.)

| AGE | GROSS MOTOR SKILL |
| --- | --- |
| **Standing Cont.** | |
| 6-12 mo | Pulls to standing position at furniture |
| 8-9 mo | Rotates the trunk over the lower extremities<br>Lower extremities are more active in pulling to a standing position<br>Pulls to a standing position by kneeling, then half-kneeling |
| 9-13 mo | Pulls to standing position with legs only, no longer needs arms<br>Stands alone momentarily |
| 12 mo | Equilibrium reactions are present in standing |
| **Walking** | |
| 8 mo | Cruises sideways |
| 8-18 mo | Walks with two hands held |
| 9-10 mo | Cruises around furniture, turning slightly in intended direction |
| 9-17 mo | Takes independent steps, falls easily |
| 10-14 mo | Walking: stoops and recovers in play |
| 11 mo | Walks with one hand held<br>Reaches for furniture out of reach when cruising<br>Cruises in either direction, no hesitation |
| 15 mo | Able to start and stop in walking |
| 18 mo | Seldom falls<br>Runs stiffly with eyes on ground |
| **Release** | |
| 0-1 mo | No release; grasp reflex is strong |
| 1-4 mo | Involuntary release |
| 4 mo | Mutual fingering in midline |
| 4-8 mo | Transfers object from hand to hand |
| 5-6 mo | Two-stage transfer; taking hand grasps before releasing hand lets go |
| 6-7 mo | One-stage transfer; taking hand and releasing hand perform actions simultaneously |
| 7-9 mo | Volitional release |
| 7-10 mo | Presses down on surface to release |
| 8 mo | Releases above a surface with wrist flexion |
| 9-10 mo | Releases into a container with wrist straight |
| 10-14 mo | Clumsy release into small container; hand rests on edge of container |
| 12-15 mo | Precise, controlled release into small container with wrist extended |

Modified from Bly, L. (1993). *Normal development in the first year of life.* Tucson, AZ: Therapy Skill Builders; Illingworth, R. S. (1991). *The normal child: Some problems of the early years and their treatment* (10th ed.). Edinburgh: Churchill-Livingstone; Knobloch, H., & Pasamanick, B. (1974). *Gesell and Amatruda's developmental diagnosis: The evaluation and management of normal and abnormal neuropsychological development in infancy and early childhood.* Hagerstown, MD: Harper and Row; Gilfoyle, E., Grady, A., & Moore, J. (1990). *Children adapt.* Thorofare, NJ: Slack.

Case-Smith, J., Allen, A.S., & Pratt, P.N. (1996). *Occupational therapy for children* (3rd ed., pp. 49-50). St. Louis, MO: Mosby-Year Book. Reprinted with permission.

c. Releasing skills: initially, involuntary dropping, then object is pulled out of one hand by the other hand. (Table 5-2).
  (1) Development progresses from no release (0 -1 month) to involuntary release (1 – 4 months) to two-stage transfer, (5 -6 months) one-stage transfer (6 – 7 months) to voluntary release (7 – 9 months).
  (2) By 9 months, release by full arm extension.
  (3) Refinement continues up to age four with the attainment of graded release.
d. Carrying skills: involves a combination of movements of the shoulder, body and distal joints of the wrist and hand to hold the item, making appropriate adjustments as necessary to maintain this hold.
e. Bilateral hand use: asymmetric movements prevail until 3 months, and then symmetric movements emerge until 10 months.

## TABLE 5-3 - DEVELOPMENT OF STAIR CLIMBING AND JUMPING/HOPPING SKILLS

| AGE | SKILL |
| --- | --- |
| **Stair Climbing** | |
| 15 mo | Creeps up stairs |
| 18-24 mo | Walks up stairs while holding on<br>Walks down stairs while holding on |
| 18-23 mo | Creeps backwards down stairs |
| 2-2½+ yr | Walks up stairs without support, marking time<br>Walks down stairs without support, marking time |
| 2-2½-3 yr | Walks up stairs, alternating feet |
| 3-3½ yr | Walks down stairs, alternating feet |
| **Jumping and Hopping** | |
| 2 yr | Jumps down from step |
| 2½+ yr | Hops on one foot, few steps |
| 3 yr | Jumps off floor with both feet |
| 3-5 yr | Jumps over objects |
| 3½-5 yr | Hops on one foot |
| 3-4 yr | Gallops, leading with one foot and transferring weight smoothly and evenly |
| 5 yr | Hops in straight line |
| 5-6 yr | Skips on alternating feet, maintaining balance |

Modified from Gesell, A., & Amatruda, C.S. (1947). *Developmental diagnosis.* New York, NY: Harper and Row; Bayley, N. (1993). *Bayley scales of infant development* (rev ed.). New York, NY: Psychological Corporation; Knobloch, H. & Pasamanick, B. (1974). *Gesell and Amatruda's developmental diagnosis: The evaluation and management of normal and abnormal neuropsychological development in infancy and early childhood.* Hagerstown, MD: Harper and Row.

Case-Smith, J., Allen, A.S., & Pratt, P.N. (1996). *Occupational therapy for children* (3rd ed., p. 59). St. Louis, MO: Mosby-Year Book. Reprinted with permission.

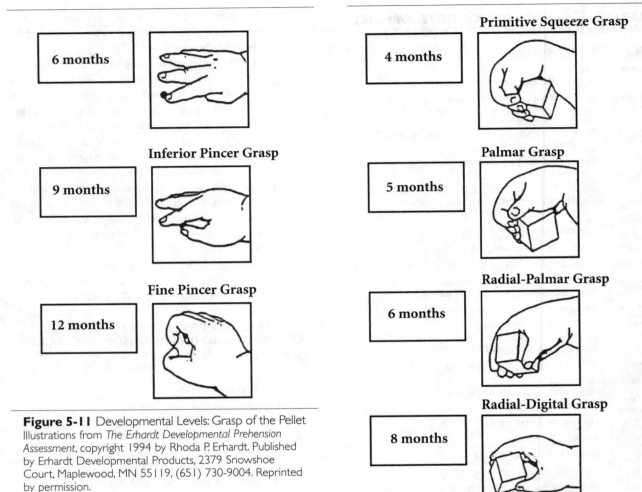

**Figure 5-11** Developmental Levels: Grasp of the Pellet
Illustrations from *The Erhardt Developmental Prehension Assessment*, copyright 1994 by Rhoda P. Erhardt. Published by Erhardt Developmental Products, 2379 Snowshoe Court, Maplewood, MN 55119, (651) 730-9004. Reprinted by permission.

(1) By 12 to 18 months, the baby uses both hands for different functions.

(2) At 18 to 24 months, manipulation skills emerge.

(3) The ability to use two different hands for two very different functions emerges at age 2½.

f. Manipulating skills according to Exner's Classification System.

(1) Finger-to-palm translation: a linear movement of an object from the fingers to the palm of the hand, e.g., picking up coins (12 - 15 months).

(2) Palm-to-finger translation: with stabilization, a linear movement of an object from the palm of the hand to the fingers, e.g., placing coins in a slot (2 – 2½ years).

(3) Shift: a linear movement of an object on the finger surfaces to allow for repositioning of the object relative to the finger pads, e.g., separating 2 pieces of paper (3 – 3½ years).

(4) Simple rotation: the turning or rolling of an object held at the finger pads approximately 90 degrees or less, e.g., unscrewing a small bottle cap (2 – 2½ years).

(5) Complex rotation: the rotation of an object 360 degrees, e.g., turning a pencil over to erase (6 - 7 years).

**Figure 5-12** Developmental Levels: Grasp of the Cube
Illustrations from *The Erhardt Developmental Prehension Assessment*, copyright 1994 by Rhoda P. Erhardt. Published by Erhardt Developmental Products, 2379 Snowshoe Court, Maplewood, MN 55119, (651) 730-9004. Reprinted by permission.

(6) In-hand manipulation with stabilization: several objects are held in the hand and manipulation of one object occurs, while simultaneously stabilizing the others, e.g., picking up pennies with thumb and forefinger while storing them in the ulnar side of the same hand (6 - 7 years).

g.  Pre-writing skills.

(1) Palmar-supinate grasp: held with fisted hand, wrist slightly flexed and slightly supinated away from mid-position; arm

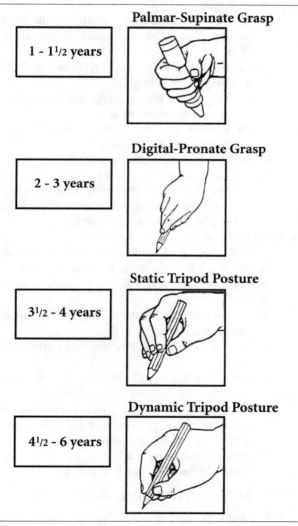

### Palmar-Supinate Grasp

1 - 1½ years

### Digital-Pronate Grasp

2 - 3 years

### Static Tripod Posture

3½ - 4 years

### Dynamic Tripod Posture

4½ - 6 years

**Figure 5-13** Developmental Levels: Pre-Writing Skills Illustrations from *The Erhardt Developmental Prehension Assessment*, copyright 1994 by Rhoda P. Erhardt. Published by Erhardt Developmental Products, 2379 Snowshoe Court, Maplewood, MN 55119, (651) 730-9004. Reprinted by permission.

moves as a unit (1 – 1½ years).

(2) Digital-pronate grasp: held with fingers, wrist neutral with slight ulnar deviation, and forearm pronated; arm moves as a unit (2 - 3 years).

(3) Static tripod posture: held with crude approximation of thumb, index, and middle fingers, ring and little fingers only slightly flexed, grasped proximally with continual adjustments by other hand, no fine localized movements of digit components; hand moves as a unit (3½ - 4 years).

(4) Dynamic tripod posture: held with precise opposition of distal phalanges of thumb, index, and middle fingers, ring and little fingers flexed to form a stable arch, wrist slightly extended, grasped distally, MCP joints stabilized during fine, localized movements of PIP joints (4½ - 6 years).

(5) Refer to Figure 5-13.

h.  Scissor use skills.

(1) Prerequisite skills for scissors use include the ability to:

(a) Open and close a hand.

(b) Isolate or combine the movements of the thumb, index and middle fingers.

(c) Use hands bilaterally; one hand to use the scissors, one to stabilize the item being cut.

(d) Coordinate arm, hand, and eye movements.

(e) Stabilize the wrist, elbow, and shoulder joints so that movement can occur at the distal joints.

(f) Interact with the environment in the constructive developmental play stage.

(2) Stages of development in scissor use, the child sequentially:

(a) Shows an interest in scissors, 2-3 years.

(b) Holds and snips with scissors, 2-3 years.

(c) Opens and closes scissors in a controlled fashion, 2-3 years.

(d) Manipulates scissors in a forward motion, 3-4 years.

(e) Coordinates the lateral direction of the scissors, 3-4 years.

(f) Cuts a straight forward line, 3-4 years.

(g) Cuts simple geometric shapes, 3-4 years.

(h) Cuts circles, 3½ - 4½ years.

(i) Cuts simple figure shapes, 4-6 years.

(j) Cuts complex figure shapes, 6-7 years.

# III. Psychosocial Development and Major Theorists

## A. Relationship to the Exam.

1. It is not likely that the NBCOT exam will ask direct questions about psychosocial theories of development.

    a. This information is provided because an understanding of typical development will be helpful for selecting an answer that is developmentally appropriate.

## B. Erik Erikson

1. Ego adaptation is the adaptive response of the ego in the development of the personality.

2. Eight stages of development are identified and include a critical personal-social crisis that when resolved by the individual gives the individual a sense of mastery and results in the acquisition of a personality quality.

    a. Basic trust vs. mistrust: the infant/baby realizes that survival and comfort needs will be met; hope is integrated into the personality (birth to 18 months).

    b. Autonomy vs. doubt and shame: the child realizes that he/she can control bodily functions; self-controlled will is integrated into the personality (2 to 4 years).

    c. Initiative vs. guilt: the child gains social skills and a gender role identity; a sense of purpose is integrated into the personality (preschool age).

    d. Industry vs. inferiority: the child gains a sense of security through peers and gains mastery over activities of his/her age group; a feeling of competency is integrated into the personality (elementary school age).

    e. Self-identity vs. role diffusion: the teenager begins to make choices about adult roles, and with the resolution of this identity crisis a sense of fidelity or membership with society is integrated into the personality (teenage years).

    f. Intimacy and solidarity vs. isolation: the young adult establishes an intimate relationship with a partner and family; the capacity to love is achieved (young adulthood).

    g. Generativity vs. self-absorption: the adult finds security in the contribution of his/her chosen personal/professional roles; the capacity to

care is achieved (middle adulthood).

    h. Integrity vs. despair: the mature adult reflects on his/her own value, and shares with the younger generation the knowledge gained; wisdom is acquired (maturity).

## C. Lawrence Kohlberg

1. Stages of Moral Development.

    a. Level 1, preconventional morality: occurs up until the age of 8.

        (1) Stage 1, punishment and obedience: the child is obedient in order to avoid punishment.

        (2) Stage 2, instrumental relativism: the child makes moral choices based on the benefit to self and sometimes to others.

    b. Level 2, conventional morality: occurs at about 9 or 10 years of age.

        (1) Stage 1, social conformity: the child desires to gain the approval of others.

        (2) Stage 2, law and order: rules and social norms are internalized.

    c. Level 3, postconventional morality: age range can vary, and not all will achieve this level.

        (1) Social contracts: the young adult has social awareness and an awareness of the legal implications of decisions/actions.

## D. Abraham Maslow

1. Maslow developed a hierarchy of basic human needs, proposing that if the lower-level needs are not met, the individual is unable to work on higher-level pursuits.

    a. Philosophic: basic survival needs (i.e., food, water, rest, warmth).

    b. Safety: the need for physical and physiologic security.

    c. Love and belonging: the need for affection, emotional support and group affiliation.

    d. Self-esteem: the need to believe in one's self as a competent and valuable member of society.

    e. Self-actualization: the need to achieve one's personal goals, after attaining all of the psychosocial developmental milestones.

# IV. Cognitive Development

## A. Jean Piaget

1. Described the process of cognitive development from birth to adolescence.

2. Major constructs.

    a. Adaptation: responding to environmental challenges as they occur.

b. Mental schemes: organizing experiences into concepts.

c. Operations: the cognitive methods used by the child to organize schemes and experiences to direct subsequent actions.

d. Adapted intelligence or cognitive competence.

e. Equilibrium: the balance between what the child knows and can act on and what the environment provides.

f. Assimilation: the ability to take a new situation and change it to match an existing scheme or generalization.

g. Accommodation: the development of a new scheme in response to the reality of a situation, or discrimination.

3. Hierarchical development of cognition.

   a. Sensorimotor period, ages birth to 2 years.
   
   (1) Reflexive stage: schemes begin in response to reflexes (1 month).
   
   (2) Primary circular reactions: child learns about cause and effect as a result of reflexive sensorimotor patterns that are repeated for enjoyment (2 to 4 months).
   
   (3) Secondary circular reactions: voluntary movement patterns emerge due to coordination of vision and hand function, and an early awareness of cause and effect develops (5 to 8 months).
   
   (4) Coordination of secondary schemata: voluntary movement in response to stimuli that cannot be seen such as in object permanence, and early development of decentered thought (9 to 12 months).
   
   (5) Tertiary circular reactions: the child seeks out new schemes, with improved gross and fine motor abilities; tool use begins (12 to 18 months).
   
   (6) Inventions of new means through mental combinations: the child demonstrates insight and purposeful tool use, and explores problem solving options. The ability to represent concepts without direct manipulation emerges (18 months to 2 years).
   
   (7) Child progresses from reflexive activity to mental representation to cognitive functions of combining and manipulating objects in play.

   b. Preoperational period, ages 2 to 7 years.
   
   (1) Classification: categorizing objects according to similarities and differences.
   
   (2) Seriation: the relationship of one object or classification of objects to another.
   
   (3) Conservation: the end product of the preoperational period. The child is able to recognize the continuities of an object or class of objects in spite of apparent changes.
   
   (4) The preoperational period is divided into two phases.
   
      (a) Preconceptual: the child expands vocabulary and symbolic representations (2 to 4 years).
      
      (b) Intuitive thought phase: the child imitates, copies or repeats what is seen or heard and bases conclusions on what he/she believes to be true rather than on logic. Inductive reasoning denotes a transition to the next stage (4 to 7 years).
   
   (5) Child progresses from dependence on perception, as opposed to logic, and egocentric orientation to logical thought, for solving problems. Child enjoys verbal and symbolic play.

   c. Concrete operations, ages 7 to 11 years.
   
   (1) Reversibility: an expansion of conservation, leads to increased spatial awareness.
   
   (2) Rules: as rules are better understood, they are also applied.
   
   (3) Empiric-inductive thinking: the child solves problems with the information that is obvious and present.
   
   (4) Child uses logical thinking on observed or mentally represented objects, enjoying games with rules which help the child adjust to social demands.

   d. Formal operations, ages 11 through the teen years.
   
   (1) Hypothetic-deductive thinking, the ability to analyze and plan.
   
   (2) Child uses logic to hypothesize many ways to solve problems, and can draw from past and present experiences to imagine what can have an effect on future situations.

4. Piaget stated that maturation of cognition is dependent upon:

   a. Organic growth, especially the maturation of the nervous system and endocrine glands.
   
   b. Experience in the actions performed on objects.

c. Social interaction and transmission.

d. A balance of opportunities for both assimilation and accommodation.

**B. Major Milestones in Cognitive Development**

1. Early object use.

    a. Child focuses on action performed with objects, e.g., banging, shaking (3 - 6 months).

    b. Child explores characteristics of objects and expands the range of schemes, e.g., pulling, turning, poking, tearing (6 - 9 months).

    c. Child combines objects in relational play, such as objects in containers (8 - 9 months).

    d. Child notices the relation between complex actions and consequences such as opening doors, placing lids on containers, and differential use of schemes based on the toy being played with, e.g., pushing a train or rolling a ball (9 - 12 months).

    e. Child acts on objects with a variety of schemes (12 months +).

    f. Child links schemes in simple combinations, e.g., placing a baby in carriage and then pushing the carriage (12 - 15 months).

    g. Child links multi-scheme combinations into a meaningful sequence, e.g., putting food in a bowl, scooping the food using a spoon, and feeding a doll (24 - 36 months).

    h. Child links schemes into a complex script (36 - 42 months).

2. Problem-solving skills.

    a. 6 - 9 months.

        (1) Child finds object after watching it disappear, e.g., toy covered by cloth.

        (2) Child uses movement as a means to an end, e.g., rolling to secure toy.

        (3) Child anticipates movement of objects in space, e.g., looking toward trajectory of object circling his/her head.

        (4) Child attends to consequences of actions, e.g., banging toy and realizing it makes noise.

        (5) Child repeats actions to repeat consequences, e.g., banging toy to hear noise.

    b. 9 - 12 months.

        (1) Child is able to use a tool after demonstration, e.g., using a stick to secure a toy that is out of reach.

        (2) Child's behavior becomes more goal directed.

        (3) Child performs an action to produce a response.

    c. 12 - 15 months.

        (1) Child recruits the help of an adult to achieve a goal.

        (2) Child attempts to activate a simple mechanism.

        (3) Child turns and inspects objects.

        (4) Child uses a trial and error approach to new challenges.

    d. 18 - 21 months.

        (1) Child attends to shapes of things and uses them appropriately.

        (2) Child begins to think before acting.

        (3) Child uses tool to obtain a favored object.

        (4) Child begins to replace trial and error with a thought process in order to attain a goal.

        (5) Child can operate a mechanical toy, e.g., an on-off switch.

        (6) Child can predict effects or presume causes.

    e. 21 - 24 months.

        (1) Child recognizes operations of several mechanisms.

        (2) Child matches circles, squares, triangles, and manipulates objects into small openings, e.g., shape sorters.

    f. 24 - 27 months.

        (1) Child discriminates sizes.

    g. 24 - 30 months.

        (1) Child can build with blocks horizontally and vertically.

    h. 27 - 30 months.

        (1) Child begins to relate experiences to one another, based on logic and knowledge of previous experiences.

        (2) Child can make a mental plan of actions without acting it out.

        (3) Child can see relationships between experiences, e.g., if the balloon is popped, it will make a loud noise.

    i. 36 - 48 months.

        (1) Child can build a tower of nine cubes, demonstrating balance and coordination.

        (2) Child can organize objects by size, and builds a structure from a mental image.

    j. 48 - 60 months.

        (1) Child can build involved structures combining various planes, along with symmetrical designs.

        (2) Child is able to utilize spatial awareness, cause-and-effect, and mental images in problem solving.

3. Symbolic play.
   a. 12 - 16 months.
      (1) Basic "make believe" play, primarily involving self, e.g., eating, sleeping.
   b. 12 - 18 months.
      (1) Child can project "make believe" play on objects and others.
      (2) Child uses a variety of schemes in imitating familiar activities.
   c. 18 - 24 months.
      (1) Child increases the use of non-realistic objects in pretending, e.g., substituting a block for a train.
      (2) Child can have inanimate objects perform actions, e.g., a doll washing itself.
   d. 24 -48 months.
      (1) See Section V.A.2 below.

# V. Development of Play

## A. Categories of Play

1. Exploratory play, 0 - 2 years.
   a. Child engages in play experiences through which he/she develops a body scheme.
   b. Sensory integrative and motor skills are also developed as the child explores the properties and effects of actions on objects and people.
   c. Child plays mostly with parents/caregiver(s).
2. Symbolic play, 2 - 4 years.
   a. Child engages in play experiences through which he/she formulates, tests, classifies, and refines ideas, feelings, and combined actions.
   b. This form of play is associated with language development.
   c. Objects that are manageable for the child in terms of symbolization, control, and mastery are preferred by the child.
   d. Child is mostly involved in parallel play with peers, and begins to become more cooperative over time.
3. Creative play, 4 - 7 years.
   a. Child engages in sensory, motor, cognitive, and social play experiences in which he/she refines relevant skills.
   b. Child explores combinations of actions on multiple objects.
   c. Child begins to master skills that promote performance of school and work related activities.
   d. Child participates in cooperative peer groups.
4. Games, 7 - 12 years.
   a. Child participates in play with rules, competi-

tion, social interaction, and opportunities for development of skills.
   b. Child begins to participate in cooperative peer groups with a growing interest in competition.
   c. Friends become important for validation of play items and performance, while parents assist and validate in the absence of peers.

# VI. Self-Care Development

## A. Feeding

1. Oral-motor development.
   a. Prior to 33 weeks of gestation an infant is fed by non-oral means.
   b. 35 weeks of gestation or after: jaw and tongue movements are strong enough to allow for feeding.
   c. 40 weeks of gestation: rooting reflexes, gag and cough reflex are present for up to four months, protecting the airway and decreasing the chances of aspiration.
   d. 4-5 months: munching occurs consisting of a phasic bite and release of a soft cookie.
   e. 6 months: strong up and down movement of the tongue.
   f. 7-8 months: beginning of mastication of soft and mashed foods with diagonal jaw movement.
   g. 9 months: lateral tongue movements make mastication of soft and mashed table food effective; able to drink from a cup; however, jaw is not firm.
   h. 12 months: jaw is firm, there is rotary chewing allowing for a good bite on a hard cookie.
   i. 24 months: able to chew most meats and raw vegetables.
2. Intervention for oral motor control.
   a. Appropriate positioning to allow for neutral pelvic alignment and trunk stability either in caregiver's lap or chair (infant seat or wheelchair); avoid head extension to prevent asphyxiation as a result of closing of the airway.
   b. Hand positioning of the caregiver: place the index finger longitudinally under the child's lip, middle finger under the jaw, and place the thumb on the lateral end of the mandible.
   c. Facilitate lip closure by applying slight upward pressure of the index finger under the child's lip.
   d. Facilitate jaw closure by firm upper pressure of the middle finger under the jaw.

e. Hand positioning of the index and middle fingers to assist in inhibiting tongue thrust.
  (1) Press bowl of spoon downward and hold on tongue.
f. Facilitate swallow by lip closure, and by placement and slight downward pressure of the spoon on the middle aspect of the tongue.
g. Facilitate chewing by placement of foods, such as long soft cooked vegetables, between the gum and teeth.
h. Integrate preventive measures to work out of abnormal patterns.

## TABLE 5-4
## DEVELOPMENTAL CONTINUUM IN SELF-FEEDING AND ASSOCIATED COMPONENT AREAS

| AGE (mo) | EATING AND FEEDING PERFORMANCE | CONCURRENT CHANGES IN PERFORMANCE COMPONENTS | | |
| --- | --- | --- | --- | --- |
| | | SENSORIMOTOR | COGNITION | PSYCHOSOCIAL |
| 5-7 | Takes cereal or poured baby food from spoon. | Has good head stability and emerging sitting abilities; reaches and grasps toys; explores and tolerates various textures (e.g., fingers, rattles); puts objects in mouth. | Attends to effect produced by actions, such as hitting or shaking. | Plays with caregiver during meals and engages in interactive routines. |
| 6-8 | Attempts to hold bottle but may not retrieve it if it falls; needs to be monitored for safety reasons. | | Object permanence is emerging and infant anticipates spoon or bottle. | Is easily distracted by stimuli (especially siblings) in the environment. |
| 6-9 | Holds and tries to eat cracker but sucks on it more than bites it; consumes soft foods that dissolve in the mouth; grabs at spoon but bangs it or sucks on either end of it. | Good sitting stability emerges; able to use hands to manipulate smaller parts of rattle; guided reach and palmer grasp applied to hand-to-mouth actions with objects. | Uses familiar actions initially with haphazard variations; seeks novelty and is anxious to explore objects (may grab at food on adult's plate). | Recognizes strangers; emerging sense of self. |
| 9-13 | Finger-feeds self a portion of meals consisting of soft table foods (e.g., macaroni, peas, dry cereal) and objects if fed by an adult. | Uses various grasps on objects of different sizes; able to isolate radial fingers on smaller objects. | Has increased organization and sequencing of schemes to do desired activity; may have difficulty attending to events outside visual space (e.g., position of spoon close to mouth). | Prefers to act on objects than be passive observer. |
| 12-14 | Dips spoon in food, brings spoonful of food to mouth, but spills food by inverting spoon before it goes into mouth. | Begins to place and release objects; likely to use pronated grasp on objects like crayon or spoon. | Recognizes that objects have function and uses tools appropriately; relates objects together, shifting attention among them. | Has interest in watching family routines. |
| 15-18 | Scoops food with spoon and brings it to mouth. | Shoulder and wrist stability demonstrate precise movements. | Experiments to learn rules of how objects work; actively solves problems by creating new action solutions. | Internalizes standards imposed by others for how to play with objects. |
| 24-30 | Demonstrates interest in using fork; may stab at food such as pieces of canned fruit; proficient at spoon use and eats cereal with milk or rice with gravy with utensil. | Tolerates various food textures in mouth; adjusts movements to be efficient (e.g., forearm supinated to scoop and lift spoon). | Expresses wants verbally; demonstrates imitation of short sequence of occupation (e.g., putting food on plate and eating it). | Has increasing desire to copy peers; looks to adults to see if they appreciate success in an occupation; interested in household routines. |

Shepherd, J. (2005). Activities of daily living and adaptations for independent living. In J. Case-Smith, (Ed.), *Occupational therapy for children* (5th ed., p., 489). St. Louis, MO: Elsevier Mosby. Reprinted with permission.

(1) Provide firm downward pressure, using a spoon, on the middle aspect of the tongue in presence of a tonic bite reflex.

(2) Prevent tongue retraction to avoid choking.

(3) Facilitate lip closure for a tongue thrust that can result in loss of liquid and food, drooling, and failure to thrive.

(4) Decrease tactile sensitivity prior to feeding as well as at other times, by providing firm pressure; encourage sucking/chewing on a cloth; rub gums, palate, tongue; promote oral exploration of toys; use a NUK tooth-brush; and vary texture of foods, gradually introducing mashed potatoes mixed with other vegetables and soft meats.

i. Consider and utilize the appropriate texture of foods as related to the child's feeding problems. Thick foods are easier to swallow and manage, especially if a tongue thrust is present.

j. A major role of the occupational therapist or OTA is to assist the caregiver in considering and promoting a pleasant social atmosphere for feeding by utilizing positioning and handling techniques to promote eye contact and bonding in a relaxed environment.

k. Consider the developmental sequence of feeding skills.

   (1) Refer to Table 5-4.

**B. Development of Dressing Skills**

  1. Refer to Table 5-5.

**C. Development of Toileting Skills**

  1. Refer to Table 5-6.

**D. Development of Home Management Skills**

  1. Refer to Table 5-7.

## TABLE 5-5 - DEVELOPMENT OF SELF-DRESSING SKILLS

| AGE (yrs) | SELF-DRESSING SKILL |
|---|---|
| 1 | Cooperates with dressing (holds out arms and feet)<br>Pulls off shoes, removes socks<br>Pushes arms through sleeves and legs through pants |
| 2 | Removes unfastened coat<br>Removes shoes if laces are untied<br>Helps pull down pants<br>Finds armholes in over-the-head shirt |
| 2 1/2 | Removes pull-down pants with elastic waist<br>Assists in pulling on socks<br>Puts on front-button coat or shirt<br>Unbuttons large buttons |
| 3 | Puts on over-the-head shirt with minimal assistance<br>Puts on shoes without fasteners (may be on wrong foot)<br>Puts on socks (may be heel on top)<br>Independently pulls down pants<br>Zips and unzips jacket once on track<br>Needs assistance to remove over-the-head shirt<br>Buttons large front buttons |
| 3 1/2 | Finds front of clothing<br>Snaps or hooks front fastener<br>Unzips front zipper on jacket, separating zipper<br>Puts on mittens<br>Buttons series of three or four buttons<br>Unbuckles shoe or belt<br>Dresses with supervision (needs help with front and back) |
| 4 | Removes pullover garment independently<br>Buckles shoes or belt<br>Zips jacket zipper<br>Puts on socks correctly<br>Puts on shoes with assistance in tying laces<br>Laces shoes<br>Consistently identifies the front and back of garment |
| 4 1/2 | Puts belt in loops |
| 5 | Ties and unties knots<br>Dresses unsupervised |
| 6 | Closes back zipper<br>Ties bow now, buttons back buttons<br>Snaps back snaps |

Shepherd, J. (2005). Activities of daily living and adaptations for independent living. In J. Case-Smith, (Ed.), *Occupational therapy for children* (5th ed., p., 547). St. Louis, MO: Elsevier Mosby. Reprinted with permission.

## TABLE 5-6 - TYPICAL DEVELOPMENTAL SEQUENCE OF TOILETING SKILLS

| APPROX. AGE (yr) | TOILETING SKILL |
|---|---|
| 1 | • Indicates discomfort when wet or soiled<br>• Has regular bowel movements |
| 1 1/2 | • Sits on toilet when placed there and supervised (short time) |
| 2 | • Urinates regularly |
| 2 1/2 | • Achieves regulated toileting with occasional daytime accidents<br>• Rarely has bowel accidents<br>• Tells someone that he or she needs to go to the bathroom<br>• May need reminders to go to the bathroom<br>• May need help with getting on the toilet |
| 3 | • Goes to bathroom independently; seats self on toilet<br>• May need help with wiping<br>• May need help with fasteners or difficult clothing |
| 4-5 | • Is independent in toileting (e.g., tearing toilet paper, flushing, washing hands, managing clothing) |

Shepherd, J. (2005). Activities of daily living and adaptations for independent living. In J. Case-Smith, (Ed.), *Occupational therapy for children* (5th ed., p., 543). St. Louis, MO: Elsevier Mosby. Reprinted with permission.

## VII. Lifespan and Occupational Therapy Developmental Theorists

### A. Relationship to Exam

1. It is not likely that the NBCOT exam will ask direct questions about these theories.
   a. This information is provided because an understanding of typical development will be helpful for selecting an answer that is developmentally appropriate.

### B. Havighurst

1. Proposed that people need to develop certain skills at different ages to meet social standards.

### TABLE 5-7 - DEVELOPMENTAL SEQUENCE FOR HOME MANAGEMENT TASKS

| AGE | TASK |
|-----|------|
| 13 months | Imitates housework |
| 2 years | Picks up and puts away toys with parental reminders<br>Copies parent's domestic activities |
| 3 years | Carries things without dropping them<br>Dusts with help<br>Dries dishes with help<br>Gardens with help<br>Puts toys away with reminders<br>Wipes spills |
| 4 years | Fixes dry cereal and snacks<br>Helps with sorting laundry |
| 5 years | Puts toys away neatly<br>Makes a sandwich<br>Takes out trash<br>Makes bed<br>Puts dirty clothes away<br>Answers telephone correctly |
| 6 years | Does simple errands<br>Does household chores without redoing<br>Cleans sink<br>Washes dishes with help<br>Crosses street safely |
| 7-9 years | Begins to cook simple meal<br>Puts clean clothes away<br>Hangs up clothes<br>Manages small amounts of money<br>Uses telephone correctly |
| 10 - 12 years | Cooks simple meal with supervision<br>Does simple repairs with appropriate tools<br>Begins doing laundry<br>Sets table<br>Washes dishes<br>Cares for pet with reminders |
| 13 - 14 years | Does laundry<br>Cooks meals |

Shepherd, J. (2005). Activities of daily living and adaptations for independent living. In J. Case-Smith, (Ed.), *Occupational therapy for children* (5th ed., p., 558). St. Louis, MO: Elsevier Mosby. Reprinted with permission.

2. Believed that these developmental tasks rely on biologic, psychologic, and sociologic conditions.
   a. Proposed that there are certain sensitive periods, when biologic, psychologic, and sociologic conditions are optimal for the accomplishment of a developmental task.
   b. Described "teachable moments", referring to the sensitive periods when conditions are optimal for integration of previous knowledge and the accomplishment of new developmental tasks with assistance.
3. Six stages of development are described along with specific developmental tasks for each stage.
4. In current society, the tasks of some stages may occur later than described by Havighurst.
5. Tasks of infancy and childhood.
   a. Walk.
   b. Take solid food.
   c. Talk.
   d. Control elimination of body wastes.
   e. Develop sex differences and sexual modesty.
   f. Develop physiologic stability.
   g. Understand concepts of social and physical reality.
   h. Develop emotional ties with parents, siblings, and others.
   i. Understand right from wrong, conscience evolves.
6. Tasks of middle childhood.
   a. Develop physical skills needed for games.
   b. Establish healthy self-concept.
   c. Make friends with children of the same age.
   d. Read, write, and calculate.
   e. Acquire a fund of information necessary for everyday life.
   f. Develop morality and values.
   g. Formulate opinions about social groups and institutions.
7. Tasks of adolescence.
   a. Establish relationships with male and female friends of same age, increasing in quantity and quality.
   b. Develop masculine/feminine social role.
   c. Become comfortable with and respect one's changing body.
   d. Decrease emotional reliance on parents/other adults.
   e. Prepare for marriage and family life.
   f. Prepare for economic career.
   g. Develop a value system to shape behavior or

develop one's own philosophy.

   h. Behave in a socially responsible manner.

8. Tasks of early adulthood.
   a. Choose a partner.
   b. Adjust to a partner.
   c. Start a family.
   d. Raise children.
   e. Manage a home.
   f. Pursue an occupation.
   g. Develop civic responsibility.
   h. Join/form a compatible social group.

9. Tasks of middle adulthood.
   a. Guide adolescents toward becoming responsible and well adjusted adults.
   b. Engage in adult civic and social responsibility.
   c. Progress in an occupational career.
   d. Pursue leisure-time activities.
   e. Relate to partner as a person.
   f. Deal with and accept physiologic changes of middle age.
   g. Accept aging parents.

10. Tasks of later maturity.
    a. Cope with decreasing physical strength and health.
    b. Adjust to retirement and reduced income.
    c. Adjust to death of a spouse/partner.
    d. Affiliate with one's age-group.
    e. Change social roles.
    f. Arrange for the most appropriate and appealing living environment.

## C. Lela Llorens

1. Individual is viewed from two perspectives.
   a. Specific period of time, referred to as horizontal development.
   b. Over the course of time, referred to as longitudinal/chronological development.
2. Both of these perspectives occur simultaneously.
3. The integration of these two aspects is critical to normal development.
4. The role of occupational therapy is to facilitate development and assist in the mastery of life tasks and the ability to cope with life expectations.
5. Lloren's frame of reference integrated many of the concepts of Gesell, Amatruda, Erikson, Havighurst, and Freud.

## D. Anne Mosey

1. Recapitulation of ontogenesis.
   a. The development of adaptive skills, which are essential learned behaviors, is considered critical for successful participation in occupational performance.
2. Six major adaptive skills along with subskills are delineated.
   a. Sensory integration of vestibular, proprioceptive, and tactile information for functional use.
      (1) Integration of the tactile subsystems (0-3 months).
      (2) Integration of primitive postural reflexes (3-9 months).
      (3) Maturation of righting and equilibrium reactions (9-12 months).
      (4) Integration of two sides of the body, awareness of body parts and their relationship, and motor plan gross movements (1-2 years).
      (5) Motor plan fine movements (2-3 years).
   b. Cognitive skill: the ability to perceive, represent and organize sensory information to think and problem solve.
      (1) Utilization of inborn behavioral patterns for environmental interaction (0-1 month).
      (2) Interrelation of visual, manual, auditory, and oral responses (1-4 months).
      (3) Early exploration of the environment and interest in outcomes of actions: remembers action responses, believes that own actions cause responses, and has an awareness of the relation of these actions and events (4-9 months).
      (4) Utilization of deliberate actions to achieve a goal: object permanence begins, anticipation of familiar events, imitation, interest in sizes/shapes, and perception of other objects as partially causal (9-12 months).
      (5) Utilization of a trial and error approach to problem solving: tool use, begins to realize that alternate routes can be used, remembers the order of a simple sequence, and realizes that others can cause events to happen (12-18 months).
      (6) Formulation of mental pictures: pretends, early cause and effect, manipulates objects in space, has a clearer understanding that others can manipulate the environment (18 months - 2 years).
      (7) Representation of objects in terms of felt experiences: understands that there are consequences to actions that others cannot read his/her mind, and recognizes that events have causes (2-5 years).

(8) Representation of objects by name: begins to understand that other people may have differing opinions (6-7 years).

(9) Comprehension that different labels can be used for the same object, use of formal logic and speculation (11-13 years).

c. Dyadic interaction skill: the ability to participate in a variety of dyadic relationships.

(1) Family relationships (8-10 months).

(2) Playmate relationships (3-5 years).

(3) Superior/authority relationship interactions (5-7 years).

(4) Friend relationships (10-14 years).

(5) Peer-superior relationships (15-17 years).

(6) Intimate/sharing/committed relationships (18-25 years).

(7) Caring/unselfish relationships (20-30 years).

d. Group interaction skill: the ability to engage in a variety of primary groups.

(1) Parallel group: minimal awareness of or interaction with others (18 months-2 years).

(2) Project group: limited in duration, cooperation, and sharing (2-4 years).

(3) Egocentric group: cooperation, competition, longer in duration, builds self-esteem (9-12 years).

(4) Cooperative group: compatible group, members concerned with meeting the needs of fellow members (9-12 years).

(5) Mature group: differing roles, concerned with completion of task as well as meeting the needs of fellow members (15-18 years).

e. Self-identity skill: the ability to perceive the self as a relatively autonomous, holistic, and acceptable person who has permanence and continuity over time.

(1) Self as a valued person (9-12 months).

(2) Assets and limitations of the self (11-15 years).

(3) Self as self-directed (20-25 years).

(4) Self as a productive, contributing member of a society (30-35 years).

(5) Self identity as an independent individual (35-50 years).

(6) Understanding the aging process of one's self and eventual death as part of the life cycle (45-60 years).

f. Sexual identity skill: the ability to feel comfortable about one's sexual nature and to engage in continued sexual relationship that takes into account mutual satisfaction of sexual needs.

(1) Act on the basis of one's pregenital sexual nature (4-5 years).

(2) Sexually mature as a positive growth experience (12-16 years).

(3) Give and receive sexual gratification (18-25 years).

(4) Sustain sexual relationship with mutual satisfaction of sexual needs (20-30 years).

(5) Accept sex-related physiological changes that occur as a natural part of the aging process (40-60 years).

## VIII. Role of the OTA in Pediatric Evaluation

1. The OTA contributes to the evaluation process.

a. The OTA can assist with the collection of data for the evaluation once service competency has been established.

b. The level of supervision required will be determined by the OTA's experience and established service competency.

c. The OTA cannot independently evaluate or interpret evaluation results

2. Evaluation methods can include parent/family/teacher interview, medical and developmental history, formal and informal observations, and standardized developmental assessments.

3. Primary purposes of parent/family/teacher interviews and home/classroom observations.

a. To explore environmental characteristics related to the child's development.

b. To identify family supports and community resources.

c. To understand cultural values.

4. Developmental considerations in the evaluation of children.

a. Consider appropriate developmental levels in selecting assessments, toys, and other evaluation media.

b. Observe symmetries/asymmetries, stability of trunk, pelvis, hips, and shoulders, at rest and during movement.

c. Observe transitional movement in and out of prone, supine, side-lying, quadruped, sitting, standing, kneeling, half-kneel, and in various sitting positions such as tailor, long, heel, or side-sitting.

d. Assess the quality of movement in and out of

the above positions.

e. Assess fine motor coordination.

f. Consider proper positioning and adaptive equipment, seating, and technology needs.

g. Assess cognition in the context of play and other occupations.

5. Assess psychosocial skills such as the child's coping style, frustration tolerance, and social interaction.

6. Consider visual and auditory status and aides.

## IX. Role of the OTA in Pediatric Intervention

1. The OTA implements intervention with OT supervision.

   a. The level of supervision required depends upon the OTA's experience and established service competency.

   b. During the implementation of intervention, the OTA informs the supervising OT of any change in the child's status and any other relevant information that may affect treatment.

2. Developmental considerations in interventions with children.

   a. All activities, toys, and other intervention media must be appropriate to the child's developmental level.

   b. Play activities should be the primary occupation intervention.

   c. Family education is essential.

      (1) Identify environmental characteristics that facilitate the child's development.

      (2) Provide advocacy training to link families to community.

      (3) Identify psychosocial factors that promote the child's development.

      (4) Teach avoidance of behaviors that may interfere with learning.

      (5) Consider and respect the family's cultural background.

   d. Provide consultation or direct intervention to facilitate school performance and achieve educational goals.

   e. Provide intervention to facilitate sensorimotor, cognitive, and psychosocial development.

   f. Fabricate or requisition positioning equipment and technological aides for home and/or school.

   g. Ensure the proper visual and auditory aides are used during intervention sessions.

   h. See Section III of this text for information on pediatric and developmental clinical conditions and diagnostic-specific interventions.

## X. Child Abuse[2]

### A. Facts and Figures

1. In the United States, child abuse is a major social justice crisis. The below facts and figures are provided to highlight the need for OTAs to be vigilant about the potential of child abuse and neglect in all interactions with children and adult survivors. These statistics will not be on the NBCOT examination.

   a. A report of child abuse is made every ten seconds.

   b. In 2007, an estimated 3.2 million child abuse reports and allegations were made involving approximately 5.8 million children.

   c. Almost five children die each day as a result of child abuse.

      (1) More than 75% of these deaths are children under the age of 4.

      (2) The death of children as a result of maltreatment is thought to be significantly underreported with the majority (60-85%) of child fatalities caused by maltreatment not recorded as such on death certificates.

2. Child abuse can occur in any family. It is evident at all socio-economic levels, in all ethnicities, cultural groups, and religions and at all levels of education.

3. Females make up 58% of abusers and are more likely to be involved in neglect or physical abuse.

4. Males make up 42% of abusers and are more likely to be involved in sexual abuse.

5. 79% of the cases involved abuse by one or both of the parents.

6. The effects of child abuse and neglect continue into adulthood.

   a. It is estimated that the cycle of abuse is continued by 30% of abused and neglected children who as parents abuse their own children,

   b. Approximately 80% of 21 year olds who survived child abuse have at least one diagnosed psychological disorder.

   c. Thirty-one percent of women in prison and 14% of men in prison in the United States are survivors of child abuse.

   d. Over 60% of adults in drug rehabilitation centers report being survivors of child abuse or neglect.

[2]Janice Romeo contributed this section on child abuse.

## B. Definition of Child Abuse

1. Any behavior directed toward a child by a parent, guardian, caregiver, other family member, or other adult that endangers or impairs a child's physical or emotional health and development.

## C. Types of Child Abuse

1. Physical.
2. Emotional or mental.
3. Sexual.
4. Neglect.

## D. Signs of Abuse

1. General signs of abuse.
   a. Withdrawal.
   b. Nightmares.
   c. Running away.
   d. Anxiety or depression.
   e. Guilt.
   f. Mistrust of adults.
   g. Fear.
   h. Aggressiveness.
2. Signs and symptoms of physical abuse.
   a. The child reports being physically mistreated.
   b. Unexplained injuries.
   c. Repeated injuries.
   d. Abrasions and lacerations.
   e. Small circular burns such as cigarette or cigar burns.
   f. Burns with a "doughnut" shape on the buttocks that may indicate scalding, or any burn that shows the pattern of an object used to inflict injury, such as an iron.
   g. Friction burns such as those from a rope.
   h. Unexplained fractures.
   i. Denial, unlikely explanations, or delays in treatment on the part of the caregiver.
   j. Unconsciousness and/or symptoms of a traumatic brain injury due to shaken baby syndrome.
3. Signs and symptoms of emotional or mental abuse.
   a. The child reports being verbally and/or emotionally mistreated.
   b. Aggressive or acting out behavior such as lying or stealing.
   c. Shy, dependent, or defensive appearance.
   d. Verbally abuses others with language that appears to have been directed toward them.
4. Signs and symptoms of sexual abuse.
   a. The child reports being inappropriately approached, touched, and/or assaulted.
   b. Abuse may be physical (e.g., touching), non-physical (e.g., indecent exposure), or violent (e.g., rape), so signs may include emotional and physical indicators.
   c. Precocious sexual behavior or knowledge.
   d. Copying adult sexual behavior.
   e. Inappropriate sexual behavior (e.g., putting tongue in other's mouth when kissing).
   f. Soreness or injury around the genitals.
   g. Reluctance or refusal to let caregivers wash parts of the body.
   h. Sexual play.
5. Signs and symptoms of neglect.
   a. Poorly nourished appearance or inadequately clothed.
   b. Consistently tired or listless behavior.
   c. Inconsistent attendance at school.
   d. Poor hygiene or obsession with cleanliness.
   e. Left alone in dangerous situations, for long periods of time and/or at an inappropriate young age.
   f. Unable to relate well to adults or form friendships.

## E. Role of Occupational Therapy

1. Mandatory reporting.
   a. The federal Child Abuse Prevention and Treatment Act (CAPTA) defined child abuse and neglect and established mandates for professionals to report abuse and neglect to law enforcement officials. See Chapter 4 Section IX C.
   b. All states must have child abuse and neglect reporting laws to qualify for federal funding under CAPTA.
   c. All states require reporting of known or suspected cases of child abuse or neglect by healthcare providers.
      (1) Standards for reporting may vary.
      (2) Reporting to the OTA's direct supervisor may/may not be sufficient.
         (a) The OTA should immediately report any and all concerns to his/her OT supervisor but he/she must be prepared to follow-up as necessary.
   d. Failure to report suspected child abuse may be considered a crime.
   e. In most states, good faith reporting is immune from liability.
   f. All states require reporting to be made to a law enforcement agency or child protective services.
2. Occupational therapy intervention.

a. Treat physical injuries, emotional injuries, and developmental delays.

b. Develop a trusting relationship with child and non-abusive caregivers.

c. Provide support to non-abusive caregivers.

d. Refer to appropriate disciplines and agencies.

# XI. Aging

## A. General Concepts and Definitions

1. Aging: the process of growing old.
   a. Describes a wide array of physiological changes in the body systems.
   b. A complex and variable process.
   c. Common to all members of a given species.
   d. Aging is developmental, occurs across the life span.
   e. Progressive with time.
   f. Evidence of aging.
      (1) Decline in homeostatic efficiency.
      (2) Decline in reaction time.
   g. Varies among and within individuals.
2. Aging changes.
   a. Cellular changes.
      (1) Increase in size; fragmentation of Golgi apparatus and mitochondria.
      (2) Decrease in cell capacity to divide and reproduce.
      (3) Arrest of DNA synthesis and cell division.
   b. Tissue changes.
      (1) Accumulation of pigmented materials, lipofuscins.
      (2) Accumulation of lipids and fats.
      (3) Connective tissue changes: decreased elastic content, degradation of collagen; presence of pseudoelastins.
   c. Organ changes.
      (1) Decrease in functional capacity.
      (2) Decrease in homeostatic efficiency.
3. Gerontology: the scientific study of the factors impacting the normal aging process and the effects of aging.
4. Geriatrics: the branch of medicine concerned with the illnesses of old age and their care.
5. Ageism: discrimination and prejudice leveled against individuals on the basis of their age.
   a. Isolates elders socially.
   b. Permits attitudes and policies that discourage elders from full participation in work, leisure and other meaningful occupations.
   c. Perpetuates fears of aging.
   d. Diminishes quality of life.

## B. Demographics, Mortality, and Morbidity

1. Life span: maximum survival potential, the inherent natural life of the species; in humans 110-120 years.
2. Senescence: the weakening of the body at a gradual but steady pace during the last stages of adulthood through death.
3. Life expectancy: the number of years of life expectation from year of birth.
   a. 77.8 years in U.S.; women live 5.2 years longer than men.
   b. Current trends are contributing to increased life expectancy.
      (1) Advances in health care, improved infectious disease control.
      (2) Advances in infant/child care, decreased mortality rates.
      (3) Improvements in nutrition and sanitation.
4. Categories of elderly.
   a. Young elderly: ages 65-74.
   b. Old elderly: ages 75-84.
   c. Old, old elderly or old & frail elderly: ages > 85.
   d. Young elderly represents 60% of elderly population; old elderly and old, old elderly represent 40% of elderly population.
5. Persons over 65: represents a rapidly growing segment with lengthening of life expectancy.
6. Non-institutionalized elderly: most live in family setting.
7. Institutionalized elderly: about 5% of persons over 65 reside in nursing homes; percentage increases dramatically with age (22% of persons over 85).
8. Most older persons (60-80%) report having one or more chronic conditions.

## B. Muscular System Changes and Adaptation in the Older Adult

1. Age-related changes.
   a. Changes may be due more to decreased activity levels (hypokinesis) and disuse than from the aging process.
   b. Loss of muscle strength: peaks at age 30, remains fairly constant until age 50; after which there is an accelerating loss, 20-40% loss by age 65 in the non-exercising adult.
   c. Loss of power (force/unit time): significant declines, due to losses in speed of contraction, changes in nerve conduction and synaptic transmission.
   d. Loss of skeletal muscle mass (atrophy): both size and number of muscle fibers decrease, by age 70 lose 33% of skeletal muscle mass.

e. Changes in muscle fiber composition: selective loss of Type II, fast twitch fibers, with increase in proportion of Type I fibers.
f. Changes in muscular endurance: muscles fatigue more readily.
   (1) Decreased muscle tissue oxidative capacity.
   (2) Decreased peripheral blood flow, oxygen delivery to muscles.
   (3) Altered chemical composition of muscle: decreased myosin ATPase activity, glycoproteins and contractile protein.
   (4) Collagen changes: denser, irregular due to cross-linkages, loss of water content and elasticity; affects tendons, bone, cartilage.

2. Clinical implications.
   a. Movements become slower.
   b. Increased complaints of fatigue.
   c. Connective tissue becomes denser and stiffer.
      (1) Increased risk of muscle sprains, strains, tendon tears.
      (2) Loss of range of motion: highly variable by joint and individual's activity level.
      (3) Increased tendency for fibrinous adhesions, contractures.
   d. Decreased functional mobility, limitations to movement.
   e. Gait may become unsteady due to changes in balance, strength; increased need for assistive devices.
   f. Increased risk of falls.

3. Strategies to slow or reverse changes.
   a. Improve health.
      (1) Correct medical problems that may cause weakness.
      (2) Improve nutrition.
      (3) Address alcoholism/substance abuse.
   b. Increase levels of physical activity, stress functional activities, and activity programs.
      (1) Gradually increase intensity of activity to avoid injury.
      (2) Plan and include adequate warm-ups and cool downs; appropriate pacing and rest periods.
   c. Provide strength training to increase/maintain muscle strength required for functional activity.
      (1) Significant increases in strength are noted in older adults with isometric and progressive resistive exercise regimes.
      (2) High-intensity training programs (70-80% of one-repetition maximum) produce quicker and more predictable results than moderate intensity programs; both have been successfully used with the elderly.
      (3) Age not a limiting factor; significant improvements noted in 80 and 90 year-old elders who were frail and institutionalized.
      (4) Improvements in strength can improve functional abilities and occupational performance.
      (5) Maintain newly gained and existing strength and incorporate into functional activities.
   d. Provide flexibility and range of motion exercises to increase range of motion needed for functional activity.
      (1) Utilize slow, prolonged stretching, maintained for 20-30 seconds.
      (2) Tissues heated prior to stretching are more distensible, e.g., warm pool.
      (3) Maintain newly gained range: incorporate into functional activities.
      (4) Mobility gains are slower with older adults.

4. See Chapter 6 for additional information on musculoskeletal system disorders and Chapter 11 for information on biomechanical evaluation and intervention approaches.

**C. Skeletal System Changes and Adaptations in the Older Adult**

1. Age-related changes.
   a. Cartilage changes: decreased water content, becomes stiffer, fragments, and erodes; by age 60 more than 60% of adults have degenerative joint changes, cartilage abnormalities.
   b. Loss of bone mass and density: peak bone mass at age 40; between 45 and 70 bone mass decreased (women by about 25%; men 15%); decreases another 5% by age 90.
      (1) Loss of calcium, bone strength: especially trabecular bone.
      (2) Decreased bone marrow red blood cell production.
   c. Intervertebral discs: flatten, less resilient due to loss of water content (30% loss by age 65) and loss of collagen elasticity; trunk length, overall height decreases.
   d. Senile postural changes.
      (1) Forward head.
      (2) Kyphosis of thoracic spine.
      (3) Flattening of lumbar spine.
      (4) With prolonged sitting, tendency to develop

hip and knee flexion contractures.

2. Clinical implications.

a. Maintenance of weight bearing is important for cartilaginous/joint health and mobility.

b. Increased risk of falls and fractures.

3. Strategies to slow or reverse changes.

a. Postural exercises: stress components of good posture.

b. Weight bearing (gravity-loading) exercise can decrease bone loss in older adults, e.g., walking, stair climbing, all activities that are performed in standing.

c. Nutritional, hormonal and medical therapies.

d. See Chapter 15 for information on fall prevention.

4. See Chapter 6 for additional information on musculoskeletal system disorders and Chapter 11 for information on biomechanical evaluation and intervention approaches.

### D. Neurological System Changes and Adaptations in the Older Adult

1. Age-related changes.

a. Atrophy of nerve cells in cerebral cortex.

b. Changes in brain morphology.

(1) Gyral atrophy: narrowing and flattening of gyri with widening of sulci.

(2) Ventricular dilation.

(3) Generalized cell loss in cerebral cortex: especially frontal and temporal lobes, association areas (prefrontal cortex, visual).

(4) Presence of lipofuscins, senile or neuritic plaques, and neurofibrillary tangles (NFT): significant accumulations associated with pathology, e.g., Alzheimer's disease.

(5) More selective cell loss in basal ganglia (substantia nigra and putamen), cerebellum, hippocampus, locus coeruleus; brain stem minimally affected.

c. Decreased cerebral blood flow and energy metabolism.

d. Changes in synaptic transmission.

(1) Decreased synthesis and metabolism of major neurotransmitters, e.g., acetylcholine, dopamine.

(2) Slowing of many neural processes, especially in polysynaptic pathways.

e. Changes in spinal cord/peripheral nerves.

(1) Neuronal loss and atrophy.

(2) Loss of motoneurons results in increase in size of remaining motor units (development of macro motor units).

(3) Slowed nerve conduction velocity: sensory

greater than motor.

(4) Loss of sympathetic fibers: may account for diminished, autonomic stability, increased incidence of postural hypotension in older adults.

f. Age-related tremors (essential tremor, ET).

(1) Occur as an isolated symptom, particularly in hands, head, and voice.

(2) Characterized as postural or kinetic, rarely resting.

(3) Benign, slowly progressive; in late stages may limit function.

(4) Exaggerated by movement and emotion.

2. Clinical implications.

a. Effects on movement.

(1) Overall speed and coordination are decreased; increased difficulties with fine motor control.

(2) Slowed recruitment of motoneurons contributes to loss of strength.

(3) Both reaction time and movement time are increased.

(4) Older adults are affected by the speed/accuracy trade off.

(a) The simpler the movement, the less the change.

(b) More complicated movements require more preparation, longer reaction and movement times.

(c) Faster movements decrease accuracy, increase errors.

(5) Older adults typically shift in motor control processing from open to closed loop: e.g., demonstrate increased reliance on visual feedback for movement.

(6) Demonstrate increased cautionary behaviors, an indirect effect of decreased capacity.

b. General slowing of neural processing: learning and memory may be affected.

c. Problems in homeostatic regulation: stressors (heat, cold, excess exercise) can be harmful, even life-threatening.

3. Strategies to slow or reverse changes.

a. Correct medical problems: improve cerebral blood flow.

b. Improve health: diet, smoking cessation.

c. Increase levels of physical activity: may encourage neuronal branching, slow rate of neural decline, and improve cerebral circulation.

d. Provide effective strategies to improve motor learning and control.

(1) Allow for increased reaction and movement times: will improve motivation, accuracy of movements.

(2) Allow for limitations of memory: avoid long sequences of movements.

(3) Allow for increased cautionary behaviors: provide adequate explanation, demonstration when teaching new movement skills.

(4) Stress familiar, well-learned skills; repetitive movements.

4. See Chapter 7 for additional information on neurological system disorders and Chapter 12 for information on neurological evaluation and intervention approaches.

## E. Sensory Systems Changes and Adaptations in the Older Adult

1. Age-related changes: older adults experience a loss of function of the senses.

   a. May lead to sensory deprivation, isolation, disorientation, confusion, appearance of senility and depression.

   b. May strain social interactions and decrease ability to interact socially and with the environment.

   c. May lead to decreased functional mobility and increased risk of injury.

   d. Alters quality of life.

2. Vision.

   a. Aging changes: there is a general decline in visual acuity; gradual prior to sixth decade, rapid decline between ages 60 and 90; visual loss may be as much as 80% by age 90; changes include:

      (1) Presbyopia: visual loss in middle and older ages characterized by inability to focus properly and blurred images, due to loss of accommodation, elasticity of lens.

      (2) Decreased ability to adapt to dark and light.

      (3) Increased sensitivity to light and glare.

      (4) Loss of color discrimination, especially for blues and greens.

      (5) Decreased pupillary responses, size of resting pupil increases.

      (6) Decreased sensitivity of corneal reflex: less sensitive to eye injury or infection.

      (7) Oculomotor responses diminished: restricted upward gaze, reduced pursuit eye movements; ptosis may develop.

   b. Additional vision loss with pathology.

      (1) Cataracts: opacity, clouding of lens due to changes in lens proteins; results in gradual loss of vision: central first, then peripheral; increased problems with glare; general darkening of vision; loss of acuity, distortion.

         (a) Surgery is an effective treatment.

      (2) Glaucoma: increased intraocular pressure, with degeneration of optic disc, atrophy of optic nerve; results in early loss of peripheral vision (tunnel vision).

         (a) If untreated, it can progress to total blindness.

         (b) If diagnosis is made early, surgery and/or medications are effective treatments.

      (3) Macular degeneration: loss of central vision associated with age-related degeneration of the macula compromised by decreased blood supply or abnormal growth of blood vessels under the retina; typically individuals retain some peripheral vision; increased sensitivity to glare, and difficulty adjusting to light changes; may progress to total blindness.

      (4) Diabetic retinopathy: damage to retinal capillaries, growth of abnormal blood vessels and hemorrhage leads to retinal scarring and finally retinal detachment; central vision is impaired, vision is blurred; complete blindness is rare.

         (a) A complication of diabetes mellitus.

      (5) CVA, homonymous hemianopsia: loss of ½ visual field in each eye (nasal half of one eye and temporal half of other eye); produces an inability to receive information from right or left side; corresponds to side of sensorimotor deficit.

      (6) Medications: impaired or fuzzy vision may result with antihistamines, anti-psychotics, anti-depressants, steroids.

   c. Clinical implications/compensatory strategies.

      (1) Assess for visual deficits: acuity, peripheral vision, light and dark adaptation, depth perception; diplopia, eye fatigue, eye pain.

      (2) Maximize visual function: assess for use of glasses, need for environmental adaptations. Refer to Chapter 15.

      (3) Sensory thresholds are increased: allow extra time for visual discrimination and response.

      (4) Work in adequate light, increase intensity,

reduce glare; avoid abrupt changes in light, e.g., light to dark.

(5) Use large, high contrast print for written materials.

(6) Provide magnifying glasses (either portable or attached to a stand/work table) to view objects and complete tasks.

(7) Provide an eye patch for diplopia.

(8) Decreased peripheral vision may limit social interactions; therefore, stand directly in front of the person at eye level when communicating with him/her.

(9) Assist in color discrimination: use warm colors (yellow, orange, red) for identification and color coding.

(10) Provide other sensory cues when vision is limited, e.g., verbal descriptions to new environments, touching to communicate you are listening, "talking" clocks and watches.

(11) Provide safety education; reduce fall risk.

3. Hearing.

a. Aging changes: occur as early as fourth decade; affects a significant number of elderly (23% of individuals aged 65-74 have hearing impairments and 40% over age 75 have hearing loss; rate of loss in men is twice the rate of women, also starts earlier).

(1) Outer ear: buildup of cerumen (ear wax) may result in conductive hearing loss; common in older men.

(2) Middle ear: minimal degenerative changes of bony joints.

(3) Inner ear: significant changes in sound sensitivity, understanding of speech, and maintenance of equilibrium may result with degeneration and atrophy of cochlea and vestibular structures, loss of neurons.

b. Types of hearing loss.

(1) Conductive: mechanical hearing loss from damage to external auditory canal, tympanic membrane or middle ear ossicles; results in hearing loss (all frequencies); tinnitus (ringing in the ears) may be present.

(2) Sensorineural: central or neural hearing loss from multiple factors, e.g., noise damage, trauma, disease, drugs, arteriosclerosis, etc.

(3) Presbycusis: sensorineural hearing loss associated with middle and older ages;

characterized by bilateral hearing loss, especially at high frequencies at first, then all frequencies; poor auditory discrimination and comprehension, especially with background noise; tinnitus.

c. Additional hearing loss with pathology.

(1) Otosclerosis: immobility of stapes results in profound conductive hearing loss.

(2) Paget's disease.

(3) Hypothyroidism.

d. Clinical implications/compensatory strategies.

(1) Assess for hearing: acuity, speech discrimination/comprehension; tinnitus, dizziness, vertigo, pain.

(2) Assess for use of hearing aids; check for proper functioning.

(3) Minimize auditory distractions, work in quiet environment.

(4) Speak slowly and clearly, directly in front of person at eye level.

(5) Use nonverbal communication to reinforce your message, e.g. gesture, demonstration.

(6) Provide written and demonstrated directions/guidelines for activities.

(7) Orient person to topics of conversation he/she cannot hear to reduce paranoia, isolation.

(8) Provide assistive devices to compensate for functional effects of hearing loss and to ensure person's safety, e.g., vibrating and flashing smoke alarms, telephones, doorbells, and clocks.

4. Vestibular/balance control.

a. Aging changes: degenerative changes in otoconia of utricle and saccule; loss of vestibular hair-cell receptors; decreased number of vestibular neurons; vestibular ocular reflex (VOR) gain decreases; begins at age 30, accelerating decline at ages 55-60 resulting in diminished vestibular sensation.

(1) Diminished acuity, delayed reaction times, longer response times.

(2) Reduced function of VOR; affects retinal image stability with head movements, produces blurred vision.

(3) Altered sensory organization: older adults more dependent upon somatosensory inputs for balance.

(4) Less able to resolve sensory conflicts when presented with inappropriate visual or pro-

prioceptive inputs due to vestibular losses.

(5) Postural response patterns for balance are disorganized: characterized by diminished ankle torque, increased hip torque, increased postural sway.

b. Additional loss of vestibular sensitivity with pathology.

(1) Mèniére's disease: episodic attacks characterized by tinnitus, dizziness, and a sensation of fullness or pressure in the ears; may also experience sensorineural hearing loss.

(2) Benign paroxysmal positional vertigo (BPPV): brief episodes of vertigo (less than 1 minute) associated with position change; the result of degeneration of the utricular otoconia that settle on the cupula of the posterior semicircular canal; common in older adults.

(3) Medications: antihypertensives (postural hypotension); anticonvulsants; tranquilizers, sleeping pills, aspirin, NSAIDS.

(4) Cerebrovascular disease: vertebrobasilar artery insufficiency (TIAs, strokes); cerebellar artery stroke, lateral medullary stroke.

(5) Cerebellar dysfunction: hemorrhage, tumors (acoustic neuroma, meningioma); degenerative disease of brain stem and cerebellum; progressive supranuclear palsy.

(6) Migraine.

(7) Cardiac disease.

c. Clinical implications/compensatory strategies.

(1) Increased incidence of falls in older adults.

(2) Refer to Chapter 15 for information on fall prevention.

5. Somatosensory.

a. Aging changes.

(1) Decreased sensitivity of touch associated with decline of peripheral receptors, atrophy of afferent fibers: lower extremities more affected than upper.

(2) Proprioceptive losses, increased thresholds in vibratory sensibility, beginning around age 50: greater in lower extremities than upper extremities, greater in distal extremities than proximal.

(3) Loss of joint receptor sensitivity; losses in lower extremities, cervical joints may contribute to loss of balance.

(4) Cutaneous pain thresholds increased:

greater changes in upper body areas (upper extremities, face) than for lower extremities.

b. Additional loss of sensation with pathology.

(1) Diabetes, peripheral neuropathy.

(2) CVA, central sensory losses.

(3) Peripheral vascular disease, peripheral ischemia.

c. Clinical implications/compensatory strategies.

(1) Assess carefully: check for increased thresholds to stimulation, sensory losses by modality, area of body.

(2) Allow extra time for responses with increased thresholds.

(3) Use touch to communicate: maximize physical contact, e.g., rubbing, stroking, tapping.

(4) Provide augmented feedback through appropriate sensory channels, e.g., using kitchen utensils with wide textured grips may be easier than narrow smooth handles.

(5) Teach compensatory strategies to prevent injury to anesthetic limbs.

(6) Provide assistive devices and environmental modifications as needed for fall prevention. See Chapter 15 for further information.

(7) Provide biofeedback devices as appropriate (e.g., limb load monitor).

6. Taste and smell.

a. Aging changes.

(1) Gradual decrease in taste sensitivity.

(2) Decreased smell sensitivity.

b. Conditions resulting in additional loss of sensation.

(1) Smoking.

(2) Chronic allergies, respiratory infections.

(3) Dentures.

(4) CVA, involvement of hypoglossal nerve.

c. Clinical implications/compensatory strategies.

(1) Assess for identification of odors, tastes (sweet, sour, bitter, salty); somatic sensations (temperature, touch).

(2) Decreased taste, enjoyment of food leads to poor diet and nutrition.

(3) Older adults frequently increase use of taste enhancers: e.g. salt or sugar.

(4) Decreased home safety: e.g., inability to sense gas leaks, smoke.

**F. Cognitive Changes and Adaptations in the Older Adult**

1. Age-related changes.

a. No uniform decline in intellectual abilities throughout adulthood.
   (1) Changes do not typically show up until mid 60s; significant declines affecting everyday life do not show up until early 80s.
   (2) Most significant decline in measures of intelligence occurs in the years immediately preceding death (termed terminal drop).
b. Tasks involving perceptual speed show early declines (by age 39); require longer times to complete tasks.
c. Numeric ability (tests of adding, subtracting, multiplying): abilities peak in mid-40s, well maintained until 60s.
d. Verbal ability: abilities peak at age 30, well maintained until 60s.
e. Memory.
   (1) Impairments are typically noted in short-term memory; long-term memory retained.
   (2) Impairments are task dependent, e.g., deficits primarily with novel conditions, new learning.
f. Learning: all age groups can learn. Factors affecting learning in older adults.
   (1) Increased cautiousness.
   (2) Anxiety.
   (3) Sensory deficits.
   (4) Pace of learning: fast pace is problematic.
   (5) Interference from prior learning.
2. Clinical implications.
   a. Older adults utilize different strategies for memory: context-based strategies vs. memorization (young adults).
3. Strategies to slow or reverse changes.
   a. Improve health.
      (1) Correct medical problems: imbalances between oxygen supply and demand to CNS, e.g., cardiovascular disease, hypertension, diabetes, hypothyroidism.
      (2) Assess needed pharmacological changes: drug reevaluation; decrease use of multiple drugs; monitor closely for drug toxicity.
      (3) Reduce chronic use of tobacco and alcohol.
      (4) Correct nutritional deficiencies.
   b. Increase physical activity.
   c. Increase mental activity.
      (1) Keep mentally engaged, "Use it or Lose it"; e.g., chess, crossword puzzles, book discussion groups, reading to children.
      (2) Maintain an engaged lifestyle: socially active, e.g., clubs, travel, work, volunteerism; allow for personal choice in activity.
      (3) Use cognitive training activities.
   d. Provide multiple sensory cues to compensate for decreased sensory processing and sensory losses and to maximize learning, e.g., provide visual demonstrations, written instructions, verbal cues.
   e. Provide stimulating, "enriching" environment; avoid environmental dislocation, e.g., hospitalization or institutionalization may produce disorientation and agitation in some elderly.
   f. Reduce stress; provide counseling and family support.

**G. Cardiopulmonary System Changes and Adaptations in the Older Adult**
1. Cardiovascular age-related changes.
   a. Changes due more to inactivity and disease than aging.
   b. Degeneration of heart muscle.
   c. Decreased coronary blood flow.
   d. Cardiac valves thicken and stiffen.
   e. Changes in conduction system: loss of pace maker cells in SA node.
   f. Changes in blood vessels: arteries thicken, less distensible; slowed exchange capillary walls; increased peripheral resistance.
   g. Resting blood pressures rise: systolic greater than diastolic.
   h. Decreased blood volume, hemopoietic activity of bone.
   i. Increased blood coagulability.
2. Clinical implications for cardiovascular changes.
   a. Changes at rest are minor: resting heart rate and cardiac output relatively unchanged; resting blood pressures increase.
   b. Cardiovascular responses to exercise: blunted, decreased heart rate acceleration, decreased maximal oxygen uptake and heart rate; reduced exercise capacity, increased recovery time.
   c. Decreased stroke volume due to decreased myocardial contractility.
   d. Maximum heart rate declines with age.
   e. Cardiac output decreases, 1% per year after age 20: due to decreased heart rate and stroke volume.
   f. Orthostatic hypotension: common problem in elderly due to reduced baroreceptor sensitivity and vascular elasticity.
   g. Increased fatigue; anemia common in elderly.

h. Systolic ejection murmur common in elderly.

i. Possible ECG changes: loss of normal sinus rhythm; increased arrhythmias.

3. Pulmonary system age-related changes.

a. Chest wall stiffness, declining strength of respiratory muscles results in increased work of breathing.

b. Loss of lung elastic recoil, decreased lung compliance.

c. Changes in lung parenchyma: alveoli enlarge, become thinner; fewer capillaries for delivery of blood.

d. Changes in pulmonary blood vessels: thicken, less distensible.

e. Decline in total lung capacity: residual volume increases, vital capacity decreases.

f. Forced expiratory volume (air flow) decreases.

g. Altered pulmonary gas exchange: oxygen tension falls with age (at a rate of 4mmHg/decade; $PaO_2$ at age 70 is 75, versus 90 at age 20).

h. Blunted ventilatory responses of chemoreceptors in response to respiratory acidosis: decreased homeostatic responses.

i. Blunted defense/immune responses: decreased ciliary action to clear secretions, decreased secretory immunoglobulins.

4. Clinical implications for pulmonary changes.

a. Respiratory responses to exercise: similar to younger adult at low and moderate intensities; at higher intensities, responses include increased ventilatory cost of work, greater blood acidosis, increased likelihood of breathlessness, and increased perceived exertion.

b. Clinical signs of hypoxia are blunted; changes in mentation and affect may provide important cues.

c. Cough mechanism is impaired.

d. Gag reflex is decreased, increased risk of aspiration.

e. Recovery from respiratory illness: prolonged in the elderly.

f. Significant changes in function with chronic smoking, exposure to environmental toxic inhalants.

5. Strategies to slow or reverse changes in cardiopulmonary systems.

a. Complete a cardiopulmonary assessment prior to commencing an exercise program.

(1) This is essential in older adults due to the high incidence of cardiopulmonary pathologies.

(2) Select an appropriate graded exercise testing protocol.

(3) Standardized test batteries and norms for elderly are not available.

(4) Many elderly cannot tolerate maximal testing; submaximal testing commonly used.

(5) Testing and training modes should be similar.

b. Individualized exercise prescription is essential.

(1) Choice of training program is based on: fitness level, presence or absence of cardiovascular disease, musculoskeletal limitations, individual's goals, roles, and activity interests.

(2) Prescriptive elements (frequency, intensity, duration, mode) are the same as for younger adults.

(3) Walking, chair and floor exercises, Yoga, Tai-Chi, and modified strength/flexibility calisthenics are well-tolerated by most elderly.

(4) Consider pool programs (exercises, Ai-Chi, walking, swimming) for persons with musculoskeletal and neurological impairments.

(5) Consider multiple modes of exercise on alternate days to maintain interest and reduce likelihood of muscle injury, joint overuse, pain, fatigue, and boredom.

c. Aerobic training programs can significantly improve cardiopulmonary function in the elderly.

(1) Decreases heart rate at a given submaximal power output.

(2) Improves maximal oxygen uptake ($VO_2$max).

(3) Greater improvements in peripheral adaptation, muscle oxidative capacity then central changes.

(4) Improves recovery heart rates.

(5) Decreases systolic blood pressure, may produce a small decrease in diastolic blood pressure.

(6) Increases maximum ventilatory capacity: vital capacity.

(7) Reduces breathlessness, lowers perceived exertion.

(8) Psychological gains, improves sense of well-being, self-image.

(9) Improves functional capacity.

d.  Improve overall daily activity levels for independent living.

(1)  Lack of exercise/activity is an important risk factor in the development of cardiopulmonary diseases.

(2)  Lack of exercise/activity contributes to problems of immobility and disability in the elderly.

6.  See Chapter 8 for additional information on cardiovascular and pulmonary system disorders and cardiopulmonary evaluation and intervention approaches.

## H.  Other Systems Changes and Adaptations in the Older Adult

1.  Integumentary changes.

a.  Changes in skin composition.

(1)  Dermis thins with loss of elastin.

(2)  Decreased vascularity; vascular fragility results in easy bruising (senile purpura).

(3)  Decreased sebaceous activity and decline in hydration.

(4)  Appearance: skin appears dry, wrinkled, yellowed, and inelastic; aging spots appear (clusters of melanocyte pigmentation); increased with exposure to sun.

(5)  General thinning and graying of hair due to vascular insufficiency and decreased melanin production.

(6)  Nails grow more slowly, become brittle and thick.

b.  Loss of effectiveness as protective barrier.

(1)  Skin grows and heals more slowly, less able to resist injury and infection.

(2)  Inflammatory response is attenuated.

(3)  Decreased sensitivity to touch, perception of pain and temperature; increased risk for injury from concentrated pressures or excess temperatures.

(4)  Decreased sweat production with loss of sweat glands results in decreased temperature regulation and homeostasis.

2.  Gastrointestinal changes.

a.  Decreased salivation, taste, and smell along with inadequate chewing (tooth loss, poorly fitting dentures); poor swallowing reflex may lead to poor dietary intake, nutritional deficiencies.

b.  Esophagus: reduced motility and control of lower esophageal sphincter; acid reflux and heartburn, hiatal hernia common.

c.  Stomach: reduced motility, delayed gastric emptying; decreased digestive enzymes and hydrochloric acid; decreased digestion and absorption; indigestion common.

d.  Decreased intestinal motility; constipation common.

3.  Renal, urogenital changes.

a.  Kidneys: loss of mass and total weight with nephron atrophy, decreased renal blood flow, decreased filtration.

(1)  Blood urea rises.

(2)  Decreased excretory and reabsorptive capacities.

b.  Bladder: muscle weakness; decreased capacity causing urinary frequency; difficulty with emptying causing increased retention.

(1)  Urinary incontinence common (affects over 10 million adults; over half of nursing home residents and one third of community dwelling elders); affects older women with pelvic floor weakness and older men with bladder or prostate disease.

(2)  Increased likelihood of urinary tract infections.

## I.  Nutrition and the Elderly

1.  Many older adults have primary nutrition problems.

a.  Nutritional problems in the elderly are often linked to health status and poverty rather than to age itself.

(1)  Chronic diseases alter the overall need for nutrients, the abilities to take in and utilize nutrients, energy demands, and overall activity levels (e.g., Alzheimer's disease, CVA, diabetes).

(2)  Limited, fixed incomes severely limit food choices and availability.

b.  There is an age-related slowing in basal metabolic rate and a decline in total caloric intake; most of the decline is associated with a concurrent reduction in physical activity.

(1)  Both undernourishment and obesity exist in the elderly and contribute to decreased levels of vitality and fitness.

c.  Contributing factors to poor dietary intake.

(1)  Decreased sense of taste and smell.

(2)  Poor teeth or poorly fitting dentures.

(3)  Reduced gastrointestinal function.

(a)  Decreased saliva.

(b)  Gastromucosal atrophy.

(c)  Reduced intestinal mobility; reflux.

(4)  Loss of interest in foods.

(5)  Isolation, lack of social support, no social-

ization during meals, loss of spouse, loss of friends.

    (6) Lack of functional mobility.

      (a) Inability to get to a grocery store to shop.

      (b) Inability to prepare foods.

  d. Dehydration is common in the elderly, resulting in fluid and electrolyte disturbances.

    (1) Thirst sensation is diminished.

    (2) May be physically unable to acquire/maintain fluids.

    (3) Environmental heat stresses may be life threatening and should be treated as medical emergencies.

  e. Diets are often deficient in nutrients, especially vitamins A and C, B12, thiamine, protein, iron, calcium, vitamin D, folic acid, and zinc.

  f. Increased use of alcohol or taste enhancers (e.g., salt and sugar) influences nutritional intake.

  g. Drug/dietary interactions influence nutritional intake (e.g., reserpine, digoxin, anti-tumor agents, excessive use of antacids).

2. Assessment.

  a. Dietary history: patterns of eating, types of foods.

  b. Psychosocial: mental status, desire to eat, depression, grief, social isolation, social supports.

  c. Body composition.

    (1) Weight/height measures.

    (2) Skin fold measurements: triceps/subscapular skin fold thickness.

    (3) Upper arm circumference.

  d. Olfactory and gustatory sensory function.

  e. Dental and periodontal disease, fit of dentures.

  f. Ability to feed self: mastication, swallowing, hand/mouth control, posture, physical weakness and fatigue.

  g. Integumentary: skin condition, edema.

  h. Compliance to special diets.

  i. Functional assessment: basic activities of daily living, feeding; overall exercise/activity levels.

3. Goals and interventions.

  a. Assist in monitoring adequate nutritional intake.

  b. Assist in maintaining nutritional support.

    (1) Refer to dietitian, nutritional consultants and/or nutritional education programs as needed.

    (2) Make recommendations for home health

aide to assist with grocery shopping and meal preparation.

    (3) Refer to elderly food programs: home delivered, i.e., "meals on wheels"; congregate meals/senior center daily meal programs; federal food stamp programs.

  c. Maintain physical function and promote adequate activity levels.

  d. Maintain independence in food preparation and self feeding.

    (1) Teach work simplification and energy conservation techniques to maximize function.

    (2) Modify the environment and adapt activities to enhance mastery and ensure safety.

    (3) See Chapters 14 and 15 for more details.

**J. Elder and Vulnerable Adult Abuse[3]**

1. Facts and figures.

  a. Statistics are difficult to accurately assess due to limited reporting. In the United States, the abuse of vulnerable and older adults is a social justice and health care crisis. The below facts and figures are provided to highlight the need for OTAs to be vigilant about the potential of abuse, neglect, and exploitation in all interactions with vulnerable and older adults. These statistics will not be on the NBCOT examination.

  b. According to the best available estimates, in the United States between 1 and 2 million older adults (age 65 or older) are victims of abuse, neglect, and/or exploitation.

  c. Nationally, Adult Protective Services (APS) investigated 565,747 reports of elder and vulnerable adult abuse in 2004. This represents a 19.7% increase from the APS 2000 Survey

  d. Nationally, APS substantiated 191,908 reports of elder and vulnerable adult abuse.

  e. Most (65.7%) reported elder abuse victims were female.

  f. Many (42.8%) were 80 years of age and older.

  g. The vast majority (89.3%) of reported elder abuse was about incidences in private homes.

2. Definitions vary; however, there are three basic categories.

  a. Domestic elder abuse.

  b. Institutional elder abuse.

  c. Self-neglect or self-abuse.

3. Signs and symptoms of elder abuse.

  a. Physical abuse signs and symptoms.

    (1) An elder's report of being physically mistreated.

[3]Janice Romeo contributed this section on elder abuse.

(2) Bruises, black eyes, welts and/or lacerations.

(3) Rope marks and/or other signs of restraint.

(4) Bone and skull fractures, sprains and/or dislocations.

(5) Open wounds, cuts, and untreated injuries in various stages of healing.

(6) Internal injuries/bleeding.

(7) Broken eyeglasses.

(8) Under- or overdosing of prescribed drugs.

(9) A sudden change in behavior.

(10) The caregiver's refusal to allow visitors to see an elder alone.

b. Sexual abuse signs and symptoms.

(1) An elder's report of sexual assault or rape.

(2) Bruises around the breasts or genital area.

(3) Unexplained venereal disease or genital infection.

(4) Unexplained vaginal or anal bleeding.

(5) Torn, stained, or bloody underclothing.

c. Emotional/psychological abuse signs and symptoms.

(1) An elder's report of being verbally or emotionally mistreated.

(2) Emotionally upset or agitated behavior.

(3) Extremely withdrawn and non-communicative or non-responsive behavior.

(4) Unusual behavior such as sucking, biting, or rocking.

d. Neglect signs and symptoms.

(1) An elder's report of being mistreated.

(2) Dehydration, malnutrition, untreated bedsores, and poor personal hygiene.

(3) Unattended or untreated health problems.

(4) Hazardous or unsafe living conditions.

e. Financial or material exploitation signs and symptoms.

(1) An elder's report of financial exploitation.

(2) Sudden changes in bank account or banking practice.

(3) The inclusion of additional names on an elder's bank signature card.

(4) Unauthorized withdrawal using an ATM card.

(5) Abrupt changes in a will or other financial documents.

(6) Substandard care or unpaid bills despite the availability of funds.

(7) Discovery of a forged signature.

(8) Sudden appearance of relatives claiming rights to decisions, money, or possessions.

(9) Unexplained transfer of funds.

(10) The provision of unnecessary services.

4. Role of occupational therapy.

a. Mandatory reporting.

(1) Elder abuse per se may or may not be designated as a specific crime in a state; however, most physical, sexual, and financial/material abuse are crimes in all states.

(2) Healthcare workers are required to report suspected or observed cases of elder abuse.

(3) Failure to report may be considered a crime.

(4) In most states Adult Protective Services, the area Agency on Aging, or the county Department of Social Services is designated to provide investigation and services.

b. Occupational therapy intervention.

(1) Treat for physical and emotional injuries.

(2) Develop a trusting relationship.

(3) Assist in developing a support system.

(4) Refer to appropriate disciplines and/or agencies.

# References

Abrams, W., Beers, M., & Berkow, R. (Eds.). (1995). *The Merck manual of geriatrics* (2nd ed.). Whitehouse Station, NJ: Merck and Co.

*Abuse of children: The signs and symptoms.* (2001). Cyber-parent, Available: www.cyberparent.com/abuse/childabuse.

Ayres, A.J. (1998). *Sensory integration and the child* (13th ed.). Los Angeles: Western Psychological Services.

Bottomley JM, Lewis CB (2003). *Geriatric rehabilitation – A clinical approach,* 2nd ed. Upper Saddle River NJ, Pearson Education.

Bundy, A.C., & Murray, E.A., (2002). Sensory integration: A. Jean Ayres' theory revisited. In A. C., Bundy, S.J. Lane, & E. A. Murray, (Eds.) *Sensory integration: Theory and practice* (2nd ed., pp. 3-33). Philadelphia: F.A. Davis.

Case-Smith, J. (Ed.). (2001). *Occupational therapy for children* (4th ed). St. Louis, MO: Mosby.

Case-Smith, J. & Humphry, R. (2005). Feeding intervention. In J. Case-Smith Ed.), *Occupational therapy for children* (5th ed., pp. 485-520). St. Louis, MO: Elsevier Mosby.

Case-Smith, J. & Shortridge, S. (1996). The developmental process. In J. Case-Smith, A. Allen, & P.N. Pratt (Eds.), *Occupational therapy for children,* 3rd ed, (44-66). St Louis, MO: Mosby.

*Child help. (2010). National Child Abuse Statistics.* Retrieved February 19, 2010, from http://www.childhelp.org/resources/learning-center/statistics .

Child Welfare Information Gateway. (2006). *Child abuse and neglect fatalities: Statistics and interventions.* Washington DC: Author.

Dunbar, S.B. (2007). Theory, frame of reference and model: A differentiation for practice considerations. In S.B. Dunbar (Ed.), *Occupational therapy models for intervention with children and families* (pp.1-9). Thorofare, NJ: Slack.

Erhardt, R.P. (1994). *The Erhardt Developmental Prehension Assessment.* Maplewood, MN: Erhardt Developmental Products.

Escolar, D.M. & Toisi, L.L. (2005). Muscles, bones and nerves. In M.L. Batshaw, L. Pellegrino, & N.J. Roizen (Ed.), *Children with disabilities* (6th ed., pp. 203-215). Baltimore, MD: Paul H. Brooks.

Kaplan, J.I., & Sadock, B.J. (2007). *Synopsis of psychiatry* (10th ed.). Philadelphia: Mosby

Klein, M. (1987). *Pre-scissor skills* (Rev. ed.). Tuscon, AZ: Therapy Skill Builders.

Lane, S.J. (2002). Structure and function of the sensory systems. In A.C., Bundy, Lane, S.J. & E.A. Murray, (Eds.), *Sensory integration: Theory and practice,* 2nd ed. (35-68). Philadelphia: F.A. Davis.

Lane, S.J. (2002). Sensory modulation. In A.C., Bundy, S.J. Lane, & E.A. Murray, (Eds.), *Sensory integration: Theory and practice*, 2nd ed. (101-122). Philadelphia: F.A. Davis.

Law, M, Missiuna, C., Pollock, N. & Stewart, D. (2005,). Foundations for occupational therapy practice with children. In J. Case-Smith, J. (Ed). *Occupational therapy for children, 5th ed.* (pp. 53-87). St. Louis, MO: Elsevier Mosby..

Miller, L.J. (2006). *Sensational kids hope and help for children with sensory processing disorders* (SPD). NY: G.P. Putnam's Sons.

Mosey, A.C. (1996). *Psychosocial components of occupational therapy.* Philadelphia: Lippincott-Raven.

National Center on Elder Abuse. (2005). *Fact sheet: Elder abuse prevalence and incidence.* Washington, DC.

Parham, L. D. & Mailoux, Z. (2005). Sensory integration. In J, Case-Smith (Ed.), *Occupational therapy for children,* 5th ed. (356-409). St. Louis, MO: Elsevier Mosby.

Parks, S. (1994). *Hawaii Early Learning Profile (HELP) manual.* Palo Alto, CA: Vort Corporation.

Reeves, G.D. & Cermak, S.A. (2002). Disorders of praxis. In A.C., Bundy, S.J. Lane, & E.A. Murray, (Eds.), *Sensory integration: Theory and practice* (2nd ed., pp. 71-100). Philadelphia: F.A. Davis.

Rogers, S. (2005). Common conditions that influence children's participation. In J. Case-Smith (Ed). *Occupational therapy for children* (5th ed., pp.160-215). St. Louis, MO: Elsevier Mosby.

Shepherd, J. (2005). Activities of daily living and adaptations for independent living. In J. Case-Smith, (Ed.), *Occupational therapy for children,* 5th ed. (521-570). St. Louis, MO: Elsevier Mosby.

Smith, S.K. *Mandatory reporting of child abuse and neglect* (2001). Available: www.smithlawfirm.com

Teaster, P., Dugar, T. Mendiondo, M., Abner, E.Cecil, K. & Otto, J. (2006). *The 2004 Survey of State Adult Protective Services: Abuse of Adults 60 Years and Older.* Washington DC: National Center on Elder Abuse.

Vergara, E. (1993). *Foundations for practice in the neonatal intensive care unit and early intervention.* (Volume 2, pp. 34-35). Baltimore, MD: American Occupational Therapy Association.

# CHAPTER 6

# MUSCULOSKELETAL SYSTEM DISORDERS

## Colleen Maher

## I. Anatomy of the Musculoskeletal System

### A. Relationship to the Examination

1. It is not likely that the NBCOT exam will ask direct questions about anatomy or physiology.
2. As a result, this chapter does not provide a complete anatomy and physiology review[1].
3. Major structures and functions of the musculoskeletal system are outlined because knowledge of these can help determine the best answer. For example, damage to the opponens pollicis would result in the need to use activities that do not require opposition.

### B. Anatomy of the Hand

1. Intrinsic muscles innervated by the median nerve (Figure 6-1).
   a. Abductor pollicis brevis.
      (1) Origin: scaphoid, trapezium, flexor retinaculum, and tendon of the abductor pollicis longus.
      (2) Insertion: base of proximal phalanx, radial side of thumb.
      (3) Function: palmar abduction.
   b. Opponens pollicis.
      (1) Origin: trapezium and flexor retinaculum.
      (2) Insertion: first metacarpal.
      (3) Function: opposition.
   c. Flexor pollicis brevis: superficial head.
      (1) Origin: trapezium, trapezoid, capitate and flexor retinaculum.
      (2) Insertion: base of proximal phalanx, radial side of thumb.
      (3) Function: thumb MCP flexion, deep head innervated by ulnar nerve.
   d. Lumbricals (radial side).
      (1) Origin: tendons of flexor digitorum profundus, index and middle fingers (radial and palmar sides).

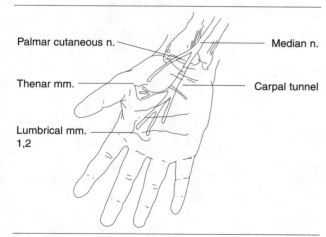

**Figure 6-1** Median Nerve
Malick, M. and Kasch, M. (1984). *Manual on management of specific hand problems.* Pittsburgh, PA: AREN. Reprinted with permission.

Palmar cutaneous n.

Median n.

Thenar mm.

Carpal tunnel

Lumbrical mm. 1,2

---

[1] This anatomy section focuses on prime movers. It is unlikely that knowledge of secondary movers will be required for success on the NBCOT examination. In addition, the examination does not directly test knowledge of origins and insertions. This information is included because some individuals find visualizing a muscle's location helpful to remembering its function.

(2) Insertion: radial side of digits II and III into extensor expansion.

(3) Function: MCP flexion and extension of IP joints.

2. Intrinsic muscles innervated by the ulnar nerve (Figure 6-2).

   a. Abductor digiti minimi.

     (1) Origin: pisiform and tendon of flexor carpi ulnaris.

     (2) Insertion: proximal phalanx of the 5th digit.

     (3) Function: abduction of the 5th digit.

   b. Opponens digiti minimi.

     (1) Origin: hook of hamate and flexor retinaculum.

     (2) Insertion: fifth metacarpal.

     (3) Function: opposition of the fifth digit.

   c. Flexor digiti minimi.

     (1) Origin: hook of hamate and flexor retinaculum.

     (2) Insertion: proximal phalanx of fifth digit.

     (3) Function: flexion of MCP joint and opposition of the fifth digit.

   d. Lumbricals (ulnar side).

     (1) Origin: tendons of flexor digitorum profundus for digits IV and V.

     (2) Insertion: radial side of digits IV and V into extensor expansion.

     (3) Function: MCP flexion and extension of IP joints of digits IV and V.

   e. Palmar interossei.

     (1) Origin: first palmar; ulnar surface of 2nd metacarpal. Second palmar; radial surface of 4th metacarpal. Third palmar; radial surface of 5th metacarpal.

     (2) Insertion: first palmar; ulnar surface of 2nd proximal phalanx. Second palmar; radial surface of 4th proximal phalanx. Third palmar; radial surface of 5th proximal phalanx.

     (3) Function: adduction and assistance with MCP flexion and extension of IP joints of digits II through V.

   f. Dorsal interossei.

     (1) Origin: all four muscles arise from the adjacent sides of the metacarpals.

     (2) Insertion: proximal phalanx on the radial aspect of the index, radial and ulnar sides of middle finger, and ulnar side of ring finger (all into extensor digitorum).

     (3) Function: abduction and assists with MCP flexion and extension of IP joints of digits II through V.

3. Extrinsic flexor muscles of the hand innervated by the median nerve (Figure 6-3).

   a. Flexor digitorum superficialis (sublimis) (FDS).

     (1) Origin: medial epicondyle.

     (2) Insertion: middle phalanx (two slips).

     (3) Function: flexion of PIP joints.

   b. Flexor digitorum profundus (FDP).

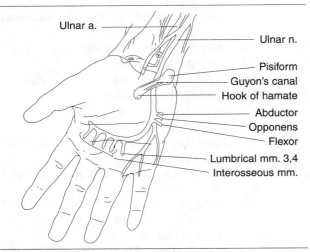

**Figure 6-2** Ulnar Nerve
Malick, M. and Kasch, M. (1984). *Manual on management of specific hand problems.* Pittsburgh, PA: AREN. Reprinted with permission.

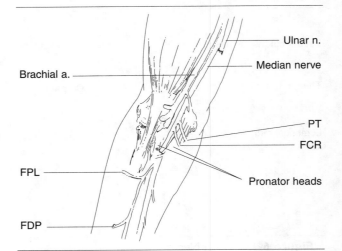

**Figure 6-3** Median Nerve
Malick, M. and Kasch, M. (1984). *Manual on management of specific hand problems.* Pittsburgh, PA: AREN. Reprinted with permission.

(1) Origin: proximal ²/₃ of the ulna and interosseous membrane.

(2) Insertion: distal phalanx.

(3) Function: flexion of DIP joints to digits II and III. (See ulnar nerve for digits IV and V).

c. Flexor pollicis longus (FPL).

(1) Origin: radius, middle ¹/₃.

(2) Insertion: distal phalanx of thumb.

(3) Function: flexion of IP joint of thumb.

4. Extrinsic flexors of the hand innervated by the ulnar nerve (Figure 6-4).

a. Flexor digitorum profundus (FDP).

(1) Origin: proximal ²/₃ of the ulna and interosseous membrane.

(2) Insertion: distal phalanx.

(3) Function: flexion of DIP joints to digits IV and V.

5. Extrinsic extensor muscles of the hand innervated by the radial nerve (Figure 6-5).

a. Extensor digitorum communis (EDC).

(1) Origin: lateral epicondyle.

(2) Insertion: medial band to middle phalanx and lateral band to distal phalanx.

(3) Function: extension of MCP joints and contributes to extension of the IP joints.

b. Extensor digiti minimi (EDM).

(1) Origin: lateral epicondyle.

(2) Insertion: inserts into EDC at MCP level of the 5th digit.

(3) Function: extension of MCP joint of the 5th digit and contributes to extension of the IP joints.

c. Extensor indicis proprius (EIP).

(1) Origin: ulna, middle ¹/₃.

(2) Insertion: inserts into EDC at MCP level.

(3) Function: extension of MCP joint of the 2nd digit and contributes to extension of the IP joints.

d. Extensor pollicis longus (EPL).

(1) Origin: ulna, middle ¹/₃.

(2) Insertion: distal phalanx of thumb.

(3) Function: extension of IP joint of thumb.

e. Extensor pollicis brevis (EPB).

(1) Origin: radius, middle ¹/₃.

(2) Insertion: proximal phalanx of thumb.

(3) Function: extension of MCP and CMC joints of thumb.

f. Abductor pollicis longus (APL).

(1) Origin: middle ¹/₃ of ulna and radius.

(2) Insertion: first metacarpal, radial side.

(3) Function: abduction and extension of CMC joint.

**C. Anatomy of the Wrist**

1. Wrist flexors innervated by the median nerve (Figure 6-3).

a. Flexor carpi radialis (FCR).

(1) Origin: medial epicondyle.

(2) Insertion: 2nd and 3rd metacarpal, base.

(3) Function: flexion of wrist and radial deviation.

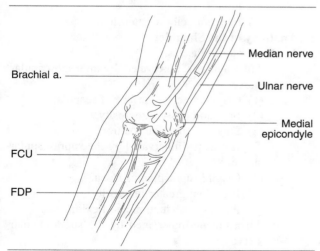

**Figure 6-4** Ulnar Nerve
Malick, M. and Kasch, M. (1984). *Manual on management of specific hand problems.* Pittsburgh, PA: AREN. Reprinted with permission.

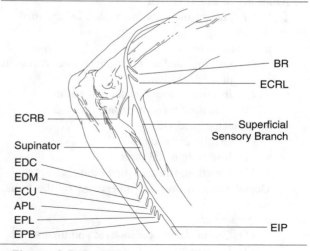

**Figure 6-5** Radial Nerve
Malick, M. and Kasch, M. (1984). *Manual on management of specific hand problems.* Pittsburgh, PA: AREN. Reprinted with permission.

b. Palmaris longus (PL).
   (1) Origin: medial epicondyle.
   (2) Insertion: palmar aponeurosis.
   (3) Function: flexion of wrist.
2. Wrist flexors innervated by the ulnar nerve (Figure 6-4).
   a. Flexor carpi ulnaris (FCU).
      (1) Origin: medial epicondyle and proximal $^2/_3$ of the ulna.
      (2) Insertion: pisiform and 5th metacarpal.
      (3) Function: flexion of wrist and ulnar deviation.
3. Wrist extensors innervated by the radial nerve (see Figure 6-5).
   a. Extensor carpi radialis brevis (ECRB).
      (1) Origin: lateral epicondyle.
      (2) Insertion: 3rd metacarpal, base.
      (3) Function: extension of wrist and radial deviation.
   b. Extensor carpi radialis longus (ECRL).
      (1) Origin: supracondylar ridge of the humerus.
      (2) Insertion: 2nd metacarpal, base.
      (3) Function: extension of wrist and radial deviation.
   c. Extensor carpi ulnaris (ECU).
      (1) Origin: lateral epicondyle.
      (2) Insertion: fifth metacarpal.
      (3) Function: extension of wrist and ulnar deviation.

**D. Anatomy of the Forearm**
1. Volar forearm muscles innervated by the median nerve.
   a. Pronator teres.
      (1) Origin: medial epicondyle and coronoid process of ulna.
      (2) Insertion: lateral surface of radius.
      (3) Function: forearm pronation.
   b. Pronator quadratus.
      (1) Origin: distal ulna.
      (2) Insertion: distal radius.
      (3) Function: forearm pronation.
2. Dorsal forearm muscles innervated by the radial nerve.
   a. Supinator.
      (1) Origin: lateral epicondyle and ulna.
      (2) Insertion: radius.
      (3) Function: forearm supination.

**E. Anatomy of the Elbow**
1. Elbow flexion: biceps and brachialis innervated by musculocutaneus nerve; brachioradialis innervated by radial nerve.
   a. Biceps.
      (1) Origin: coracoid process and supraglenoid tubercle.
      (2) Insertion: radial tuberosity.
      (3) Function: elbow flexion with forearm supinated.
   b. Brachialis.
      (1) Origin: distal $^2/_3$ of humerus.
      (2) Insertion: ulnar tuberosity.
      (3) Function: elbow flexion with forearm pronated.
   c. Brachioradialis.
      (1) Origin: supracondylar ridge.
      (2) Insertion: distal radius.
      (3) Function: elbow flexion with forearm neutral.
2. Elbow extension: triceps and anconeus innervated by radial nerve.
   a. Triceps.
      (1) Origin: long head; infraglenoid tuberosity. Lateral head; posterior humerus. Medial head; distal to lateral head.
      (2) Insertion: olecranon.
      (3) Function: elbow extension.
   b. Anconeus.
      (1) Origin: lateral epicondyle and capsule of elbow joint.
      (2) Insertion: olecranon and upper $^1/_4$ of dorsal ulna.
      (3) Function: elbow extension.

**F. Anatomy of the Shoulder**
1. Rotator cuff muscles.
   a. Subscapularis innervated by the subscapular nerve.
      (1) Origin: anterior surface of scapula.
      (2) Insertion: lesser tuberosity.
      (3) Function: internal rotation.
   b. Supraspinatus innervated by the suprascapular nerve.
      (1) Origin: supraspinatus fossa.
      (2) Insertion: greater tuberosity.
      (3) Function: abduction and flexion.
   c. Infraspinatus innervated by the suprascapular nerve.
      (1) Origin: infraspinatus fossa.
      (2) Insertion: greater tuberosity.
      (3) Function: external rotation.
   d. Teres minor innervated by the axillary nerve.

(1) Origin: axillary border of scapula.

(2) Insertion: greater tuberosity.

(3) Function: external rotation.

2. Shoulder flexion muscles.

  a. Anterior deltoid innervated by axillary nerve.

    (1) Origin: clavicle.

    (2) Insertion: deltoid tuberosity.

  b. Coracobrachialis innervated by the musculocutaneus nerve.

    (1) Origin: coracoid process.

    (2) Insertion: medial aspect of deltoid.

  c. Supraspinatus (as above).

3. Shoulder abduction muscles.

  a. Middle deltoid innervated by the axillary nerve.

    (1) Origin: acromion.

    (2) Insertion: deltoid tuberosity.

  b. Supraspinatus (as above).

4. Horizontal abduction muscles.

  a. Posterior deltoid innervated by the axillary nerve.

    (1) Origin: spine of scapula.

    (2) Insertion: deltoid tuberosity.

5. Horizontal adduction muscles.

  a. Pectoralis major innervated by the lateral pectoral nerve.

    (1) Origin: medial clavicle, sternum and ribs 1-7.

    (2) Insertion: greater tuberosity.

6. Shoulder extension muscles.

  a. Latissimus dorsi innervated by the thoracodorsal nerve.

    (1) Origin: T6 – T12, L1 – L5, sacral vertebrae, ribs 9 – 12, iliac crest and inferior angle of scapula.

    (2) Insertion: intertubercular groove of the humerus.

  b. Teres major innervated by the subscapular nerve.

    (1) Origin: inferior angle of scapula.

    (2) Insertion: intertubercular groove of the humerus.

  c. Posterior deltoid (as above).

## G. Anatomy of the Scapula

1. Upward rotation muscles.

  a. Trapezius (upper, middle, and lower) innervated by the spinal accessory nerve (CNXI).

    (1) Origin.

      (a) Upper fibers: occiput and ligamentum nuchae.

      (b) Middle fibers: spinous processes of T1 to T5.

      (c) Lower fibers: spinous processes of T6 to T12.

    (2) Insertion.

      (a) Upper fibers: lateral ⅓ of the clavicle.

      (b) Middle fibers: acromion and spine of scapula.

      (c) Lower fibers: medial end of spine of scapula.

  b. Serratus anterior innervated by the long thoracic nerve.

    (1) Origin: ribs 1 – 8 and aponeurosis of intercostals.

    (2) Insertion: superior and inferior angles of scapula and vertebral border of scapula.

2. Downward rotation muscles.

  a. Levator scapulae innervated by C3-C4 nerves.

    (1) Origin: C1-C4 transverse processes.

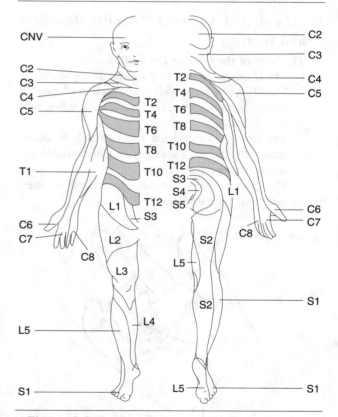

**Figure 6-6** Dermatomes

McCormack, G. (1996). The Rood approach to treatment of neuromuscular dysfunction. In J.W. Pedretti (Ed.). *Occupational therapy: Practice skills for physical dysfunction*, 4th ed, (p. 383). St. Louis, MO: Mosby. Reprinted with permission.

(2) Insertion: vertebral border of scapula.
b. Rhomboids (major and minor) innervated by the dorsal scapular nerve.
(1) Origin: C7 – T5 spinous processes.
(2) Insertion: spinous process.
c. Serratus anterior (as above).
d. Latissimus dorsi (as above).
3. Scapula adduction muscles.
a. Middle trapezius (as above).
b. Rhomboid major (as above).
4. Scapula abduction muscles.
a. Serratus anterior (as above).
5. Scapula elevation muscles.
a. Trapezius (upper), (as above).
b. Levator scapulae (as above).
6. Scapula depression muscles.
a. Trapezius (lower), (as above).

## H. Dermatome Distribution
1. (Figure 6-6).

# II. Hand and Upper Extremity Disorders and Injuries

## A. The Role of the OTA in Evaluation
1. The OTA contributes to the evaluation process.
2. The OTA can assist with the collection of data for the evaluation once service competency has been established.
3. The level of supervision required will be determined by the OTA's experience and established service competence.
4. The OTA cannot independently evaluate or interpret evaluation results.

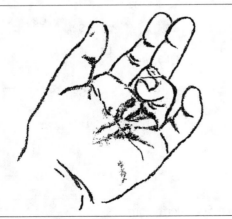

**Figure 6-7** Dupuytren's Contractures
Falkenstein, N. & Weiss-Lessard, S. (1999). *Hand rehabilitation: A quick reference guide and review* (p. 109). St. Louis, MO: Mosby. Reprinted with permission.

## B. The Role of the OTA in Intervention
1. The OTA implements intervention with OT supervision.
2. The level of supervision required depends upon the OTA's experience and established service competence.
3. During the implementation of intervention, the OTA informs the supervising occupational therapist of any change in the individual's status and any other relevant information that may affect treatment.

## C. Dupuytren's Disease
1. Disease of the fascia of the palm and digits.
a. The fascia becomes thick and contracted.
b. Results in flexion deformities of the involved digits (Figure 6-7).
2. Etiology: unknown.
3. Conservative treatment has not been successful.
4. Surgical release is required.
5. Occupational therapy intervention.
a. Wound care: dressing changes. Whirl pool if infection is suspected
(1) The OTA may be asked to assist with maintaining a sterile field.
b. Edema control: elevation above the heart.
c. Extension splint: initially at all times except to remove for ROM and bathing.
(1) The OTA may asked to assist with modifying the splint (especially extension as ROM improves).
d. A/PROM, and progress to strengthening when wounds are healed.
e. Scar management (massage, scar pad, and compression garment).
f Purposeful and occupation-based interventions that emphasize flexion (gripping) and extension (release) of the digits.

## D. Complex Regional Pain Syndrome (CRPS)
1. Type I formerly known as reflex sympathetic dystrophy (RSD).
2. Type II formerly known as causalgia.
3. Vasomotor dysfunction as a result of an abnormal reflex.
4. It can be localized to one specific area or spread to other parts of the extremity.
5. Etiology: may follow trauma (e.g., Colles' fracture) or surgery, but actual cause is unknown.
6. Symptoms include severe pain, edema, discoloration, osteoporosis, sudomotor changes, temperature changes, trophic changes, and vasomotor instability.
7. Occupational therapy intervention.

a. Modalities to decrease pain: fluidotherapy, hot packs, and TENS.

b. AROM to involved joints.

c. Edema control: manual edema mobilization (developed by Sandra Artzberger), elevation, compression gloves and massage.

    (1) Caution should be used when performing massage.

        (a) Avoid aggressive massage as this may exacerbate the symptoms.

d. ADL to encourage pain-free active use.

e. Desensitization to address hypersensitivity.

    (1) May include various textures, fluidotherapy (control fan and heat), and gentle tapping.

f. Stress loading (weight bearing and joint distraction activities, including scrubbing and carrying activities).

g. Splinting to prevent contractures and enable ability to engage in leisure/productive activities.

h. Interventions to avoid include passive range of motion, passive stretching, joint mobilization, dynamic splinting, and casting.

i. Encourage self management.

## E. Fractures

1. Types of fractures.

    a. Intraarticular versus extraarticular.

    b. Closed versus open.

    c. Dorsal displacement versus volar displacement.

    d. Midshaft versus neck versus base.

    e. Complete versus incomplete.

    f. Transverse versus spiral versus oblique.

    g. Comminuted.

2. Medical treatment.

    a. Closed reduction: types of stabilization include short arm cast (SAC), long arm cast (LAC), splint, sling or fracture brace.

    b. Open reduction internal fixation (ORIF): types include nails, screws, plates, or wire.

    c. External fixation.

    d. Arthrodesis: fusion.

    e. Arthroplasty: joint replacement.

3. Most common UE fractures.

    a. Colles' fracture: fracture of the distal radius with dorsal displacement.

    b. Smith's fracture: fracture of the distal radius with volar displacement.

    c. Carpal fractures: most common is scaphoid fracture (60% of carpal fractures). The proximal scaphoid has a poor blood supply and may become necrotic.

    d. Metacarpal fractures: classified according to location (head, neck, shaft or base). A common complication is rotational deformities.

    e. Proximal phalanx fractures: most common with thumb and index. A common complication is loss of PIP A/PROM.

    f. Middle phalanx fractures: not commonly fractured.

    g. Distal phalanx fracture: most common finger fracture. May result in mallet finger (which involves terminal extensor tendon).

    h. Elbow fracture: involvement of the radial head may result in limited rotation of the forearm.

    i. Humerus fractures: nondisplaced vs. displaced fractures.

        (1) Etiology: fall onto an outstretched upper extremity.

        (2) Fractures of the greater tuberosity may result in rotator cuff injuries.

        (3) Humeral shaft fractures may cause injury to the radial nerve resulting in wrist drop.

4. Occupational therapy evaluation.

    a. Occupational profile.

    b. History should include mechanism of injury and fracture management.

    c. Results of special tests (X-rays, MRI, and CT scan).

    d. Edema.

    e. Pain.

    f. AROM.

        (1) Do not assess PROM or strength until ordered by physician.

        (2) Exceptions are humerus fractures which often begin with PROM or AAROM.

    g. Sensation.

    h. Roles, occupations, ADL, and activities related to roles.

5. Occupational therapy intervention.

    a. Immobilization phase: stabilization and healing are the goals.

        (1) AROM of joints above and below the stabilized part.

        (2) Edema control: elevation, retrograde massage, and compression garments.

        (3) Light ADL and role activities with no resistance, progress as tolerated.

    b. Mobilization phase: consolidation is the goal.

        (1) Edema control: elevation, retrograde massage, contrast baths and compression garments.

(2) AROM.

    (a) Progress to PROM when approved by physician (4 to 8 weeks).

    (b) Exceptions are humerus fractures which often begin with PROM or AAROM.

(3) Light functional/purposeful activities.

    (a) Progress to occupation-based activities.

(4) Pain management: positioning and physical agent modalities.

(5) Strengthening: begin with isometrics when approved by physician.

## F. Cumulative Trauma Disorders (CTD)

1. Also known as repetitive strain injuries (RSI) and/or overuse syndromes, and/or musculoskeletal disorders.

2. Risk factors: repetition, static position, awkward postures, forceful exertions and vibration.

3. Non-work risk factors: acute trauma, pregnancy, diabetes, arthritis, and wrist size and shape.

4. Most common types.

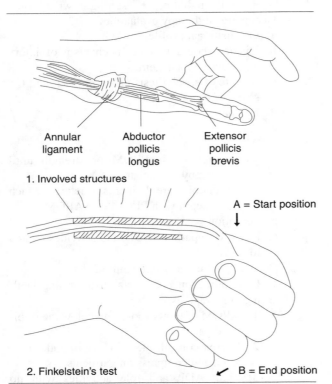

Annular ligament    Abductor pollicis longus    Extensor pollicis brevis

1. Involved structures

A = Start position

2. Finkelstein's test      B = End position

**Figure 6-8** DeQuervain's
Falkenstein, N. & Weiss-Lessard, S. (1999). *Hard rehabilitation: A quick reference guide and review.* St. Louis, MO: Mosby. Reprinted with permission.

    a. DeQuervains.

    (1) Stenosing tenosynovitis of the abductor pollicis longus (APL) and the extensor pollicis brevis (EPB). (Figure 6-8).

    (2) Pain and swelling over the radial styloid.

    (3) Positive Finkelstein's Test.

    (4) Conservative treatment.

        (a) Thumb spica splint (IP joint free).

        (b) Activity/work modification.

        (c) Ice massage over radial wrist.

        (d) Gentle AROM of wrist and thumb to prevent stiffness.

    (5) Post operative treatment.

        (a) Thumb spica splint and gentle AROM (0–2 weeks).

        (b) Strengthening, ADL, and role activities (2–6 weeks).

        (c) Unrestricted activity (6 weeks).

    b. Lateral and medial epicondylitis.

    (1) Lateral epicondylitis: overuse of wrist extensors, especially the extensor carpi radialis brevis. Also called tennis elbow.

    (2) Medial epicondylitis: overuse of wrist flexors. Also called golfer's elbow.

    (3) Conservative treatment.

        (a) Elbow strap, wrist splint.

        (b) Ice and deep friction massage.

        (c) Stretching.

        (d) Activity/work modification.

        (e) As pain decreases, begin strengthening.

    c. Trigger finger.

    (1) Tenosynovitis of the finger flexors: most commonly is the A1 Pulley.

    (2) Caused by repetition and the use of tools that are placed too far apart.

    (3) Conservative treatment.

        (a) Trigger finger splint (MCP extended, IP joints free).

        (b) Scar massage.

        (c) Edema control.

        (d) Tendon gliding.

        (e) Activity/work modification: avoid repetitive gripping activities and using tools with handles too far apart.

    d. Nerve compressions: See Section G.

## G. Peripheral Nerve Compressions

1. Three major nerves: median, ulnar and radial.

2. Carpal tunnel syndrome (CTS): a median nerve compression at the wrist.

    a. Etiology: repetition, awkward postures, vibration, anatomical anomalies, and pregnancy.

b. Symptoms: numbness and tingling of the thumb, index, middle, and radial half of the ring fingers.

  (1) Paresthesias usually occur at night.

  (2) Person will complain of dropping things.

  (3) Positive Tinel's sign at wrist. Positive Phalen's sign.

  (4) Advanced stage of CTS can result in muscle atrophy of the thenar eminence.

c. Conservative treatment.

  (1) Wrist splint in neutral: should be worn at night and during the day if performing repetitive activity.

  (2) Activity modification: avoid activities with extreme positions of wrist flexion, wrist flexion with repetitive finger flexion and wrist flexion with a static grip.

  (3) Ergonomics: appropriate workstation design. CTS is the most common work related injury of the upper extremity.

d. Surgical intervention: carpal tunnel release (CTR).

e. Post-operative treatment of CTR.

  (1) Edema control: elevation, retrograde massage, compression glove and/or contrast bath.

  (2) AROM.

  (3) Nerve gliding exercises.

  (4) Sensory reeducation.

  (5) Strengthening of thenar muscles.

  (6) Work/activity modification.

3. Cubital tunnel syndrome: an ulnar nerve compression at the elbow.

  (1) Etiology: second most common compression; pressure at elbow (leaning on elbow) and extreme elbow flexion.

  (2) Symptoms.

    (a) Numbness and tingling along ulnar aspect of forearm and hand.

    (b) Pain at elbow with extreme position of elbow flexion.

    (c) Weakness of power grip.

    (d) Positive Tinel's sign at elbow.

    (e) Advanced stages can lead to atrophy of FCU, FDP to digits IV and V and ulnar nerve innervated intrinsic muscles of the hand.

  (3) Conservative treatment.

    (a) Elbow splint to prevent positions of extreme flexion (especially at night).

    (b) Elbow pad to decrease compression of nerve when leaning on elbows.

    (c) Activity/work modification.

  (4) Surgical intervention: decompression or transposition.

  (5) Post-operative treatment.

    (a) Edema control.

    (b) Scar management.

    (c) AROM and nerve gliding (2 weeks post-operative).

    (d) Strengthening (4 weeks post-operative).

    (e) MCP flexion splint if clawing noted.

4. Radial nerve palsy: a radial nerve compression.

  (1) Etiology: Saturday night palsy, a term used to describe sleeping in a position that places stress on the radial nerve. Also, compression as a result of a humeral shaft fracture.

  (2) Symptoms: weakness or paralysis of extensors to the wrist, MCPs and thumb; wrist drop.

  (3) Conservative treatment.

    (a) Dynamic extension splint.

    (b) Work/activity modification.

    (c) Strengthening wrist and finger extensors when motor function returns.

  (4) Surgical intervention: decompression.

  (5) Post-operative treatment.

    (a) ROM.

    (b) Nerve gliding.

    (c) Strengthening (6-8 weeks post-operative).

    (d) ADL and meaningful role activities.

**H. Nerve and Tendon Repairs**

1. These are diagnoses that are more commonly treated by the occupational therapist in the acute phase following surgery.

a. With established service competency, the OTA may work collaboratively with the occupational therapist to treat these more complex hand injuries in the late phase of healing.

**I.  Rotator Cuff Tendonitis**

1. Anatomy of rotator cuff.

a. Supraspinatus.

  (1) Function: abduction and flexion.

b. Infraspinatus and teres minor.

  (1) Function: external rotation.

c. Subscapularis.

  (1) Function: internal rotation.

d. The rotator cuff functions together to control the head of the humerus in the glenoid fossa.

e. Site of impingement: coracoacromial arch (acromion, coracoacromial ligament and coracoid process).

2. Etiology.
   a. Repetitive overuse.
   b. Curved or hook acromion.
   c. Weakness of rotator cuff.
   d. Weakness of scapula musculature.
   e. Ligament and capsule tightness.
   f. Trauma.

3. Occupational therapy conservative intervention.
   a. Activity modification: avoid above shoulder level activities until pain subsides.
   b. Educate in sleeping posture: avoid sleeping with arm overhead or combined adduction and internal rotation.
   c. Decrease pain: positioning, modalities and rest.
   d. Restore pain free ROM.
   e. Strengthening: below shoulder level.
   f. Purposeful and occupation-based activities.

4. Surgical interventions.
   a. Arthroscopic surgery.
   b. Open repair: small, medium, large and massive tears.

5. Occupational therapy post-operative intervention.
   a. PROM (0 to 6 weeks); progress to AA/AROM.
   b. Decrease pain: begin with ice, progress to heat.
   c. Strengthening (6 weeks post-operative): begin with isometrics, progress to isotonic (below shoulder level).
   d. Activity modification: light ADL and meaningful role activities; progress as tolerated.
   e. Leisure and work activities (8 to 12 weeks post-operative).

**J. Adhesive Capsulitis**
1. Also known as frozen shoulder.
2. Restricted passive shoulder range of motion.
   a. Greatest limitation is external rotation, then abduction, internal rotation and flexion.
3. Anatomy: glenohumeral ligaments and joint capsule.
4. Etiology.
   a. Inflammation and immobility.
   b. Linked to diabetes mellitus and Parkinson's disease.
5. Occupational therapy conservative intervention.
   a. Encourage active use through ADL and role activities.
   b. PROM.

c. Modalities.

6. Surgical interventions: manipulation and arthroscopic surgery.

7. Occupational therapy post-operative intervention.
   a. PROM immediately following surgery.
   b. Pain relief: modalities.
   c. Encourage use of extremity for all ADL and role activities.

**K. Shoulder Dislocations**
1. Anterior dislocation most common.
2. Etiology.
   a. Trauma.
   b. Repetitive overuse.
3. Occupational therapy intervention.
   a. Regain ROM: avoid combined abduction and external rotation with anterior dislocation.
   b. Pain free ADL and role activities.
   c. Strengthen rotator cuff.

## III. Arthritis

**A. Definition**
1. An inflammation of a joint or joints.

**B. Types**
1. Rheumatoid arthritis.
   a. Systemic, symmetrical and affects many joints.
      (1) Most commonly attacks the small joints of the hands.

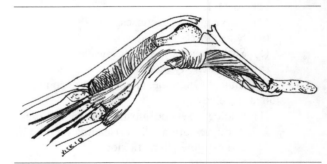

**Figure 6-9** Boutonniere Deformity
Darlington, Vicki, OTR/L, CHT with permission.

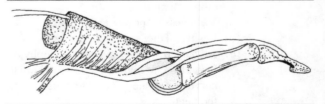

**Figure 6-10** Swan Neck Deformity
Darlington, Vicki, OTR/L, CHT with permission.

(2) Characterized by remissions and exacerbations.

(3) Begins in the acute phase as an inflammatory process of the synovial lining.

b. Etiology is unknown but there are two main theories.

(1) Infection theory.

(2) Autoimmune theory.

c. Symptoms.

(1) Pain.

(2) Stiffness.

(3) Limited range of motion.

(4) Fatigue.

(5) Weight loss.

(6) Limited activities of daily living status, diminished ability to perform role activities.

(7) Swelling.

(8) Deformities.

d. Types of deformities common with rheumatoid arthritis.

(1) Ulnar deviation and subluxation of the wrists and MCP joints.

(2) Boutonniere deformity: flexion of PIP joint and hyperextension of DIP joint. (Figure 6-9).

(3) Swan neck deformity: hyperextension of PIP joint and flexion of DIP joint. (Figure 6-10).

2. Osteoarthritis.

a. Degenerative joint disease.

(1) Not systemic but wear and tear.

(2) Commonly affects large weight bearing joints.

(3) Attacks hyaline cartilage.

b. Etiology.

(1) Genetic.

(2) Trauma.

(3) Inflammation.

(4) Cumulative trauma.

(5) Endocrine and metabolic diseases.

c. Symptoms.

(1) Pain.

(2) Stiffness.

(3) Limited range of motion.

(4) Bone spurs.

d. Types of bone spurs.

(1) Heberden's nodes at the DIP joints.

(2) Bouchard's nodes at the PIP joints.

**C. Occupational Therapy Evaluation**

1. Role of the OTA in the evaluation process.

a. The OTA can assist with the collection of data

for the evaluation once service competency has been established.

b. The level of supervision required will be determined by the OTA's experience and established service competence.

c. The OTA cannot independently evaluate or interpret evaluation results.

2 Occupational profile.

3 ROM: focus on AROM.

a. PROM should be avoided, especially in the inflammatory stage.

b. Note deformities and nodules.

4. Muscle strength.

a. Avoid muscle testing unless requested by physician.

b. Document strength in relation to function.

5. Grip strength: use sphygmomanometer.

6. ADL and role activities: note if ADL and role activity deficits are related to pain, limitation in motion, deformity, weakness, or fatigue.

7. Pain: use pain scales.

8. Edema: volumeter or tape measure.

**D. Occupational Therapy Intervention**

1. Role of the OTA.

a. The OTA implements intervention with OT supervision.

(1) The level of supervision required depends upon the OTA's experience and established service competence.

(2) During the implementation of intervention, the OTA informs the supervising occupational therapist of any change in the individual's status and any other relevant information that may affect treatment.

2. Splinting.

a. Resting hand splints in the acute stage.

b. Wrist splint only if arthritis specific to wrist.

c. Ulnar drift splint to prevent deformity.

d. Silver ring splints to prevent boutonniere and swan neck deformities.

e. Dynamic MCP extension splint with radial pull for post-operative MCP arthroplasties.

f. Hand base thumb splint for CMC arthritis.

3. Joint protection techniques.

4. Energy conservation techniques.

5. ROM: focus on AROM.

a. Gentle PROM if person unable to perform AROM.

b. All exercises should be pain free.

6. Heat modalities.

a. Hot packs can be used before exercise.
   (1) An exception is during the acute inflammatory stage when heat should be avoided.
b. Paraffin is recommended for the hands.
7. Strengthening.
   a. Avoid during inflammatory stage.
   b. Gentle strengthening while avoiding positions of deformity.
8. ADL and role activities.
   a. Joint protection and energy conservation techniques should be incorporated.
   b. Adaptive equipment should be provided to prevent deformity, decrease stress on small joints, and extend reach.
   c. Refer to Chapter 11.

## IV. Osteogenesis Imperfecta[1]

### A. Etiology
1. An autosomal dominant inherited disorder.

### B. Signs and Symptoms
1. Fractures in utero, and during the birth process in the most severe cases.
2. Brittle bones that fracture easily.
3. Multiple fractures as the child grows.
4. Deformities of the arms and legs.
5. Developmental growth problems.
6. Eye abnormalities, i.e., blue sclera, cataracts.
7. Risk of hearing impairments.

### C. Medical Management
1. Casts and braces.
2. Pain management.
3. Audiological consultation.
4. Activity restrictions due to high risk of fractures and actual fracture occurrence.
5. See this chapter's section on the medical treatment of fractures.

### D. Occupational Therapy Evaluation
1. Role of the OTA in the evaluation process.
   a. The OTA can assist with the collection of data for the evaluation once service competency has been established.
   b. The level of supervision required will be determined by the OTA's experience and established service competence.
   c. The OTA cannot independently evaluate or interpret evaluation results.
2. Activity interests that can be safely pursued.
3. Environmental risk factors.
4. See this chapter's section on occupational therapy evaluation for fractures.

### E. Occupational Therapy Intervention
1. Role of the OTA
   a. The OTA implements intervention with OT supervision.
      (1) The level of supervision required depends upon the OTA's experience and established service competence.
      (2) During the implementation of intervention, the OTA informs the supervising occupational therapist of any change in the individual's status and any other relevant information that may affect treatment.
2. Activity adaptation and assistive device prescription to facilitate safe participation in daily occupations.
3. Environmental modifications to maintain safety.
4. Preventive positioning and protective splinting/padding.
5 Activities to increase muscle strength.
6. Weight bearing activities to facilitate bone growth.
7. Family, caregiver and teacher education regarding proper handling, positioning, safety and activity/environmental modification.
8. See this chapter's section on occupational therapy intervention for fractures.

## V. Hip Fractures

### A. Etiology
1. Trauma.
2. Osteoporosis.
3. Pathological fractures (i.e., cancer).

### B. Types
1. Femoral neck fracture.
2. Intertrochanteric fracture.
3. Subtrochanteric fracture.

### C. Medical Management
1. Closed reduction for minimally displaced fractures.
2. Open reduction internal fixation (ORIF).
3. Joint replacement.

### D. Occupational Therapy Evaluation.
1. Role of the OTA in the evaluation process.
   a. The OTA can assist with the collection of data for the evaluation once service competency has been established.
   b. The level of supervision required will be determined by the OTA's experience and established service competence.
   c. The OTA cannot independently evaluate or interpret evaluation results.
2. Review precautions and weight bearing status

[1]Marge E. Moffett Boyd contributed this section on osteogenesis imperfecta.

before initiating evaluation.

3. Occupational role requirements and expectations.
4. ADL: focus on dressing, bathing, and transfers.
5. ROM and strength of upper extremities.
6. Conduct other assessments as needed, (e.g., cognitive).

**E. Occupational Therapy Intervention.**
1. Role of the OTA.
   a. The OTA implements intervention with OT supervision.
      (1) The level of supervision required depends upon the OTA's experience.
      (2) During the implementation of intervention, the OTA informs the supervising OT of any change in the individual's status and any other relevant information that may affect treatment.
2. Bed mobility and bedside ADL.
3. Upper extremity strengthening.
4. Functional ambulation and transfers with appropriate weight bearing status and appropriate ambulation device (i.e., walker, crutches).
   a. The type of ambulation device is determined by the person's weight bearing status.
5. Instruct in and practice use of assistive devices for use in the home (e.g., shower chair, elevated commode seat).
6. Practice role activities (e.g., small meal preparation) using proper weight bearing status and ambulatory device.

**F. Precautions**
1. Weight bearing status and the amount of ROM allowed at the hip will be determined by the surgeon.
2. Time frames for beginning OT intervention are

also determined by the surgeon.

**G. Complications**
1. Avascular necrosis.
2. Non-union.
3. Degenerative joint disease.
4. The result of complications can be the need for a total hip replacement.

# VI. Total Hip Replacement/Total Hip Arthroplasty

**A. Etiology**
1. Trauma, from hip fracture.
2. Disease, most often arthritis, surgery is then elective.

**B. Types**
1. Total hip joint implant: replaces acetabulum and femoral head.
2. Austin Moore: partial hip replacement. Replaces femoral head.
3. (Figure 6-11).

**C. Surgical Procedures**
1. Cemented or uncemented.
2. Anterolateral or posterolateral (more common).

**D. Occupational Therapy Evaluation**
1. Role of the OTA in the evaluation process.
   a. The OTA can assist with the collection of data for the evaluation once service competency has been established.
   b. The level of supervision required will be determined by the OTA's experience and established service competence.
   c. The OTA cannot independently evaluate or interpret evaluation results.
2. Review precautions and weight bearing status before initiating evaluation.

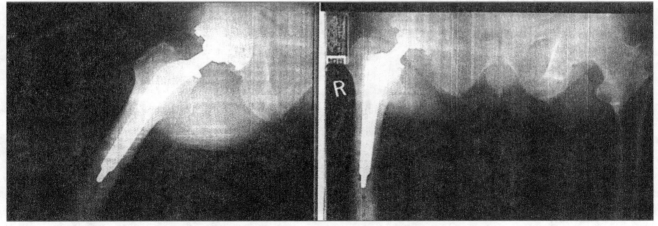

**Figure 6-11** Hybrid cemented total hip arthroplasty (Biomet Integral Design, Warsaw, IN)
From Maxey, L. & Magnussen, J. *Rehabilitation for the postsurgical orthopedic patient*, p. 173. Mosby Publications. Reprinted with permission.

3. Occupational role requirements and expectations.
4. ADL: focus on dressing, bathing, and transfers while maintaining precautions.
5. ROM and strength of upper extremities.
6. Conduct other assessments as needed, (e.g., cognitive).

### E. Occupational Therapy Intervention

1. Role of the OTA
   a. The OTA implements intervention with OT supervision.
      (1) The level of supervision required depends upon the OTA's experience and established service competence.
      (2) During the implementation of intervention, the OTA informs the supervising OT of any change in the individual's status and any other relevant information that may affect treatment.
2. Educate the individual in hip precautions.
   a. Do not flex beyond 90°.
   b. Do not adduct or cross legs.
      (1) Avoid extension for antereolateral approach.
   c. Do not rotate the hip.
      (1) Avoid internal rotation for postereolateral approach and external rotation for antereolateral approach.
   d. Do not pivot at hip.
   e. Sit only on raised chair and raised toilet seat.
   f. Transfer sit-to-stand by keeping operated hip in slight abduction and extended out in front.
3. Instruct in and practice use of long handled equipment.
4. Provide transfer training.
   a. Practice with tub bench, raised toilet seat.
   b. Practice car transfers.
   c. Practice bed to chair transfers.
5. Practice role activities (e.g., small meal preparation) using proper weight bearing status and ambulatory device.

## VII. Amputations

### A. Etiology

1. Congenital, peripheral vascular disease, trauma, cancer, and infection.

### B. Classification of Amputations

1. Upper extremity level of amputation.
   a. Forequarter: loss of clavicle, scapula and entire upper extremity.
   b. Shoulder disarticulation: loss of entire upper extremity.
   c. Above-elbow (AE) (long or short): amputation above the elbow at any level on the upper arm.
   d. Elbow disarticulation: amputation of the upper extremity distal to the elbow joint.
   e. Below-elbow (BE) (long or short): amputation below the elbow at any level of the forearm.
   f. Wrist disarticulation: amputation distal to the wrist joint. Loss of entire hand.
   g. Finger amputation: amputation of digit(s) at any level.
   h. (Figure 6-12).
2. Lower extremity level of amputation.
   a. Hemipelvectomy: amputation of half of pelvis and entire lower extremity.
   b. Hip disarticulation: amputation at the hip joint.

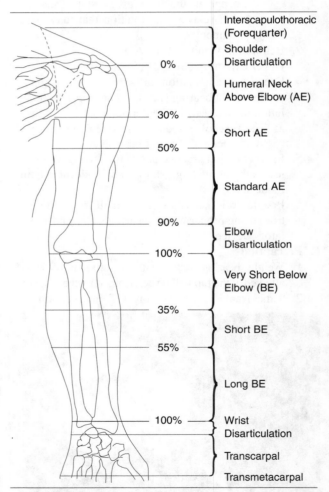

**Figure 6-12** Levels of Amputation
Celikyol, F. (1995). Amputation and prosthetics. In C.A. Trombly (Ed.). *Occupational therapy for physical dysfunction*, (p. 850). Baltimore, MD: Williams and Wilkins. Reprinted with permission.

Loss of the entire lower extremity.

   c. Above-knee amputation (transfemoral): amputation above knee at any level on the thigh.

   d. Knee disarticulation: amputation at the knee joint.

   e. Below-knee amputation (transtibial): amputation below knee at any level on the calf. Most common.

   f. Complete tarsal: amputation at the ankle.

   g. Partial tarsal: amputation of metatarsals and phalanges.

   h. Complete phalanges: amputation of toe(s).

## C. Terminal Devices

1. Functions to grasp and maintain hold on an object.
2. The two main types of TDs are the hook and the hand.
   a. Voluntary opening (VO): hook remains closed until tension is placed on cable and then it opens.
   b. Voluntary closing (VC): hook remains opened until tension is placed on cable and then it closes.
   c. Cosmetic device: minimal function.
3. Determination of the most appropriate TD is based upon the person's interests, roles, and preferences.
   a. TDs can be interchangeably used with a prosthesis if the shaft size is the same.

## D. Complications

1. Neuromas: nerve endings adhered to scar tissue.
   a. These can be very painful and hypersensitive.
2. Skin breakdown.
3. Phantom limb syndrome: sensation of the presence of the amputated limb.
4. Phantom limb pain: sensation of the presence of the amputated limb but is also painful.
5. Infection.
6. Knee flexion contractures in transtibial amputation.

## E. Preprosthetic Treatment

1. Change of dominance activities, if needed.
2. ROM of uninvolved joints.
3. Prepare limb for a prosthesis
4. Desensitization.
5. Wrapping to shape and shrink the residual limb.
   a. Wrap distal to proximal.
   b. Tension should decrease with proximal wrapping.
6. ADL training, including education in skin care.

## F. Prosthetic Treatment

1. Functional training with prosthesis.

   a. Practice engagement in activities of interest and occupational role activities.

2. Donning and doffing the prosthesis.
3. Increase prosthetic wearing tolerance.
4. Individualize treatment to enhance physical and psychological adjustment.

## G. Treatment for LE Amputations

1. Wrapping to shape residual limb and decrease swelling.
2. Desensitization
3. Strengthening (UE) with the focus on triceps.
4. Transfer training, stand pivot.
5. ADL training; LE dressing is the most difficult.
6. Standing tolerance.
7. W/C mobility.

# VIII. Burns

## A. Classification

1. Superficial (first degree burn) involves the epidermis only.
   a. Minimal pain and edema, but no blisters.
   b. Healing time is 3 to 7 days.
2. Superficial partial thickness burn.
   a. Second degree burns involve the epidermis and upper portion of dermis (e.g., sunburn).
   b. Appearance: red, blistering and wet.
   c. Painful, no grafting necessary, heals on its own.
   d. Healing time is 7 to 21 days.
3. Deep partial thickness burn.
   a. Deep second degree burn involving the epidermis and deep portion of dermis; hair follicles and sweat glands.
   b. Appearance: red, white and elastic.
   c. Sensation may be impaired.
   d. Potential to convert to full thickness burn due to infection.
      (1) May require a skin graft.
   e. Healing time is 21 to 35 days.
4. Full thickness burn.
   a. Third degree burn involving the epidermis and dermis; hair follicles, sweat glands, and nerve endings.
   b. Appearance: white, waxy, leathery, and non-elastic.
   c. Pain free, requires skin graft.
   d. Hypertrophic scar.
   e. Healing time can take months.
5. Fourth degree burn.
   a. Involves fat, muscle, and bone.
   b. Electrical burn: destruction of nerve along

pathway.
6. Rule of nines is a method of assessing burn wound size.
   a. (Figure 6-13).

**B. Occupational Therapy Evaluation and Intervention**
1. Role of the OTA in the evaluation process.
   a. The OTA can assist with the collection of data for the evaluation once service competency has been established.
   b. The level of supervision required will be determined by the OTA's experience and established service competence.
   c. The OTA cannot independently evaluate or interpret evaluation results.
2. Role of the OTA.
   a. The OTA implements intervention with OT supervision.
      (1) The level of supervision required depends upon the OTA's experience and established service competence.
      (2) During the implementation of intervention, the OTA informs the supervising OT of any change in the individual's status and any other relevant information that may affect treatment.
      (3) During intervention, the psychosocial impact of burns on the person's body image, personal identity, emotional regulation skills, and social participation must be considered and integrated into the intervention process.
3. Superficial partial-thickness burns.
   a. Evaluation.
      (1) Occupational profile.
      (2) ROM, 72 hours post-operative.
      (3) Sensation, when wounds are healed.
      (4) Strength, when wounds are healed.
      (5) Observe ADL and meaningful role activities, as soon as possible.
   b. Intervention.
      (1) Wound care and debridement, sterile whirlpool and dressing changes.
      (2) Gentle AROM and PROM to individual's tolerance.
      (3) Edema control.
      (4) Splinting, if necessary.
      (5) ADL and role activities.
4. Deep partial-thickness burns.
   a. Evaluation.
      (1) Same as superficial partial-thickness burns.
   b. Intervention.
      (1) Wound care and debridement, sterile whirlpool and dressing changes.
      (2) Gentle AROM and PROM to individual's tolerance.
      (3) Edema control.
      (4) Splinting.
      (5) Occupational role activities and ADL.
      (6) Strengthening (when wounds are healed).
5. Full thickness burn – requires grafting.
   a. Evaluation.
      (1) ROM (5 to 7 days post-operative).
      (2) All other evaluations same as above.
   b. Post-operative intervention.
      (1) 72 hours: dressing changes, splint at all times.
      (2) Five to seven days: begin AROM, light ADL and meaningful activities, sterile whirlpool.
      (3) Over seven days: PROM as tolerated, ADL and meaningful activities.
      (4) When wounds are healed, use massage.
      (5) Order compression garments.
      (6) Provide otoform/elastomer inserts.
      (7) Strengthening.

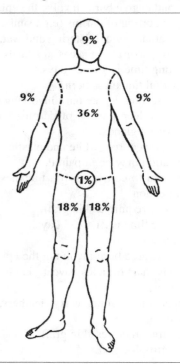

**Figure 6-13** Rule of Nines - Adult
Pedretti, L.W. (1996). *Occupational therapy: Practice skills for physical dysfunction* (4th ed.) p. 615. St. Louis, MO: Mosby. Reprinted with permission.

**C. Antideformity Positions Following Burn Injury**
1. Neck: neutral to slight extension.
2. Chest/abdomen: trunk extension and scapula retraction.
3. Axilla: shoulder abduction 90 degrees and external rotation (airplane splint). Avoid stressing brachial plexus.
4. Elbow: 0-10 degrees of extension.
5. Forearm: neutral to supination.
6. Wrist: 30-45° extension.
7. Hand: MCPs 70° flexion, IP extension and thumb abducted.
8. Hip: 10-15° abduction.
9. Knee: knee extension, anterior burn: mild flexion.
10. Ankle: 5° dorsiflexion.

**D. Hand Splints**
1. Burns to the hand.
   a. Wrist in 20 to 30 degrees extension.
   b. MCP joints in 50 to 70 degrees flexion.
   c. IP joints in full extension.
   d. Thumb abducted and extended.
2. If burns to volar surface of hand.
   a. Wrist in 0 to 30 degree extension.
   b. MCP joints in neutral and abducted.
   c. IP joints in full extension.
   d. Thumb abducted and extended.

**E. Hypertrophic Scar**
1. Most common with deep second and third degree burns.
2. Appears six to eight weeks after wound closure.
3. One to two years to mature.
4. Compression garments should be worn 24 hours daily.
   a. Applied when wounds are healed.
   b. Recommendation is to wear 24 hours a day for 1-2 years until scar is matured.
5. Additional interventions include ROM, skin care, ADL, role activities and patient/family support.

# IX. Pain

**A. Definition**
1. Personal sensation of hurt that can significantly affect an individual's quality of life.

**B. Types of Pain**
1. Acute pain has a recent onset and usually lasts for a short duration.
2. Chronic pain is of a long duration and can lead to depression.
3. Myofascial pain is specific to muscles, tendons, or fascia.
   a. Myofascial pain syndrome (MPS).
      (1) Persistent, deep aching pains in muscle, nonarticular in origin.
      (2) Characterized by well-defined, highly sensitive tender spots (trigger points).
4. Fibromyalgia syndrome (FMS) is a musculoskeletal pain and fatigue disorder that can vary in intensity.
   a. Widespread pain accompanied by tenderness of muscles and adjacent soft tissues.
   b. A nonarticular rheumatic disease of unknown origin.
5. Low back pain.
   a. Most common work related injury.
   b. Location: lumbar lordosis.
   c. Etiology.
      (1) Poor posture: seated and standing.
      (2) Repetitive bending using poor body mechanics.
      (3) Heavy lifting.
      (4) Sleeping with poor posture.
   d. Symptoms.
      (1) Pain.
      (2) Difficulty with self care activities and other role activities (especially lower extremity activities).
      (3) Difficulty sleeping.

**C. Assessment of Pain**
1. Role of the OTA in the evaluation process.
   a. The OTA can assist with the collection of data for the evaluation once service competency has been established.
   b. The level of supervision required will be determined by the OTA's experience and established service competence.
   c. The OTA cannot independently evaluate or interpret evaluation results.
2. Determine location of pain.
   a. Localized or diffuse.
3. Evaluate intensity of pain.
   a. Pain intensity scale of 0-10 is most commonly used.
      (1) Drawings of different facial expressions depicting pain intensity can also be used.
   b. Identify the time of day, positions, and activities during which the pain is most intense.
4. Determine the onset and duration of pain.
   a. Gradual or sudden onset.
   b. The length of time pain has been experienced.
5. Description of pain.

a. Common descriptors include sharp, throbbing, tender, burning, and shooting.

6. Functional assessment of pain.
   a. Pain scales that commonly address function.
      (1) McGill Pain Questionnaire.
      (2) Pain Disability Index.
      (3) Functional Interference Estimate.
   b. Refer to pain management section in Chapter 7.

**D. Occupational Therapy Intervention**
1. Role of the OTA.
   a. The OTA implements intervention with OT supervision.
      (1) The level of supervision required depends upon the OTA's experience and established service competence.
      (2) During the implementation of intervention, the OTA informs the supervising OT of any change in the individual's status and any other relevant information that may affect treatment.
2. Utilize physical agent modalities (TENS and superficial heat) and massage in preparation for purposeful and occupation-based activities.
3. Client education.
   a. Teach proper positioning techniques and proper body mechanics.
4. Splint in the resting position.
5. Gentle ROM.
6. Teach relaxation exercise.
7. Utilize proper body mechanics during self-care, leisure, and work activities.
8. Environmental modifications in the home and at work. See Chapter 15.
9. Work programs: Work hardening, work conditioning and ergonomics. See Chapter 14.
10. Correct standing and seated posture.
11. Modify activities and provide ADL training and adaptive equipment, as needed.
11. Provide alternative exercise programs (e.g., aquatic therapy, Ai-Chi, Tai-Chi).

# References

American Occupational Therapy Association. (1995). *Standards of practice,* Bethesda, MD: Author.

American Society of Hand Therapists. (1992). *Clinical assessment recommendations*, (2nd ed.). Chicago, IL: Author.

Bracciano, A.G. (2008). *Physical agent modaliites: Theory and application for the occupational therapist (2nd ed.).* Thorofare, NJ: SLACK Inc.

Clark, G., Wilgis, E. F., Aiello, B., Eckhaux, D., & Eddington, L. (1993). *Hand rehabilitation: A practical guide.* Orlando, FL: Churchill Livingstone.

Clarkson, H.M. (2000). *Musculoskeletal assessment: Joint range of motion and manual muscles strength, (2nd ed.).* Philadelphia: Lippincott Williams and Wilkins.

Cooper, C. (2007). *Fundamentals of hand therapy: Clinical reasoning and treatment guidelines for common diagnoses of the upper extremity.* Philadelphia: Elsevier.

Escolar, D., Tosi, L. Rocha, A., & Kennedy, A. (2007). Muscles, bones, and nerves. In M. Batshaw, L. Pellegrino, & N. Roizen (Eds.) *Children with disabilities*, 6th ed. (pp. 203-215). Baltimore, MD: Paul Brookes.

Falkenstein, N. & Weiss-Lessard, S. (1999). *Hand rehabilitation: A quick reference guide and review,* St. Louis, MO: Mosby.

Greene, D.P. & Roberts, S.L. (2005). *Kinesiology: Movement in the context of activity* (2nd ed.), St Louis: Mosby.

Hislop, H. & Montgomery, J. (1995). *Daniel's and Worthingham's muscle testing.* (6th ed.). Orlando, FL: W.B. Saunders.

Hopkins, H., & Smith, H. (1993). *Willard and Spackman's occupational therapy.* (8th ed.). Philadelphia: P.A. Lippincott.

Hunter, J., Mackin, E. & Callahan, A. (1995). *Rehabilitation of the hand: surgery and therapy.* (4th ed.). St. Louis, MO: Mosby.

Jacobs, K. (1997). *Quick reference dictionary for occupational therapy.* Thorofare, NJ: Slack.

Kendall, F. (1995). *Muscle testing and function.* (4th ed.). Baltimore, MD: Williams and Wilkins.

Malick, M. & Kasch, M. (1984). *Manual on management of specific hand problems.* Pittsburgh, PA: AREN.

Manning, D.C. (2000). Reflex sympathetic dystrophy, sympathetically maintained pain and complex regional pain syndrome: diagnosis of inclusion, exclusion, or confusion? *Journal of Hand Therapy*, 13(4), 260-268.

Michlovitz S.L.& Nolan T.P.(2005), *Modalities for therapeutic intervention*, (4th ed.). Philadelphia: F.A. Davis Company.

Neer, C. (1990). *Shoulder reconstruction*. Orlando, FL: W.B. Saunders.

Norkin, C.C. & White, D.J. (1995). *Measurement of joint range of motion*. (2nd ed.). Philadelphia: F.A. Davis.

Pendleton, H. M. & Schultz-Krohn, W. (2006). *Pedretti's occupational therapy: Practice skills for physical dysfunction* (6th ed.). St. Louis: Mosby.

Radomski. M.V. & Trombly Latham, C.A. (2008). *Occupational therapy for physical dysfunction* (6th ed.). Baltimore: Lippincott Williams and Wilkins.

Sladyk K., Jacobs, K. & MacRae, N. (2010). *Occupational therapy essentials for clinical competence*. Thorofare, NJ: Slack.

Stoykov, M.E. (2001, August 20). OT treatment for complex regional pain syndrome, *OT Practice*, 10-14.

Weiss, S. & Falkenstein, N. (2005). *Hand rehabilitation a quick reference guide and review*. 2nd ed, St. Louis: Elsevier Mosby.

# CHAPTER 7

# NEUROLOGICAL SYSTEM DISORDERS

Glen Gillen • Susan B. O'Sullivan • Jan G. Garbarini

## I. Anatomy and Physiology of the Nervous System

### A. Relationship to the Examination

1. It is not likely that the NBCOT exam will ask direct questions about anatomy or physiology.
   a. As a result, this chapter does not provide a complete anatomy and physiology review.
2. Major structures and functions of the nervous system are outlined because knowledge of these can help determine the best answer. For example, damage to the temporal lobe would result in the need to communicate nonverbally.

### B. Brain

1. Cerebral hemispheres (telencephalon).
   a. Convolutions of gray matter composed of gyri (crests) and sulci (fissures).
      (1) Lateral central fissure (Sylvian fissure) separates temporal lobe from frontal and parietal lobes.
      (2) Longitudinal cerebral fissure separates the two hemispheres.
      (3) Central sulcus separates frontal lobe from the parietal lobe.
   b. Paired hemispheres, consisting of 6 lobes on each side: frontal, parietal, temporal, occipital, insular, limbic.
      (1) Frontal lobe.
         (a) Precentral gyrus: primary motor cortex for voluntary muscle activation.
         (b) Prefrontal cortex: controls emotions, judgments.
         (c) Premotor cortex related to planning of movements including Broca's area which controls motor aspects of speech.
      (2) Parietal lobe.
         (a) Postcentral gyrus: primary sensory cortex for integration of sensation.
         (b) Receives fibers conveying touch, proprioceptive, pain and temperature sensations from opposite side of body.
      (3) Temporal lobe.
         (a) Primary auditory cortex: receives/ processes auditory stimuli.
         (b) Associative auditory cortex: processes auditory stimuli.
         (c) Wernicke's area: language comprehension.
      (4) Occipital lobe.
         (a) Primary visual cortex: receives/processes visual stimuli.
         (b) Visual association cortex: processes visual stimuli.
      (5) Insula: deep within lateral sulcus, associated with visceral functions.
      (6) Limbic system.
         (a) Consists of the limbic lobe (cingulate, parahippocampal, and subcallosal gyri),

hippocampal formation, amygdaloid nucleus, hypothalamus, anterior nucleus of thalamus.

    (b) Phylogenetically oldest part of the brain, concerned with instincts and emotions contributing to preservation of the individual.

    (c) Basic functions include feeding, aggression, emotions, endocrine aspects of sexual response.

  c. White matter: myelinated nerve fibers located centrally.

    (1) Transverse (commissural) fibers: interconnect the two hemispheres, including the corpus callosum (the largest), anterior commissure, and hippocampal commissure.

    (2) Projection fibers: connect cerebral hemispheres with other portions of the brain and spinal cord.

    (3) Association fibers: connect different portions of the cerebral hemispheres, allowing cortex to function as an integrated whole.

  d. Basal ganglia.

    (1) Masses of gray matter deep within the cerebral hemispheres, including the corpus striatum (caudate nucleus and lenticular nuclei), amygdaloid nucleus, and claustrum. The lenticular nuclei are further subdivided into the putamen and globus pallidus.

    (2) Forms an associated motor system (extrapyramidal system) with other nuclei in the subthalamus and midbrain.

    (3) Has numerous fiber interconnections.

      (a) Caudate loop (complex loop) functions in association with association cortex in the formation of motor plans.

      (b) Putamen loop (motor loop) functions in association with sensorimotor cortex to scale and adjust movements.

2. Cerebellum.

  a. Located behind dorsal pons and medulla in posterior fossa.

  b. Structure.

    (1) Joined to brain stem by 3 pairs of peduncles: superior, middle, and inferior.

    (2) Comprised of 2 hemispheres and midline vermis; have cerebellar cortex, underlying white matter, and 4 paired deep nuclei.

**C. Spinal Cord**

1. General structure.

  a. Cylindrical mass of nerve tissue extending from the foramen magnum in skull continuous with medulla to the lower border of first lumbar vertebra in the conus medullaris.

  b. Divided into 30 segments: 8 cervical, 12 thoracic, 5 lumbar, 5 sacral, a few coccygeal segments.

2. Central gray matter contains: 2 anterior (ventral) and 2 posterior (dorsal) horns united by gray commissure with central canal.

  a. Anterior horns contain cell bodies that give rise to efferent (motor) neurons: alpha motor neurons to effect muscles and gamma motor neurons to muscle spindles.

  b. Posterior horns contain afferent (sensory) neurons with cell bodies located in the dorsal root ganglia.

  c. Two enlargements, cervical and lumbosacral, for origins of nerves of upper and lower extremities.

  d. Lateral horn is found in thoracic and upper lumbar segments for preganglionic fibers of the autonomic nervous system.

3. White matter: anterior (ventral), lateral, and posterior (dorsal) white columns or funiculi.

  a. Ascending fiber systems (sensory pathways).

  b. Descending fiber systems (motor pathways).

4. Autonomic nervous system (ANS).

  a. Concerned with innervation of involuntary structures: smooth muscle, heart, glands; helps maintain homeostasis (constant internal body environment).

  b. Divided into 2 divisions: sympathetic and parasympathetic; both have afferent and efferent nerve fibers; preganglionic and postganglionic fibers.

    (1) Sympathetic (thoracolumbar) division: prepares body for fight or flight, emergency responses, raises heart rate and blood pressure, constricts peripheral blood vessels and redistributes blood; inhibits peristalsis.

    (2) Parasympathetic (craniosacral) division: conserves and restores homeostasis; slows heart rate and reduces blood pressure, increases peristalsis and glandular activity.

**D. Neurons**

1. Structure.

  a. Neurons vary in size and complexity.

    (1) Cell bodies (genetic center) with dendrites (receptive surface area to receive information via synapses).

(2) Axons conduct impulses away from the cell body (one-way conduction).

(3) Synapses allow communication between neurons; chemical neurotransmitters are released (chemical synapses) or electrical signals pass directly from cell to cell (electrical synapses).

b. Neuron groupings and types.

(1) Nuclei are compact groups of nerve cell bodies; in the peripheral nervous system these groups are called ganglia.

(2) Projection neurons carry impulses to other parts of the CNS.

(3) Interneurons are short relay neurons.

(4) Axon bundles are called tracts or fasciculi; in spinal cord, collections of tracts are called columns, or funiculi.

2. Lower motor neuron system and upper motor neuron system.

a. See Table 7-1.

### E. Peripheral Nervous System

1. Peripheral nerves are referred to as lower motor neurons (LMN): functional components may vary, including:

a. Motor (efferent) fibers originate from motor nuclei (cranial nerves) or anterior horn cells (spinal nerves).

b. Sensory (afferent) fibers originate in cells outside of brain stem or spinal cord with sensory ganglia (cranial nerves) or dorsal root ganglia (spinal nerves).

c. Autonomic nervous system fibers: sympathetic fibers at thoracolumbar spinal segments and parasympathetic fibers at craniosacral segments.

### TABLE 7-1

| LOWER MOTOR NEURON SYSTEM | UPPER MOTOR NEURON SYSTEM |
|---|---|
| Structures: cell bodies in the anterior horn of the spinal cord, spinal nerves, the cranial nerve fibers that travel to target muscles. | Structures: any nerve cell body or nerve fiber in the spinal cord (except the anterior horn cells), all superior structures (gray and white matter affecting motor function and descending nerve tracts), cranial nerve nuclei. |
| Symptoms of a lesion: flaccidity, decreased or absent deep tendon reflexes, atrophy. | Symptoms of a lesion: increased deep tendon reflexes, spasticity, clonus, emergence of primitive reflexes including Babinski's sign, exaggerated cutaneous reflexes, autonomic dysreflexia, flaccidity may occur at the level of the lesion. |

2. Cranial nerves: 12 pairs of cranial nerves, all nerves are distributed to head and neck except C.N. X which is distributed to thorax and abdomen.

3. Spinal nerves: 31 pairs of spinal nerves; spinal nerves are divided into groups (8 cervical, 12 thoraces, 5 lumbar, 5 sacral, coccygeal) and correspond to vertebral segments; each has a ventral root and a dorsal root.

a. Ventral (anterior) root: efferent (motor) fibers to voluntary muscles (alpha motoneurons, gamma motoneurons), and to viscera, glands and smooth muscles (preganglionic ANS fibers).

b. Dorsal (posterior) root: afferent (sensory) fibers from sensory receptors from skin, joints, and muscles; each dorsal root possesses a dorsal root ganglion (cell bodies of sensory neurons); there is no dorsal root for C1.

c. The term dermatome refers to a specific segmental skin area innervated by sensory spinal axons. Refer to Chapter 6.

## II. Cerebral Vascular Accident (CVA)

### A. Specific Types and Etiology

1. The term CVA or stroke applies to clinical syndromes that accompany ischemic or hemorrhagic lesions.

a. Cerebral insufficiency: due to transient disturbances of blood flow, e.g., transient ischemic attack (TIA).

b. Cerebral infarction: due to either embolism or thrombosis of the intra or extracranial arteries.

c. Cerebral hemorrhage: bleed secondary to hypertension or aneurysm.

d. Cerebral arteriovenous malformation (AVM): abnormal, tangled collections of dilated blood vessels that result from congenitally malformed vascular structures.

### B. Prevalence, Onset, and Prognosis

1. Stroke is the third largest cause of death, a leading cause of chronic long-term disability, and the most common neurologic condition in the U.S.

2. 795,000 persons have a stroke each year. Approximately 600,000 are first time strokes.

3. 66% of stroke survivors are age 65 or older.

### C. Symptoms of CVA

1. Abrupt onset of unilateral neurological signs (weakness, vision loss, sensory changes, etc.).

2. Symptoms progress over several hours to 2 days.

3. Specific symptoms are determined by the site of the infarct and the involved artery.

a. Refer to Table 7-2 for hemispheric specialization information which is based on lateralization in most individuals.

    (1) Hemispheric asymmetry and functional localization can vary in individuals.

**D. Risk Factors**

1. Modifiable risk factors.
   a. Hypertension.
   b. Cardiac disease.
   c. Atrial fibrillation.
   d. Diabetes mellitus.
   e. Smoking.
   f. Alcohol abuse.
   g. Hyperlipidemia.
2. Nonmodifiable risk factors.
   a. Age: relative risk increases with age.
   b. Gender: males are at higher risk.
   c. Race: African-American and Latino are at greater risk.
   d. Heredity.

**E. Diagnosis**

1. Usually diagnosed clinically using symptoms as a guide to lesion location.
2. Infarction visualized via computerized axial tomography (CT) scan (may initially read as negative).
3. Arteriography.
4. Positron emission tomography (PET) and single photon emission computerized tomography (SPECT) scanning to distinguish between infarcted and noninfarcted tissue.

5. Magnetic resonance imaging (MRI) to rule out other conditions and screen for acute bleeding.
6. Diagnostic testing.
   a. Transcranial and carotid Doppler for noninvasive visualization of plaque or occlusion of the cerebral vessels.
   b. Electrocardiogram (ECG) to detect arrhythmias.
   c. Echocardiography to evaluate presence of cardiac emboli and cardiac disease.
   d. Blood work to rule out metabolic abnormalities.

**F. Medical Management**

1. Immediate care.
   a. Airway maintenance.
   b. Adequate oxygenation.
   c. Nutritional intervention (IV fluids, alternative feeding routes).
   d. Decubiti prevention.
   e. Treatment of underlying cardiac dysfunction (dysrhythmias).
2. Pharmacologic therapies.
   a. Antithrombotic therapy (antiplatelet and anticoagulation) is used for rapid recanalization and reperfusion of occluded vessels to reduce infarction area, e.g., aspirin, heparin.
   b. Thrombolytic therapy is used in acute strokes to open occluded cerebral vessels and restore blood flow to ischemic areas, e.g., t-PA.

## III. Trauma

**A. Traumatic Brain Injury**

1. Etiology.
2. Damage results from penetration of the skull or from rapid acceleration or deceleration of the brain.
   a. Injury occurs in the tissue at the point of impact, at the opposite pole (contrecoup), and diffusely along the frontal and temporal lobes.
   b. Injury can result from a variety of occurrences.
      (1) Skull fractures.
      (2) Closed head injuries.
      (3) Penetrating wounds of the skull and brain.
      (4) Traumatic injury to extracranial blood vessels.
      (5) Nerve tissues, blood vessels, and meninges are sheared, torn, or ruptured, resulting in hemorrhage, edema, and ischemia.
3. Prevalence, onset, and prognosis.
   a. Responsible for more deaths and disabilities than any other neurologic cause in the population under age 50.
   b. Males are twice as likely to incur a TBI with

## TABLE 7-2 - HEMISPHERIC SPECIALIZATION*

| LEFT HEMISPHERE | RIGHT HEMISPHERE |
| --- | --- |
| Movement of right side of body | Movement of left side of body |
| Processing of sensory information from right side of body | Processing of sensory information from left side of body |
| Visual reception from right field | Visual reception from left field |
| Visual verbal processing | Visual spatial processing |
| Bilateral motor praxis | Left motor praxis |
| Verbal memory | Nonverbal memory |
| Bilateral auditory reception | Attention to incoming stimuli |
| Speech | Emotion |
| Processing of verbal auditory information | Processing of nonverbal auditory information |
| | Interpretation of abstract information |
| | Interpretation of tonal inflections |

*Based on hemispheric lateralization in most clients. It must be recognized that hemispheric asymmetry and functional localization varies in individuals.

the highest risk group being 15 to 29 year-olds.

   c. 400,000 new head injuries are reported each year.

4. Symptoms.
   a. Concussion characterized by post-traumatic loss of consciousness and memory disturbances.
   b. Cerebral contusion/laceration/edema accompanied by surface wounds and skull fractures.
   c. A variety of symptoms can result.
      (1) Hemiplegia or monoplegia and abnormal reflexes.
      (2) Decorticate or decerebrate rigidity.
      (3) Fixed pupils.
      (4) Coma.
      (5) Changes in vital signs.

5. Diagnostic testing.
   a. Administration of the Glasgow Coma Scale (rating of eye opening, motor responses, and verbal responses). The scale ranges from 3 (deep coma or death) to 15 (fully awake person). See Table 7-3.
   b. Administration of the Rancho Los Amigos Levels of Cognitive Functioning. See Table 7-4.
   c. CT scan and MRI to visualize intracranial structure damage.

6. Medical management.
   a. Resuscitation.
   b. Management of respiratory dysfunction.
   c. Cardiovascular monitoring.
   d. Surgical, pharmacologic, or mechanical means to decrease intracranial pressure.
   e. Neurosurgery to manage lacerated vessels and depressed skull fractures.
   f. Pharmacologic interventions.
      (1) Antibiotics.
      (2) Anticonvulsants.
      (3) Sedatives.
      (4) Antidepressants.

## B. Spinal Cord Injury (SCI)

1. Etiology.
   a. Trauma to the spinal cord as a result of compression, shearing force, contusion secondary to motor vehicle accident, diving accident, penetration wound (gunshot or knife), sports injury, or fall.
   b. Non-traumatic cord injuries may be a result of tumor, progressive degenerative disease.

2. Classification of injury/signs and symptoms.
   a. Degree of impairment and severity of injury is graded using the ASIA Impairment Scale:
      (1) A = complete, no sensory or motor function

is preserved in the sacral segments S4-S5.
      (2) B = incomplete, sensory but no motor function is preserved below the neurological level and extends through the sacral segments.
      (3) C = incomplete, motor function is preserved below the neurological level, and the majority of key muscle groups below the neurological level have a muscle grade less than 3/5.
      (4) D = incomplete, motor function is preserved below the neurological level, and the majority of key muscle groups below the level have a muscle grade greater than or equal to 3/5.
      (5) E = normal, sensory and motor function are normal.

### TABLE 7-3 - GLASGOW COMA SCALE

| | | |
|---|---|---|
| Best eye response (E) | Eyes opening spontaneously | 4 |
| | Eyes opening to speech | 3 |
| | Eyes opening in response to pain | 2 |
| | No eye opening | 1 |
| Best verbal response (V) | Oriented (patient responds coherently and appropriately to questions such as the patient's name and age, where they are and why, the year, month, etc.) | 5 |
| | Confused (patient responds to questions coherently but there is some disorientation and confusion) | 4 |
| | Inappropriate words (random or exclamatory speech, but not conversational exchange) | 3 |
| | Incomprehensible sounds (Moaning but no words) | 2 |
| | None | 1 |
| Best motor response (M) | Obeys commands (the person does simple things as asked.) | 6 |
| | Localizes to pain. (purposeful movements towards changing painful stimuli) | 5 |
| | Withdraws from pain (pulls part of body away when pinched) | 4 |
| | Flexion in response to pain (decorticate response) | 3 |
| | Extension to pain (decerebrate response) | 2 |
| | No motor response | 1 |

Reprinted from *The Lancet*, 304., Teasdale G, Jennett B. Assessment of coma and impaired consciousness. A practical scale, 281-284. Copyright 1974, with permission from Elsevier.

# TABLE 7-4 - RANCHO LEVEL OF COGNITIVE FUNCTIONING

**Level I - No Response: Total Assistance**
- Complete absence of observable change in behavior when presented visual, auditory, tactile, proprioceptive, vestibular or painful stimuli.

**Level II - Generalized Response: Total Assistance**
- Demonstrates generalized reflex response to painful stimuli.
- Responds to repeated auditory stimuli with increased or decreased activity.
- Responds to external stimuli with physiological changes generalized, gross body movement and/or not purposeful vocalization.
- Responses noted above may be same regardless of type and location of stimulation.
- Responses may be significantly delayed.

**Level III - Localized Response: Total Assistance**
- Demonstrates withdrawal or vocalization to painful stimuli.
- Turns toward or away from auditory stimuli.
- Blinks when strong light crosses visual field.
- Follows moving object passed within visual field.
- Responds to discomfort by pulling tubes or restraints.
- Responds inconsistently to simple commands.
- Responses directly related to type of stimulus.
- May respond to some persons (especially family and friends) but not to others.

**Level IV - Confused/Agitated: Maximal Assistance**
- Alert and in heightened state of activity.
- Purposeful attempts to remove restraints or tubes or crawl out of bed.
- May perform motor activities such as sitting, reaching and walking but without any apparent purpose or upon another's request.
- Very brief and usually non-purposeful moments of sustained alternatives and divided attention.
- Absent short-term memory.
- May cry out or scream out of proportion to stimulus even after its removal.
- May exhibit aggressive or flight behavior.
- Mood may swing from euphoric to hostile with no apparent relationship to environmental events.
- Unable to cooperate with treatment efforts.
- Verbalizations are frequently incoherent and/or inappropriate to activity or environment.

**Level V - Confused, Inappropriate Non-Agitated: Maximal Assistance**
- Alert, not agitated but may wander randomly or with a vague intention of going home.
- May become agitated in reponse to external stimulation, and/or lack of environmental structure.
- Not oriented to person, place or time.
- Frequent brief periods, non-purposeful sustained attention.
- Severely impaired recent memory, with confusion of past and present in reaction to ongoing activity.
- Absent goal directed, problem solving, self-monitoring behavior.
- Often demonstrates inappropriate use of objects without external direction.

- May be able to perform previously learned tasks when structured and cues provided.
- Unable to learn new information.
- Able to respond appropriately to simple commands fairly consistently with external structures and cues.
- Responses to simple commands without external structure are random and non-purposeful in relation to command.
- Able to converse on a social, automatic level for brief periods of time when provided external structure and cues.
- Verbalizations about present events become inappropriate and confabulatory when external structure and cues are not provided.

**Level VI - Confused, Appropriate: Moderate Assistance**
- Inconsistently oriented to person, time and place.
- Able to attend to highly familiar tasks in non-distracting environment for 30 minutes with moderate redirection.
- Remote memory has more depth and detail than recent memory.
- Vague recognition of some staff.
- Able to use assistive memory aide with maximum assistance.
- Emerging awareness of appropriate response to self, family and basic needs.
- Moderate assist to problem solve barriers to task completion.
- Supervised for old learning (e.g. self care).
- Shows carry over for relearned familiar tasks (e.g. self care).
- Maximum assistance for new learning with little or nor carry over.
- Unaware of impairments, disabilities and safety risks.
- Consistently follows simple directions.
- Verbal expressions are appropriate in highly familiar and structured situations.

**Level VII - Automatic, Appropriate: Minimal Assistance for Daily Living Skills**
- Consistently oriented to person and place, within highly familiar environments. Moderate assistance for orientation to time.
- Able to attend to highly familiar tasks in a non-distraction environment for at least 30 minutes with minimal assist to complete tasks.
- Minimal supervision for new learning.
- Demonstrates carry over of new learning.
- Initiates and carries out steps to complete familiar personal and household routine but has shallow recall of what he/she has been doing.
- Able to monitor accuracy and completeness of each step in routine personal and household ADLs and modify plan with minimal assistance.
- Superficial awareness of his/her condition but unaware of specific impairments and disabilities and the limits they place on his/her ability to safely, accurately and completely carry out his/her household, community, work and leisure ADLs.
- Minimal supervision for safety in routine home and community activities.
- Unrealistic planning for the future.
- Unable to think about consequences of a decision or action.
- Overestimates abilities.
- Unaware of others' needs and feelings.
- Oppositional/uncooperative.
- Unable to recognize inappropriate social interaction behavior.

## TABLE 7-4 - RANCHO LEVEL OF COGNITIVE FUNCTIONING  CONTINUED

### Level VIII - Purposeful, Appropriate: Stand-By Assistance

- Consistently oriented to person, place and time.
- Independently attends to and completes familiar tasks for 1 hour in distracting environments.
- Able to recall and integrate past and recent events.
- Uses assistive memory devices to recall daily schedule, "to do" lists and record critical information for later use with stand-by assistance.
- Initiates and carries out steps to complete familiar personal, household, community, work and leisure routines with stand-by assistance and can modify the plan when needed with minimal assistance.
- Requires no assistance once new tasks/activities are learned.
- Aware of and acknowledges impairments and disabilities when they interfere with task completion but requires stand-by assistance to take appropriate corrective action.
- Thinks about consequences of a decision or action with minimal assistance.
- Overestimates or underestimates abilities.
- Acknowledges others' needs and feelings and responds appropriately with minimal assistance.
- Depressed.
- Irritable.
- Low frustration tolerance/easily angered.
- Argumentative.
- Self-centered.
- Uncharacteristically dependent/independent.
- Able to recognize and acknowledge inappropriate social interaction behavior while it is occurring and takes corrective action with minimal assistance.

### Level IX - Purposeful, Appropriate: Stand-By Assistance on Request

- Independently shifts back and forth between tasks and completes them accurately for at least two consecutive hours.
- Uses assistive memory devices to recall daily schedule, "to do" lists and record critical information for later use with assistance when requested.
- Initiates and carries out steps to complete familiar personal, household, work and leisure tasks independently and unfamiliar personal, household, work and leisure tasks with assistance when requested.

- Aware of and acknowledges impairments and disabilities when they interfere with task completion and takes appropriate corrective action but requires stand-by assist to anticipate a problem before it occurs and take action to avoid it.
- Able to think about consequences of decisions or actions with assistance when requested.
- Accurately estimates abilities but requires stand-by assistance to adjust to task demands.
- Acknowledges others' needs and feelings and responds appropriately with stand-by assistance.
- Depression may continue.
- May be easily irritable.
- May have low frustration tolerance.
- Able to self monitor appropriateness of social interaction with stand-by assistance.

### Level X - Purposeful, Appropriate: Modified Independent

- Able to handle multiple tasks simultaneously in all environments but may require periodic breaks.
- Able to independently procure, create and maintain own assistive memory devices.
- Independently initiates and carries out steps to complete familiar and unfamiliar personal, household, community, work and leisure tasks but may require more than usual amount of time and/or compensatory strategies to complete them.
- Anticipates impact of impairments and disabilities on ability to complete daily living tasks and takes action to avoid problems before they occur but may require more than usual amount of time and/or compensatory strategies.
- Able to independently think about consequences of decisions or actions but may require more than usual amount of time and/or comempensatory strategies to select the appropriate decision or action.
- Accurately estimates abilities and independently adjusts to task demands.
- Able to recognize the needs and feelings of others and automatically respond in appropriate manner.
- Periodic periods of depression may occur.
- Irritability and low frustration tolerance when sick, fatigued and/or under emotional stress.
- Social interaction behavior is consistently appropriate.

Reprinted with permission from the author Chris Hagen.

---

3. Specific symptoms.
   a. Spinal shock (4-8 weeks), all reflex activity is obliterated below the level of the injury presenting as flaccid paralysis.
   b. Sensory deficits may be partial loss or complete.
   c. Loss of bowel/bladder control.
   d. Loss of temperature control below the lesion.
   e. Decreased respiratory function.
   f. Sexual dysfunction.
   g. Changes in muscle tone.
      (1) Spasticity in upper motor neuron lesions.
      (2) Flaccidity in lesions below L1.
   h. Loss of motor function resulting in tetraplegia (quadriplegia) or paraplegia; may be complete or incomplete.
4. Complications.
   a. Respiratory complications, decreased vital capacity, pneumonia.
   b. Decubitus ulcer formation.
   c. Orthostatic hypotension: an excessive fall in blood pressure upon assuming the upright position.
   d. Deep vein thrombosis.

e. Autonomic dysreflexia: an abnormal response to a noxious stimulus (catheter blockage, sitting on a sharp object) that results in extreme rise in blood pressure, pounding headache, and profuse sweating. This complication is deemed a medical emergency if not reversed (by removing the stimulus) quickly.

f. Urinary tract infection.

g. Heterotopic ossification, the formation of bone in abnormal anatomical locations.

5. Medical management.

a. Prevention of further cord damage via stabilization.

b. Traction and rest for unstable injuries.

c. Surgery with internal fixation.

d. Diuretic prescription to decrease inflammation.

e. Bladder care.

f. Decubiti prevention.

g. Control of autonomic dysreflexia and orthostatic hypotension.

h. Prevention of thrombus formation.

i. Treatment for heterotopic ossification.

C. **Cerebral Palsy (CP)**

1. Etiology.

a. Caused by an injury and/or disease prior to, during, or shortly after birth resulting in brain damage and secondary neurological and muscular deficits.

b. Common causes during the perinatal period include lack of oxygen, intracranial hemorrhage, meningitis, chronic alcohol abuse, toxicosis, infections, genetic factors, endocrine and metabolic disorders.

2. Onset, prevalence, and prognosis.

a. Occurs in 1.5 to 2 per 1,000 births.

b. Prognosis is dependent on the severity of the brain injury and the location.

c. It is nonprogressive; however, deformities and contractures may develop depending on the level of involvement.

d. It may be accompanied with seizure, intellectual and/or behavioral disorders.

e. The individual can have normal intelligence, which is masked by significant motor deficits.

f. An increase in the number of infants surviving prematurely and an increase in low birth weight have resulted in a higher incidence of the spastic diplegia type of CP.

3. Diagnosis.

a. Detected usually by 12 months of age.

b. Sometimes diagnosis may not be identified in early infancy.

(1) An infant may initially present with hypotonia.

(2) As the child's neuromotor status evolves spasticity may develop.

(3) The child may present with primitive reflexes and automatic reactions, hyperresponsive reflexes, clonus, variable tone, asymmetry, involuntary movements, feeding difficulties due to oral motor impairments, cognitive and other developmental delays.

c. Persistence of primitive reflexes contributes to diagnosis, and these may extend into adulthood.

d. The location and severity of the lesion determines the type of cerebral palsy.

(1) A lesion of the motor cortex will result in spasticity with flexor and extensor imbalance.

(2) A lesion in the basal ganglia results in fluctuations in muscle tone causing dyskinesia, dystonia, or athetosis; characterized by choreoathetosis with jerky involuntary movements more proximal than distal and lack of cocontractions; or writhing involuntary movements more distal than proximal.

(3) A lesion in the cerebellum results in ataxic movements and is characterized by a lack of stability so coactivation is difficult resulting in more primitive total patterns of movement.

e. The distribution of the disorder in limbs determines the classification.

(1) Monoplegia involves one extremity.

(2) Hemiplegia involves the upper and lower extremity on the same side.

(3) Paraplegia involves the lower extremities.

(4) Quadriplegia involves all extremities.

(5) Diplegia involves less upper extremity involvement and greater lower extremity functional impairment.

4. Complications.

a. Language and intellectual deficits occur in 50 to 75% of children with cerebral palsy.

b. Seizures occur in 50% of children with cerebral palsy.

c. Visual impairments occur in 40 to 50% of children with cerebral palsy.

d. Feeding disturbances.

5. Medical management.

a. Antispasticity drugs.

b. Orthopedic management to address development of scoliosis and joint contractures.

c. Surgery may be indicated to decrease contractures and improve functional movement.

d. Medications for seizures if present.

e. Dietary interventions and special feeding techniques for regularity in elimination and/or other medical complications.

# IV. Disorders of Movement/Neuromuscular Diseases

## A. Classification of Symptoms

1. Tremor: rhythmic, alternating, oscillatory movements produced by repetitive patterns of muscle contraction and relaxation.

   a. Tremors are classified by rate, rhythm, distribution.

   b. Tremors are identified as to whether they occur at rest (resting tremor) or during activity (action or intention tremor).

2. Dyskinesias: involuntary, nonrepetitive, but occasionally stereotyped movements affecting distal, proximal, and axial musculature in varying combinations. Most dyskinesias are representative of basal ganglia disorders.

3. Myoclonus: a brief and rapid contraction of a muscle or group of muscles.

4. Tics: brief, rapid, involuntary movements, often resembling fragments of normal motor behavior. They tend to be stereotyped and repetitive, but not rhythmic.

5. Chorea: brief, purposeless, involuntary movements of the distal extremities and face. Usually considered to be a manifestation of dopaminergic overactivity in the basal ganglia.

6. Dystonia: results in sustained abnormal postures and disruptions of ongoing movement resulting from alterations of muscle tone. Dystonias may be generalized or focal.

## B. Parkinson's Disease

1. Etiology: a hypokinetic CNS movement disorder that is idiopathic, slowly progressive, and degenerative.

2. Prevalence, onset, and prognosis.

   a. Onset of the disease is usually after age 40, with increasing incidence in older age groups.

   b. Occurs in 1% of the population over 50.

   c. Rate of deterioration ranges from 2 to 20 years.

3. Symptoms.

   a. Begins insidiously with a resting "pill-rolling" tremor of one hand.

   b. Cardinal signs include tremor, rigidity, resist-

ance to passive motion that is not velocity dependent (cogwheel or leadpipe), akinesia, postural instability, festinating gait, falling backwards (retropulsion) or forwards (propulsion), mask face, micrographia.

4. Diagnostic testing.

   a. Presence of cardinal signs.

   b. Degeneration in dopaminergic pathways in the basal ganglia, primarily in the substantia nigra.

   c. Positive response to Sinemet (Levodopa/ Carbidopa).

   d. Stage of disease progression is diagnosed using Hoehn and Yahr's five stage scale.

      (1) Stage I = unilateral tremor, rigidity, akinesia, minimal or no functional impairment.

      (2) Stage II = bilateral tremor, rigidity or akinesia, with or without axial signs, independent with ADL, no balance impairment.

      (3) Stage III = worsening of symptoms, first signs of impaired righting reflexes, onset of disability in ADL performance, can lead independent life.

      (4) Stage IV = requires help with some or all ADL, unable to live alone without some assistance, able to walk and stand unaided.

      (5) Stage V= confined to a wheelchair or bed, maximally assisted.

5. Medical management.

   a. Surgical interventions: thalamotomy, pallidotomy, fetal tissue transplant, deep brain stimulators.

   b. Pharmacology: Levodopa (the metabolic precursor of dopamine), Sinemet (Levodopa/ Carbidopa), dopamine agonists, anticholinergics (Benadryl, Artane, Cogentin) for rigidity and tremors, dopamine releasers (Amantadine).

## C. Spina Bifida

1. Etiology is unknown.

   a. Genetic, intrauterine, and/or environmental factors contribute to the neural tube defect involving the vertebral arches and the spinal column.

   b. Some studies suggest certain medications and a lack of folic acid may induce neural tube defects.

2. Onset, prevalence, and prognosis.

   a. Occurs in about 1 in every 1,000 births.

   b. The prognosis and degree of impairment is dependent on the level of the lesion and the extent of the neural tube defect of the vertebral arches and the spinal column.

(1) Lesions usually occur in the thoracic or lumbar spine.
3. Diagnosis.
   a. Detected prenatally through amniocentesis for levels of alpha-fetoprotein and acetylcholinesterase, and ultrasound if indicated.
   b. A less reliable means of prenatal detection involves determining the amount of alpha-fetoprotein in the mother's blood.
4. Classification of spina bifida.
   a. Spina bifida occulta: a bony malformation with separation of vertebral arches of one or more vertebrae with no external manifestations.
      (1) Occult spinal dysraphism (OSD): when external manifestations such as a red birthmark (hemangioma or flame nervus), patch of hair, a dermal sinus (opening in skin), a fatty benign tumor (lipoma), or dimple covering the site are present.
      (2) Spina bifida cystica: an exposed pouch.
   b. Spina bifida with meningocele: protrusion of a sac through the spine, containing cerebral spinal fluid and meninges; however, does not include the spinal cord.
   c. Spina bifida with myelomeningocele: protrusion of a sac through the spine, containing cerebral spinal fluid and meninges as well as the spinal cord or nerve roots.
5. Specific symptoms.
   a. Spina bifida occulta usually does not result in any symptoms.
      (1) Occasionally slight instability and neuromuscular impairments, such as mild gait involvement and bowel or bladder problems may occur.
   b. Occult spinal dysraphism may result in the spinal cord being split (diplomyelia) or being tied down and tethered (diastematomyelia) which may lead to neurological damage and developmental abnormality as the child grows.
   c. Spina bifida meningocele usually does not present with symptoms impacting on function as the spinal cord itself is not entrapped.
      (1) Occasionally slight instability and neuromuscular impairments, such as mild gait involvement and bowel or bladder problems may occur.
   d. Spina bifida with a myelomeningocele results in sensory and motor deficits occurring below the level of the lesion, and may result in lower extremity paralysis and/or deformities, and bowel and bladder incontinence.
      (1) The level of lesions impact leg movements.
      (2) Lesions of S2 - S4 results in bladder and bowel problems.
         (a) A neurogenic bladder impacts on the sensation to urinate and the control of the urinary sphincter.
         (b) Incomplete emptying of the bladder results; this often leads to infections.
         (c) A neurogenic bowel causes constipation and incontinence.
6. Medical management.
   a. During the neonatal period precautions are taken to protect the sac from rupturing and from infection which may result in meningitis.
      (1) All or part of the sac may be removed 24 to 48 hours after birth.
   b. A ventriculoperitoneal or other type of shunt is indicated should the complication of hydrocephalus occur, in which the cerebral spinal fluid is not absorbed resulting in an increase in size of the ventricles and the infant's head.
      (1) Brain damage as a result of increased intercranial pressure can cause mental retardation.
      (2) Increased pressure may also result in Arnold-Chiari Syndrome in which a portion of the cerebellum and medulla oblongata slip down through the foramen magnum to the cervical spinal cord.
      (3) Shunts can become blocked resulting in increased intra-cranial pressure.
         (a) Signs and symptoms during the first year of life include extreme head growth and often a soft spot on the forehead.
         (b) Signs and symptoms by the second year of life include severe headache, vomiting, and/or irritability.
         (c) Intracranial pressure can possibly lead to paralysis of the sixth cranial nerve resulting in visual impairments.
         (d) Intracranial pressure may contribute to seizure disorders and deterioration of physical and/or cognitive functioning.
      (4) Shunts can become infected.
         (a) Signs and symptoms include vomiting, lethargy, and/or fever.
         (b) Seizures and deterioration of physical and/or cognitive functioning may result.

(5) Early identification is vital, as these conditions are life threatening.

    (a) Immediate notification of signs and symptoms to the child's/facility's neurosurgeon is required.

    (b) Blocked shunts are revised by removing the blocked section and replacing it with a catheter.

    (c) Infections are treated by withdrawing fluid through or replacing the tubing. Intravenous antibiotics are also administered.

    (d) Medications to reduce cerebrospinal fluid production and intra-cranial pressure are sometimes used as an interim measure.

b. Urological management, and if indicated intermittent catheterization.

c. Orthopedic management for motor deficits.

d. Surgical intervention may be indicated for Tethered Cord Syndrome.

    (1) Tethered Cord Syndrome occurs in the tail end of the spinal cord when it is stretched as a result of compression, being trapped with a fatty mass, or a developmental abnormality.

    (2) Visible signs include a hairy patch of skin, a hemangioma, and/or a dimple of the lower spine.

    (3) Difficulties with bowel and bladder, gait disturbances, and/or deformities of the feet may result.

### D. Muscular Dystrophies/Atrophies

1. Etiology: a group of degenerative disorders due to a hereditary disease process.

    a. Duchenne muscular dystrophy is due to an absent muscle protein product, dystrophin.

2. Onset, prevalence, and prognosis.

    a. Muscular dystrophies/atrophies can begin in infancy, childhood, or adulthood.

    b. Progress may be rapid and fatal, or may remain stable throughout life.

        (1) Those starting early in life tend to be more severe and to progress more rapidly.

3. Diagnosis.

    a. Detection is confirmed by blood tests for muscle enzymes or muscle proteins, nerve conduction velocity, electromyography, and, if indicated muscle or nerve biopsy.

    b. Common symptoms include hypotonia, muscle weakness, and atrophy.

4. Major types.

    a. Duchenne's muscular dystrophy is the most common form of muscular dystrophy.

        (1) It is detected between two and six years of age.

        (2) It is inherited, sex-linked and recessive occurring in males 1 per 3,500 births.

        (3) Symptoms include enlargement of calf muscles and at times enlargement of the forearm and thigh muscles giving an appearance the child is healthy.

            (a) This enlargement is due to fibrosis and formation of adipose tissues, which causes weakness.

            (b) It is known as pseudohypertrophy.

        (4) Weakness of the proximal joints progresses to the point that the child has to crawl up his thighs with his hands to stand from a kneeling position known as Gower's sign.

        (5) Weakness occurs in all voluntary muscles, including the heart and diaphragm.

        (6) Individuals rarely survive beyond their early 20s due to respiratory problems, infections, and/or cardiovascular complications.

    b. Arthrogryposis multiplex congenita.

        (1) It is detected at birth and associated with loss of anterior horn cells.

        (2) Presence of weakness, deformities, and associated joint contractures.

        (3) Position of rest for the upper extremities tends to be internal rotation of the shoulders, extension of the elbows, and flexion of the wrists; for the lower extremities, there is flexion and internal rotation of the hips and clubfeet.

        (4) It may be stable, mildly progressive, or may improve.

        (5) Related problems include congenital heart defects, spinal defects, torticollis, and involvement of the diaphragm.

    c. Limb-girdle muscular dystrophy.

        (1) Onset begins between the first and third decades of life.

        (2) Proximal muscles of the pelvis and shoulder are initially affected.

        (3) Typically slowly progressive.

    d. Facioscapulohumeral muscular dystrophy.

        (1) Occurs in early adolescence.

(2) Involves the face, upper arms, and scapular region, causing masking and decreased mobility of the face and the inability to lift the arms above shoulder level.

  e. Spinal muscular atrophy.

    (1) The infantile form known as Werdnig-Hoffman disease, has a life expectancy up to approximately two years of age.

    (2) The intermediate form is detected six months to three years of age and progresses rapidly with a life expectancy of early childhood.

  f. Congenital myasthenia gravis.

    (1) A disorder involving transmission of impulses in the neuromuscular junction.

    (2) Onset starting near birth and occurring more frequently in males.

  g. Charcot-Marie-Tooth disease.

    (1) A disease involving the peripheral nerves marked by progressive weakness, primarily in peroneal and distal leg muscles.

    (2) Typically occurs in the teenage years or earlier.

  h. Myopathies.

    (1) Symptoms are similar to dystrophies; however, myopathies progress slowly; resulting in a better prognosis.

    (2) Weakness of the face, neck and limbs is characteristic.

5. Specific symptoms.

  a. Low muscle tone and weakness contributes to abnormal movement patterns and delayed developmental milestones.

  b. There may be difficulty with oral motor feeding, necessitating a nasogastric or gastrostomy tube.

  c. Weakness contributes to deformities of the extremities and spine.

  d. Difficulty with breathing may require tracheostomies or mechanical ventilators, and frequently results in death.

6. Medical management.

  a. Prescribed medications to decrease pulmonary complications, prolong life.

  b. Nutritional management for difficulties with feeding and the tendency to gain weight secondary to inactivity.

  c. Prevention of skin breakdown and decubitus ulcers.

  d. Steroids to help delay or reverse muscle weakness; however, the undesirable side effects associated with steroids bring their use into question.

**E. Progressive Supranuclear Palsy**

1. Etiology: manifested by loss of voluntary, but preservation of reflexive eye movements, bradykinesia, rigidity, axial dystonia, pseudobulbar palsy, and dementia.

2. Onset, prevalence, and prognosis.

  a. Occurs in later middle life.

  b. Affects 6.5/100,000 people.

  c. Death occurs approximately 15 years after onset.

**F. Huntington's Chorea**

1. Etiology: an autosomal dominant disorder.

2. Onset, prevalence, and prognosis.

  a. Begins in middle-age.

  b. Onset of this disease process is insidious.

  c. Occurs in 1 in 10,000.

  d. Characterized by choreiform movements and progressive intellectual deterioration.

  e. Psychiatric disturbance (personality change, manic-depressive symptoms, and schizophreniform illness) may precede the onset of the movement disorder.

**G. Cerebellar/Spinocerebellar Disorders**

1. Etiology: characterized by ataxia, dysmetria, dysdiadochokinesia, hypotonia, movement decomposition, tremor, dysarthria, and nystagmus.

**H. Structural Cerebellar Lesions**

1. Etiology: includes vascular lesions (stroke) and tumor deposits, producing symptoms and signs appropriate to their locus within the cerebellum.

  a. Demyelinating plaques of multiple sclerosis may also arise in the cerebellum white matter and give rise to cerebellar symptoms.

  b. Alcoholism and nutritional deprivation can cause degeneration of the vermis and anterior cerebellum.

**I. Spinocerebellar Degenerations**

1. Etiology: a group of degenerative disorders, characterized by progressive ataxia due to the degeneration of the cerebellum, brain stem, spinal cord, peripheral nerves, and the basal ganglia.

2. These disorders are grouped as spinal ataxias, cerebellar ataxias, and multiple system degeneration.

  a. Friedreich's ataxia.

    (1) Etiology: autosomal recessive inheritance.

    (2) Onset occurs in childhood or early adolescence.

    (3) Symptoms: the prototype of spinal ataxia.

      (a) This process is characterized by gait

unsteadiness, upper extremity ataxia, and dysarthria.
(b) Tremor may be a minor feature.
(c) Presentation also includes areflexia and loss of large fiber sensory modalities.
(d) As the disease progresses, scoliosis and cardiomyopathy are common.
b. Cerebellar cortical degeneration.
(1) Etiology: pathologic changes are seen in the cerebellum and the inferior olives.
(2) Onset begins between ages 30 and 50.
(3) Symptoms: cerebellar symptoms are the only signs detectable.
c. Multiple systems degeneration (olivoponto-cerebellar atrophies).
(1) Etiology: characterized by spasticity, extra-pyramidal, sensory, lower motor neuron, and autonomic dysfunction.
(2) Onset occurs in young to middle life.
3. Medical management for movement disorders is limited in many cases.
a. Pharmacologic intervention may be able to dampen effects of the movement disorders.
b. Agents utilized for this population include pro-pranolol, clonazepam, clonidine, and anti-cholinergic agents depending upon symptoma-tology.

## V. Disorders of the Peripheral Nervous System/ Neuromuscular Diseases

### A. Amyotrophic Lateral Sclerosis (ALS)
1. Etiology: motor neuron disease of unknown etiol-ogy characterized by progressive degeneration of corticospinal tracts and anterior horn cells or bul-bar efferent neurons.
2. Onset, prevalence, and prognosis.
a. The disease is more prevalent in men than women at a ratio of 1.2:1.
b. Onset occurs at an average age of 57.
c. Death usually occurs in 2-5 years.
3. Symptoms.
a. Muscle weakness and atrophy, evidence of anterior horn cell destruction, often begins dis-tally and asymmetrically.
b. Cramps and fasciculations precede weakness.
c. Signs usually begin in the hands.
d. Lower motor neuron signs are soon accompa-nied by spasticity, hyperactive deep tendon reflexes, and evidence of corticospinal tract involvement.

e. Dysarthria and dysphagia are evident.
f. Sensory systems, eye movements, and urinary sphincters are often spared.
4. Diagnosis.
a. Usually clinical, with generalized motor involvement unaccompanied by sensory abnor-malities.
b. Electromyography can support the diagnosis.
c. Other processes such as spinal cord tumors and myopathies must be ruled out.
5. Medical management.
a. There is no specific treatment to slow the dis-ease process.
b. Treatment is aimed at treating secondary com-plications such as spasticity (treated with anti-spasmodics), and prevention of aspirations (gastrostomy and modified diets), etc.

### B. Brachial Plexus Disorder
1. Etiology: secondary to traction during birth, inva-sion of metastatic cancer, after radiation treatment secondary to fibrosis, or traction injury.
2. Symptoms.
a. Mixed motor and sensory disorders of the cor-responding limb.
b. Rostral injuries produce shoulder dysfunction while caudal injuries produce dysfunction in the hand.
3. Diagnosis.
a. Made via CT scanning of the plexus in cases where a mass is present.
b. EMG/nerve conduction velocities are used to localize the plexus lesion.

### C. Peripheral Neuropathies
1. Etiology: peripheral neuropathy of a single nerve may be the result of trauma, pressure paralysis, forcible overextension of a joint, hemorrhage into a nerve, exposure to cold or radiation, or ischemic paralysis.
a. Multiple nerves may be affected in cases of collagen vascular disease, metabolic diseases (diabetes mellitus), or infectious agents (Lyme disease).
b. Other causes include nutritional deficiency, malignancy, microorganisms, exposure to toxic agents, and chronic alcohol abuse.
2. Diagnosis.
a. Focused on the cause of the symptoms.
b. Specific tests utilized include electromyography, nerve conduction velocity, muscle biopsy, and examinations to identify systemic disorders.

3. Symptoms.
   a. A syndrome of sensory, motor, reflex, and vasomotor symptoms.
   b. Symptoms include pain, weakness, and paresthesias in the distribution of the affected nerve.
4. Medical management.
   a. Guided by the underlying disease process, not the symptoms of the neuropathy.
   b. Treatment of the underlying systemic disorder (diabetes, tumor, multiple myeloma), may slow progression, although recovery is slow.

### D. Guillain-Barré Syndrome
1. Etiology is unknown. May occur after an infectious disorder, surgery, or an immunization.
2. Onset prevalence, and prognosis.
   a. Affects both sexes at any age.
   b. Onset of recovery is 2 - 4 weeks after first symptoms.
   c. Long-term prognosis.
      (1) 50% exhibit mild neurological deficits.
      (2) 15% exhibit residual functional deficits.
      (3) 80% are ambulatory in 6 months.
      (4) 5% die of complications.
3. Diagnosis.
   a. Diagnosis is based on clinical symptoms.
   b. Lumbar puncture reveals increased protein without cells in the cerebrospinal fluid.
   c. Electromyography and nerve conduction studies may support the diagnosis.
   d. Segmental demyelination is apparent and in severe cases, axonal degeneration accompanies the demyelination.
4. Symptoms.
   a. Acute, rapidly progressive form of polyneuropathy characterized by symmetric muscular weakness and mild distal sensory loss/paresthesias.
   b. Weakness is always more apparent than sensory findings and is at first more prominent distally.
   c. Deep tendon reflexes are lost and sphincters are spared.
   d. Respiratory failure and dysphagia may be seen in some cases.
5. Medical management.
   a. Severe cases constitute a medical emergency requiring constant monitoring of vital signs.
   b. Respiratory support may be necessary in some cases.
   c. Plasmapheresis may be utilized to slow symptoms or halt progression.
   d. Intravenous immunoglobulin has been utilized effectively.

### E. Myasthenia Gravis
1. Etiology: the disease is caused by an autoimmune attack on the acetylcholine receptor of the postsynaptic neuromuscular junction.
   a. This process is considered a disorder of neuromuscular transmission.
   b. The initiating event leading to antibody production is unknown.
2. Onset, prevalence, and prognosis.
   a. Occurs at any age but most often affects younger women and older men.
   b. Occurs in 14 per 100,000.
   c. Prognosis varies, but usually is a progressive disabling process.
   d. Death may occur from respiratory complications.
3. Diagnosis.
   a. Diagnosis is often missed because of the rarity of the disease and the vagueness of symptoms.
   b. Characterized by episodic muscle weakness, chiefly in muscles innervated by cranial nerves.
   c. The possibility of myasthenia gravis is suggested by any of the below symptoms and is confirmed by response to anticholinesterase drugs.
4. Symptoms.
   a. Common symptoms include ptosis, diplopia, muscle fatigue after exercise, dysarthria, dysphagia, and proximal limb weakness.
   b. Sensation and deep tendon reflexes are intact.
   c. Symptoms fluctuate over the course of the day.
   d. In relapsing periods, quadriparesis may develop.
   e. Life threatening respiratory muscle involvement may occur.
5. Medical management.
   a. Treatment includes cholinesterase inhibitors, corticosteroids, immunosuppressive agents, and plasmapheresis.
   b. The anticholinergics and plasmapheresis treat current symptoms.
   c. Corticosteroids and immunosuppressives may alter the disease course by interfering with autoimmune pathogenesis.

### F. Post-Polio Syndrome (PPS)
1. Etiology: some motor neurons infected with the polio virus die (leaving paralyzed muscle cells), others survive. Recovered motor neurons develop new terminal axon sprouts that reinnervate muscle

cells. After years of stability, these motor units break down, causing new muscle weakness.

    a. Degeneration of the axon sprouts explains the new weakness and fatigue, but the mechanism remains controversial.

    b. A current explanation is related to the overuse of individual motor neurons over time.

2. Onset, prevalence, and prognosis.

    a. 250,000 people live with post-polio syndrome.

    b. Onset is typically 15 years after recovery from polio.

    c. Progress is slow with a good prognosis unless breathing or swallowing difficulties occur.

3. Diagnosis.

    a. Based on clinical symptoms.

    b. Characterized by the onset of new muscle weakness after years of stable functioning.

    c. Disuse weakness should be ruled out.

4. Symptoms.

    a. New onset of weakness.

    b. Easily fatigued.

    c. Muscle pain.

    d. Joint pain.

    e. Cold intolerance.

    f. Atrophy.

    g. Loss of functional skills.

5. Medical management.

    a. Bracing with orthoses and pacing daily activity.

    b. Stretching programs.

    c. Exercise program.

    d. Low doses of tricyclic antidepressants to relieve muscle pain.

    e. Pyridostigmine to reduce fatigue and improve strength.

## VI. Demyelinating Disease

### A. Multiple Sclerosis (MS)

1. Etiology: the exact cause is unknown.

    a. The myelin damage is probably mediated by the immune system.

    b. Postulated etiologies include infection by a slow or latent virus and the possibility of environmental factors contributing to the disease.

2. Onset, prevalence, and prognosis.

    a. More prevalent in areas further north of the equator.

    b. Occurs in 100/100,000 in northern U.S.; 30/100,000 in southern U.S.

    c. Occurs between the ages of 15 and 50; it is most often diagnosed when persons are in their 30s.

    d. Overall prognosis is variable with an unpredictable disease course.

3. Diagnosis.

    a. Diagnosis is largely based on symptoms.

    b. Slowly progressive CNS disease characterized by patches of demyelination in the brain and spinal cord.

    c. Basic diagnostic criteria are evidence of multiple CNS lesions and evidence of at least two episodes of neurological disturbance in an individual between 10 and 59 years.

    d. Diagnostics may include MRI to detect lesions, evoked potentials to measure conduction along sensory pathways, and cerebrospinal fluid examination.

4. Symptoms.

    a. Multiple and varied neurologic symptoms and signs, usually with remissions and exacerbations.

    b. Onset of symptoms is usually insidious.

    c. Paresthesias in one or more extremities, on the trunk, or in the face.

    d. Weakness or clumsiness in the leg or hand is common.

    e. Visual disturbance (diplopia, partial blindness, nystagmus, eye pain, etc.).

    f. Emotional disturbances (lability, euphoria, and reactive depression).

    g. Vertigo.

    h. Bladder dysfunction.

    i. Cognitive features may include apathy, memory loss, lack of judgment, and inattention.

    j. Sensorimotor findings may include: spasticity, increased reflexes, ataxia, weakness, gait instability, easy fatigue, hemiplegia or quadriplegia.

    k. The course of the symptoms is highly variable and may follow one of three patterns.

        (1) Exacerbations and remissions.

        (2) Relapse and remission.

        (3) Chronic and progressive.

5. Medical management is symptom-specific.

    a. During acute exacerbation, anti-inflammatory drugs are used to control symptoms.

    b. Antispasmodics (Baclofen) may be effective to counteract spasticity.

    c. Management of bowel and bladder dysfunction may require pharmacologic intervention. Catheterization (indwelling or intermittent) is necessary in many cases of bladder dysfunction.

## VII. Occupational Therapy Evaluation and Intervention for Neurological System Disorders

**A. Role of the OTA in Evaluation**

1. The OTA contributes to the evaluation process.
   a. The OTA can assist with the collection of data for the evaluation once service competency has been established.
   b. The level of supervision required will be determined by the OTA's established service competency.
   c. The OTA cannot independently evaluate or interpret evaluation results.

**B. Client Factors and Performance Component/Skill Evaluation**

1. Sensory and motor dysfunction.
   a. Extent of paralysis/weakness.
   b. Severity and distribution of spasticity.
   c. Gross and fine motor coordination loss.
   d. Evaluation of sensory modalities: light touch, pain, pressure, proprioception, kinesthesia, temperature, gustatory, olfactory, auditory.
   e. Postural control evaluation.
   f. Range of motion testing.
   g. Manual muscle testing.
   h. Skin integrity.
2. Cognitive/perceptual dysfunction.
   a. Evaluation of foundation visual skills: acuity, visual fields, ocular range of motion, accommodation, pursuits, saccades.
   b. Evaluation of pervasive impairments: decreased arousal, decreased alertness, loss of selective/sustained attention, concrete thinking, decreased insight, impaired judgment, confusion, disorientation, language dysfunction, impaired motivation, and impaired initiative.
   c. Evaluation of the impact of specific deficits on basic and instrumental activities of daily living and mobility including: apraxia, spatial neglect, body neglect, perseveration, spatial relations dysfunction, various agnosias, organization and sequencing dysfunction, and memory loss.
3. Psychosocial dysfunction.
   a. Evaluation of emotional/affective disturbances: lability, euphoria, apathy, depression, aggression, irritability, frustration tolerance.
   b. Coping mechanisms.
   c. Adaptation to change in occupational role

functioning or to difficulty in assuming occupational roles.

4. See subsequent evaluation chapters for more information on each of the above areas.

**C. Areas of Occupation Evaluation**

1. Basic activities of daily living.
2. Instrumental activities of daily living.
3. Durable medical equipment evaluation.
4. School/work and return to school/work issues.
5. Play/leisure interests.
6. Mobility needs.
7. Social participation interests.
8. See Chapter 14 on the evaluation of performance in areas of occupation.

**D. Performance Context Evaluation**

1. Cultural barriers.
2. Architectural barriers.
3. Societal limitations.
   a. Financial barriers.
   b. Stigma.
4. Home evaluation.
5. School/work site evaluations.
6. See chapter on mastery of the environment.

**E. General Intervention/Treatment Guidelines**

1. Role of the OTA.
   a. The OTA implements intervention with OT supervision.
      (1) The level of supervision required depends upon the OTA's experience and established service competency.
      (2) During the implementation of intervention, the OTA informs the supervising therapist of any change in the individual's status and any other relevant information that may effect treatment.
2. Positioning.
   a. Seating and wheeled mobility prescription.
   b. Bed positioning.
   c. Pressure reduction and pressure relief techniques.
3. Postural control training for seated and standing activities.
4. Motor learning approaches.
5. Motor control retraining/relearning for functional integration of affected limbs.
6. Specific ADL training/retraining/adaptation.
7. Prescription of assistive devices and technology.
8. Splinting for contracture prevention and/or enhancement of function (e.g., tenodesis splint).
9. Family/caregiver education.

10. Cognitive-perceptual retraining/compensation in the context of functional activities.
11. Visual skills retraining and/or adaptation (e.g., an eye patch for diplopia).
12. Intervention for sexual dysfunction.
13. Bowel and bladder training with adaptive techniques and equipment.
14. Skin care education.
15. Durable medical equipment prescription.
16. Sensory re-education.
17. Assistance with the development of coping strategies.
18. Community re-integration.
19. Work hardening programs for adults.
20. Collaboration with educational team for children.
21. See chapters in Section IV for more information on each of the above areas.

## VIII. Pain

### A. Definition
1. The sensory and emotional experience associated with actual or potential tissue damage.

### B. Acute Pain
1. Pain provoked by noxious stimulation.
2. Associated with an underlying pathology (injury or acute inflammation/disease).
3. Signs include sharp pain and sympathetic changes (increased heart rate, increased blood pressure, pupillary dilation, sweating, hyperventilation, anxiety, protective/escape behaviors).

### C. Chronic Pain
1. Pain that persists beyond the usual course of healing.
2. Symptoms present for greater than 6 months for which an underlying pathology is no longer identifiable or may never have been present.

### D. Pain Syndromes
1. Neuropathic pain: pain as a result of lesions in some part of the nervous system (central or peripheral); usually accompanied by some degree of sensory deficit.
   a. Thalamic pain: continuous, intense pain occurring on the contralateral hemiplegic side; the result of a stroke involving the ventral posterolateral thalamus; poor rehabilitation potential.
   b. Complex Regional Pain Syndrome Type I (formerly known as reflex sympathetic dystrophy, [RSD]): pain maintained by efferent activity of sympathetic nervous system.
      (1) Characterized by abnormal burning pain (causalgia), hypersensitivity to light touch, and sympathetic hyperfunction (coldness, sweating, etc.).
      (2) Usually associated with traumatic injury.
   c. Disorders of peripheral roots and nerves.
      (1) Complex Regional Pain Syndrome Type II (formerly known as neuralgia): pain occurring along the branches of a nerve; frequently paroxysmal.
      (2) Radiculalgia: neuralgia of nerve roots.
      (3) Paresthesias, allodynia: with nerve injury or transection.
   d. Herpes Zoster (shingles): an acute, painful mono-neuropathy caused by the varicella-zoster virus.
      (1) Characterized by vesicular eruption and marked inflammation of the posterior root ganglion of the affected spinal nerve or sensory ganglion of the cranial nerve; ventral root involvement (motor weakness) in 5%-10% of cases.
      (2) Infection can last from 10 days to 5 weeks.
      (3) Pain may persist for months (post-herpetic neuralgia).
   e. Phantom limb pain: pain in a limb following amputation of that limb; differentiated from far more common phantom limb sensation.
   f. Musculoskeletal pain. Refer to Chapter 6.
   g. Psychosomatic pain: the origin of the pain experience is due to mental or emotional disorders.
   h. Headache and craniofacial pain, e.g., temporomandibular joint syndrome (TMJ).
   i. Referred pain: pain arising from deep visceral tissues that is felt in a body region remote from the site of pathology, resulting in tenderness and cutaneous hyperalgesia; e.g., medial left arm pain with heart attack; right subscapular pain from gallbladder attack.

### E. Assessment of Chronic Pain
1. Role of the OTA in evaluation.
   a. The OTA can assist with the collection of data for the evaluation once service competency has been established.
   b. The level of supervision required will be determined by the OTA's experience and established service competency.
   c. The OTA cannot independently evaluate or interpret evaluation results.
2. Evaluation focus.
   a. History: determine chief complaints, description of onset, and mechanism of injury.
   b. Determine localization: chronic pain is poorly localized, not well defined.

c. Identify nature of pain: constant, intermittent.

d. Determine irritating stimuli/activities.

e. Determine subjective assessment using pain intensity rating scales.

  (1) Simple descriptive scales: verbal report, (e.g., select the words that best describe your pain).

  (2) Semantic differentiation scales (e.g., McGill Pain Questionnaire).

  (3) Numerical rating scales (rate pain on a scale of 1 to 10, e.g., 8/10).

  (4) Visual analog scale (e.g., bisect line where · your pain falls, from mild to severe pain).

  (5) Spatial distribution of pain: using drawings to plot location, type of pain.

f. Physical examination: identification of underlying pathology (cause of pain); objective physical findings are usually not readily identified.

  (1) Assess all systems: musculoskeletal, neurologic, and cardiopulmonary. Check for muscle guarding.

  (2) Check for postural stress syndrome (PSS): chronic muscle lengthening and/or shortening that causes postural malalignment and stress to soft tissues.

  (3) Check for movement adaptation syndrome (MAS): habituated movement dysfunction.

  (4) Check for autonomic changes (sympathetic activity): typically present with acute pain but not with chronic pain.

  (5) Assess for abnormal movements.

g. Assess degree of suffering.

  (1) Verbal complaints are out of proportion to degree of underlying pathology; include emotional content.

  (2) The person exhibits a stooped posture, antalgic gait.

  (3) The person exhibits facial grimacing.

h. Assess for functional changes.

  (1) Check for self-imposed limited activity; disrupted lifestyle; disuse syndrome.

  (2) Check for avoidance of work, home management, leisure, social, and/or sexual activity.

i. Assess for consequences of pain, behavioral impact, secondary gains.

  (1) Monetary benefits (malingering, insurance claims).

  (2) Sympathy and attention.

  (3) Avoidance of undesirable tasks.

j. Assess for depression, anxiety.

k. Assess for prescription drug misuse.

l. Assess for dependence on health care system: multiple health care providers, clinical services; "shopping around" behaviors.

m. Determine responsiveness of pain to physiological interventions/treatments: chronic pain is often unresponsive.

n. Determine motivational/affective components.

  (1) Previous experience with pain.

  (2) Learned responses to pain.

  (3) Perception of control over pain.

  (4) Ethnic/cultural aspects of pain.

  (5) Familial response to pain behavior.

**F. Occupational Therapy Intervention**

1. Role of the OTA in intervention.

  a. The OTA implements intervention with OT supervision.

    (1) The level of supervision required depends upon the OTA's experience and established service competency.

    (2) During the implementation of intervention, the OTA informs the supervising therapist of any change in the individual's status and any other relevant information that may effect treatment.

2. Intervention focus.

  a. Educate the individual about contributing factors.

  b. Assist the individual in identifying and responding adaptively to pain behaviors.

    (1) Remove behavioral reinforcers.

    (2) Establish a behavior contract.

    (3) Provide positive reinforcers, educational support.

    (4) Demonstrate change, allow person to experience success.

    (5) Practice well behaviors.

  c. Assist the individual in developing strategies and using techniques to manage pain.

    (1) Teach coping skills/stress management/ assertive communication.

    (2) Provide relaxation training.

      (a) Progressive relaxation techniques (e.g., Jacobson's), deep breathing exercises.

      (b) Guided imagery.

      (c) Yoga, Tai Chi, Ai Chi.

      (d) Biofeedback.

  d. Refer to other professionals for direct pain/symptom control interventions.

e. Establish a realistic daily activity program.
(1) Improve overall level of conditioning: daily walking program.
(2) Improve overall functional capacity, independence in functional mobility skills, activities of daily living and meaningful occupations.
(3) Prescribe assistive devices as appropriate.
(4) Teach energy conservation techniques.
(5) Provide meaningful diversional activities.
f. Provide family education.

# IX. Sensory Processing Disorders

## A. Etiology
1. Unknown.
2. Subtle, primarily subcortical, neural dysfunction with impaired processing of sensory information and modulation of multisensory systems.
3. Symptoms are classified under the categories of:
   a. Sensory modulation disorder (SMD).
   b. Sensory-based motor disorder (SBMD).
   c. Sensory discrimination disorder (SDD).

## B. Presenting Signs and Symptoms
1. Stress and frustration demonstrated in performance of everyday activities.
2. Difficulties with play, learning, social situations, and other developmental functions.
3. Difficulty with planning and sequencing motor tasks (dyspraxia).
   a. Tendency to avoid or reject simple motor challenges.
4. Poor initiation of activities as demonstrated in some children due to difficulty generating ideas (ideation).
5. Difficulty with goal directed action on the environment, known as an adaptive response.
6. Responses may present along a continuum of under-responsivity (hyposensitivity) to over-responsivity (hypersensitivity) of multisensory processing and sensory seeking.
7. Tactile processing dysfunction manifestations.
   a. Deficits in modulation (regulation and organization).
      (1) Tactile defensiveness: over-responsivity/hypersensitivity to ordinary touch sensations.
         (a) The individual may demonstrate irritation and discomfort from a variety from textures such as clothing, sand, grass, glue, water, paint and/or food.
         (b) The individual may dislike brushing his/her teeth or hair.
         (c) The individual may demonstrate various behavioral responses including distractibility, anger, hostility, temper tantrums, fear, and/or distress.
      (2) Under-responsivity/hyposensitivity to tactile stimuli as demonstrated by diminished sensory registration and responsiveness.
         (a) The individual may not respond to normal levels of tactile input and may seek disproportionate amounts of stimuli to gain environmental information (e.g., excessive touching of people or objects).
   b. Deficits in tactile discrimination.
      (1) Difficulty interpreting tactile information in a precise and efficient manner.
         (a) Contributes to impaired body scheme and somatodyspraxia (a disorder in motor planning due to poor tactile perception and proprioception).
         (b) Contributes to awkwardness in fine and gross motor tasks, impaired manipulation skills, visual perception, and eye-hand coordination.
         (c) Hinders ability to learn about properties and substances.
      (2) Difficulty with localizing tactile stimuli.
   c. Impaired stereognosis and decreased fine motor and eye-hand coordination skills may be demonstrated in difficulties with writing and cutting with a scissors and knife.
8. Proprioceptive processing dysfunction manifestations.
   a. Deficits in modulation.
   b. Discrimination deficits demonstrated by poor awareness of position of body, body parts, and body schema.
   c. Clumsiness, awkwardness.
   d. Distractibility.
   e. Motor planning and movement difficulties
   f. Reliance on visual cues or other cognitive strategies to motor plan, guide movements, and perform tasks.
   g. Use of too much or too little force, e.g., stomping when walking, breaking objects unintentionally.
   h. Poor awareness of personal space.
   i. Seek heavy resistance and pressure.
9. Vestibular processing dysfunction manifestations.

a.  Deficits in modulation.
   (1)  Over-responsivity/hypersensitivity to movement, characterized by aversion to movement impacting on the sympathetic system.
   (2)  Hyposensitivity to movement characterized by the individual seeking intense vestibular stimulation without complaints of feeling dizzy, and by a tendency to be a thrill seeker unaware of potential danger.
   (3)  Gravitational insecurity characterized by excessive fear during typical activities when the head is not upright, especially when the individual's feet are off the ground, when moving backwards or upwards in space, walking on uneven terrain, jumping, getting on/off elevators, using any playground equipment involving movement, and when handling even minimal heights.

b.  Vestibular discrimination deficits, characterized by the above symptoms; however, symptoms are demonstrated on a subtle level.
c.  Low muscle tone.
d.  Postural-ocular deficits
e.  Decreased balance and equilibrium reactions.
f.  Poor bilateral coordination.
g.  Poor endurance.
h.  Poor motor planning and sequencing.
i.  Behavior responses include difficulty with attention, organization of behavior, communication.

10. Sensory-based motor disorder.
   a.  Deficits in proprioceptive and vestibular systems.
   b.  Dyspraxia: difficulty with planning movements, particularly those that are complex or new.
   c.  Postural disorders: decreased muscle tone impacting on stability.

**C.  Medical Management**
1.  Possible pharmacology intervention to decrease activity level.

**D.  Occupational Therapy Evaluation**
1.  Parent interview regarding medical and developmental history.
2.  Teacher interview regarding school performance, play, and behaviors.
3.  Informal observations of performance and behavior in a variety of settings, e.g., classroom, playground, home.
4.  Formal assessment of clinical observations using

Ayres unpublished and nonstandardized tool.
   a.  Items to be observed include specific reflexes, crossing body midline, bilateral coordination, muscle tone.
5.  Assess using standardized tests for tactile processing, vestibular-proprioceptive processing, visual perception, practic ability and their impact on occupational functioning.
6.  Role of the OTA in Evaluation.
   a.  The OTA contributes to the evaluation process.
      (1)  The OTA can assist with the collection of data for the evaluation once service competency has been established.
      (2)  The level of supervision required will be determined by the OTA's established service competency.
      (3)  The OTA cannot independently evaluate or interpret evaluation results.

**E.  Occupational Therapy Intervention**
1.  Role of the OTA.
   a.  The OTA implements intervention with OT supervision.
      (1)  The level of supervision required depends upon the OTA's experience and established service competency.
      (2)  During the implementation of intervention, the OTA informs the supervising therapist of any change in the individual's status and any other relevant information that may effect treatment.
2.  See Chapter 10 for information on the sensory integration (SI) frame of reference and intervention approaches.

# X.  Seizure Disorders[1]

**A.  Etiology**
1.  Abnormal bursts of electricity interfere with normal brain function.
2.  Seizures are usually idiopathic; they can be hereditary.
3.  Seizures are often associated with conditions that involve scarring in the brain.
   a.  Severe head injuries or brain hemorrhage.
   b.  Cerebral palsy.
   c.  Hydrocephalus.
   d.  Metabolic disorders.
   e.  Infections, meningitis, encephalitis, congenital infections.
   f.  Rubella.

---

[1]Marge E. Moffett Boyd contributed to this section on seizure disorders.

**B. Presenting Signs and Symptoms for Specific Classifications of Seizures**

1. Epilepsy is a chronic state of recurrent seizures.
2. Generalized seizures.
   a. Tonic-clonic seizures/grand mal seizures.
      (1) Most common type of seizure disorder in children.
      (2) A brief warning/aura such as numbness, taste, smell, or other sensation occurs.
      (3) Tonic phase includes a loss of consciousness, stiffening of the body, heavy and irregular breathing, drooling, skin pallor, and occasional bladder and bowel incontinence for a few seconds before the clonic phase begins.
      (4) Clonic phase includes alternating rigidity and relaxation of muscles.
      (5) Postictal state follows the clonic phase, and includes a period of drowsiness, disorientation or fatigue.
   b. Myoclonic-akinetic seizure.
      (1) Myoclonic seizures are not the same as infantile myoclonic seizures.
      (2) Myoclonic seizures are brief, involuntary jerking of the extremities, with or without loss of consciousness.
      (3) Akinetic seizures include a loss of tone.
      (4) Myoclonic-akinetic seizures are difficult to control.
   c. Absence seizures or petit mal seizures.
      (1) Typically occur between ages of 4 and 12 years.
      (2) A loss of consciousness without loss of muscle tone occurs.
      (3) The child does not fall down, but does not recall the episode or any lapse in time.
3. Partial focal seizures.
   a. Simple partial seizures.
      (1) Abnormal electrical impulses occur in a localized area of the brain, often in the motor strip of the frontal lobe.
      (2) Involuntary, repetitive jerking of the left hand and arm occurs, but the individual can maintain interaction with his/her environment.
      (3) Focal seizures may become generalized, and result in a loss of consciousness.
   b. Complex partial or psychomotor seizures.
      (1) Symptoms vary.
      (2) There are alterations in consciousness and unresponsiveness.
      (3) Automatic motions, such as lip smacking, chewing and swallowing, and nervous movement of the hands/fingers, and repetitive movements occur.
      (4) Visual or auditory sensations occur just before the seizure.
4. Selected seizure syndromes.
   a. Infantile spasms or West syndrome, infantile myoclonic seizures or jackknife epilepsy.
      (1) Begins at 3 to 9 months of age.
      (2) Dropping of the head and flexion of the arms occurs.
      (3) Seizures may occur hundreds of times per day.
      (4) Prognosis is generally poor.
      (5) Spasms sometimes decrease after several years, but are often replaced by other seizure disorders.
      (6) These seizures often indicate an underlying disorder such as tuberous sclerosis.
   b. Lennax-Gastaut syndrome.
      (1) Children with severe seizures, mental retardation, and a specific EEG pattern.
      (2) Seizures of different types begin during the first three years of life and are difficult to control.
      (3) Associated with various brain disorders from structural abnormalities to birth asphyxia.
      (4) A regression of developmental status can occur in some cases.
5. Simple febrile seizures.
   a. Most common type of seizure, occurring in 5 to 10% of children under the age of five, precipitated by a fever.
   b. The seizure lasts less than 10 minutes and it includes a loss of consciousness and involuntary, generalized jerking of a grand mal seizure.
   c. These seizures usually do not cause damage and they do not lead to epilepsy.

**C. Diagnostic Criteria**

1. Clinical observations of the obvious manifestations associated with the specific seizure disorder.
2. The EEG alone is not sufficient to diagnose a seizure disorder since the disorder does not always show up on the EEG and conversely abnormal EEG patterns may appear when there is no clinical evidence of seizures.

**D. Impact on Occupational Performance**

1. The seizure disorder and/or the anticonvulsive

medication(s) prescribed to control the seizures may affect the individual's alertness and learning potential.

2. The amount of brain damage incurred by the seizures and associated conditions and the effects of medication can influence performance in all areas of occupation.

**E. Medical Management**

1. A neurologist is most often required to medically manage seizures.

2. Seizure disorders are treated with anticonvulsive medications.

   a. Phenobarbital (Luminal), carbamazepine (Tegretol), Phenytoin (Dilantin) and valproic acid (Depakene) are used with grand mal seizures.

   b. Ethosuximide (Zarontin) is used with petit mal seizures.

   c. Carbamazepine and primidone are used with psychomotor seizures.

   d. Clonazepam (Clonopin), steroids, and CTH (hormone secreted by the pituitary gland) are used with myoclonic seizures.

**F. Intervention for Seizure Disorders**

1. First aid procedures for seizures.

   a. Remain calm.

   b. Remove dangerous objects and protect the individual from harm, without interfering with his or her movements.

   c. If the individual is upright, gently guide them to the floor and loosen clothing.

   d. Turn the individual on his/her side to prevent choking.

   e. Do not insert anything between the individual's teeth.

   f. Do not be alarmed if the individual seems to stop breathing momentarily.

   g. If the individual's breathing actually stops, use standard rescue breathing techniques.

2. Post-seizure care.

   a. Allow the individual to rest or sleep after the seizure.

   b. Call a physician if this is the individual's first seizure, if the seizure is followed by another seizure (status epilepticus), or if the seizure lasts more than 5 minutes.

   c. Notify the parents/guardians/caregivers or designated emergency contact person that a seizure has occurred.

   d. Observe safety precautions if the individual seems groggy, confused, or weak following the seizure.

3. Occupational therapy evaluation and intervention.

   a. Assess and intervene for developmental delays as necessary.

   b. Observe all medical and safety precautions.

   c. Document and report any seizure activity, medication side effects, or behavioral changes.

# References

Blackman, J.A. (1997) Spina bifida. In J.A. Blackman. *Medical aspects of developmental disabilities in children birth to three, 3rd ed.* (pp. 36-39). Gaithersberg, MD: Aspen.

Blackman, J.A. (1997). Seizure disorders. In J.A. Blackman. *Medical aspects of developmental disabilities in children birth to three, 3rd ed.* (238-246). Gaithersberg, MD: Aspen.

Case-Smith, J. (Ed.). (2005). *Occupational therapy for children, 5th ed.* St. Louis, MO: Elsevier Mosby.

Escolar, D.M. & Toisi, L.L. (2005). Muscles, bones and nerves. In M.L. Batshaw, L. Pellegrino, & N.J. Roizen (Ed.), *Children with disabilities, 6th ed.* (pp. 203-215). Baltimore, MD: Paul H. Brooks.

Cohen, H. (Ed.). (1999). *Neuroscience for rehabilitation, 2nd ed.* Philadelphia: J.B. Lippincott.

Fisher, A.G., Murray, E.A., & Bundy, A.C. (1991). *Sensory integration.* Philadelphia: F.A. Davis.

Gillen, G., & Burkhardt, A. (Eds.). (2004). *Stroke rehabilitation: A function-based approach. 2nd ed.* St. Louis, MO: Mosby/Elsevier.

Gutman, S. A., & Schonfeld, A. B. (2003). *Screening adult neurologic populations: A step-by-step instruction manual.* Bethesda, MD: American Occupational Therapy Association.

Kandell, E.R., Schwartz, T.H., & Tessel, T.M. (Eds.). (2000). *Principles of neural science (4th ed.).* Norwalk, CT: Appleton and Lange.

Lane, S.J. (2002). Structure and function of the sensory systems. In A. C., Bundy, S.J. Lane, & E. A. Murray, (Eds.), *Sensory integration: Theory and practice, 2nd ed.* (pp. 35-68). Philadelphia, PA: F.A. Davis.

Lane, S.J. (2002). Sensory modulation. In A.C., Bundy, S.J. Lane, & E.A. Murray, (Eds.), *Sensory integration: Theory and practice, 2nd ed.* (pp. 101-122). Philadelphia: F.A. Davis.

Liptak, G.S., Gregory (2005) Neural tube defects. In M.L. Batshaw, L. Pellegrino, & N.J. Roizen (Ed.), *Children with disabilities, 6th ed.* (pp. 419- 438). Baltimore, MD: Paul H. Brooks.

Madsen, J.H. *Tethered cord syndrome: Questions and answers,* Retrieved 7/30/01 from www.boston-neurosurg.org/amphitheater/tetheredcord.html

Miller, L.J. (2006). *Sensational kids hope and help for children with sensory processing disorders (SPD).* NY: G.P. Putnam's Sons.

Parham, L.D. & Mailoux, Z. (2005). Sensory integration. In J, Case-Smith (Ed.), *Occupational therapy for children 5th ed.* (pp. 356-409). St. Louis, MO: Elsevier Mosby.

Pendleton, H., & Schultz-Krohn, W. (Eds.) (2006). *Occupational therapy: Practice skills for physical dysfunction, 6th ed.* St. Louis, MO: Elsevier Mosby.

Reeves, G.D. & Cermak, S.A. (2002). Disorders of praxis. In A.C., Bundy, S.J. Lane, & E.A. Murray, (Eds.), *Sensory integration: Theory and practice, 2nd ed.* (pp. 71-100). Philadelphia: F.A. Davis.

Rogers, S. (2005). Common conditions that influence children's participation. In J. Case-Smith (Ed). *Occupational therapy for children, 5th ed.* (pp.160-215). St. Louis, MO: Elsevier Mosby.

Schultz-Krohn, W. & Pendleton, H. (eds.) (2006). *Occupational therapy: practice skills for physical dysfunction, 6th ed.,* Elsevier Mosby, St. Louis.

Shaf, R. & Lane, S. (2009). Neuroscience foundations of vestibular, proprioceptive, and tactile sensory strategies. *OT Practice, 14*(22), CE1-CE8.

Vining-Radomski, M. & Trombly-Latham, C.A. (2007). *Occupational therapy for physical dysfunction, 6th ed.* Baltimore: Williams & Wilkins.

Weinstein, S.L. & Gaillard, W.D. (2005). Epilepsy. In M. L. Batshaw, L. Pellegrino, & N.J. Roizen (Eds.), *Children with disabilities, 6th ed.* (439-460). Baltimore, MD: Paul H. Brooks.

# CHAPTER 8

# CARDIOVASCULAR AND PULMONARY SYSTEM DISORDERS

Regina M. Lehman • Susan B. O'Sullivan • Julia Ann Starr • Josephine Dolera

## I. Cardiovascular System

### A. Function
1. Delivers oxygen to organs and tissues.
2. Removes carbon dioxide and other by-products from body.
3. Assists in the regulation of core body temperature.

### B. Cardiovascular Anatomy and Physiology
1. Relationship to the examination.
   a. It is not likely that the NBCOT exam will ask direct questions about anatomy and physiology.
   b. As a result, this chapter does not provide a complete anatomy and physiology review.
   c. Major structures and functions are outlined because knowledge of these can increase understanding of cardiovascular function.
2. Heart tissue.
   a. Pericardium: fibrous protective sac enclosing heart.
   b. Epicardium: inner layer of pericardium.
   c. Myocardium: heart muscle, the major portion of the heart.
   d. Endocardium: smooth lining of the inner surface and cavities of the heart.
3. Heart chambers.
   a. Four chambers arranged in pairs, functioning as two pumps working in sequence.
      (1) Right atrium (RA): receives blood from systemic circulation (from the superior and inferior vena cavae); during systole (contraction) blood is sent into right ventricle.
      (2) Right ventricle (RV): pumps blood via the pulmonary artery to the lungs for oxygenation; the low pressure pulmonary pump.
      (3) Left atrium (LA): receives oxygenated blood from the lungs (from the pulmonary veins); during systole, blood is sent into the left ventricle.
      (4) Left ventricle (LV): pumps blood via the aorta throughout the entire systemic circulation; walls of left are thicker and stronger than right ventricle; the high-pressure systemic pump.
   b. Blood flow.
      (1) Systemic circulation to RA to RV then to lungs for oxygenation.
      (2) LA receives oxygenated blood from the lungs, sends blood to LV.
      (3) LV pumps blood to the body via the aorta.
4. Valves: provide one-way flow of blood into, out of, and within heart.
5. Coronary circulation.
   a. Right coronary artery (RCA): supplies right atrium, most of right ventricle, and in most individuals the inferior wall of left ventricle, atrioventricular (AV) node and bundle of His; 60% of time supplies the sinoatrial (SA) node.

b. Left coronary artery (LCA): supplies most of the left ventricle; has two main divisions - left anterior descending (LAD) and circumflex.

c. Veins: parallel arterial system.

6. Conduction: specialized tissue allows rapid transmission of electrical impulses in the myocardium; includes nodal tissue and Purkinje fibers.

   a. Sinoatrial (SA) node: main pacemaker of the heart; initiates sinus rhythm; has sympathetic and parasympathetic innervation affecting both heart rate and strength of contraction.

   b. Atrioventricular (AV) node: has sympathetic and parasympathetic innervation; merges with bundle of His.

   c. Purkinje tissue: specialized conducting tissue of the ventricles.

   d. Conduction of heart beat.
      (1) Impulse originates in SA node and spreads throughout both atria which contract together.
      (2) Impulse stimulates AV node, is transmitted down bundle of His to the Purkinje fibers.
      (3) Impulse spreads throughout the ventricles which contract together.

7. Myocardial fibers: striated muscle tissue/fibers which exhibit rhythmicity of contraction as fibers contract as a functional unit; myocardial metabolism is primarily aerobic, sustained by continuous O2 delivery.

8. Peripheral circulation.

   a. Arteries: transport oxygenated blood from areas of high pressure to lower pressures in the body tissues.

   b. Capillaries: minute blood vessels that connect the ends of arteries (arterioles) with the beginning of veins (venules); forms an anastomosing network.

   c. Veins: transport dark, unoxygenated blood from tissues back to the heart.

9. Neural control of heart rate and blood vessels.

   a. Parasympathetic control (cholinergic): cardioinhibitory center.

   b. Sympathetic control (adrenergic): cardioacceleratory center.

   c. Additional control mechanisms.
      (1) Baroreceptors: main mechanism controlling heart rate; respond to changes in blood pressure.
      (2) Chemoreceptors: sensitive to changes in blood chemicals ($O^2$, $CO^2$, lactic acid).

(3) Body temperature: heart rate changes analogously to temperature.

(4) Ion concentrations.
   (a) Hyperkalemia: increased potassium ions, decreases the rate and force of contraction, and produces EKG changes.
   (b) Hypokalemia: decreased potassium ions, produces EKG changes; arrhythmias, may progress to ventricular fibrillation.
   (c) Hypercalcemia: increased calcium concentration; increases heart rate.
   (d) Hypocalcemia: decreased calcium concentration; depresses heart action.

d. Cardiac output: amount of blood ejected from the heart per minute; dependent upon heart rate and stroke volume.

e. Stroke volume: average amount of blood ejected per heart beat.

f. Peripheral resistance.
   (1) Increased peripheral resistance increases arterial blood volume and pressure.
   (2) Decreased peripheral resistance decreases arterial blood volume and pressure.
   (3) Influenced by arterial blood volume: viscosity of blood and diameter of arterioles and capillaries.

## II. Coronary Artery Disease (CAD)

### A. Definition

1. Atherosclerotic disease process that narrows the lumen of coronary arteries resulting in ischemia to the myocardium.

### B. Atherosclerosis

1. Etiology: characterized by thickening of the intimal layer of the blood vessel wall from the focal accumulation of lipids.

2. Onset: variable depending upon presence or absence of risk factors.

3. Prevalence: increases with age and presence of risk factors.

4. Prognosis: good with early detection and treatment.

5. Multiple risk factors.

   a. Non-modifiable risk factors: age, sex, race, significant family history.

   b. Modifiable risk factors: cigarette smoking, high blood pressure, elevated cholesterol levels, inactivity.

   c. Contributing risk factors: diabetes, obesity, stress.

   d. Two or more risk factors increase the risk of CAD.

## C. Main Clinical Syndromes of CAD

1. Angina pectoris: clinical manifestation of ischemia characterized by mild to moderate substernal chest pain/discomfort most commonly felt as pressure or dull ache in the chest and left arm but may be felt anywhere in the upper body including neck, jaw, back, arm, epigastric area.
   a. Usually lasts less than 20 minutes due to transient ischemia.
   b. Represents an imbalance in myocardial oxygen supply and demand; brought on by:
      (1) Increased demands on heart: exertion/exercise, emotional upsets, smoking, extremes of temperature (especially cold), overeating, tachyarrhythmias.
      (2) Vasospasm: symptoms may be present at rest.
   c. Types of angina.
      (1) Stable angina: classic exertional angina; relieved with rest and/or sublingual nitroglycerin.
      (2) Unstable angina (preinfarction, crescendo angina): coronary insufficiency with risk for myocardial infarction or sudden death; pain is difficult to control; presents with low level activity or rest.
2. Myocardial infarction (MI): prolonged ischemia, injury, and death of an area of the myocardium caused by occlusion of one or more of the coronary arteries; results in necrosis of heart tissue.
   a. Precipitating factors: atherosclerotic heart disease with thrombus formation, coronary vasospasm or embolism; cocaine toxicity.
   b. Symptomology/presenting signs and symptoms.
      (1) Severe substernal pain of more than 20 minutes duration which may radiate to neck, jaw, arm, epigastric area.
      (2) Dyspnea, rapid respiration, shortness of breath.
      (3) Indigestion, nausea, and vomiting.
      (4) Pain may be misinterpreted as indigestion.
      (5) Pain unrelieved by rest and/or sublingual nitroglycerin.
   c. Infarction sites.
      (1) Transmural (Q wave infarction); full thickness of myocardium.
      (2) Nontransmural (non Q wave infarction); subendocardial, subepicardial, intramural infarctions.
      (3) Coronary artery occlusion.
         (a) Inferior MI, right ventricle infarction, disturbances of upper conduction system: right coronary artery.
         (b) Lateral MI, ventricular ectopy: circumflex artery.
         (c) Anterior MI, disturbances of lower conduction system: left anterior descending artery.
   d. Results of impaired ventricular function.
      (1) Decreased stroke volume, cardiac output and ejection fraction.
      (2) Increased end diastolic ventricular pressure.
   e. Electrical instability, arrhythmias, present in injured and ischemia areas.
3. Congestive heart failure (CHF): cardiac failure.
   a. A condition in which the heart is unable to maintain adequate circulation of the blood to meet the metabolic needs of the body.
   b. Etiology: may be caused by coronary artery disease, valvular disease, congenital heart disease, hypertension, infections.
   c. Physiological abnormalities: decreased cardiac output, elevated end diastolic pressures (preload); increased heart rate; impaired ventricular contractility.
   d. Left heart failure: blood is not adequately pumped into systemic circulation; due to an inability of left ventricle to pump blood out of lungs, increases in ventricular end-diastolic pressure and left pressures with pulmonary signs and symptoms including:
      (1) Dyspnea: exertional, orthopnea (in supine), paroxysmal nocturnal (sudden shortness of breath at night).
      (2) Cough, rales, wheezing.
      (3) Weakness, fatigue.
      (4) Tachycardia, change in heart sounds.
      (5) Chest pain.
      (6) Table 8-1.
   e. Right heart failure: blood is not adequately returned from the systemic circulation to the heart; due to failure of right ventricle, increased pulmonary artery pressures with:
      (1) Peripheral edema: weight gain, dependent edema, venous stasis.
      (2) Nausea, anorexia.
      (3) Change in heart sounds.
      (4) Table 8-1.

### D. Classification of Heart Disease

1. The American Heart Association has classified heart disease according to the patient's activity level based on METs (metabolic equivalents).
   a. Basal metabolic rate equals 3.5 ml of oxygen per kilogram of body weight per minute.
2. Class I.
   a. Heart disease; no limits to activity; no complaints.
   b. Max MET 6.5.
3. Class II.
   a. Slight activity limit; comfort at rest; ordinary activity results in fatigue, pain, dyspnea, palpitations.
   b. Max MET 4.5.
4. Class III.
   a. Marked limitation; comfort at rest; less than ordinary activity - fatigue, palpitations, dyspnea, and angina pain.
   b. Max MET 3.0.

### TABLE 8-1 - POSSIBLE CLINICAL MANIFESTATIONS OF CARDIAC FAILURE

#### SIGNS ASSOCIATED WITH RIGHT-SIDED HEART FAILURE

| | |
|---|---|
| Nausea | Increase in RAP, CVP |
| Anorexia | Jugular venous distention |
| Weight gain | + hepatojugular reflex |
| Ascites | Right ventricular heave |
| Right upper quadrant pain | Murmur of tricuspid insufficiency Hepatomegaly Peripheral edema |

#### SIGNS ASSOCIATED WITH LEFT-SIDED HEART FAILURE

| | |
|---|---|
| Fatigue | Tachycardia |
| Cough | $S_3$ gallop |
| Shortness of breath | Crackles |
| DOE | Increased PAP, PAWP, SVR |
| Orthopnea | Laterally displaced PMI |
| PND | Left ventricular heave |
| Diaphoresis | Pulsus Alternans Confusion Decreased urine output Cheyne-Stokes respirations (advanced failure) Murmur of mitral insufficiency |

RAP, right atrial pressure. CVP, central venous pressure. PAP, pulmonary artery pressure. PAWP, pulmonary artery wedge pressure. SVR, systemic vascular resistance. DOE, dyspnea on exertion. PND, paroxysmal nocturnal dyspnea. PMI, point of maximal impulse.

From Pocket Guide to Cardiovascular Care, 1990 by Susan Stillwell and Edith Randall, CV Mosby Company, p19, with permission.

5. Class IV.
   a. Inability to carry out physical activity without discomfort; symptoms of cardiac insufficiency present at rest; increased discomfort with any activity.
   b. Max MET 1.5.
6. As the person can perform the same activity at a lower pulse rate, they can be reclassified.

### E. Medical and Surgical Management/Relevant Pharmacology

1. Diagnostic procedures.
   a. Chest x-ray: done to evaluate evidence of congestion in lungs, heart chamber hypertrophy, and structural abnormalities.
   b. Electrocardiogram (ECG): done to identify cardiac arrhythmias, assess amount and location of damage to myocardium, determine adequacy of oxygenation of myocardium.
   c. Holter monitor: records ECG signals over a 24 hour period while person engages in normal daily routine to determine heart function during various activities.
   d. Echocardiogram: ultrasound used to record size, structure, and motion of the heart and vessels; reveals valvular defects and structural abnormalities.
   e. Cardiac stress test: records cardiac activity during graded exercise; used to determine the extent to which cardiac disease affects functional capacity; provides guidelines related to the type and amount of physical activity that a person can engage in safely.
   f. Cardiac catheterization: invasive procedure used to visualize coronary circulation to determine the degree of CAD, congenital heart defect, valvular disease, myocardial damage.
   g. Pulmonary function test: used to determine cause of dyspnea, degree of lung disease; provides information related to endurance potential for functional activities.
2. Dietary interventions: low salt, low cholesterol, weight reduction.
3. Medical therapy: drugs aimed at reducing oxygen demand on the heart and increasing coronary blood flow.
   a. ACE inhibitors/nitrates/vasodilators (nitroglycerin, Notorstat, Minoxidil, Vasotec, Monopril): improve coronary blood flow, relieve chest pain/angina.
   b. Beta blockers (Inderal, propranolol): control

arrhythmias, chest pain; reduce blood pressure.

c. Calcium channel blockers (Cardizem, Procardia): reduce BP, control arrhythmias, chest pain.

d. Antihypertensives (Inderol, Lopressor): control hypertension/blood pressure.

e. Diuretics (Lasix): control hypertension.

4. All medications have possible side effects.

a. If any unusual symptoms occur during treatment they could be associated with an adverse drug reaction.

(1) In these cases, the OTA should alert the occupational therapist, cardiologist, or attending physician.

5. Surgical interventions include the following procedure presented in order of invasiveness. Surgical procedures may result in deconditioning and impact on the patient's ability to carryout both BADL and IADL.

a. Percutaneous transluminal coronary angioplasty (PCTA): surgical dilation of a blood vessel using a small balloon-tipped catheter inflated inside the lumen; relieves obstructed blood flow; improves coronary blood flow; relieves angina.

b. Intravascular stents: implanted post PCTA to prevent restenosis and occlusion in coronary or peripheral arteries.

c. Revascularization surgery (coronary artery bypass grafting, CABG): surgical circumvention of an obstruction in a coronary artery using an anastomosing graft (saphenous vein, internal mammary artery)

d. Ventricular assistive devices (VADs): implanted device (accessory pump) used with severely involved patients, those awaiting transplant.

e. Transplantation: used in end-stage myocardial disease.

6. Thrombolytic therapy for acute myocardial infarction.

a. Medications administered to activate body's fibrinolytic system, dissolve clot, and restore coronary blood flow.

**F. Peripheral Vascular Disease (PVD)**

1. Arterial disease.

a. Arteriosclerosis obliterans.

(1) Chronic, occlusive arterial disease of medium and large-sized vessels.

(2) Associated with hypertension, hyperlipidemia, CAD, diabetes.

(3) Affects primarily lower extremities.

b. Thromboangiitis obliterans (Buerger's disease): chronic inflammatory vascular occlusive disease.

(1) Most common in young males who smoke.

(2) Begins distally and progresses proximally in both lower and upper extremities.

(3) Symptoms include pain, paresthesias, cold extremities, diminished temperature sensation, fatigue; risk of ulceration and gangrene.

c. Diabetic angiopathy: inappropriate elevation of blood glucose levels and accelerated atherosclerosis; neuropathies a major problem; ulcers may lead to gangrene and amputation.

d. Raynaud's phenomenon: abnormal vasoconstriction reflex exacerbated by exposure to cold or emotional stress; affects largely females.

2. Venous disease.

a. Varicose veins: distended, swollen superficial veins.

b. Deep vein thrombosis (DVT): inflammation of a vein in association with the formation of a thrombus; usually occurs in lower extremities.

(1) May be a contributing factor to or a complication of cerebral vascular accident (CVA) or the result of prolonged bed rest during serious illness.

(2) Signs and symptoms include a change in lower extremity temperature, color circumference, appearance, or tenderness/pain. These require immediate medical attention.

c. Chronic venous insufficiency.

d. Lymphatic disease (lymphedema): excessive accumulation of fluid due to obstruction of lymphatics, causes swelling of soft tissues in arms and legs.

## III. Pulmonary System

### A. Function

1. Respiration, delivers oxygen to cardiovascular system.

2. Removes carbon dioxide and other by-products from body.

### B. Anatomy and Physiology

1. Bony thorax: anterior border is the sternum, lateral border is the ribcage, posterior border is the vertebral column; shoulder girdle can affect the motion of the thorax.

2. Airways.

a. Upper airways: nose, pharynx, larynx.

b. Lower airways: conducting airways (trachea to terminal bronchioles) and the respiratory unit (respiratory bronchioles, alveolar ducts, alveolar sacs and alveoli).

3. Lungs.
4. Pleura.
5. Muscles of ventilation.
   a. Primary muscles of inspiration: diaphragm, intercostals.
   b. Accessory muscles of inspiration: used when a more rapid or deeper inhalation is required or in disease; include sternocleidomastoid, scalenes, levator costarum, serratus, trapezius, and pectorals.
   c. Expiratory muscles.
      (1) Resting expiration: done by passive relaxation of inspiratory muscles and elastic recoil tendency of lungs.
      (2) Expiratory muscles used when quicker, fuller expiration is desired or in disease; include quadratus lumborum, intercostals, rectus abdominis, triangularis sterni.
6. Mechanics of breathing: forces acting upon the rib cage include elastic recoil of lungs, bony thorax, muscles.
7. Ventilation and perfusion: the movement of gas in and out of the pulmonary system.
   a. Measurements include volumes, capacities, flow rates.
   b. Optimal respiration occurs when ventilation and perfusion (blood flow to lungs) are matched.
   c. Body position/gravity affects distribution of ventilation and perfusion.
8. Respiration: diffusion of gas across the alveolo-capillary membrane.
9. Control of ventilation.
   a. Receptors: baroreceptors, chemoreceptors, irritant receptors, stretch receptors.
   b. Central control centers: brain and autonomic nervous system.
   c. Ventilatory muscles.

## IV. Pulmonary Dysfunction

### A. Acute Diseases

1. Bacterial pneumonia: an intra-alveolar bacterial infection.
   a. Gram positive bacteria usually acquired in the community; pneumococcal pneumonia (streptococcal) is the most common type.
   b. Gram negative bacteria usually develops in host who has underlying chronic condition, acute illness, recent antibiotic therapy; usually results in early tissue necrosis and abscess formation.
2. Viral pneumonia: an interstitial or interalveolar inflammatory process caused by viral agents.
3. Aspiration pneumonia: aspirated material causes an acute inflammatory reaction within the lungs; usually found in patients with impaired swallowing ability (dysphagia).
4. Tuberculosis: See Section B below
5. Pneumocystis Carinii pneumonia: pulmonary infection caused by a protozoan in immunocompromised hosts, most often found in patients following transplantation, neonates, those infected with HIV.

### B. Tuberculosis (TB) [1]

1. Etiology: an airborne infection caused by a bacterium (Mycobacterium tuberculosis).
2. Risk factors.
   a. A person with TB of the throat or chest can pass the infection by sneezing or coughing.
   b. People most at risk for infection are those who live around or are in close contact with an infected individual every day (e.g., family members, friends, coworkers, health care personnel).
   c. People who have weakened immune systems are at greater risk for rapid onset of TB disease.
   d. People who have had a TB infection within 2 years of treatment are at high risk for re-infection.
   e. Babies, young children, and elderly people have a higher risk.
   f. Intravenous drug users have a higher risk.
3. Signs and symptoms of TB.
   a. A bad cough for more than 2 weeks.
   b. Chest pain.
   c. Blood tinged sputum or phlegm.
   d. Weakness or fatigue.
   e. Weight loss.
   f. Loss of appetite.
   g. Chills/fever.
   h. Night sweats.
4. Medical treatment.
   a. Drug therapy is frequently used to treat TB infection or prevention after an exposure.
   b. Persons who have TB disease may need to take several different drugs to do a better job of killing the bacteria.

[1] This section was completed by Ann Burkhardt.

c. If a person stops taking the drugs before the prescribed interval, the drugs may become ineffective in fighting the infection.

d. Development of multi-drug resistant TB (MDR TB) can occur.

e. Types of drugs.

    (1) Isoniazid (INH) which must be taken for 6 months.

        (a) People with weakened or undeveloped immune systems may have to take INH longer.

        (b) All of the INH pills prescribed must be taken.

        (c) A person on INH must see the doctor/nurse regularly or they may develop a resistance to the drug therapy.

        (d) Side effects of INH therapy include loss of appetite, nausea, vomiting, jaundice, and fever lasting more than 3 days, abdominal pain, tingling in the fingers or toes.

        (e) A person receiving INH should avoid alcoholic beverages while receiving drug therapy.

    (2) Rifampin.

        (a) Side effects include orange tint to urine, saliva, or tears; inability to wear contact lenses; sun sensitivity.

        (b) Affects birth control pills and implants, rendering them ineffective.

        (c) Lessens effectiveness of methadone therapy for drug addiction.

    (3) Pyrazinamide.

    (4) Ethambutol.

    (5) Streptomycin.

f. Serious side effects of all of the above drug therapies.

    (1) No appetite.

    (2) Nausea, vomiting.

    (3) Jaundice.

    (4) Fever lasting more than 3 days.

    (5) Abdominal pain.

    (6) Tingling in the fingers or toes.

    (7) Easy bruising.

    (8) Blurred vision.

    (9) Tinnitus, hearing loss.

**C. Chronic Obstructive Diseases**

1. Chronic obstructive pulmonary disease (COPD): a disorder characterized by poor expiratory flow rates.

   a. Peripheral airways disease: inflammation of the distal conducting airways; association with smoking.

   b. Chronic bronchitis: chronic inflammation of the tracheobronchial tree with cough and sputum production lasting at least 3 months for 2 consecutive years.

   c. Emphysema: permanent abnormal enlargement and destruction of air spaces distal to terminal bronchioles.

2. Asthma: an increased reactivity of the trachea and bronchi to various stimuli (allergens, exercise, cold).

   a. Manifests by widespread narrowing of the airways due to inflammation, smooth muscle constriction, and increased secretions.

   b. Reversible in nature.

3. Cystic fibrosis. (refer to pediatric pulmonary disease section).

4. Hyaline membrane disease/respiratory distress syndrome. (see pediatric pulmonary disease section).

**D. Chronic Restrictive Diseases**

1. Etiologies vary.

2. Diseases are all characterized by difficulty expanding the lungs causing a reduction in lung volumes.

**E. Carcinomas**

   1. Refer to Chapter 9.

**F. Pulmonary Edema**

1. Excessive seepage of fluid from the pulmonary vascular system into the interstitial space.

2. May eventually cause alveolar edema.

# V. Occupational Therapy Cardiopulmonary Assessment

**A. Role of the OTA**

1. Contribute to the evaluation process in collaboration with the occupational therapist.

2. Conduct specific assessments with OT supervision upon establishment of service competency.

   a. The level of supervision required will be determined by the OTA's experience and established service competency.

3. The OTA cannot independently evaluate or interpret evaluation results.

4. Recognize and report presenting symptoms.

   a. Pain/angina: note location, severity, type. See Tables 8-3 Common Angina and Dyspnea Rating Scale and 8-4 Intermittent Claudication

Scale.

b. Dyspnea (shortness of breath): note severity, position, or times at which discomfort is experienced. See Table 8-3.

c. Fatigue/perceived exertion: note severity, time of occurrence, association with activities. See Table 8-5 Borg Scale for Rating Perceived Exertion.

d. Palpitations: note person's awareness of heart rhythm abnormalities including pounding, fluttering, racing heart beat, skipped beats.

e. Dizziness: note time of occurrence and association with postural changes during activity.

f. Edema.
   (1) Fluid retention may be identified by swelling, especially in the lower extremities, or sudden weight gain.
   (2) Note location, measurements, time of day when edema is most prominent, resolution with activity.

**B. Vital Signs**

1. Specific training and establishment of service competency are required to enable the OTA to assess vital signs (pulse/heart rate, auscultation, blood pressure, respiration).

2. Important and reliable indicator of activity tolerance/response to evaluation and treatment.
   a. See Table 8-2 for normal vital sign values for infants and adults.

3. Parameters are established by the primary physician or cardiologist.
   a. Parameters require modification over the course of treatment to reflect increases or decreases in functional capacity,
   b. Ongoing communication between the OTA, occupational therapist, and primary physician is important.

4. Vital signs must be monitored pre-activity, during activity, and post-activity to ensure compliance with parameters.

5. The OTA should report any abnormalities to the OT and physician to determine the appropriate

course of action.

6. Pulse/heart rate: rhythmical throbbing of arterial wall as a result of each heartbeat; influenced by force of contraction, volume and viscosity of blood, diameter and elasticity of vessels; emotions, exercise, blood temperature, hormones.

a. Assessment: done by palpation of peripheral pulses; with normal rhythm palpate 30 seconds; with irregular rhythm palpate 1-2 minutes; taken prior to activity, during activity, and

---

### TABLE 8-3 - COMMON ANGINA AND DYSPNEA RATING SCALES

**5-GRADE ANGINA SCALE**

| | |
|---|---|
| 0 | No angina |
| 1 | Light, barely noticeable |
| 2 | Moderate, bothersome |
| 3 | Severe, very uncomfortable |
| 4 | Most pain ever experienced |

**5- GRADE DYSPNEA SCALE**

| | |
|---|---|
| 0 | No dyspnea |
| 1 | Mild, noticeable |
| 2 | Mild, some difficulty |
| 3 | Moderate difficulty, but can continue |
| 4 | Severe difficulty, cannot continue |

**10-GRADE ANGINA/DYSPNEA SCALE**

| | |
|---|---|
| 0 | Nothing |
| 0.5 | Very, very slight |
| 1 | Very slight |
| 2 | Slight |
| 3 | Moderate |
| 4 | Somewhat severe |
| 5 | Severe |
| 6 | |
| 7 | Very severe |
| 8 | |
| 9 | |
| 10 | Very, very severe |
| | Maximal |

Reprinted, with permission, from American Association of Cardiovascular and Pulmonary Rehabilitation, 2004. *Guidelines for cardiac rehabilitation and secondary prevention programs*, 4th ed, (Champaign, IL: Human Kinetics), 32, 81.

---

### TABLE 8-4 – INTERMITTENT CLAUDICATION RATING SCALE

| | |
|---|---|
| 0 | No claudication pain |
| 1 | Initial, minimal pain |
| 2 | Moderate, bothersome pain |
| 3 | Intense pain |
| 4 | Maximal Pain, cannot continue |

Reprinted, with permission, from American Association of Cardiovascular and Pulmonary Rehabilitation, 2004. *Guidelines for cardiac rehabilitation and secondary prevention programs*, 4th ed, (Champaign, IL: Human Kinetics), 32, 81.

---

### TABLE 8-2 - NORMAL VALUES FOR INFANTS AND ADULTS

| PARAMETER | INFANT | ADULT |
|---|---|---|
| Heart Rate | 120 bpm | 60-80 bpm |
| Blood Pressure | 75/50 mmHg | 120/80 mmHg |
| Respiratory Rate | 40 br/min | 12-18 br/min |

post activity.
b. Palpation sites.
   (1) Radial: most common monitoring site; radial artery, radial wrist at base of thumb.
   (2) Temporal: superior and lateral to eye.
   (3) Carotid: on either side of anterior neck between sternocleidomastoid muscle and trachea; best reflects cardiac function.
   (4) Brachial: medial aspect of the antecubital fossa; used to monitor blood pressure.
   (5) Femoral.
   (6) Popliteal.
   (7) Pedal.
7. Pulse/heart rate (HR) parameters:
a. Normal adult HR is 70 beats per minute (bpm); range 60-80 bpm.
   (1) As an individual ages, the normal resting heart rate range may increase up to 100 bpm.
b. Pediatric: newborn is 120 bpm; range 70-170 bpm.
c. Tachycardia: greater than 100 bpm.
d. Bradycardia: less than 60 bpm.
e. Irregular: force and frequency vary; may be due to arrhythmia, myocarditis.
f. Weak, thready pulse.
g. Bounding, full pulse.
h. Bruit: abnormal sound or murmur; associated with atherosclerosis.
8. Auscultation of heart: done with stethoscope to assess heart sounds. Note the addition of extra, abnormal heart sounds.
9. Blood pressure (BP).
a. Monitor at rest, during evaluation/activity, post activity.
b. Normal adult BP is <120/<80mm HG (systolic/diastolic); range between 110-140 systolic, 60-80 diastolic.
c. Pediatric: 1 month - 80 systolic, 45 diastolic, 6 years - 105-125 systolic, 60-80 diastolic.
d. Increased BP may be related to stress, pain, hypoxia, drugs, and disease.
e. Decreased BP may be related to bed rest, drugs, arrhythmias, blood loss/shock, and myocardial infarction.
f. Hypertension: BP above 120/80.
10. Respiration.
a. Monitor at rest, during evaluation/activity, post activity.
b. Rate and depth of breathing: normal is 12-18 breaths per minute.
c. Auscultation of lungs/respiratory sounds.
   (1) Normal: soft, rustling sound heard throughout all inspiration and start of expiration.
   (2) Abnormal: crackles/rales.
     (a) Rattling, bubbling sounds; may be due to secretions in lungs.
     (b) Wheezes, whistling sounds.

**C. Condition of Extremities**
1. Diaphoresis: excessive sweating associated with decreased cardiac output.
2. Pulses: decreased or absent pulses associated with peripheral vascular disease (PVD).
3. Skin color and vascular status.
a. Cyanosis: bluish color related to decreased cardiac output or cold; especially lips, fingertips, nail beds.
b. Pallor: absence of rosy color in light skinned individuals, associated with decreased peripheral blood flow, PVD.
c. Rubor: dependent redness with PVD.
d. Temperature.
e. Skin changes: clubbing of fingernails; pale, shiny, dry, abnormal pigmentation; ulceration, dermatitis; gangrene.
f. Intermittent claudication: pain, cramping, fatigue occurring during exercise and relieved by rest, associated with PVD; pain is typically in calf.
g. Edema.

**D. Mobility Assessment**
1. Evaluation is ongoing during activity performance.
a. The OTA contributes to the evaluation process to assess:
   (1) Bed mobility.
   (2) Transfers.
   (3) Wheelchair mobility.
   (4) Ambulation status.
2. The OTA observes and reports any overt signs/symptoms of distress, the optimal position(s) for activities and the person's endurance.
3. Refer to Chapter 15.

**E. Activities of Daily Living/Instrumental Activities of Daily Living**
1. The OTA contributes to the evaluation process to assess:
a. Self care.
b. Household management tasks.
c. Leisure activities.
d. Community activities.

e. Note level of function and type of assistance required.

2. The OTA observes and reports any overt signs/symptoms of distress, the optimal position(s) for activities and the person's endurance.

3. Note level of dyspnea and angina reported during activities. See Table 8-3.

4. Refer to Chapter 14.

**F. Cognition**

1. The OTA contributes to the evaluation process by providing information related to person's baseline ability to understand, process, retain, and apply information taught during rehabilitation.

2. The OTA contributes to the evaluation process to assess:
   a. Orientation.
   b. Memory.
   c. Concentration.
   d. Judgment.

3. Refer to Chapters 12 and 13.

**G. Activity Tolerance**

1. The OTA contributes to the evaluation process by observing and monitoring vital signs (BP, HR, respiration, level of dyspnea, angina, claudication pain, and perceived exertion). See Tables 8-3, 8-4, and 8-5.

2. Metabolic equivalent levels (METs). (Tables 8-6 and 8-7.)
   a. The use of METs during the assessment of activity tolerance must take into consideration the physical status of the patient and their pattern of activities prior to the cardiac event.

**H. Environmental Assessment**

1. Accomplished via a visit to the discharge environment and completion of an on-site assessment.

2. The OTA contributes to the evaluation process. Focus of assessment includes:
   a. Accessibility issues related to safety, risk for falls, environmental barriers in the discharge environment.
      (1) Barriers may include stairs, clutter, spatial limitations.
   b. Physical demands of the discharge environment, i.e., presence of stairs, airborne irritants.

3. Refer to Chapter 15.

**I. Psychosocial Assessment**

1. The OTA contributes to the evaluation process. Focus of assessment includes:
   a. Signs and symptoms of depression, anxiety, and/or stress and the potential effects on the individual's ability to complete/engage in activities.

---

## TABLE 8-5 – BORG SCALE FOR RATING PERCEIVED EXERTION

**15-GRADE SCALE**

| 6 | No exertion at all | How you feel when lying in bed or sitting in a chair relaxed. |
|---|---|---|
| 7 | Extremely light | |
| 8 | | |
| 9 | Very light | Little or no effort. |
| 10 | | |
| 11 | Light | |
| 12 | | Target range: How you should feel with exercise or activity. |
| 13 | Somewhat hard | |
| 14 | | |
| 15 | Hard (heavy) | |
| 16 | | |
| 17 | Very hard | How you feel with the hardest work you have ever done. |
| 18 | | |
| 19 | Extremely hard | |
| 20 | Maximal exertion | Don't work this hard. |

**PATIENT INSTRUCTIONS:**
This is a scale for rating perceived exertion.

**Perceived exertion is the overall effort or distress of your body during exercise.**
The number 6 represents no perceived exertion or leg discomfort and 20 represents the greatest amount of exertion that you have ever experienced.

At various times during the exercise test you will be asked to select a number that indicates your rating of perceived exertion at the time.

Do you have any questions?

Borg, G. (1998). *Borg's perceived exertion and pain scales.* Champaign, IL: Human Kinetics. Reprinted with permission.

b. Stress management, coping styles and psychosocial family/caregiver and spiritual supports.
2. Refer to Chapters 10 and 13.

# VI. Occupational Therapy Cardiopulmonary Rehabilitation

A. **Phase 1: Inpatient Rehabilitation/Hospitalization Stage**
  1. Program focus.
     a. Patient education regarding disease process and recovery.
        (1) Increase knowledge of energy conservation and work simplification principles and techniques. Refer to Chapter 11.
        (2) Increase knowledge of the approximate metabolic cost of activities (Table 8-6).
     b. Improve ability to carry out self care and low level functional activities.
     c. Decrease anxiety.
     d. Support smoking cessation and dietary modification efforts if warranted.

## TABLE 8-6 - SUGGESTED INTERDISCIPLINARY STAGES FOR PATIENTS WITH CARDIOPULMONARY HISTORY AND/OR PRECAUTIONS

| STAGE/MET LEVEL | ADL AND MOBILITY | EXERCISE | RECREATION |
|---|---|---|---|
| Stage I (1.0-1.4 MET) | Sitting: Self-feeding, wash hands and face, bed mobility[c] <br> Transfers <br> Progressively increase sitting tolerance | Supine: (A)[a] or (AA)[b] exercise to all extremities (10-15 times per extremity) <br> Sitting: (A) or (AA) exercise to only neck and lower extremities <br> Include deep breathing exercises | Reading, radio, table games (noncompetitive), light handwork |
| Stage II (1.4-2.0 MET) | Sitting: Self-bathing, shaving, grooming, and dressing in hospital <br><br> Unlimited Sitting <br> Ambulation: At slow pace, in room as tolerated | Sitting: (A) exercise to all extremities, progressively increasing the number of repetitions[c] <br> NO ISOMETRICS | Sitting: Crafts, e.g., painting, knitting, sewing, mosaics, embroidery <br><br> NO ISOMETRICS |
| Stage III (2.0-3.0 MET) | Sitting: Showering in warm water, homemaking tasks with brief standing periods to transfer light items, ironing | Sitting: Wheelchair mobility, limited distances <br> Standing: (A) exercise to all extremities and trunk, progressively increasing the number of repetitions[c] <br> May include (1) balance exercises and (2) light mat activites without resistance. <br> Ambulation: Begin progressive ambulation at 0% grade and comfortable pace. | Sitting: Card playing, crafts, piano, machine sewing, typing[c] |
| Stage IV (3.0-3.5 MET) | Standing: Total washing, dressing, shaving, grooming, showering in warm water; kitchen/homemaking activities while practicing energy conservation (e.g., light vacuuming, dusting and sweeping, washing light clothes) <br><br> Ambulation: unlimited distance walking at 0% grade, in and/or outside[c] | Standing: Continue all previous exercise, progressively increasing: <br> 1. Number of repetitions <br> 2. Speed of repetitions <br> May include additional exercises to increase workload up to 3.5 MET, balance and mat activities with mild resistance <br> Ambulation: Unlimited on level surfaces in and/or outside[c] progressively increasing speed and/or duration for periods up to 15-20 minutes or until target heart rate is reached[c] <br> Stairs: May begin slow stair climbing to patient's tolerance up to two flights <br> Treadmill: 1 mph at 1% grade, progressing to 1.5 mph at 2% grade[c] <br> Cycling: Up to 5.0 mph without resistance | Candlepin bowling <br> Canoeing - slow rhythm, pace <br> Golf putting <br> Light gardening (weeding and planting) <br> Driving[c] |

(A)[a] = active.  (AA)[b] = active assistive.  c, Please refer to physician's guidelines.

e. Discharge to home.

2. Intervention.

  a. The OTA implements intervention with OT supervision.

  b. If person is pain free, exhibits no arrhythmia and has regular pulse of 100 or less, an activity program is initiated.

  c. Intense monitoring during activity especially in CCU.

  d. Beginning activities at MET level = 1-2.

    (1) Bed mobility, static standing.

    (2) Transfer from bed to chair/bedside commode.

    (3) Bed bath, feeding, grooming at sink in sitting.

    (4) AROM/warm-up exercises.

    (5) Wheelchair mobility/ambulation in room.

  e. All activities use energy conservation techniques. General principles of energy conservation and work simplification include:

    (1) Pace oneself.

    (2) Monitor body position during activities.

    (3) Organize daily activities and work areas.

    (4) Delegate responsibilities.

  f. Breathing exercises.

    (1) Specific training needed to establish OTA service competence.

    (2) Abdominal diaphragmatic breathing: strengthens diaphragm, decreases need to use neck and shoulder muscles, decreases energy required for activity.

    (3) Pursed lip breathing: controls respiratory rate; decreases rate of breathing, helps remove trapped air from lungs.

    (4) Techniques are done during all exercises and activities.

  g. Vital signs (BP, HR, rate of respiration, oxygen saturation) and exertion scales are monitored prior to each activity, at peak of each activity, immediately upon cessation of activity, and 4-5

---

## TABLE 8-6 - SUGGESTED INTERDISCIPLINARY STAGES FOR PATIENTS WITH CARDIOPULMONARY HISTORY AND/OR PRECAUTIONS (CONT.)

| STAGE/MET LEVEL | ADL AND MOBILITY | EXERCISE | RECREATION |
|---|---|---|---|
| Stage V (3.5-4.0MET) | Standing: Washing dishes, washing clothes, ironing, hanging light clothes, and making beds | Standing: Continue exercises as in stage IV progressively increasing: 1. Number of repetitions 2. Speed of repetitions May add additional exercises to increase workload up to 4.0 MET Ambulation: As in stage IV, increasing speed up to 2.5 mph on level surfaces[c] Stairs: As in stage IV and progressively increasing to patient's tolerance. Treadmill: 1.5 mph at 2% grade, progressing to 1.5 mph at 4% grade up to 2.5 mph at 0% grade[c] Cycling: Up to 8 mph without resistance[c] May use up to 7-10 lb of weight for upper and lower extremity exercise in sitting | Swimming (slowly) Light carpentry Golfing (using power cart) Light home repairs |
| Stage VI | Standing: Showering in hot water, hanging and/or wringing clothes, mopping, stripping and making beds, raking | Standing: As in stage V Ambulation: As in stage V, increasing speed to 3.5 mph on level surfaces[c] Stairs: As in stage V Treadmill: 1.5 mph at 5-6% grade, progressing to 3.5 mph at 0% grade[c] Cycling: Up to 10 mph without resistance May use up to 10-15 lb of weight in upper and lower extremity exercises in sitting | Swimming (no advanced strokes) Slow dancing Ice or roller skating (slowly) Volleyball Badminton Table tennis (noncompetitive) Light calisthenics |

(A)[a] = active.
(AA)[b] = active assistive.
c, Please refer to physician's guidelines.

Atchison, B. (1995). Cardiopulmonary diseases. In Trombly, C.A. (Ed.). *Occupational therapy for physical dysfunction* (4th ed., pp.884-885). Baltimore, MD: Williams & Wilkins. Reprinted with permission.

minutes post activity.

h. As person's activity tolerance improves, more strenuous, higher MET level activities are added in progression from basic ADL to instrumental ADL (Table 8-6).

i. Observe any contraindications/precautions as per physician orders.

   (1) Observe/monitor for shortness of breath, (SOB), chest pain, nausea, vomiting, dizziness, and/or fatigue.

   (2) Adhere to activity guidelines and MET levels.

   (3) Observe for decrease in systolic BP greater than 120 mm/Hg.

   (4) Monitor heart rate (some facilities have specific guidelines).

     (a) Max HR 100 very light activity - very high risk.

     (b) Max HR 120 light activity - less than 6 weeks after MI, surgery.

     (c) Max HR 130 recent bypass surgery, cardiomyopathy, CHF.

     (d) Target HR 60-80% patient's max HR - treadmill test.

## TABLE 8-7 - APPROXIMATE METABOLIC COST OF ACTIVITIES[a]

| ENERGY LEVEL | OCCUPATIONAL | RECREATIONAL |
|---|---|---|
| 1.5-2 MET[b]<br>4-7 mL $O^2$/min/kg<br>2-2.5 kcal/min[d] | Desk work<br>Auto driving[c]<br>Typing<br>Electric calculating machine operation | Standing<br>Walking (strolling 1.6 km or 1 mile/hr)<br>Flying,[c] motorcycling[c]<br>Playing cards[c]<br>Sewing, knitting |
| 2-3 MET<br>7-11 mL $O^2$/min/kg<br>2.5-4 kcal/min[d] | Auto repair<br>Radio, TV repair<br>Janitorial work<br>Typing, manual<br>Bartending | Level walking (3.25 km or 2 miles/hr)<br>Level bicycling (8 km or 5 miles/hr)<br>Riding lawn mower<br>Billiards, bowling<br>Skeet,[c] shuffleboard<br>Woodworking (light)<br>Powerboat driving[c]<br>Golf (power cart)<br>Canoeing (4 km or 2.5 miles/hr)<br>Horseback riding (walk)<br>Playing piano and many muscial instruments |
| 3-4 MET<br>11-14 mL $O^2$/min/kg<br>4-5 kcal/min[d] | Brick laying, plastering<br>Wheelbarrow (220 lb or 100 kg load)<br>Machine assembly<br>Trailer-truck in traffic<br>Welding (moderate load)<br>Cleaning windows | Walking (5 km or 3 miles/hr)<br>Cycling (10 km or 6 miles/hr)<br>Horseshoe pitching<br>Volleyball (6 person noncompetitive)<br>Golf (pulling bag cart)<br>Archery<br>Sailing (handling small boat)<br>Fly fishing (standing in waders)<br>Horseback (sitting to trot)<br>Badminton (social doubles)<br>Pushing light power mower<br>Energetic musician |
| 4-5 MET<br>14-18 mL $O^2$/min/kg<br>5-6 kcal/min[d] | Painting, masonry<br>Paperhanging<br>Light carpentry | Walking (5.5 km or 3.5 miles/hr)<br>Cycling (13 km or 8 miles/hr)<br>Table tennis<br>Golf (carrying clubs)<br>Dancing (foxtrot)<br>Badminton (singles)<br>Tennis (doubles)<br>Raking leaves<br>Hoeing<br>Many calisthenics |

## TABLE 8-7 - APPROXIMATE METABOLIC COST OF ACTIVITIES[a] CONT.

| ENERGY LEVEL | OCCUPATIONAL | RECREATIONAL |
|---|---|---|
| 5-6 MET<br>18-21 mL $O^2$/min/kg<br>6-7 kcal/min[d] | Digging garden<br>Shoveling light earth | Walking (6.5 km or 4 miles/hr)<br>Cycling (16 km or 10 miles/hr)<br>Canoeing (6.5 km or 4 miles/hr)<br>Horseback (posting to trot)<br>Stream fishing (walking in light current in waders)<br>Ice or roller skating (15 km or 9 miles/hr) |
| 6-7 MET<br>21-25 mL $O^2$/min/kg<br>7-8 kcal/min[d] | Shoveling 10 min (22 lb or 10 kg) | Walking (8 km or 5 miles/hr)<br>Cycling (17.5 km or 11 miles/hr)<br>Badminton (competitive)<br>Tennis (singles)<br>Splitting wood<br>Snow shoveling<br>Manual lawn mowing<br>Folk (square) dancing<br>Light downhill skiing<br>Ski touring (4 km or 2.5 miles/hr), loose snow<br>Water skiing |
| 7-8 MET<br>25-28 mL $O^2$/min/kg<br>8-10 kcal/min[d] | Digging ditches<br>Carrying 175 lb or 80 kg<br>Sawing hardwood | Jogging (8 km or 5 miles/hr)<br>Cycling (19 km or 12 miles/hr)<br>Horseback (gallop)<br>Vigorous downhill skiing<br>Basketball<br>Mountain climbing<br>Ice hockey<br>Canoeing (8 km or 5 miles/hr)<br>Touch football<br>Paddleball |
| 8-9 MET<br>28-32 mL $O^2$/min/kg<br>10-11 kcal/min[d] | Shoveling 10 min (31 lb or 14 kg) | Running (9 km or 5.5 miles/hr)<br>Cycling (21 km or 13 miles/hr)<br>Ski touring (6.5 km or 4 miles/hr), loose snow<br>Squash (social)<br>Handball (social)<br>Fencing<br>Basketball (vigorous) |
| 10+ MET<br>32+ mL $O^2$/min/kg<br>11+ kcal/min[d] | Shoveling 10 min (35 lb or 16 kg) | Running<br>  6 mph = 10 MET<br>  7 mph = 11.5 MET<br>  8 mph = 13.5 MET<br>  9 mph = 15 MET<br>  10 mph = 17 MET<br>Ski touring (8+ km or 5+ miles/hr), loose snow<br>Handball (competitive)<br>Squash (competitive) |

a  includes resting metabolic needs.

b  1 MET is the energy expenditure at rest, equivalent to approximately 3.5 mL $O^2$/kg body weight/min.

c  A major increase in metabolic requirements may occur because of excitement, anxiety, or impatience, which are common responses during some activities. The patient's emotional reactivity must be assessed when prescribing or sanctioning certain activities.

d  Based on a 70 kg person.

Atchison, B. (1995). Cardiopulmonary diseases. In Trombly, C.A. (Ed.). *Occupational therapy for physical dysfunction* (4th ed., pp.881-882). Baltimore, MD: Williams & Wilkins. Reprinted with permission.

(5) Avoid isometric muscle work (i.e., activities that involve holding muscle contractions), straining, and breath holding (Valsalva).

(6) Avoid holding UEs over head for extensive time periods.

(7) Monitor BP also for resting diastolic BP 120 mm/Hg; systolic 200 mm/Hg.

(8) Avoid lateral arm movements and exercises that stretch chest and pull incision.

(9) Observe for facial changes.

(10) Evidence and/or complaint of pain.

(11) Avoid lateral arm movements and exercises that stretch and pull chest and pull incision.

(12) Exercise may be contraindicated for unstable angina.

j. There may be clinical signs/symptoms or diagnoses for which therapy should either be stopped or is contraindicated.

(1) Uncontrolled atrial/ventricular arrhythmias.

(2) Recent embolism/thrombophlebitis.

(3) Dissecting aneurysm.

(4) Severe aortic stenosis.

(5) Acute systemic illness.

(6) Acute MI.

(7) Digoxin toxicity.

(8) Acute hypoglycemia or metabolic disorder.

(9) Third degree heart block.

(10) Unstable angina

k. Patients are generally discharged to Phase 2 when they are able to carry out activities at MET level 3.5 - 4 (Tables 8-6 and 8-7). Tables should be used as a general reference to determine the approximate level of energy required to perform an activity.

l. Keep in mind that MET levels are used to quantify the amount of energy required to perform an activity and to provide the practitioner with a guideline for grading activities used in treatment.

(1) Selection of activities based on MET level must take into consideration the patient's physical status and activity patterns prior to the cardiac or pulmonary event, as well as the patient's subjective report of level of exertion during activity performance.

m. Educate individual about heart disease and the recovery process, provide emotional support.

3. Length of stay 5-14 days.

**B. Phase 2: Outpatient Rehabilitation.**

1. Program focus.

a. Educate patient on the importance of continued exercise.

b. Build up activity tolerance.

c. Improve ability to carry out IADL and community tasks.

d. Improve ability to perform work activities.

e. Support person's efforts in smoking cessation and lifestyle changes as needed.

2. Intervention.

a. The OTA implements intervention with OT supervision.

b Intervention focus includes:

(1) Consumer and family education.

(2) Graded exercise program with slow and gradual increase of weight.

(3) Practice of functional activities in the discharge environment.

(4) Use of energy conservation techniques and compensatory techniques in daily tasks.

(5) Engagement in community activities.

c. The OTA needs to establish service competence to monitor status.

d. The OTA observes and reports any overt signs/symptoms of distress, the optimal position(s) for activities and the person's endurance.

3. Length of program is dependent upon person's progress through MET levels, activity tolerance and prognosis.

a. Outpatient program up to 12 weeks post cardiac event, surgery, or pulmonary disease exacerbation.

b. Outpatient/home program begins with 4-5 METs activities.

c. During 6 months of rehabilitation increase gradually to 7.0 METs activities.

d. Sexual activity as per physician, usually at 5-6 MET level.

**C. Phase 3: Maintenance/Training Stage**

1. Maintenance gym program.

a. Weight training to maintain upper and lower body strength.

b. Cardiovascular training to maintain cardiopulmonary health.

2. May begin as early as 4 weeks post cardiac event, surgery, or pulmonary disease exacerbation.

3. See Table 8-8 for the recommended continuum of care for cardiac rehabilitation services and lifelong maintenance

## TABLE 8-8 – RECOMMENDED CONTINUUM OF CARE FOR CARDIAC REHABILITATION

| | | | | | | Weeks | | | | | | | | |
|---|---|---|---|---|---|---|---|---|---|---|---|---|---|---|
| 0 | 1 | 2 | 3 | 4 | 5 | 6 | 7 | 8 | 9 | 10 | 11 | 12 | Beyond | |

Inpatient – hospital
  clinical pathway

Transitional care – subacute facility,
  home care, pretraining at home

Outpatient programming – cardiac rehabilitation center

Maintenance – lifelong – community facility or at home

Reprinted, with permission, from American Association of Cardiovascular and Pulmonary Rehabilitation, 2004. *Guidelines for cardiac rehabilitation and secondary prevention programs*, 4th ed, (Champaign, IL: Human Kinetics), 32, 81.

## VII. Pediatric Pulmonary Disorders[1]

A. **Cystic Fibrosis (CF)**
  1. Etiology.
     a. Genetically inherited autosomal recessive trait, gene mutation.
     b. Both parents must be carriers. Neither parent will have the disease.
  2. Diagnosis.
     a. Chronic, progressive lung disease (production of abnormal mucus).
     b. Salt concentration in the sweat.
     c. Decreased release of certain enzymes by the pancreas.
     d. Certain abnormalities revealed on x-rays.
     e. Failure to grow properly.
  3. Complications.
     a. Reduced life expectancy of up to 26 years.
     b. Cardiac symptoms are a possible complication of CF.
     c. Diabetes, cirrhosis, and rectal prolapse are rare complications of CF.
     d. Five to ten percent of children with CF present with intestinal blockage.
  4. Medical management/relevant pharmacology.
     a. Aerosol (mist).
     b. Chest physical therapy to loosen secretions that block lung airways.
     c. Vitamin and mineral supplements, enzymes.
     d. Antibiotics.
  5. Effect on function.
     a. Exercise intolerance.
     b. Poor nutrition due to malabsorption may contribute to developmental delays.

  6. Occupational therapy evaluation.
     a. The OTA contributes to the evaluation process in collaboration with the occupational therapist.
        (1) The OTA can assist with the collection of data for the evaluation once service competency has been established.
        (2) The level of supervision required will be determined by the OTA's experience and established service competence.
     b. The OTA cannot independently evaluate or interpret evaluation results.
     c. The aims of this process are to:
        (1) Assess for developmental delays related to decreased strength and endurance and decreased attention due to pain.
        (2) Assess the environment to determine adaptations for energy conservation and possible equipment needs.
        (3) Assess psychosocial status.
           (a) Child and family stress related to frequent hospitalizations, school absences, social isolation, and constant home treatment.
           (b) Fatigue related to the level of care that is required.
           (c) Emotional stress related to the pain and prognosis
  7. Occupational therapy intervention.
     a. The OTA implements intervention with OT supervision.
        (1) The level of supervision required depends upon the OTA's experience and established competency.

[1] Marge E. Moffett Boyd contributed this section on pediatric pulmonary disorders.

(2) During the implementation of intervention, the OTA informs the supervising therapist of any change in the individual's status and any other relevant information that may affect treatment.

b. Intervention focus includes:
(1) Energy conservation.
(2) Environmental adaptations to enhance performance.
(3) Positioning to promote postural drainage.
(4) Neurodevelopmental treatment to improve endurance and postural stability.
(5) Facilitation of fine, gross, visual motor, cognitive, and psychosocial development.
(6) Parent education.
  (a) Treatment protocols for the above interventions.
  (b) Advocacy skills to obtain necessary services and equipment for the child.
  (c) Advocacy skills to obtain respite services.
(7) Observation of medical precautions during occupational therapy sessions (i.e., respiratory/cardiac contraindications).

**B. Respiratory Distress Syndrome (RDS)**
1. Etiology.
   a. Premature birth.
   b. Insufficient production of surfactant to keep alveoli (air pockets of the lungs) open.
2. Diagnosis.
   a. Lungs collapse after each breath.
   b. X-ray of lungs reveals "ground glass" appearance.
   c. Collapsed alveoli are dense and appear white on the X-ray as opposed to the black appearance on an X-ray of air filled alveoli.
   d. RDS is also called Hyaline Membrane Disease (HMD).
3. Prenatal management.
   a. To stimulate surfactant production and to reduce the risk of RDS, the mother is treated prophylactically with steroid medication 24-36 hours before delivery of a premature infant.
4. Medical management/relevant pharmacology.
   a. Mild case.
      (1) Supplemental oxygen alone, or in combination with positive airways pressure (CPAP), a mixture of oxygen and air provided under pressure through short, two-pronged tubes placed in the nose.

b. Severe case.
   (1) Intubation and a mixture of oxygen and air provided by a ventilator under positive end expiration pressure (PEEP).
c. To reduce the severity of RDS and the risk of chronic lung disease, a single dose of surfactant replacement is given within 6 hours of development of RDS.
5. Complications/secondary diagnosis.
   a. Risk of severe intracranial hemorrhage (approximately 35%).
   b. Risk of bronchopulmonary dysplasia (BPD) (approximately 35%).
   c. Risk for developmental delay, severe developmental delay (less than 15%).
   d. The risk for these complications is far greater for infants who do not receive the above mentioned treatments.
6. Effect on function.
   a. The future intellectual development of the premature infant who had RDS and who received the latest treatments appears to be good.
   b. The functional effects for infants who develop BPD or who incur a severe intracranial hemorrhage may include motor, sensory, cognitive, and/or language impairments.
   c. For premature infants with RDS, functional effects may include visual defects, hypotonia, and other health issues that can impact on development.
7. Occupational therapy evaluation.
   a. The OTA contributes to the evaluation process in collaboration with the occupational therapist.
      (1) The OTA can assist with the collection of data for the evaluation once service competency has been established.
      (2) The level of supervision required will be determined by the OTA's experience and established service competence.
   b. The OTA cannot independently evaluate or interpret evaluation results.
   c. The aims of this process are to:
      (1) Assess for developmental delays.
      (2) Assess the environment.
8. Occupational therapy intervention.
   a. The OTA implements intervention with OT supervision.
      (1) The level of supervision required depends upon the OTA's experience.

(2) During the implementation of intervention, the OTA informs the supervising occupational therapist of any change in the child's status and any other relevant information that may affect treatment.

   b. Intervention includes:

     (1) Monitoring development.

     (2) Facilitating sensori-motor and cognitive development.

     (3) Addressing psychosocial issues that arise.

     (4) Providing parent education regarding handling, positioning, energy conservation, and methods to facilitate normal development.

     (5) Adapting environment as needed.

     (6) Observing medical precautions.

     (7) Referral as necessary to ophthalmologist and other relevant services.

## C. Bronchopulmonary Dysplasia (BPD)

1. Etiology.
   a. Respiratory disorder often as a result of barotrauma.
      (1) High inflating pressures.
      (2) Infection.
      (3) Meconium aspiration.
      (4) Asphyxia.
   b. A complication of prematurity.
   c. The walls of the immature lungs thicken, making the exchange of oxygen and carbon dioxide more difficult.
   d. The mucous lining of the lung is reduced along with the airway diameter.
2. Diagnosis.
   a. Infant must work harder than normal to obtain sufficient oxygen for survival.
3. Medical management /relevant pharmacology.
   a. Months or years of oxygen therapy and artificial ventilation.
   b. Bronchodilators and diuretics to keep the airways and lungs dry.
4. Complications.
   a. Greater risk for hypotonia and gross motor delays.
   b. Feeding problems can lead to poor nutrition.
      (1) Malabsorption problems.
      (2) Fragile bones with an increased risk of fractures.
   c. Central nervous system problems, such as damage to parts of the brain, can lead to delays or impairments in motor, sensory, speech, and cognitive function.
   d. Recurrent otitis media can lead to conductive hearing loss that can affect the development of speech and language as well as cognition.
5. Effect on function.
   a. Poor autonomic and sensory state regulation, can impact on the alert state which is necessary for proper feeding.
   b. Poor exercise/activity tolerance due to illness and compromised respiration.
   c. Reduced ability to socialize due to long periods of poor health and the increased susceptibility to infection.
   d. Isolation and stress on the child and family members can lead to psychosocial problems.
   e. Greater risk for attachment disorder, affecting the child's ability to relate to others due to isolation and dependence on technological equipment.
6. Occupational therapy evaluation.
   a. The OTA contributes to the evaluation process in collaboration with the occupational therapist.
      (1) The OTA can assist with the collection of data for the evaluation once service competency has been established.
      (2) The level of supervision required will be determined by the OTA's experience and established service competence.
   b. The aims of this process are to:
      (1) Assess for developmental delays/deficits.
      (2) Assess the environment to determine adaptations related to energy conservation, positioning, and enhanced occupational performance.
7. Occupational therapy intervention.
   a. The OTA implements intervention with OT supervision.
   b. Intervention includes:
      (1) Facilitating sensori-motor and cognitive development.
      (2) Addressing psychosocial issues that arise.
      (3) Adapting environment.
      (4) Providing parent education regarding handling, positioning, feeding, energy conservation and appropriate environmental adaptations.
      (5) Supporting parent advocacy related to acquiring necessary services and equipment.
      (6) Observing all medical precautions.

# References

Atchison, B. (1995). Cardiopulmonary diseases. In Trombly, C.A. (Ed.). *Occupational therapy for physical dysfunction* (4th ed., pp. 884-885). Baltimore: Williams & Wilkins.

Batshaw, M.L., & Perret, Y.M. (2002). *Children with disabilities: A medical primer* (5th ed.). Baltimore: Paul H. Brookes.

Blackman, J.A. (1997) Cystic fibrosis. In J.A. Blackman. *Medical aspects of developmental disabilities in children birth to three* 3rd ed., (pp. 88-90). Gaithersberg, MD: Aspen.

Blackman, J.A. (1997) Chronic lung disease. In J.A. Blackman. *Medical aspects of developmental disabilities in children birth to three* (3rd ed., pp. 59-63). Gaithersberg, MD: Aspen.

Centers for Disease Control and Prevention: Division of Tuberculosis Elimination (2007). Retrieved February 15, 2008 from http://www.cdc.gov/TB/pubs/tbfactsheets/TBTrends.htm.

Ciccone, C. (2004). Medication. In W. Turk & L. Cahalin (Eds.). *Cardiovascular and pulmonary physical therapy: An evidence-based approach* (pp. 189-218). New York: McGraw-Hill.

Collins, S. & Cocanour, B. (2004). Anatomy of the cardiopulmonary system. In W. Turk & L. Cahalin (Eds.). *Cardiovascular and pulmonary physical therapy: An evidence-based approach* (pp. 73-94). New York: McGraw-Hill.

McIntyre, M. (2007, March 5). Keeping VAD patients functional *Advance for Occupational Therapy Practitioners*. pp.43-44, 56.

Rais-Bahrami, K. & Short, B.L. (2007) Premature and small-for-dates infants. In M.L. Batshaw, L. Pellegrino, & N.J. Roizen (Eds.), *Children with disabilities*. 6th ed., (pp.107-122). Baltimore, MD: P.H. Brooks.

Rogers, S. L. (2005). Common conditions that influence children's participation. In J. Case-Smith (Ed.), *Occupational Therapy for children*, 6th ed., (pp. 160-215). St. Louis, MO: Elsevier Mosby.

Vining-Radomski, M. & Trombly-Latham, C.A. (2007). *Occupational therapy for physical dysfunction* 6th ed., Baltimore: Williams & Wilkins.

Williams, M. (Ed.): AACVPR: (2004). *Guidelines for cardiac rehabilitation and secondary prevention programs,* 4th ed. Champaign, IL: Human Kinetics.

# CHAPTER 9

# GASTROINTESTINAL, RENAL-GENITOURINARY, ENDOCRINE, IMMUNOLOGICAL, AND INTEGUMENTARY SYSTEMS DISORDERS

Ann Burkhardt

## I. Gastrointestinal System

### A. Dysphagia and Swallowing Disorders

1. Structures involved.
   a. Oral facial musculature.
   b. Pharyngeal and laryngeal structures.
   c. Piriform sinuses.
   d. Vocal folds.
   e. Bronchioles / bronchi.
   f. Lungs.
   g. Esophagus.
2. Facial paralysis.
   a. Incomplete closure of the mouth.
   b. Loss of the bolus out of the front of the oral cavity.
3. Praxis/motor planning deficits.
   a. Inability to effectively chew and coordinate tongue movements to propel the bolus toward the base of the tongue.
   b. Residual food centrally located in the oral cavity.
   c. Difficulty forming a bolus with smoother consistencies.
4. Sensory impairment of the oral cavity.
   a. Lack of awareness of residual food on the side of the mouth that has decreased sensation.
      (1) Pocketing of food.
      (2) Spillage of residual food into the airway at a time when the vocal cords are open; tim-

ing of the swallow sequence is off.
5. Weakness of the tongue/base of tongue structures.
   a. Inefficient propulsion of bolus at an efficient rate of speed past the base of the tongue into the pharyngeal cavity.
   b. Lack of closure at the cricopharyngeal junction.
      (1) Sub-optimal propulsion of the bolus.
      (2) Interference with the normal timing of the swallow sequence.
      (3) Failure to trigger closure of the vocal folds during swallow; aspiration.
6. Weakness of the elevation of the pharynx during swallow.
   a. Incomplete triggering (diminished neural stimulation) of the pharyngeal phase of swallowing.
7. Vocal cord paralysis.
   a. Inefficient closure of the vocal folds during the pharyngeal phase of swallow.
      (1) Vocal cords are in paramedian position; swallow may be safe.
      (2) Vocal cords fail to meet/close to protect airway; aspiration may occur.
8. Penetration of the bronchioles/bronchi by the bolus when aspiration occurs.
   a. Food enters the lung; true aspiration occurs.
      (1) Bacteria can cause pneumonia (aspiration pneumonia).

(2) If the person's immune system is functioning well, he/she may not experience pneumonia.

9. Clinical aspiration.
   a. Food enters the airway.
      (1) Person can clear airway by coughing (reflex intact).
      (2) Person silently aspirates.
         (a) Bolus enters lung and person does not react.
         (b) Bolus enters the lung and person experiences respiratory distress without a cough.
         (c) Person coughs too weakly to raise the bolus in order to expel it.

10. Diminished esophageal motility.
    a. Bolus sits in the esophagus and can slowly either move toward the stomach or upward toward the pharynx.
       (1) Person may feel that food is stuck in the esophagus.
       (2) Person aspirates when food propels upward and he/she cannot swallow it.

11. Clinical exams and functional findings.
    a. Staff report questioning swallowing dysfunction.
       (1) Person coughs during or after drinking water or other thin liquid.
    b. The person's face changes color during or after eating.
       (1) Flushed/reddened color, ashened appearance for persons with darker skin.
       (2) Blanches.
    c. Person gasps for breath, but has a partial or complete airway obstruction.
       (1) Heimlich maneuver.
    d. Swallowing assessment.
       (1) The OTA can contribute to the evaluation process in collaboration with the OT.
          (a) Supervision is required.
          (b) The level of supervision required will be determined by the OTA's experience.
       (2) Service competency must be established.
       (3) The OTA cannot independently evaluate or interpret evaluation results.

12. Relationship of swallowing dysfunction to occupation.
    a. Disruption of role relative to family unit, ability to comfortably eat at the dinner table.

(1) Modified diet could be infantilizing.
(2) Tube feeding may preempt person's ability to partake in the family meal in cultural/social context.
   b. Disruption of ability/comfort level for eating out in public.
      (1) Person may choose not to dine in a public social context.
      (2) If business lunches or dinners are part of a vocational role, the person may not be able to resume his/her vocation without modification of expectations regarding how participation in social meals relates to vocational performance.
   c. Alteration of self-concept concerning life roles and appearance.
      (1) If person is tube fed, how does that alter how he/she perceives self?
         (a) Sex appeal can be questioned.
         (b) Self image as it impacts on life roles (e.g., a jet-setter or fashion plate) can be altered.
      (2) If tube fed, how does that alter how others perceive him/her?
         (a) Accepted, feared, or pitied by children, grandchildren, family, and friends.

13. Intervention.
    a. Provide family-centered intervention to determine an acceptable dinner table alternative to interaction.
    b. Work with person toward developing new roles and occupations to transition from old role (i.e., head of table).
    c. Provide ongoing education and information to family regarding person's feeding/nutrition.
    d. The role of the OTA in intervention.
       (1). The OTA implements intervention with OT supervision.
       (2). The level of supervision required depends upon the OTA's experience and established service competence.
       (3) During the implementation of intervention, the OTA informs the supervising therapist of any change in the individual's status and any other relevant information that may affect treatment any the individual's status and any other relevant information that may affect treatment.
    e. Refer to Chapter 12 for further information on intervention.

## B. Gastric Esophageal Reflux Disease (GERD)

1. Structures involved include the lower esophagus and gastric sphincter.
   a. Food enters stomach and mixes with stomach acid/digestive juices.
   b. Lower esophageal sphincter inefficiently closes; stomach contraction propels acid/acidic bolus back into the esophagus.
      (1) Person reports heartburn sensation, indigestion, or dull chest pain.
   c. Positional elevation of the head above the stomach, when the person is reclined, may discourage upward retropulsion of the bolus from the stomach.
2. Frequent complaints of people who have GERD.
   a. Heartburn/indigestion.
   b. Swallowing problems.
      (1) A sensation of feeling that something is getting stuck in their "throat".
      (2) Chest pressure or pain.
      (3) Regurgitation after swallowing.
3. Intervention.
   a. Sleeping with more than one pillow (elevating the head to discourage regurgitation associated with body posture).
   b. Drug therapy.
   c. Diet modification.
      (1) Less spice.
      (2) Small meals on a more frequent basis.
   d. Stress management.

## C. Small Bowel Obstruction

1. Etiology.
   a. Secondary to scar tissue.
   b. Secondary to radiation of the abdomen (long term effect).
   c. Result of tumor obstruction.
2. Surgical treatment.
   a. Resection with open stoma (colostomy).
   b. Closed abdominal surgery.
3. Rehabilitation issues.
   a. Self-care aspects of stoma care must be addressed for persons with decreased fine motor skills (e.g., individuals with peripheral neuropathy secondary to chemotherapy treatment).
   b. Decrease mobility of gross movements that cause traction on the healing scar.
      (1) Bending.
      (2) Stooping.
      (3) Foot/lower leg related self-care.
         (a) Dressing.
         (b) Bathing.
         (c) Nail and foot care.
   c. Altered appetite in post-operative phase.

## D. Neurogenic Bowel

1. Etiology: sympathetic nerve impairment, generally occurring in persons who have spinal cord injury above the (thoracic) T-6 level.
   a. Loss of control of anal sphincter.
   b. Sensory loss resulting in a lack of awareness of feces in the bowel.
   c. Motor loss, decreased or lost ability to self-initiate or control a bowel movement.
2. Flaccidity of muscles results in incontinence.
3. Autonomic dysreflexia, an extreme rise in blood pressure can result.
   a. This is a medical emergency if not reversed.
   b. Irritants that would normally cause pain to areas below the spinal injury specific to the bowel.
      (1) Bowel irritation or over-distention.
      (2) Constipation/impaction.
      (3) Distention during bowel program (digital stimulation).
      (4) Hemorrhoids.
      (5) Infection or irritation (appendicitis).
   c. Additional irritants.
      (1) Bladder infection or over distention.
         (a) Urinary tract infection (UTI).
         (b) Urinary retention.
         (c) Blocked catheter.
         (d) Overfilled urine collection bag.
         (e) Non-compliance with intermittent catheterization program.
      (2) Skin-related disorders.
         (a) Any skin irritation below area of injury.
         (b) Decubitus ulcers.
         (c) Ingrown toenails.
         (d) Burns.
         (e) Tight or restrictive clothing or pressure to skin from clothing restrictions or wrinkles.
      (3) Sexual activity.
         (a) Over-stimulation during sex. Stimuli to the pelvic region that would be felt as pain if sensation were intact.
         (b) Menstrual cramps.
         (c) Labor and delivery.
      (4) Other.

(a) Heterotopic ossification/myositis ossificans.

(b) Skeletal fractures.

d. Management of autonomic dysreflexia.

(1) Identify the offending stimulus and relieve the underlying issue immediately.

(2) Medications, if no impact can be made.

(a) Immediate emergent (i.e., Procardia, Nitroglycerine, Clonidine, Hydralazine).

(b) Chronic (i.e., Prazosin [Minipress], Clonidine [Catapres]).

e. Prevention of autonomic dysreflexia.

(1) Teach person/caregiver frequent pressure relief principles.

(2) Ensure compliance with intermittent catheterization.

(3) Practice well balanced diet habits.

(4) Ensure medication compliance.

(5) Educate person with condition and caregivers or family members.

(a) Recognition of the cause, signs, symptoms (i.e., sweating, headache).

(b) First aid procedures to deal effectively with the occurrence.

(c) Prevention methods for this condition.

# II. Renal-Genitourinary System

## A. Kidney Disease

1. Risk factors.

a. Diabetes.

(1) 3 of every 10 individuals with diabetes develop kidney failure.

(2) 60-65% of all persons with diabetes also have high blood pressure.

(3) 10-40% of people with Type 2 diabetes develop severe kidney disease and End Stage Renal Disease (ESRD).

(4) Diabetes can contribute to development of nephrotic syndrome.

b. Hypertension (HTN).

(1) Uncontrolled or poorly controlled hypertension is the primary diagnosis for 26% of all new cases of chronic kidney failure each year.

(2) Hypertension is a serious problem among African-Americans.

(3) 65% of HTN in women and 78% of HTN in men can be directly attributed to obesity.

c. Systematic lupus erythematosus.

(1) Lupus can contribute to development of nephrotic syndrome.

2. Treatment for renal disease.

a. Prevention, early intervention, and control of hypertension.

(1) Diet.

(2) Medication.

(3) Exercise.

(4) Stress reduction.

(5) Smoking cessation.

b. Prevention, early detection, and control of diabetes. See this chapter's section on diabetes.

c. Medical treatment of lupus.

(1) Control symptoms to prevent complications.

(2) Treat with diuretics and drugs that prevent spillage of protein in the urine (angiotensin converting enzyme-ACE).

d. Medical treatment of nephrotic syndrome.

(1) Treat with diuretics and drugs that prevent spillage of protein in the urine.

(2) Drug control of fluid overload and/or spillage of protein into the urine (proteinuria).

(3) Encourage compliance with drug therapy, dietary and exercise recommendations.

e. Medical treatment of acute renal failure.

(1) Drug control of underlying medical contributory conditions.

(2) Emergent, acute dialysis.

f. Medical treatment of end stage renal disease (ESRD).

(1) Dialysis required to remain alive.

(a) Hemodialysis.

(b) Peritoneal dialysis: inpatient treatment, continuous ambulatory peritoneal dialysis (CAPD).

(2) Transplantation.

3. Impact on performance skills/client factors.

a. Motor dysfunction.

(1) Muscle pain.

(2) Edema limiting mobility.

(3) Weakness.

b. Sensory system function.

(1) Neuropathy (diabetes related, toxicity related, cyclosporin, anti-rejection drug related).

(2) Vision loss (diabetes related).

c. Cognitive dysfunction.

(1) Alteration of body image due to dialysis (tied to equipment/schedule) or post trans-

plant (foreign tissue).
    (2) Delusions due to sepsis or toxicity.
    (3) Dementia, multi-infarct or metabolic.
  d. Perceptual/neurobehavioral dysfunction.
    (1) Dementia/infarct related.
    (2) Stroke related.
  e. Psychological/emotional dysfunction.
    (1) Anxiety disorder.
    (2) Depression.
    (3) Mood/adjustment disorder.
    (4) Poor management of psychosocial disorders can increase the risk of cardiac arrest.
    (5) Supportive counseling and social support are indicated.
    (6) Drug therapy and complementary medicine.
4. Impact on occupational performance/areas of occupation.
  a. Self care.
    (1) Alteration in urination.
    (2) Need for meticulous sanitary technique with self dialysis.
    (3) Strict adherence to a disease specific/highly restrictive diet.
    (4) Alteration in sexuality.
      (a) Impotence.
      (b) Alteration of self esteem/body image.
      (c) Feeling less desirable.
    (5) Need for use of adapted equipment.
      (a) Tub/toilet bench.
      (b) Build-ups.
      (c) Reaching assistive devices.
      (d) Fine motor assistive devices (button hooks, etc.).
    (6) Energy conservation/work simplification; fatigue is an issue.
    (7) Altered mobility.
      (a) Wheeled mobility.
      (b) Use of assistive devices to walk such as an ankle-foot orthosis, walker, cane.
  b. Instrumental activities.
    (1) Housekeeping.
      (a) Need for lighter work load and housekeeping assistance.
      (b) Altered role in the family.
    (2) Community mobility.
      (a) Adapted vehicles.
      (b) Access to handicapped transit passes or parking spaces.
      (c) Special planning for long distance travel.

    (3) Meal preparation.
      (a) Training to change usual habits to cook appropriately for dietary limitations.
      (b) Planning to budget and purchase appropriate supplies.
      (c) Safety in cooking.
    (4) Management of personal finances.
      (a) Ability to do banking.
      (b) Ability to budget funds.
      (c) Ability to prioritize goals.
      (d) Ability to achieve goals or problem solve solutions.
    (5) Leisure/sports activities.
      (a) Ability to participate.
      (b) Ability to pace self/self regulate.
      (c) Choice of activities that allow participation with minimum risk.
      (d) Awareness of precautions for participation.
      (e) Access to sports facilities that have adaptive possibilities or sources for adaptations.
5. Impact on performance contexts.
  a. Social context.
    (1) How disease affects role in the family.
    (2) How disease affects role in the workplace.
    (3) How disease affects role in the community, including spiritual communities, social groups, special interests.
  b. Cultural context.
    (1) How cultural group accepts condition and/or treatment.
    (2) Relative taboo of treatment options/choices.
    (3) Acceptance of individual in view of impairment/disease.

**B. Neurogenic Bladder/UTI**
1. Refer to this chapter's gastrointestinal system section.

# III. Immunological System

## A. Cancer
1. Etiology: Unknown for some cancers, strong link to risk factors for others.
2. Risk factors for cancer.
  a. Heredity.
    (1) Some tumors seem to have a high hereditary risk.
      (a) Breast cancer.
      (b) Prostate cancer.

(c) Skin cancer.

(d) Colon cancer.

b. Environmental.

(1) Cluster patterns related to chemical pollution.

c. Habit or lifestyle related.

(1) Smoking and use of smokeless/chewing tobacco can contribute to lung cancer and head and neck cancer.

(2) Drinking alcohol contributes to some head and neck cancers.

(3) Obesity/high fat diets may be linked to an increased risk of some cancers.

3. Prevention, early intervention, and control.

a. Specific to type of cancer. For ovarian cancer should be screened by blood test and abdominal ultrasound.

b. Protecting/monitoring the environment.

c. Avoiding contributory habits.

(1) Self-regulatory behaviors/willpower.

(2) Help-seeking assistance to comply.

(a) 12-step programs.

(b) Support groups.

(c) Individual treatment.

(3) Health care professionals should coach people who want to quit or change habits.

4. Diagnostic staging of cancer.

a. Stage 1: tumor present, no perceived spread of disease.

(1) Lesion operable.

(2) Prognosis good (70-90% mean survival at 5 years).

(a) No spread of disease to the lymph nodes.

(b) No metastatic lesions.

b. Stage 2: localized spread of the tumor.

(1) Lesion is operable and can be removed with margins.

(2) Spread is limited and usually responds well to treatment (chemo/radiation/immunotherapy).

(3) Mean 5 year survival rate is 50% ± 5%.

c. Stage 3: extensive evidence of a primary tumor that has spread to other organs in the body.

(1) Tumor can be surgically debulked, but some cells may remain behind.

(2) There is deeper spread of the tumor cells in the lymphatics.

(3) Widespread evidence of cancer throughout multiple organs of the body.

(4) Mean 5 year survival rate is 20% ± 5%.

d. Stage 4: inoperable primary lesion.

(1) Survival dependent on depth and extent of the tumor spread as well as the ability to have the tumor respond to therapy (mean 5 year survival rate is <5 %).

(2) Multiple metastases.

5. Medical treatment.

a. Surgery.

(1) Lumpectomy.

(2) En bloc resection.

(3) Reconstruction.

(4) Amputation.

b. Chemotherapy.

(1) Intravenous.

(2) Shunt.

(3) Oral.

c. Radiation.

(1) External beam.

(2) Brachytherapy: seed implantation, flexible rods.

d. Immunotherapy.

(1) Interferon.

(2) Monoclonal antibodies.

e. Hormonal therapy.

f. Transplantation.

(1) Bone marrow.

6. Rehabilitation.

a. Pre-operative.

(1) Pre-operative functional assessments and preparation of the client for post-operative phase and care.

(2) Client and caregiver education concerning recovery and follow up care/functional expectations and client engagement.

b. Post-operative.

(1) Intervention planning based on a client's medical status and blood value guidelines that can affect safety during activity (platelets, hemoglobin level).

(2) Post-operative precautions related to structural change from surgery.

(a) This will be dependent on the location of the tumor and the procedure done (e.g., if a joint is replaced with an en bloc resection and shoulder indwelling prosthetic; abdominal precautions when the tumor is in the abdominal cavity; regional precautions when there is an incision near a joint, etc).

c. Convalescence.
  (1) Rehabilitation of motor impairments.
  (2) Rehabilitation of sensory impairments.
  (3) Rehabilitation of cognitive impairments.
  (4) Rehabilitation of neurobehavioral impairments.
  (5) Psychological support to enhance coping ability during recovery from cancer treatment phase.
    (a) Liminality: self recognition of vulnerability and self sense of mortality.
    (b) Occupational role and body image adjustment.
    (c) Obtainment of social support.
  (6) Development of health supporting behaviors (screening, follow-up, diet, exercise, stress management, vocational skill support or assistance to change job skills).
d. End of life care (Hospice).
  (1) Support quality of life as disease advances and functional status declines.
  (2) Provide client with as much control as they can and desire to have to their day to day life and lifestyle support.
  (3) Be present, be accountable, listen and counsel as possible concerning progression of disease and sense of liminality.
  (4) Encourage planning for death, control over goodbyes, funeral arrangements, advanced directives, etc.
  (5) Empower life celebration and life reflection (journaling, scrapbooks, phone call contact and recontact, letter writing).
  (6) Refer for legal support, if needed and requested).
  (7) See chapter 13 for additional information on psychosocial issues related to the end of life and dying.

**B. Scleroderma**
1. Rheumatic, connective tissue disease associated with impaired immune response.
2. Etiology: unknown.
  a. Three main components.
    (1) Vascular.
    (a) Raynaud's phenomenon.
    (b) Constant recurrent constriction of small blood vessels leading to pulmonary hypertension.
      (c) Decreased esophageal motility.
    (2) Fibrotic.
      (a) Scar tissue resulting from excess collagen (protein) causing thickness of skin and a burning sensation in the skin.
      (b) Fibrosis of the lungs causing restrictive lung disease.
    (3) Autoimmunity.
      (a) B Cell-produced antibodies (anti-centromere, anti-topisomerase I antibodies).
  b. Two basic types of the disease.
    (1) Limited.
      (a) Skin involvement (with a good prognosis).
      (b) Linear scleroderma (bands of thicker skin, with a good prognosis).
    (2) Systemic.
      (a) Systemic sclerosis of internal organs, which is life threatening.
      (b) CREST Syndrome with a good prognosis.
        • Calcinosis or calcium in the skin.
        • Raynaud's phenomenon.
        • Esophageal dysfunction.
        • Sclerodactyly of fingers and toes.
        • Telangiectasis or red spots covering the hands, feet, forearms, face and hips.
      (c) General morphea.
2. Risk factors: unknown, two main theories.
  a. Genetic.
  b. Environment.
3. Prevalence in the United States.
  a. 80% of scleroderma victims are women 30-50 years old at diagnosis.
  b. 300,000 cases in the U.S.
4. Prevention.
  a. Control symptoms of Raynaud's phenomenon.
  b. Have screening echocardiograms to rule out pulmonary hypertension.
  c. Smoking cessation.
5. Intervention.
  a. Raynaud's phenomenon.
    (1) Keep fingers and toes warm.
    (2) Dress in layers.
    (3) Drug therapy: vasodilators: Procardia XL, Altace, Norpace, Trental, Cardizem.
    (4) Biofeedback.
  b. Pulmonary artery problems.
    (1) Drug therapy: Procardia SL, anti-coagulation therapy.

(2) Oxygen: nasal.
c. Gastrointestinal problems.
   (1) Drug therapy: antacids, e.g., Maalox, Mylanta, Tums, Tagamet, etc.
   (2) Dietary modifications: soft diet, avoidance of alcoholic beverages and spicy foods.
   (3) Treatment of infection: erythromycin, tetracycline, doxycycline.
d. Fibrosis of the skin.
   (1) Protective gloves: cotton, insulated, mildly compressive.
   (2) Drug therapy: Cuprimine, Relaxin (under investigation).
e. Myositis: inflammatory muscle disease.
   (1) Cessation of exercise.
   (2) Drug therapy: low dose of oral steroids.
f. Fibrosis of the lungs.
   (1) Drug therapy: Cytoxan, or Cuprimine and Methotrexate.
6. Sequelae of scleroderma and recommendations.
a. Poor circulation, as in Raynaud's phenomenon.
   (1) Use of dressing in layers of clothing and clothing style modifications for neutral warmth.
   (2) Biofeedback: guided imagery to concentrate on improving distal circulation.
   (3) Education to encourage skin inspection.
   (4) Activity modifications to prevent trauma to fingers and toes.
b. Contractures.
   (1) Splinting at optimal resting length for hands/wrists to attempt to slow progressive development of contractures.
   (2) Use of silicone gel in the palms of the hands.
   (3) Use of electrical/mechanical vibration (muffled) to stimulate rapidly adapting-type A-nerve fibers and decrease burning sensation in hands.
c. Facial disfigurement and alteration in body image and self-identity.
   (1) "Look good/feel better" programs.
   (2) Work with people to help them choose adaptations and new accessories to ease their adjustment to their changing appearance.
   (3) Support groups: in person and on-line.
d. Thoracic spinal lesions can result in paraparesis, neurogenic bowel/bladder, altered mobility, and altered activity of daily living activities.

   (1) Neurorehabilitation and biomechanical approaches as indicated.
e. Space occupying lesions in the brain produce stroke-like symptoms.
   (1) Rehabilitation for functional deficits.

**C. Acquired Immunodeficiency Syndrome (AIDS)**
1. Etiology: infection by the human immunodeficiency virus (HIV).
2. Risk factors for infection.
   a. Unprotected sex.
   b. Contact with blood or body fluids.
3. Prevention.
   a. Avoid unprotected sex via abstinence or use of condoms.
   b. Avoid contact with body fluids.
      (1) Blood procedures.
      (2) Breast feeding.
      (3) Secretions of vagina/rectum, during birth (protection of baby), during sex, during hygiene.
      (4) Urine or feces.
      (5) Tears (low % of infection).
   c. Practice standard precautions with all persons Refer to Table 3-2 and Table 3-3 in Chapter 3.
4. Human immunodeficiency virus (HIV) infection.
   a. Retrovirus.
      (1) The RNA of the virus combines with recombinant RNA of human cells.
      (2) The new DNA has 1 strand of normal RNA/1 strand of virus.
      (3) The virus can eclipse into the cell, remaining dormant until stimulated by the body.
   b. HIV attacks the lymphatic system, the system that protects the body's immunity to opportunistic infections.
      (1) The T-cells (also known as CD4+ cells) attack the cells of the body including central nervous system cells, gastrointestinal tract cells, uterine/cervical cells.
   c. Four stages of infection.
      (1) Acute infection: flu-like response to initial contact with the virus.
      (2) Asymptomatic disease: HIV replicates and affects the immune system, but no visible signs other than blood abnormalities are detectable.
      (3) Symptomatic HIV: signs and symptoms appear.
      (4) Advanced disease, or AIDS: severely compromised immunity; CD4+ level drops to

below 1000/mm3.

d. Sequelae of HIV infection.

(1) Generalized lymphadenopathy/enlarged lymph nodes.

  (a) Fatigue.

  (b) Weight loss, malabsorption of nutrients (wasting syndrome).

  (c) General malaise.

(2) Fever.

(3) Diarrhea.

(4) All of the above result in decreased tolerance for activity participation and lack of energy.

(5) Neurological impairment.

  (a) Cognitive impairment (i.e., safety issues, communication and expression impairments, alteration of personality, decreased ability to engage as before in interpersonal relationships).

  (b) Affective changes.

  (c) Sensory changes (associated with dementia).

  (d) Basic ADL impairments such as inability to hold and manipulate objects for use (money, combs, tooth brushes, writing implements, feeding utensils, telephone, remote control, etc.).

  (e) Myelopathy (spinal cord pathology).

  (f) Peripheral neuropathy.

  (g) Visual impairment (i.e., peripheral: cytomegaloviral (CMV) infection, retinopathy, central: neurobehavioral loss/impairment).

e. Drug therapy.

(1) Protease inhibitors work to suppress the viral load in the bloodstream.

  (a) Must be taken consistently on time or effectiveness is lost.

  (b) Has shown a dramatic change in the management, treatment, and survivability of persons with a diagnosis of HIV/AIDS.

(2) Chemotherapy.

  (a) Less effective than protease inhibitors.

  (b) Loaded with side effects (specific to drugs used).

  (c) Drugs used related to neoplastic processes observed. Examples include Kaposi's sarcoma, lymphoma.

  (d) Drugs used to treat Hodgkin's; non-Hodgkin's (highly differentiated type, non-differentiated type).

  (e) Drugs used to treat opportunistic infections. Examples include Foscarnet.

**D. Hepatitis**

1. Etiology: a viral infection.

2. Risk factors.

a. Type A.

(1) Contaminated seafood.

(2) Protective immunization possible.

b. Type B, C, and other identified forms.

(1) Body and blood borne exposure.

(2) Protective immunization possible for type B.

c. Healthcare workers are most susceptible to hepatitis B.

3. Prevention.

a. Practice standard precautions with all persons to prevent contact with blood or body fluids. Refer to Table 3-2 and 3-3 in Chapter 3.

4. Sequelae.

a. Fever.

b. Fatigue.

c. The above contribute to decreased tolerance for activity participation and lack of energy.

**E. Tuberculosis (TB)**

1. See Section IV.B in Chapter 7.

**F. Methicillin resistant Staphylococcus aureus (MRSA)**

1. Etiology: usually mild infections (pimples or boils) on the skin; or more serious infections on skin; or infection in surgical wounds. The infection can be locally confined or systemic (entering the bloodstream and affecting primarily the lungs or the urinary tract).

2. Risk factors.

a. Having a weakened immune system.

b. Confinement in a hospital or other healthcare institutions.

c. Living in close quarters (military barracks, college dormitory, etc.).

d. Direct skin contact with an infected body part of another person (contact sports).

e. Secondary skin contact from something used by someone with an infection (e.g. shared towels during sports activities).

3. The infection resists treatment from known antibiotics, even broad spectrum antibiotics. Some antibiotics still work to fight it.

4. Signs and symptoms.

a. Redness accompanied by swelling and pain in the area of the wound.

b. Drainage such as pus in the local area of the wound
c. Fever
d. Skin abscess
e. Chest pain
f. Cough
g. Fatigue
h. Head ache
i. Muscle ache
j. Rash
k. Shortness of breath

5. Testing.
   a. Cultures of blood, sputum, skin or urine.

6. Prevention, detection and early intervention.
   a. Avoid high risk situations that contribute to possible exposure.
   b. Take preventative measures.
      (1) Wash your hands.
      (2) Avoid sharing personal items (e.g. razors or towels).
      (3) Keep any wounds or cuts covered.
      (4) Avoid communal bathing /swimming were infected persons may have been.
      (5) Assure facilities you use are clean.

7. Medical treatment for MRSA.
   a. Draining of a skin sore by a physician.
   b. Antibiotic treatment.
   c. Additional measures depending on severity and location of infection.
      (1) Intravenous fluids.
      (2) Oxygen.
      (3) Dialysis (if kidney failure occurs).

8. Sequelae of MRSA.
   a. Chance of recurrence of infection in the future.
   b. Any organ system damage that occurs as a result from untreated or unmanaged infections.

## G. Rehabilitation for Immunological System Disorders

1. Overall goals and approaches can be preventive, restorative, supportive, and/or palliative depending on treatment setting, diagnosis, stage of illness, and expected outcomes.

2. The role of the OTA in intervention.
   a. The OTA implements intervention with OT supervision.
   b. The level of supervision required depends upon the OTA's experience and established service competence.
   c. During the implementation of intervention, the OTA informs the supervising OT of any change in the individual's status and any other relevant information that may affect treatment.

3. Interventions for impairment level problems.
   a. Counsel people to be compliant with screening and treatment regimens.
   b. Set personal goals to invest behaviorally in one's health.
   c. Provide support to those dealing with immunological system disorders that are chronic illnesses (i.e., TB).
   d. Provide supportive counseling and social support for psychological disorders that can develop (e.g., anxiety disorder, depression, and/or adjustment disorders).
   e. Refer to physician for drug therapy and complementary medicine as indicated for accompanying physical and/or psychiatric disorders (e.g., kidney disease, depression).

4. Interventions for activity level problems.
   a. Self care.
      (1) Adaptations and training to do self care tasks with greatest ease while conserving energy. For example, for an individual with scleroderma:
         (a) Alter grasp and pinch patterns and level of demand and upper extremity demand.
         (b) Alter size of feeding utensils and tooth brushes to accommodate decreased ability to open mouth.
         (c) Prevent shearing forces on skin during specific personal activities of daily living tasks.
   b. Work.
      (1) Modifications to work site to allow participation in component tasks and activities.
      (2) Counseling and intervention for transition to disability status when work is no longer possible.
   c. Leisure/sports.
      (1) Modify specific tasks and activities (e.g., to protect body parts involved by sclerodermic changes).
      (2) Determine interests and skills to introduce new leisure or sports activities of interest to the person to transition to less physically demanding tasks as a disease progresses.
   d. Rest.
      (1) Monitor and intervene to maximize the ability to be well positioned during sleep.

(2) Monitor sleep habits and patterns and intervene when strategies are needed to relax and unwind or to schedule time and opportunity for relaxation.

5. Interventions for participation problems.
   a. Needs assessment to determine individual issues the person has with mobility, social, or political access to their personal, home, or community environments.
   b. Identification and facilitation of procurement of system changes to allow person access and ability to participate as a contributing member of society.

6. Acute hospitalization phase.
   a. Early mobilization.
   b. Preservation of function.
   c. Positioning.
   d. Psychological/emotional support.
   e. Prevention of long term disability.

7. Inpatient rehabilitation.
   a. Restoration of functional abilities.
      (1) Self-care, basic ADL.
      (2) Instrumental ADL.
      (3) Energy conservation and work simplification.
   b. Restoration of activity/exercise tolerance.
   c. Achievement and maintenance of quality of life.
   d. Role readjustment intervention.
   e. Planning to return to community.
      (1) Access to environment.
      (2) Participation issues.

8. Home care.
   a. Restoration of functional ability.
   b. Restoration of activity/exercise tolerance.
   c. Community mobility.
      (1) To inner and outer boundaries of home environment.
      (2) Into the street/block.
      (3) Further ability to venture out into the community (i.e., marketing, use of transportation, medical/business appointments, leisure access).

9. Community-based care.
   a. School related.
      (1) Transition from home schooling back to school for the child returning.
      (2) Transition of having student return to class for the classmates.
   b. Work related.

(1) Participatory as per Americans with Disabilities Act (ADA).
   c. Population-related intervention.
      (1) Coalition-related and grant funded initiatives for prevention and outreach programs.

# IV. Endocrine System and Metabolic System

## A. Diabetes

1. Prevalence
   a. There are 20.8 million children and adults in the United States, or 7% of the population, who have diabetes.
   b. While an estimated 14.6 million have been diagnosed, 6.2 million people (or nearly one-third) are unaware that they have the disease.

2. Types, etiology, and risk factors.
   a. Type 1 diabetes (insulin-dependent) (5-10% of all diagnosed cases of diabetes).
      (1) Autoimmune.
      (2) Genetic.
      (3) Environmental factors.
   b. Type 2 diabetes (non-insulin-dependent) (90-95% of all diabetes).
      (1) Older age.
      (2) Obesity.
      (3) Family history.
      (4) Prior history of gestational diabetes.
      (5) Impaired glucose tolerance.
      (6) Physical inactivity.
      (7) Race/ethnicity.
         (a) African-Americans.
         (b) Hispanic/Latino Americans.
         (c) American Indians.
         (d) Asian-Americans (non-Japanese).
         (e) Pacific Islanders.
   c. Gestational diabetes (2-5% of all pregnancies; 40% may go on later to develop Type 2 diabetes in later life).
      (1) Usually resolves after pregnancy.
      (2) Occurs at a greater frequency in people in race/ethnicity risk groups.
      (3) Obesity is another risk factor.
   d. Other types of Diabetes (1-2% of all cases of diabetes).
      (1) Genetic syndromes.
      (2) Surgery.
      (3) Drugs (e.g., steroids).
      (4) Malnutrition.
      (5) Infections.
   e. Signs and symptoms.

(1) Frequent urination.

(2) Excessive thirst.

(3) Unexplained weight loss.

(4) Extreme hunger.

(5) Visual changes.

(6) Sensory changes (tingling/numbness) in the hands or feet.

(7) Fatigue.

(8) Very dry skin.

(9) Slow healing wounds.

(10)Increased rate of infections.

3. Prevention.

a. Regular physical activity may reduce the risk of type 2 diabetes.

b. Maintaining normal body weight may be preventive.

4. Sequelae/complications.

a. Fatigue/decreased activity tolerance.

b. Urinary disturbance.

c. Visual loss, low vision, blindness.

d. Peripheral neuropathy.

(1) Amputations.

e. Propensity to develop wounds.

f. Poor general health/increased rate of infections disrupting life roles and activity participation.

g. Hypoglycemia.[1]

(1) Symptoms include vagueness, dizziness, tachycardia, pallor, weakness, diaphoresis, seizures and/or coma.

(2) If person is conscious, immediately provide carbohydrates in the form of hard candy, fruit juice or honey.

(3) If person is unconscious, immediately call for emergency medical care.

h. Hyperglycemic crises.[1]

(1) Ketoacidosis: signs include dehydration, rapid and weak pulse, and acetone breath.

(2) Hyperosmolar coma: signs include stupor, thirst, polyuria, and neurologic abnormalities.

(3) Call for emergency medical services as IV fluids and insulin are required.

5. Rehabilitation.

a. Preventive exercise.

b. Education concerning compliance and need for medical management of condition.

c. Psychological and emotional support to improve self care habits.

d. Lifestyle readjustment to complications when and if they occur.

(1) Low vision.

(2) Safety assessment and intervention.

(3) Physical adaptations.

e. Protective issues regarding peripheral neuropathy.

(1) Safety assessment.

(2) Education concerning risk associated with sensory loss.

(3) Skin care.

(4) Pain management.

(5) Adapted equipment/techniques to facilitate participation in lifestyle.

(6) Instrumental activities supporting compliance of self management.

f. Early attention to wound management.

(1) Teach skin care and inspection techniques.

(2) Teach person to self advocate quickly when changes are observed.

g. Assistance in problem solving and modifying self care as changes occur in the medical status of the condition.

(1) Problem solve resources for specialized treatment.

(2) Teach person to recognize changes in their functional status that warrant further attention and intervention.

**B. Obesity and Bariatric Issues[2]**

1. Obesity is defined as a condition characterized by excess body fat.

2. Body Mass Index (BMI): a formula for determining obesity. BMI is calculated by dividing an individual's weight in kilograms by the square of the person's height in meters.

a. World Health Organization Classification (adopted by National Institutes of Health):

(1) Overweight defined as BMI ranging from 25 to 29.9.

(2) Obesity defined as BMI $\geq$ 30.

(3) Morbidly obese defined as BMI $>$ 40.

3. A national health problem: overweight (65% of Americans) and obesity (31% of Americans).

a. Health risks associated with obesity: hypertension, hyperlipidemia, type 2 diabetes, cardiovascular disease, stroke, glucose intolerance, sleep apnea, gallbladder disease, menstrual irregularities and infertility, and cancer (endometrial, breast, prostate, and colon).

b. Waist circumference is used to determine distribution of body fat. Abdominal obesity (central accumulation of fat) is an independent pre-

---

[1]This section was completed by Rita P. Fleming-Castaldy.

[2]Susan O'Sullivan contributed to this section.

dictor of morbidity and mortality.
  c. Childhood obesity: most prevalent nutritional disorder affecting children in United States.
4. Etiology: health disparity; result of complex social, behavioral, cultural, environmental, physiological, and genetic factors.
  a. Social.
    (1) Education & income level.
    (2) Occupation.
    (3) Family background.
  b. Behavioral.
    (1) Eating on the run/ fast food.
    (2) Eating alone.
    (3) Eating for comfort /'comfort foods'.
    (4 Binge eating.
  c. Cultural.
    (1) 'Food and love' cultures (food given as a sign of affection).
    (2) Larger body size is more highly valued (e.g., West African cultures).
    (3) Post depression-era eating (i.e., consuming more because there is money to buy).
    (4) 'Restaurant cultures' (larger proportions/ food diversity/higher fat content).
  d. Environmental.
    (1) Lack of time to devote to meal planning and preparation.
    (2) Lack of time to develop and maintain a proper exercise routine (sandwiched generation: caregiving their parents and children simultaneously/perceived lack of time for self).
    (3) Lack of access to resources.
      (a) No facilities in which to exercise.
      (b) No exercise coach/partners.
  e. Physiological.
    (1) A nutritionally related imbalance that occurs resulting in excess body fat.
      (a) Poor diet and nutrition.
      (b) Eating processed foods.
      (c) Excessive food consumption: excess calories are consumed that are not expended by work or exercise.
        • Activity level: lack of exercise; poor choice of exercise in proportion to what is consumed.
        • Compulsive over-eating: psychiatric disorder.
    (2) Excess body fat that occurs from a metabolic imbalance.

      (a) Gestational diabetes (passively introduced to fetus: results in oversized infants at birth).
      (b) Adrenal disorders: cortisol and stress.
5. Prevention.
  a. Education.
    (1) Raising awareness of behavioral factors that contributes to obesity (e.g. sedentary lifestyle).
    (2) Community driven group intervention focused on health promotion and wellness.
  b. Habit intervention with occupations and activities that contribute to obesity (e.g. choose this/not that approaches, not eating while stressed, mindful eating).
  c. Tertiary intervention when overcoming obesity is not the issue-focus on occupational needs of the client.
6. Sequelae.
  a. Decreased ability in performance areas of occupations (BADL, IADL, mobility, social participation).
  b. Symptomatology related to larger body size: musculoskeletal pain, limited mobility, lower activity tolerance.
7. Rehabilitation.
  a. Lifestyle redesign: combination of changes in daily habits, patterns and routines to reduce body weight through nutritional changes (e.g., emphasis on fruits, vegetables, whole grains, and lean protein), changes in activity time engagement combined with increased physical activity.
    (1) Personalized plan to change lifestyle habits that contribute to obesity risk.
    (2) Personalized activity-focused exercise program combining personal interests, desired participation, goals, and positive meaning.
    (3) Instruction in self-monitoring of exercise responses (heart rate, perceived exertion).
    (4) Supportive coaching/counseling to improve compliance and make long term life altering change.
  b. Inpatient rehabilitation tertiary care.
    (1) Access devices and equipment to maximize client participation in daily activities of meaning (BADL, IADL, mobility and participation).
      (a) Bariatric equipment: wheeled mobility, assistive devices, lifters, seating adap-

tations, clothing adaptations. See Chapter 15.

(2) Activity participation to relearn lifestyle modifications and to offer practice in altering habits and patterns that require adjustment in order to maximize the individual client's participation and meaningful engagement.

c. Precautions.

(1) Cardiopulmonary compromise is typically exhibited (i.e., shortness of breath, elevated blood pressure, and angina).

(2) Altered biomechanics affects hips, knees, ankle/foot; back and joint pain.

(a) Increased risk of orthopedic injury.

(3) Increased risk of skin breakdown due to shear forces.

(4) Increased heat intolerance, risk of hyperthermia and heat exhaustion.

(5) Increased risk of practitioner injury when using poor body mechanics or inadequate assistance during transfers and lifts.

## C. Lyme Disease

1. Etiology.

a. Tick bite of the genus Ixodes that are infected with Borrelia burgdorferi or of the western black-legged tick.

2. Prevention.

a. Ticks are usually found on animals, on the tips of grasses and shrubs, in woody areas, and on the fringes of gardens, especially those surrounding new homes that were built in formerly wooded areas.

b. Avoid tick-infested areas especially in May, June, and July.

c. Wear light colored clothing, so ticks can be easily seen.

d. Tuck pants legs into socks or boots and shirt into pants.

e. Tape the area where pants and socks meet.

f. Spray insect repellent containing DEET on clothes and exposed skin, excluding the face.

g. Use permethrin (kills ticks on contact) on clothes.

h. Wear a hat and long-sleeved shirt.

i. Walk in the center of trails and avoid contact with grass and brush.

j. After being outdoors, change clothes and inspect skin for the presence of ticks.

k. Remove any ticks with tweezers, grasping the tick as close to the skin surface as possible and pull straight back.

l. Save the live tick, (if retrieved) in a plastic container and take it to a local health department for identification.

3. Sequelae.

a. Impairs the immune response and affects the neurological and orthopedic systems.

b. Early symptoms.

(1) Fatigue.

(2) Headache.

(3) Chills and fever.

(4) Muscle and joint pain.

(5) Swollen lymph nodes.

(6) Rash, erythema migrans: a circular red patch occurring 3 days-1 month after the bite from an infected tick.

(a) Commonly in the groin, thigh, trunk and armpits.

(b) The center of the rash may clear as it enlarges, resembling a bulls-eye.

c. Late symptoms.

(1) Arthritis: brief bouts of pain and swelling in one or more of the large joints.

(a) Knees are most commonly affected joints.

(2) Nervous system abnormalities.

(a) Numbness.

(b) Pain.

(c) Bell's palsy.

(d) Meningitis.

(3) Heart rate irregularities.

4. Diagnosis.

a. Presence of symptoms and signs.

b. History of exposure to ticks, especially in geographic areas where Lyme disease is known to occur.

c. Blood titer to determine whether antibodies for Lyme disease are present.

5. Medical treatment.

a. Antibiotics, oral or intravenous.

b. Management of joint-related symptoms from the accompanying arthritis.

6. Rehabilitation.

a. Joint pain and swelling.

(1) Provide education regarding acute arthritic flares.

(a) Rest.

(b) Anti-inflammatory medicine compliance.

(c) Splinting or wrapping to protect inflamed joints and prevent over-stretching of enlarged joint.

(d) Teach energy conservation and work simplification.

(2) Following flare, in sub-acute phase, provide gradual re-introduction of normal performance of daily tasks and activities.

b. Nervous system abnormalities.

(1) Numbness.

(a) Safety assessment and intervention to preserve safety and prevent injury.

(b) Management of aesthesias that are perceived as painful.

(c) Occupation-based interventions to encourage and preserve function and to cope with chronic pain conditions.

(2) Pain.

(a) Use of physical agent modalities to reduce pain.

(b) Use of stress management (complementary care) techniques to control the intensity of the pain and to increase coping ability.

(c) Use of neutral warmth to decrease intensity of pain.

(d) Use of adapted techniques to avoid triggering of movements that exacerbate pain during activity (e.g., sit on higher seat to decrease stress load in sit or stand).

(3) Bell's palsy.

(a) Make a facial splint to prevent long term asymmetry of facial muscles. Clip or pincer mold of the inside and outer lip of the mouth on the involved side. Elastic attaching mouth mold to ear piece (similar to eyeglass ear rim).

(b) Use electric stimulation to stimulate denervated muscles.

(c) Teach person to use their fingers to assist buccal closure and prevent spillage of the bolus through the lips.

(d) Provide counseling concerning alteration in body image, since the individual is coping with a facial deformity.

(4) Meningitis.

(a) Acute care: positioning, splinting, supportive care while hospitalized.

(b) Rehabilitation if there is recovery-related sequelae (i.e., neurological impairment, motor impairment, sensory impairment, cognitive impairment, or activity of daily living impairment).

(5) Heart rate irregularities.

(a) Telemetry during daily performance of tasks and activities that support role performance.

(b) Pulse oximetry measurements, if oxygenation is poor during performance of daily tasks and activities.

(c) Work simplification, adaptation, and modification to prevent further complications associated with arrhythmias.

# V. Integumentary System[3]

## A. Decubitus Ulcers

1. Etiology and risk factors.

a. Pressure that interrupts normal circulation causing localized areas of cellular necrosis.

(1) Greatest risk is over bony prominences (e.g., ischial tuberosity).

(2) Intensity and duration of the pressure determines the severity of the decubiti.

b. Conditions that predispose an individual to the formation of decubitus ulcers include immobility or altered mobility, weight loss, edema, incontinence, obesity, pathological conditions, and/or changes in skin condition due to aging.

c. The presence of substance abuse, cognitive deficits, and/or psychological impairments can jeopardize the individual's ability to understand and complete the required daily decubiti prevention regimen.

2. Types, signs, and symptoms.

a. Stage I: redness, edema, superficial epidermis and dermis involved.

b. Stage II: redness, edema, blistering and hardening (induration) of tissue, skin is open and inflammation extends to the fat layer with superficial necrosis in advanced Stage II lesions.

(1) Stages I and II are considered partial thickness ulcers.

c. Stage III: a full thickness skin lesion extending down to the muscle, the ulcer margin is thickened.

d. Stage IV: ulcer extends down to the bone and includes bone destruction.

e. Decubiti are often called pressure sores or bed-

[3]This section was completed by Rita P. Fleming-Castaldy.

sores by lay persons.

3. Intervention.

a. Prevention is the most effective intervention.

(1) Use wheelchair cushions, flotation pads, and pressure-relief bed aids to distribute pressure over a larger skin surface.

(2) Train the individual and/or caregivers in positioning and weight-shifting techniques and schedules and in proper skin care.

(a) Full push-ups, lateral leans, forward leans, or wheelchair tilt/recline options are common techniques used depending upon the abilities of the individual.

(b) Weight shifts should occur every 30 minutes for 30 seconds or every 60 minutes for 60 seconds.

(c) Integrate weight-shifting into daily activities (e.g., lean forward to pick up the phone, lean sideways when reading the mail).

(3) Train in proper skin care.

(a) Keep skin free of excessive moisture, dryness, and heat.

(b) Check skin at least two times per day for any evidence of breakdown.

• Most individuals perform this in bed in the morning before arising and in the evening before sleep.

• Target for inspection the scapula, elbows, ischia, sacrum/coccyx, trochanters, heels, ankles, and knees.

(4) Encourage adequate intake of fluids and food to maintain nutrition, promote healing, and achieve a recommended body weight.

b. Medical management including occlusive dressings, debridement, surgery and/or grafting may be needed depending upon the severity of the decubitus ulcer.

c. Encourage participation in meaningful and productive activities.

(1) Individuals who pursue active lifestyles have fewer decubiti.

# VI. Whole Body System Disorders[4]

## A. Heat Syndromes

1. Etiology and risk factors.

a. Heat production increases with infection, exercise, and/or drugs.

b. Heat loss decreases with high humidity and/or temperature, excess clothing, obesity, cardiovascular disease, dehydration, sweat gland dysfunction, lack of acclimatization, and/or drugs.

c. When an individual's heat loss is not sufficient to offset his/her heat production, his/her body will retain heat and a heat syndrome can develop.

d. Individuals who are elderly, obese, or taking drugs are at increased risk.

2. Prevention.

a. In hot weather, wear light-weight, loose-fitting clothing.

b. Avoid hot places; seek shade, use fans, and air conditioners.

c. Rest frequently.

d. Increase fluid intake.

3. Types, signs and symptoms.

a. Heat cramps are characterized by a normal body temperature, nausea, diaphoresis, muscle twitching or spasms, weakness, and/or severe muscle cramps.

b. Heat exhaustion is characterized by a rapid pulse, decreased blood pressure, nausea, vomiting, cool pallid skin, mental confusion, headache, and/or giddiness but no fever.

c. Heat stroke is characterized by hot, dry red skin; a body temperature higher than 104 degrees; slow, deep respiration; tachycardia; dilated pupils; confusion; progressing to seizures and possibly loss of consciousness.

4. Intervention.

a. Heat stroke is a medical emergency and hospitalization is required.

(1) Immediately call emergency medical services.

(2) Lower person's body temperature by placing ice packs on arterial pressure points.

(3) Hypothermia blankets, IV infusions, and medications are necessary.

b. Heat cramps and heat exhaustion usually do not require hospitalization.

(1) Loosen clothing and have the person lie in a cool place.

(2) Replace fluid and electrolytes with salt tablets and a balanced electrolyte drink. If these are not available, give fluids and seek additional medical care.

(3) Massage muscles if cramps are severe.

(4) IV infusions and oxygen may be indicated if symptoms are severe.

[4]This section was completed by Rita P. Fleming-Castaldy.

# References

AIDS Info [On-line]. Available: http://www.aidsinfo.nih.gov/

American Lyme Disease Foundation, Inc. Web page [On-line]. Available: http://www.aldf.com/Diagnosis_of_Lyme_disease.shtml.

Blanchard, S.A. (2009) Variables associated with obesity among African-American women in Omaha. *American Journal of Occupational Therapy, 63,* 58-68.

Burkhardt, A., & Joachim, J. (1996). *A therapist's guide to oncology: Medical issues affecting management.* San Antonio, TX: Therapy Skill Builders

Calibrisi, P., & Schein, P.S. (1993). *Medical oncology.* New York: McGraw-Hill.

Casale, R., Buounocore, M., and Matucci-Cerinic, M. (1997). Review article: Systemic sclerosis (scleroderma): An integrated challenge in rehabilitation. *Archives of Physical Medicine and Rehabilitation. 78* (7), 767-773.

Centers for Disease Control. (2010). *US Government Web, subsection on diabetes.* [On-line]. Available: http://www.cdc.gov/diabetes/

Centers for Disease Control update: HIV/AIDS Prevention. [On-line]. Available: http://www.cdc.gov/nchstp/hiv_aids/pubs/faq/faq11.htm.

Centers for Disease Control. (2009). *Healthcare-associated methicillin resistant staphylococcus aureus (HA-MRSA)* [On-line]. Available: http://www.cdc.gov/ncidod/dhqp/ar_MRSA.html

Centers for Disease Control Morbidity and Mortality Weekly Review (1999). *IDSA Guidelines for the prevention of opportunistic infections in persons infected with HIV.* [On-line]. Available: http://www.cdc.gov/epo/mmwr/preview/mmwrhtml/ rr4810al.htm.

Cox, M., Holm, S., Kurfuerst, S., Lynch, A., & Schuberth, L. (2007). Specialized knowledge and skills in feeding, eating, and swallowing for occupational therapy practice. *American Journal of Occupational Therapy, 61,* 686-700.

Foley, R.N. & Collins, A.J. (2007) End-stage renal disease in the United States: An update from the United States Renal Data System. *Journal of the American Society for Nephrology, 18,* 2644–2648.

Forhan M, Bhambhani Y, Dyer D, Ramos-Salas X, Ferguson-Pell M, Sharma A.(2010) Rehabilitation in bariatrics: Opportunities for practice and research. *Disability & Rehabilitation,* published ahead of date. [On-line] Available: http://informahealthcare.com/doi/abs/10.3109/09638280903483885

Logeman, J. (1983). *Evaluation and treatment of swallowing disorders* (1st ed.). Boston: Little Brown.

Melvin, J. (1994). *Scleroderma: Caring for your hands and face.* AOTA: Rockville, MD.

Poole, J.L. (2010) Musculoskeletal rehabilitation in the person with scleroderma. *Current Opinions in Rheumatology, 22,* 205-12.

National Kidney Foundation. (2010). *Nephrotic syndrome,* [On-line]. Available:http://www.kidney.org/atoz/content/nephrotic.cfm

Springhouse Corporation. (1999). *Professional guide to diseases.* (5th ed.). Springhouse, PA: Author.

Wilson, J.D., Braunwald, E., Isselbacher, K.J., Petersdorf, R.G., Martin, J.B., Fauci, A.S., & Root, R.K. (1991). *Harrison's principles of internal medicine s* (12th ed.). New York: McGraw-Hill.

# CHAPTER 10

# PSYCHIATRIC AND COGNITIVE DISORDERS

Janice L. Romeo • Rita P. Fleming-Castaldy

## I. Signs and Symptoms of Psychiatric Illness[1]

### A. Consciousness

1. A state of awareness.
2. Disturbances of consciousness.
   a. These disturbances are usually a result of brain pathology.
   b. Disorientation is a disturbance of orientation to person, place, or time. Situation is sometimes used as a fourth consideration.
   c. Delirium is a disoriented reaction with restlessness and confusion. It may be associated with fear and hallucinations.
   d. Confusion involves inappropriate reactions to environmental stimuli, manifested by a disordered orientation in relation to person, place, and time.
   e. Sundowning occurs in the late afternoon and at night in older people.
      (1) Characterized by, confusion, ataxia, and falling, agitation and sometimes aggression.
      (2) It is associated with sedation, dementia, and changes in orienting cues such as light and familiar people and objects.

### B. Attention

1. The ability to remain focused on an activity or experience or the ability to concentrate.
2. Disturbances of attention.
   a. Distractibility is the inability to concentrate one's attention without attention being drawn to unimportant or irrelevant stimuli.
   b. Selective inattention is blocking out those activities, objects, or concepts that produce anxiety.
   c. Hypervigilance is excessive attention and alertness that guards against potential danger.
   d. Trance is a sleeplike state with minimal environmental awareness, followed by amnesia for the experience.

### C. Emotion

1. A feeling state associated with affect and mood that consists of psychological and physical components (e.g., fear, anger, joy).
2. Affect is the observable component of emotions.
   a. Appropriate affect is consistent with the accompanying idea, thought, or speech.
   b. Disturbances of affect.
      (1) Inappropriate affect is inconsistent with the accompanying idea, thought, or speech.
      (2) Blunted affect is a severe lack of affect.
      (3) Restricted or constricted affect is reduced, but less so than blunted affect.
      (4) Flat affect is the absence of any affective signs of emotion.
      (5) Labile affect is rapid and abrupt changes in affect.

[1]Acknowledgments: Christine L. Hischmann MS, OTR/L, FAOTA, Director of Occupational Therapy, Clarks Summit State Hospital, Clarks Summit, PA and William Lambert, MA, OTL, Lecturer in Occupational Therapy, The University of Scranton, Scranton PA critically reviewed this chapter and provided helpful input to ensure the accuracy and currency of the chapter's content.

3. Mood is a pervasive and sustained emotion manifested by thoughts and actions (e.g., elation, anger, depression).
4. Other emotions.
   a. Anxiety is a feeling of apprehension or worry associated with anticipation of future danger.
   b. Free-floating anxiety is a pervasive anxiety that does not have a specific focus.
   c. Fear is an anxiety that is focused on a real danger.
   d. Physiological disturbances associated with mood are frequently autonomic in nature.

**D. Motor Behavior**
1. Behavioral and motoric expressions of impulses, drives, wishes, motivations, and cravings.
2. Disturbances of motor behavior.
   a. Echopraxia is the meaningless imitation of another person's movements.
   b. Catatonia is characterized by immobility or rigidity.
   c. Stereotypy is the repetition of fixed patterns of movement and speech (e.g., echolalia).
   d. Psychomotor agitation is excessive motor and cognitive activity, usually nonproductive and in response to inner tension.
   e. Hyperactivity is restless, sometimes aggressive or destructive activity, often associated with brain pathology.
   f. Psychomotor retardation is decreased or slowed motor and cognitive activity.
   g. Aggression is forceful, angry, or destructive speech or behavior.
   h. Acting out is the physical expression of thoughts and impulses.
   i. Akathisia is the state of restlessness characterized by an urgent need for movement, usually as a side effect of medication.
   j. Ataxia is the irregularity or failure of muscle coordination upon movement.

**E. Thinking**
1. A goal-directed reasoned flow of ideas and associations.
   a. When thinking follows a logical sequence, it is considered normal.
2. Disturbances in form of thought.
   a. Circumstantiality is speech that is delayed in reaching the point and contains excessive or irrelevant details.
   b. Tangentiality is the abrupt changing of focus to a loosely associated topic.

c. Perseveration is a persistent focus on a previous topic or behavior after a new topic or behavior has been introduced.
d. Flight of ideas refers to rapid shifts in thoughts from one idea to another.
e. Thought blocking is the interruption of a thought process before it is carried through to completion.
3. Disturbances in content of thought.
   a. Delusions are false beliefs about external reality without an appropriate stimulus that cannot be explained by the individual's intelligence or cultural background.
   b. Compulsions are a need to act on specific impulses to relieve associated anxiety.
   c. Obsessions constitute a persistent thought or feeling that cannot be eliminated by logical thought.
   d. Other examples of disturbances in content of thought include poverty of content, phobias, and hypochondria.

**F. Speech**
1. The expression of ideas, thoughts, and feelings through language.
2. Disturbances in speech.
   a. Pressured speech is rapid and increased in amount. It may be difficult to interrupt.
   b. Poverty of speech is limited in amount and content.
   c. Nonspontaneous speech consists of responses that are given only when spoken to directly.
   d. Stuttering consists of the repetition or prolongation of sounds or syllables.
   e. Perseveration in speech is continued repetition of a word or phrase.
3. Disturbances in language output.
   a. Expressive aphasia (Broca's) is a disturbance in which the individual knows what he/she wants to say, but cannot say it.
   b. Receptive aphasia (Wernicke's) is an organic loss of the ability to comprehend what has been said.
   c. Nominal aphasia (also known as anomial or amnestic) is the inability to name objects.
   d. Global aphasia involves all forms of aphasia.

**G. Perception**
1. The process of interpreting sensory information received from the environment.
2. Disturbances of perception.
   a. Hallucinations are false sensory perceptions

that are not in response to an external stimulus.

  b. Illusions are misperceptions or misinterpretations of real sensory events.

3. Disturbances associated with a cognitive disorder.

  a. Agnosia is the inability to understand and interpret the significance of sensory input.

  b. Astereognosis is the inability to identify objects through touch.

  c. Visual agnosia is the inability to recognize people and objects.

  d. Apraxia is the inability to carry out specific motor tasks in the absence of sensory or motor impairment.

  e. Adiadochokinesia is the inability to perform rapidly alternating movements.

4. Disturbances associated with conversion and dissociative phenomena.

  a. These disturbances are in response to repressed material and involve physical symptoms and distortions that are not under voluntary control or associated with a physical disorder.

  b. Depersonalization is a subjective sense of being unreal or inanimate.

  c. Derealization is a subjective sense that the environment is unreal.

  d. Fugue is a state of serious depersonalization, often involving travel or relocation, in which the individual takes on a new identity with amnesia for his/her old identity.

  e. Dissociative identity disorder involves the appearance that an individual has developed two or more distinct personalities.

  f. Dissociation involves the separation of a group of mental or behavioral processes from the rest of the person's psychic activity.

    (1) It may involve separating an idea from its emotional tone.

**H. Memory**

1. The ability to store and retrieve information related to past experiences.

2. Levels of memory.

  a. Immediate memory is the ability to recall material within seconds or minutes.

  b. Recent memory is the ability to recall events of the past few days.

  c. Recent past memory is the ability to recall events of the past few months.

  d. Remote memory is the ability to recall events of the distant past.

3. Disturbances of memory.

  a. Amnesia is an inability to recall past experiences or personal identity.

    (1) It may be caused by organic or emotional dysfunction.

    (2) Retrograde amnesia is the inability to remember events that occurred prior to the precipitating event.

## II. Diagnosis of Psychiatric Disorders

**A. Determination of Diagnosis by the Psychiatrist**

1. The individual's psychiatric history and physical status is reviewed.

2. A clinical interview, which includes a mental status examination, is conducted.

3. Clinical observation of the individual.

  a. Appearance.

  b. Speech.

  c. Actions.

  d. Thoughts.

**B. The Mental Status Examination**

1. General description of the individual.

  a. Appearance.

  b. Behavior and psychomotor activity.

  c. Attitude toward examiner.

2. Mood and affect.

  a. Mood (pervasive, sustained emotion).

  b. Affect (observable expression of mood).

  c. Appropriateness of mood and affect.

3. Speech.

4. Perceptual disturbances.

5. Thought.

  a. Process or form of thought.

  b. Content of thought.

6. Sensorium and cognition.

  a. Alertness and level of consciousness.

  b. Orientation to person, place, time, and situation.

  c. Memory.

  d. Concentration and attention.

  e. Capacity to read and write.

  f. Abstract thinking.

  g. Fund of information and intelligence.

7. Impulse control.

8. Judgment and insight.

9. Reliability.

**C. Current Diagnostic Information**

1. The Diagnostic and Statistical Manual of Mental Disorders, 4th edition, text revision (DSM-IV-TR) is the primary source.

2. The DSM-IV-TR uses a multiaxial format for

diagnosing mental disorders.

a. Axis I identifies the clinical disorders and other conditions that may be a focus of clinical attention.

b. Axis II includes personality disorders and mental retardation. When DSM-V is published in 2012, mental retardation will be re-classified as intellectual disorders.

c. Axis III identifies general medical conditions.

d. Axis IV lists psychosocial and environmental problems.

    (1) Problems with primary support group.

    (2) Problems related to the social environment.

    (3) Educational problems.

    (4) Occupational problems.

    (5) Housing problems.

    (6) Economic problems.

    (7) Problems with access to health care services.

    (8) Problems related to interaction with the legal system/crime.

    (9) Other psychosocial and environmental problems.

e. Axis V provides a global assessment of functioning (GAF).

    (1) The GAF is based on the clinicians' assessment of the person's psychological, social, and occupational functioning on a proposed mental health continuum that is coded from 0-100.

        (a) 0 designates there is inadequate information upon which to make an assessment.

        (b) The subsequent codes are provided in increments of 10 (e.g. 10-1, 20 -11, etc).

        (c) The code of 1-10 designates a person who has completed a serious suicide act or who presents a persistent danger to self or others. This danger can be physical harm or the complete inability to care for self.

        (d) The code of 100-91 designates a person who functions at a superior level and has no mental health symptoms.

    (2) Along the GAF's hypothetical continuum, the code descriptions include:

        (a) The functional impact of psychiatric symptoms (e.g., code 30-21: behavior is seriously influenced by hallucinations, code 90-81: anxiety impedes performance on a test).

        (b) The level of impairment in occupational functioning (e.g., code 40-31: major impairments result in inability to work or failure at school, code 70-61: some difficulties at work or school such as occasional truancy).

        (c) The level of impairment in social functioning (e.g., 20-11: severe communication impairments such as mutism, 50-41: serious impairments that result in having no friends).

    (3) The occupational therapist and the OTA can provide valuable information to the clinical team about a client's occupational and social functioning to help obtain an accurate GAF diagnostic code.

3. DSM-IV diagnoses are made when the following criteria are met.

a. The behavior is not caused by other medical conditions, substance abuse, or medications.

b. The symptoms cause significant distress and impairments in function.

c. The symptoms cannot be better accounted for by another diagnosis.

## III. Psychotic Disorders[2]

### A. Schizophrenia

1. Diagnostic criteria.

a. Criterion A: the presence of two or more of the following symptoms.

    (1) Delusions.

    (2) Hallucinations.

    (3) Disorganized speech.

    (4) Grossly disorganized or catatonic behavior (positive symptoms).

    (5) Negative symptoms (see below).

b. Criterion B: disturbance in one or more areas of function such as work, interpersonal relations, or self care.

c. Criterion C: continuous signs of the illness for 6 months including at least one month of symptoms that meet criterion A.

d. Positive symptoms are the excesses or distortions of normal function as found in criterion A.

e. Negative symptoms represent a loss or absence of function.

    (1) Restricted emotion.

    (2) Decreased thought and speech.

    (3) Lack of motivation and initiative.

[2]Often referred to as thought disorders in non-medical settings.

(4) Inability to relate to others.

2. Subtypes of schizophrenia.
   a. Paranoid type.
      (1) Characterized by preoccupation with one or more delusions of persecution or grandeur.
      (2) Auditory hallucinations are frequently present.
      (3) Individuals with paranoid type schizophrenia tend to exhibit fewer of the negative symptoms.
   b. Disorganized type.
      (1) Distinguished by marked regression demonstrating primitive, disinhibited, and disorganized behavior.
   c. Catatonic type.
      (1) Characterized by severe disturbances in motor behavior involving stupor, negativism, rigidity, excitement, or posturing.
   d. Undifferentiated type.
      (1) Used to classify those patients who do not clearly fit into one of the other categories.
   e. Residual type.
      (1) Used when there is continued evidence of schizophrenic behavior in the absence of a complete set of diagnostic criteria.

3. Onset, prevalence, and prognosis.
   a. The onset of schizophrenia is usually between early adolescence and the mid thirties with a life time prevalence of 0.6 to 1.9%.
   b. Ten to 20% of diagnosed cases have been found to sustain a good outcome.
   c. Twenty to 30% are able to lead somewhat normal lives.
   d. The prognosis is poor for over 50% of individuals with schizophrenia, resulting in repeated hospitalizations, periods of exacerbation and episodes of major mood disorders.

**B. Other Psychotic Disorders**

1. Schizophreniform disorder.
   a. The individual meets the criteria for schizophrenia; however, the episode lasts more than one month but less than the six months required for a diagnosis of schizophrenia.

2. Schizoaffective disorder.
   a. The person has an uninterrupted period of illness during which, at some time, there is a major depressive episode, a manic episode, or a mixed episode concurrent with symptoms that meet criterion A symptoms for schizophrenia.

3. Delusional disorder.
   a. The individual's predominant symptoms are non-bizarre delusions with the absence of other criterion A symptoms of schizophrenia.

4. Brief psychotic disorder.
   a. The individual experiences at least one day but less than one month with one or more criterion A symptoms of schizophrenia which result from severe psychosocial stress.

**C. Impact on Function**

1. Many individuals with psychotic disorders demonstrate deficits in cognitive-perceptual and social interaction skills that affect all areas of function.
   a. The deficits in the processing of sensory information that is experienced by some individuals makes interaction with the environment difficult and frightening.
   b. Individuals who have difficulty with their own ego boundaries often exhibit socially inappropriate, sometimes intrusive, behaviors.
   c. Some individuals have lost or failed to develop the social and communication skills necessary for effective and satisfying interpersonal interactions and relationships.
   d. Deficits in cognitive function due to thought disorders and difficulties with the performance of basic skills interfere with all occupational performance areas from self-care and use of leisure time to vocational pursuits.
   e. It is important to assess and continue to monitor the degree of assistance and structure needed to maintain optimum independence in all performance areas.

**D. Medical Management**

1. Treatment consists primarily of the use of antipsychotic medications and the provision of a structured supportive environment.

2. Pharmacology.
   a. Traditional antipsychotic medications.
      (1) Include Thorazine, Prolixin, Haldol, and Navane. Mellaril, Stelazine, and Trilafon are rarely used.
      (2) Long-acting injections are available for Haldol (once a month) and Prolixin (once every two weeks).
      (3) Side-effects may include: dry mouth, blurry vision, photosensitivity, constipation, orthostatic hypotension, Parkinsonism, dystonias (i.e., impaired tonicity), akathisias (i.e., restless, anxiety provoking

need for movement), tardive dyskinesia (slow, rhythmic, automatic, stereotyped movements), and cardiovascular disorders.

    (4) Complications may include Neuroleptic Malignant Syndrome, an autonomic emergency leading to increased blood pressure, tachycardia, sweating, convulsions, and coma.

  b. Atypical antipsychotics.

    (1) Clozaril, Risperdal, Zyprexa, Seroquel, Geodon, Abilify.

      (a) Long acting atypical injections are available for Risperdal Consta (once every 2 weeks) and Invega Sustenna (once every 4 weeks).

    (2) Side-effects vary with individual medications.

    (3) Complications of Clozaril may include agranulocytosis, which is a decrease in certain white blood cells that requires weekly blood count monitoring.

  c. Neuromuscular side-effects of antipsychotics may be treated by Cogentin, Artane, Benadryl, and Symmetrel.

    (1) Side effects include dry mouth, blurry vision, sedation, dizziness, hypotension, insomnia, and confusion.

**E. Diagnostic-Specific Considerations for Occupational Therapy**

1. When working with persons with psychotic disorders, the presence of disordered thinking requires the OTA to communicate simply, clearly, and concretely.

2. External structure to organize the individual's thinking, environment, and daily activities is often required.

3. The provision of supports and tools to enable recovery is essential (e.g., WRAP –Wellness and Recovery Action Plan).

4. See sections XV and XVI in this chapter for additional evaluation and intervention guidelines.

5. Chapter 13 provides further information on general OT psychosocial evaluation and intervention approaches and specific interventions to manage psychotic behaviors (i.e., delusions and hallucinations).

## IV. Mood Disorders

**A. Overview**

1. Mood disorders are diagnosed based on the incidence of manic, hypomanic, major depressive, and mixed episodes. (See below for descriptions of specific episodes).

2. Mood episodes are not coded diagnoses in and of themselves.

3. Treatment addresses the symptoms of the episode experienced by the patient.

  a. It will vary with shifts in mood.

**B. Diagnostic Criteria for Specific Mood Disorders**

1. Major depressive disorder.

  a. One or more depressive episodes.

  b. May be a single episode or recurrent episodes.

2. Bipolar I disorder.

  a. One or more manic episodes.

  b. May be combined with depressive episodes.

3. Bipolar II disorder.

  a. One or more major depressive episodes.

  b. There must be at least one hypomanic episode.

4. Other mood disorder diagnoses.

  a. Dysthymia is characterized by at least 2 years of a depressed mood, most days, with depressive symptoms that are not severe enough to meet the criteria for a major depressive episode.

  b. Cyclothymic disorder is characterized by at least 2 years with numerous periods of hypomanic and depressive symptoms that do not meet the criteria for a manic episode or a major depressive episode.

**C. Onset, Prevalence, and Prognosis**

1. While major depressive disorder can develop at any age, the median age at onset is 32.

2. The median age of onset for bipolar disorder is 25 years, although the illness can start in early childhood or as late as the 40's and 50's.

3. The lifetime prevalence of depressive disorders is 20 to 26% in women and 8 to 12% in men.

4. Bipolar disorders have a lifetime prevalence of 1.0 to 2.4%.

5. The prognosis for recurrences of mood disorders is poor; however, the effectiveness of medications has increased the number of individuals who are able to maintain satisfying life styles, resulting in a more favorable overall prognosis.

**D. Manic Episode**

1. Diagnostic criteria.

  a. A distinct period of abnormally and persistently elevated, expansive, or irritable mood lasting at least one week.

  b. During this period, three or more of the following symptoms have persisted.

(1) Inflated self-esteem or grandiosity.

(2) Decreased need for sleep.

(3) More talkative than usual or pressured to keep talking.

(4) Flight of ideas or feeling that thoughts are racing.

(5) Distractibility.

(6) Increase in goal-directed activity or psychomotor agitation.

(7) Excessive involvement in pleasurable activities that have a high potential for painful consequences.

  c. Behaviors often associated with a manic episode.

(1) Treatment-resistance resulting from failure to recognize illness.

(2) Suggestive or flamboyant dress.

(3) Gambling, promiscuity, excessive spending, or giving things away.

(4) Irritable, assaultive, or suicidal behavior.

2. Impact on function.

  a. The lack of inhibition experienced during a manic phase may lead to excessive spending, impulsive travel, flamboyant and promiscuous dress and/or behavior, etc.

  b. Individuals may be euphoric in early phases, but may become labile, threatening, and assaultive.

  c. Individuals may have high, often undirected, energy levels and require little sleep.

  d. Poor judgment can lead to dangerous situations, poor self care, problems in relationships, and decreased or irresponsible work performance.

  e. The incidence of substance abuse is increased.

3. Medical management.

  a. Antipsychotics (III D. 2.).

  b. Mood stabilizing medications.

(1) Lithium: Eskalith, Lithobid, and time-released forms.

   (a) Side effects include excessive thirst, tremors, excessive urination, weight gain, nausea, diarrhea, and cognitive impairment.

   (b) Precautions include the monitoring of blood levels to maintain the narrow therapeutic window.
   • High levels may cause nerve damage and death.
   • Early symptoms of toxicity include

motoric disturbances.

(2) Anticonvulsants.

   (a) Depakote, Tegretol, Lamictal, Topamax, Keppra, Lyrica, and Trileptal. Neurontin is rarely used.

   (b) Side effects include dizziness, drowsiness, ataxia, weight gain, sedation.

(3) Mood stabilizers are also used to prevent bipolar disorder.

4. Diagnostic-specific considerations for occupational therapy.

  a. Limit-setting to reduce the individual's fears of losing control, increase participation in the treatment process, and promote safety.

  b. Engagement in activities that provide for release of excess energy in a positive and therapeutic manner.

  c. Periods between manic episodes should be used to educate the individual and the family on symptom management.

  d. See sections XV and XVI in this chapter for overall evaluation and intervention guidelines.

  e. Chapter 13 provides additional information on general OT psychosocial evaluation and intervention approaches and specific intervention approaches for managing manic or monopolizing behaviors.

## E. Major Depressive Episode

1. Diagnostic criteria.

  a. A two week period of depressed mood or loss of interest or pleasure.

  b. Five or more of the following symptoms.

(1) Depressed mood most of the day.

(2) Markedly diminished interest or pleasure.

(3) Weight loss/gain, increase/decrease in appetite.

(4) Insomnia/hypersomnia.

(5) Psychomotor retardation/agitation.

(6) Fatigue, loss of energy.

(7) Feelings of worthlessness or guilt.

(8) Diminished ability to concentrate/make decisions.

(9) Recurrent thoughts of death/suicide (with or without a plan), suicide attempt.

  c. Behaviors often associated with depressive episodes.

(1) Irritability, anxiety, phobias, and obsessive thinking.

(2) Difficulties in social interactions, relationships, and sexual functioning.

(3) Self-destructive behavior including suicide and substance abuse.

(4) There may be an increased use of medical services.

2. Impact on function.

   a. Individuals are often tearful, brooding and isolative.

   b. Anxiety leads to excessive concerns about physical health, complaints of pain, and alcohol abuse.

   c. Hopelessness, lack of energy, and slow thought processing lead to limited interest in activity and difficulty performing tasks in all occupational performance areas including self care, social interaction, and productivity.

3. Medical management.

   a. Antidepressant medications.

     (1) Selective Serotonin Reuptake Inhibitors (SSRIs) include Prozac, Zoloft, Paxil, and Celexa. Lexapro and Luvox are rarely used due to potentiating effects with other medications.

       (a) Side effects include nausea, headache, sexual dysfunction, and insomnia.

     (2) Tricyclics include Elavil, Tofranil, Norpramin, and Pamelor. However, these are rarely used secondary to the success of the SSRIs and SNRIs.

       (a) Side effects include dry mouth, blurred vision, sedation, postural hypotension, and other anticholinergic effects.

     (3) Selective norepinephrine, or serotonin and norepinephrine inhibitors (SNRIs) include Effexor, Wellbutrin, and Remeron. Desyrel and Serzone are rarely used.

       (a) Side effects vary but may include hypertension, anxiety, dizziness, sedation, nervousness, weight gain, nausea, sweating.

     (4) Monoamine Oxidase Inhibitors (MAOIs) include Nardil and Parnate. These are almost never used unless the patient has had success on these in the past and is non-responsive to other medications.

       (a) Side-effects include weight gain, hypotension, insomnia, liver damage, etc.

       (b) Precautions include dietary restrictions for individuals taking MAOIs.

         • Ingesting foods or beverages that contain the amino acid tyramine can sudddenly increase blood pressure and may lead to stroke or other serious cardiac reactions.

         • Foods and beverages with tyramine must be completely avoided. These include aged cheeses, pickled foods (e.g., sauerkraut, herring), cured or smoked meats (e.g., salami, sausage, pepperoni, hot dogs), liver, yogurt, sour cream, fruits that must ripen to eat (e.g., avocados, bananas), fava beans, peapods, chocolate, beer and red wine (including non-alcoholic and alcohol-reduced), meat tenderizers, soy products (soy sauce, tofu), yeast extracts, and any product that has been improperly stored, over-ripened, not fresh, and/ or past an expiration date.

         • Many over the counter drugs also contain ingredients that can cause a serious interaction with MAOIs. These include cold, sinus, and hay fever medications, nasal decongestants, asthma inhalants, 'pep' pills, and appetite suppressants.

       (c) Severe headaches or palpitations can be the first sign of a hypertensive crisis. The medication should be stopped immediately and a physician consulted

   b. The most effective treatment involves antidepressant medication combined with psychotherapy.

   c. Cognitive approaches are helpful for those who demonstrate self-awareness, intact cognitive skills, and the ability to actively participate in the treatment process.

   d. Electroconvulsive therapy (ECT) is very effective, although how it works is not fully understood.

     (1) It often produces some memory loss for the period surrounding treatment.

4. Diagnostic-specific considerations for occupational therapy.

   a. The provision of a safe environment and the management of behaviors that threaten the safety and well being of the individual are paramount.

     (1) Individuals must be closely monitored for

self-destructive and/or suicidal behavior.
(2) The most dangerous time may be when the depression begins to lift and the person becomes mobilized.
b. See sections XV and XVI in this chapter for additional evaluation and intervention guidelines.
c. Chapter 13 provides further information on general OT psychosocial evaluation and intervention approaches and specific interventions to manage suicidal behaviors and other depressive symptoms.

**F. Mixed Episode**
1. The criteria are met for both a manic episode and a major depressive episode for at least one week.

**G. Hypomanic Episode**
1. Symptoms are the same as for a manic episode; however, they are not severe enough to cause marked impairment in social or occupational function or to require hospitalization.

## V. Substance-Related Disorders

**A. Overview**
1. Substance-related disorders are diagnosed based upon the taking of a drug of abuse (including alcohol and prescription medications), the side-effects of medication(s), and/or exposure to toxins (inhalants, lead).
2. Substance-related disorders are categorized into two groups.
   a. Substance use disorders include dependence and abuse.
   b. Substance-induced disorders include a multitude of diagnoses including intoxication, withdrawal, and substance-induced anxiety, affective, and psychotic disorders.
      (1) These disorders are generally treated medically and therefore, will not be further described.

**B. Substance Dependence**
1. Diagnostic criteria.
   a. There must be evidence of tolerance and withdrawal.
      (1) Tolerance to a substance results in diminished effects from taking the same amount of a substance and the need to use increasing amounts to experience the desired effect.
      (2) Withdrawal refers to the symptoms (specific to the substance) that occur with decrease

or discontinuation.
      (a) The substance is then used not for pleasure, but to prevent or relieve the withdrawal symptoms.
   b. Individual continues to abuse the substance despite serious consequences.

**C. Substance Abuse**
1. Diagnostic criteria.
   a. There must be continued use despite serious consequences.

**D. Onset, Prevalence, and Prognosis**
1. The onset of abuse is becoming earlier and earlier. While it often begins in adolescence, it may begin anytime from childhood through seniority.
2. Recent statistics reveal the prevalence of substance abuse or dependence.
   a. 9.3 % for adolescents aged 12 to 17 years.
   b. 19.6 % for young adults aged 18 to 25.
   c. 5.9% for adults ages 26 or older.
3. According to a 2008 study, drinking alcohol is a prevalent activity in the United States.
   a. 57.7% of males aged 12 or older were current drinkers, higher than the rate for females (45.9%).
   b. Among youths aged 12 to 17, the percentage of males who were current drinkers (14.2%) was similar to the rate for females (15.0%).
   c. Among adults aged 18 to 25, an estimated 58.0% of females and 64.3% of males reported current drinking in 2008.
4. Prognosis varies depending on several factors including motivation, substance used, and degree and type of support.

**E. Impact on Function**
1. The impact that substance use has on the individual depends on the type of substance used and on whether the individual is abusing the substance, or is dependent upon it.
2. Results of disorders of use.
   a. Disinterest and inability to care for self.
   b. Difficulty with and loss of personal relationships.
   c. Inability to be productive and/or hold a job.
   d. Involvement of the legal system.
3. Prolonged use may lead to severe physical, cognitive, and psychiatric problems and can result in death.

**F. Medical Management**
1. Treatment focus.
   a. Assist the individual to refrain from substance use through medication.

b. Assist with concrete practical services, such as obtaining social security, housing, and food stamps, as needed.

c. Support groups, including Alcoholics Anonymous, Narcotics Anonymous and others.

d. Psychotherapy.

## G. Diagnostic-Specific Considerations for Occupational Therapy

1. Due to the presence of learned "survival skills", the individual's abilities and potential may be overestimated.

    a. The OTA can apprise the team of the person's actual skills and deficits.

    b. The OTA assists the team in identifying realistic expectations and discharge plans.

2. The individual's identification of the reasons for substance use is important.

3. The development of the skills necessary to cope with life stressors without substance use is critical for a substance-free lifestyle. Skills needed include:

    a. Interpersonal relationships and socialization.

    b. Productivity, work, school.

    c. Leisure time use.

4. Life-long patterns of denial, resistance, and other defensive behaviors can make treatment challenging and difficult.

5. See sections XIV and XV in this chapter for additional evaluation and intervention guidelines.

6. Chapter 13 provides further information on general OT psychosocial evaluation and intervention approaches.

# VI. Anxiety Disorders

## A. Overview

1. Anxiety disorders include a range of disorders that include episodic periods of intense anxiety to chronic periods of lower levels anxiety.

2. Anxiety is an internal sense of apprehension and psychological distress. It may or may not have a specific focus.

## B. Panic Attacks and Agoraphobia

1. Panic attacks are symptoms of anxiety.

    a. They are not coded diagnoses.

2. Panic attacks are discrete periods of intense fear or discomfort, in which four or more symptoms develop abruptly and reach a peak within 10 minutes.

    a. Palpitations, or accelerated heart rate.

    b. Sweating.

c. Trembling or shaking.

d. Sensations of shortness of breath or smothering.

e. Feelings of choking.

f. Chest pain or discomfort.

g. Nausea or abdominal stress.

h. Feeling dizzy, unsteady, lightheaded, or faint.

i. Derealization or depersonalization.

j. Fear of losing control or going crazy.

k. Fear of dying.

l. Paresthesias.

m. Chills or hot flashes.

3. Agoraphobia associated with panic attack.

    a. Anxiety about being in places or situations from which escape may be difficult or embarrassing, or in which help may not be available if needed.

    b. Situations are avoided or endured with anxiety about having a panic attack.

## C. Selected Anxiety Disorders

1. Panic disorder.

    a. Recurrent panic attacks followed at least once by concern for recurrence.

2. Specific phobia.

    a. A clinically significant anxiety from a specific object or situation leading to avoidant behavior.

3. Social phobia.

    a. A clinically significant anxiety from certain types of social or performance situations leading to avoidance.

4. Obsessive-compulsive disorder.

    a. Obsession are recurrent and persistent thoughts, images, or impulses that are disturbing, intrusive, and inappropriate.

    b. Compulsions are repetitive behaviors that the person is driven to perform to reduce anxiety or prevent a dreaded event of situation.

    c. The obsessions or compulsions are time-consuming and distressing despite the individual's awareness of their irrationality.

5. Post-traumatic stress disorder.

    a. The persistent re-experiencing (for more than one month) of an extremely traumatic event that produces symptoms of increased arousal.

    b. Results in avoidance of stimuli associated with the traumatic event.

6. Acute stress disorder.

    a. Similar to post-traumatic stress disorder; however, it immediately follows the event.

    b. The symptoms do not persist beyond one month.

7. Generalized anxiety disorder.
   a. Consists of 6 months of persistent and excessive unfocused anxiety and worry.

**D. Onset, Prevalence, and Prognosis**
1. Anxiety disorders often begin in childhood but may develop at any time.
2. Post traumatic stress disorder and acute stress disorder follow the stressful event.
3. Prevalence and prognosis vary with the specific disorder.

**E. Impact on Function**
1. The degree of impact varies with the severity and type of anxiety disorder.
2. Reactions may vary from temporary discomfort to severely avoidant and paralyzing behavior.

**F. Medical Management**
1. Psychotherapy to explore psychodynamic issues.
2. Several types of medications may be helpful depending on the specific disorder.
   a. Anxiolytic medications include Xanax, Valium, Librium, Ativan, Klonopin, and BuSpar.
      (1) Side effects include drowsiness, ataxia, headache, nausea, depression, and dependence.
   b. Antidepressant medications are helpful in some cases.
      (1) Refer to mood disorder section for side-effect profiles.
   c. Anti-obsessional medications (Anafranil, and Paxil, Prozac, Zoloft at high doses) reduce obsessional thinking. Luvox is rarely used due to potentiating effects.
      (1) Side effects are similar to that of the Selective Serotonin Reuptake Inhibitors.
   d. In some cases hypnotic medications to induce sleep may be used briefly.
      (1) Hypnotic medications include Restoril, Dalmane, Ambien, and Benadryl.
      (2) Side effects are similar to those of the anxiolytics.

**G. Diagnostic-Specific Considerations for Occupational Therapy**
1. Skills training and cognitive behavioral approaches may reduce avoidant behavior.
2. Development of relaxation and stress management skills may decrease the incidence and severity of symptoms.
3. Graded activities designed to promote self-efficacy may increase self-confidence, motivation, and participation in treatment.

4. See sections XV and XVI in this chapter for additional evaluation and intervention guidelines.
5. Chapter 13 provides further information on general OT psychosocial evaluation and intervention approaches.

# VII. Personality Disorders

**A. Diagnostic Criteria**
1. Evidence of characteristics and patterns of inner experience and behavior that deviate markedly from the culturally accepted norms in cognition, affect, impulse control, and interpersonal relating.
2. Behavior must be inflexible and maladaptive across a broad range of personal and social situations.
3. There must be evidence of onset in late childhood or adolescence.

**B. Specific Personality Disorders**
1. Paranoid personality disorder.
   a. Persons with this disorder are characterized by long-standing suspiciousness and mistrust of people in general.
   b. They refuse responsibility for their own feelings and assign responsibility for them to others.
   c. They can often appear hostile, irritable, and angry.
2. Schizoid personality disorder.
   a. This is frequently diagnosed in individuals who display a lifelong pattern of social withdrawal.
   b. Their discomfort with human interaction, their introversion, and their bland, constricted affect are noteworthy.
   c. Persons with schizoid personality disorder are often seen by others as eccentric, isolated, or lonely.
3. Schizotypal personality disorder.
   a. Persons with this disorder appear odd or strange in their thinking and behavior to those who come in contact with them.
   b. Magical thinking, peculiar ideas, ideas of reference, illusions, and derealization are part of this individual's everyday world.
4. Antisocial personality disorder.
   a. This disorder is characterized by continual antisocial or criminal acts, but it is not synonymous with criminality.
   b. It is an inability to conform to social norms that involves many aspects of the individual's adolescent and adult development.
   c. Persons with antisocial personality disorder

have no regard for the safety or feelings of others and they lack remorse.

5. Borderline personality disorder.

   a. Individuals with borderline personality disorder experience extraordinarily unstable affect, mood, behavior, relationships, and self-image.

   b. Fear of real or imagined abandonment leads to frantic efforts to avoid it.

   c. Recurrent self-destructive or self-mutilating behavior may be threatened or carried out.

   d. Majority of patients have a history of trauma (i.e., physical, sexual, emotional abuse).

6. Histrionic personality disorder.

   a. This disorder is characterized by colorful, dramatic, extroverted behavior in excitable, emotional persons.

   b. An inability to maintain deep, long-lasting attachments with accompanying flamboyant presentation is often characteristic.

7. Narcissistic personality disorder.

   a. Persons with this disorder are characterized by a heightened sense of self-importance and a grandiose feeling that they are special in some way.

8. Avoidant personality disorder.

   a. Persons with this disorder show an extreme sensitivity to rejection, which may lead to a socially withdrawn life.

   b. These individuals are not, however, asocial. They show a great desire for companionship but consider themselves inept or unworthy.

   c. Individuals with avoidant personality disorder need unusually strong and repeated guarantees of uncritical acceptance.

   d. These persons are commonly referred to as having an inferiority complex.

9. Dependent personality disorder.

   a. Persons with this disorder subordinate their own needs to those of others and need others to assume responsibility for major areas in their lives.

   b. Individuals with dependent personality disorder lack self-confidence.

   c. They may experience discomfort when alone for more than a brief period.

10. Obsessive-compulsive personality disorder.

    a. Characterized by emotional constriction, orderliness, perseverance, stubbornness, and indecisiveness.

    b. The essential feature is a pervasive pattern of perfectionism and inflexibility.

    c. It should not be confused with obsessive-compulsive disorder.

11. Personality disorders not otherwise specified (NOS).

    a. Passive-aggressive.

    b. Depressive.

    c. Sadomasochistic.

    d. Sadistic.

## C. Onset, Prevalence, and Prognosis

1. Symptoms of personality disorders usually begin in childhood or early adolescence.

2. The prevalence of personality disorders varies with the specific disorder from rare to approximately 9.1%.

3. The prognosis for individuals with personality disorders varies, with the condition often remaining unchanged.

   a. There is an increased risk of the development of depressive disorders among persons with personality disorders.

   b. There is some evidence that the symptoms of avoidant, borderline, and antisocial personality disorders may decrease with age.

## D. Impact on Function

1. Personality disorders are grouped in clusters according to their impact on behavior.

   a. Cluster A.

      (1) Paranoid, schizoid, and schizotypal.

      (2) Individuals with these disorders are often perceived as odd and eccentric.

   b. Cluster B.

      (1) Antisocial, borderline, histrionic, and narcissistic.

      (2) Individuals with these disorders are often perceived as dramatic, emotional, and erratic.

   c. Cluster C.

      (1) Avoidant, dependent, obsessive-compulsive, and those not otherwise specified.

      (2) Individuals with these disorders are often perceived as anxious or fearful.

   d. The type and degree of impact on relationships and daily function depend on the severity and type of disorder.

## E. Medical Management

1. Psychotherapy and certain medications may reduce symptomatology for some patients.

2. Monitoring, supervision, and hospitalization may be required during periods of increased sympto-

matology, and/or aggressive or self-destructive behavior.

**F. Diagnostic-Specific Considerations for Occupational Therapy**

1. Assistance of the individual in the identification of the functional problems associated with symptoms may increase commitment to treatment and the pursuit of behavioral change.
2. Cognitive behavioral approaches (including dialectical behavioral therapy) and an increase in functional and coping skills may decrease symptomatic behavior.
3. See sections XV and XVI in this chapter for additional evaluation and intervention guidelines.
4. Chapter 13 provides further information on general OT psychosocial evaluation and intervention approaches.

# VIII. Cognitive Disorders

## A. Diagnostic Criteria

1. Conditions for which the primary symptoms are cognitive deficits. This may be from substance abuse, medical conditions, or other known or unknown causes.
2. Delirium.
   a. A disturbance of consciousness (awareness of environment) with a decreased ability to attend.
   b. There is a change from previous cognition and/or perception.
   c. It covers a short period of time (hours to days) and tends to fluctuate.
   d. There are many causes.
      (1) Brain dysfunction.
      (2) Medication.
      (3) Endocrine disorders.
      (4) Cardiac disorders.
      (5) Infections and inflammations (e.g., fever, UTI).
      (6) Liver function disorders.
      (7) See Table 10-1 for reversible causes of mental confusion.
3. Dementia.
   a. Disturbances of memory and multiple cognitive deficits.
      (1) Aphasia.
      (2) Apraxia.
      (3) Agnosia.
      (4) Disturbance of executive function (i.e., planning, organization, sequencing).
   b. Dementia often includes personality changes.
   c. Dementia must lead to functional problems.
   d. It represents a decline in the person's previous level of cognitive skills.
   e. Alzheimer's type and vascular dementia account for 75% of all cases.
   f. Other causes include AIDS, Pick's disease, Huntington's chorea, Parkinson's disease, and alcoholism.
   g. Although symptoms of Alzheimer's and vascular dementia are the same, vascular dementia requires evidence of a vascular cause.
   h. Mental confusion due to reversible causes must be ruled out. (Table 10-1).
4. Amnesic disorders.
   a. Difficulty with memory only, but sufficient to cause functional difficulty.
   b. Causes and types.
      (1) Cerebrovascular accident.
      (2) Multiple sclerosis.
      (3) Korsakoff's syndrome.
      (4) Alcoholic blackouts.
      (5) Electroconvulsive therapy.
      (6) Traumatic brain injury.
      (7) Transient global amnesia.

---

**TABLE 10.1**
**REVERSIBLE CAUSES OF MENTAL CONFUSION**

**Sensory changes and problems**
- Age-related losses in hearing, vision, touch, etc.
- Unavailable or inadequate prostheses such as hearing aids, glasses, dentures, etc.
- Sensory overload; too much, too long, too fast.
- Sensory deprivation; too little stimulation, isolation, restraints.
- Loss of cues to aid orientation and memory such as clocks, magazines, calendars, and strict adherence to routines and rituals.

**Depression**

**Drug use and misuse**
- Drug interactions, side effects, and build-up from longer absorption and elimination times.
- Over-the-counter cold, sleeping, and pain remedies; often taken without the physician's knowledge and which react with prescribed drugs.

**Infections/Inflammation**
- Viral or bacterial infections; may be accompanied by fever.
- Urinary tract infections, pneumonia, etc.
- Gallbladder disease.

**Metabolic problems caused by**
- Liver or kidney disease.
- Thyroid disorders (hyperthyroidism and hypothyroidism).
- Dehydration from diuretics, low fluid intake, hot weather.
- Poorly controlled diabetes.

**B. Onset, Prevalence, and Prognosis**
1. Delirium occurs in 10 to 60% of hospitalized individuals depending on the related medical condition.
   a. It may resolve quickly or take several days.
   b. It is more severe with advanced age.
   c. It may indicate a poor prognosis over time.
2. Dementia is present in 5% of those over 65 and increases with age.
   a. There may be periods of plateauing with a gradual decline over time.
3. The prevalence of and prognosis for amnesic disorders varies with the cause.
   a. It is most often associated with alcohol use disorders and head injury.

**C. Impact on Function**
1. The degree of impact varies according to the nature and severity of the symptoms.
2. The individual may require intervention varying from education in compensatory strategies to the need for total care.
3. Reisburg's stages of mental confusion describe the progressive impact of dementia on functional abilities. (Table 10-2).

## TABLE 10.2 - REISBURG'S STAGES FOR DEMENTIA

Stage 1: No disability is noted

Stage 2: The person complains about forgetting normal age-related information (location of objects: keys, wallet, etc.)

Stage 3: Beginning signs and deficits are noted in this stage

| THE PERSON'S STRENGTHS | THE PERSON'S WEAKNESSES |
| --- | --- |
| 1. Remains independent in IADLs | 1. Forgets important information for first time in one's life |
| 2. Can recognize challenging situations to avoid, in order to minimize manifested deficits | 2. Experiences difficulty completing complex tasks |
| 3. Can utilize compensation as an adaptive mechanism | 3. Experiences difficulty negotiating directions to new location |

Stage 4: Deficits are noted in all IADLs

| THE PERSON'S STRENGTHS | THE PERSON'S WEAKNESSES |
| --- | --- |
| 1. Can still perform simple, repetitive ADLs independently | 1. Becomes increasingly forgetful |
| 2. Can live at home with support | 2. Becomes unable to follow and sequence written cues |
| 3. Can follow simple verbal and demonstrational cues | 3. Becomes unable to perform familiar, challenging activities |
| | 4. Experiences difficulty in word finding |
| | 5. Cannot manage at home without assistance |

Stage 5: Person cannot function independently

| THE PERSON'S STRENGTHS | THE PERSON'S WEAKNESSES |
| --- | --- |
| 1. Can perform ADLs and some IADLs with correct cues and assistance | 1. Demonstrates poor judgment |
| 2. Can respond to encouragement | 2. Experiences difficulty with all decision making |
| 3. Becomes unable to safely drive an automobile | 3. Forgets to take care of hygiene |

Stage 6: Person cannot perform ADLs without cues

| THE PERSON'S STRENGTHS | THE PERSON'S WEAKNESSES |
| --- | --- |
| 1. Can perform components of familiar tasks | 1. Demonstrates significant deficits in following 2 steps of a task |
| 2. Can follow demonstration/hand over hand cues | 2. Cannot sequence steps of ADL tasks |
| | 3. Cannot speak in full sentences |
| | 4. Becomes incontinent of bowel and bladder |

Stage 7: The person can be in a vegetative state. He/she is usually bedbound and unable to respond verbally or non-verbally to questions or commands

## D. Medical Management

1. Differential diagnosis to ensure that symptoms are not pseudodementia due to a reversible cause. (Table 10-1).
2. Medical treatment involves resolution of the causes of the disorder if possible.
3. There are a limited number of newer medications that appear to maintain or slow the decline of cognitive function (e.g. Aricept, Cognex).
4. If causes of the disorder are not treatable, attempts are made to mitigate symptoms where possible.

## E. Diagnostic-Specific Considerations for Occupational Therapy

1. Maintenance of quality of life through activity adaptation and environmental modification.
2. Family education to understand the nature of the person's disorder and improve the management of its symptoms and functional effects.
3. See sections XV and XVI in this chapter for additional evaluation and intervention guidelines.
4. Chapter 13 provides further information on general OT psychosocial evaluation and intervention approaches and specific interventions to manage the effects of cognitive disorders and Alzheimer's disease.

# IX. Eating Disorders

## A. Anorexia Nervosa

1. Diagnostic criteria.
   a. Refusal to maintain body weight at or above normal weight for age and height, or failure to make expected weight gain during a period of growth leading to a body weight less than 85% of that expected.
   b. Intense fear of gaining weight or becoming fat, even though underweight.
   c. Disturbance in the way in which one's body weight or shape is experienced.
      (1) Undue influence of body weight or shape on self-evaluation.
      (2) Denial of the seriousness of the current low body weight even when hospitalized or gravely ill.
   d. In postmenarchical females, amenorrhea, the absence of at least three consecutive menstrual cycles.
   e. Anorexia includes a food restrictive type and a binge eating/purging type.
2. Onset, prevalence, and prognosis.
   a. Anorexia most commonly begins in the mid-teens.

(1) It occurs in 5% of adolescent girls.
(2) It is 10 to 20 times more common in girls.
   b. The long term prognosis may not be good, with mortality rates from 5 to 18%.
3. Behavioral characteristics.
   a. Individuals often exhibit obsessive/compulsive behavior, depression, anxiety, rigidity, perfectionism, and poor sexual adjustment.

## B. Bulimia Nervosa

1. Diagnostic criteria.
   a. Recurrent episodes of binge eating defined as a lack of control over discrete periods of excessive eating of an abnormally large amount of food.
   b. The purging type includes recurrent, inappropriate compensatory behavior in order to prevent weight gain.
      (1) Self-induced vomiting.
      (2) Use of laxatives and/or diuretics.
      (3) Fasting.
      (4) Excessive exercising.
   c. Binge eating and purging behaviors both occur, on average, at least twice a week for three months.
   d. Self-evaluation is unduly influenced by body shape and weight.
   e. The disturbance does not occur exclusively during episodes of anorexia nervosa.
2. Onset, prevalence, and prognosis.
   a. The usual age of onset of bulimia is later than that of anorexia.
      (1) It begins in adolescence or in early adulthood.
      (2) It is present in 1 to 3% of women.
      (3) It is significantly more common in women.
   b. The prognosis is better than for anorexia, with 80% of individuals not meeting the criteria for diagnosis after 10 years.
3. Behavioral characteristics.
   a. Individuals are often obsessed with their appearance and attractiveness to the opposite sex.
   b. They are likely to be sexually active and maintain a normal weight.

## C. Eating Disorders Not Otherwise Specified

1. Includes several types.
   a. Binge-eating disorder (BED) is the one that will be most typically seen in OT practice due to the co-morbidities caused by the obesity that result from this disorder (e.g., diabetes).
      (1) Recurrent episodes of binge eating until

uncomfortably full without purging.

    (a) Eating is more rapid than typical and is often initiated when not hungry and/or when alone due to embarrassment about the amount of food being consumed.

**D. Impact on Function**

1. ADL such as self care, eating, and feeding can be severely disrupted.
2. IADL such as shopping for clothing and food, meal preparation and cleanup, and health management and maintenance can be significantly affected.
3. Work skills can be intact unless food-restricting behaviors and/or medical problems interfere with work performance or prevocational/vocational skill development.
   a. Focus on weight control may interfere with pursuit of vocational goals and/or the development of prerequisite skills.
4. Leisure skills can be intact unless affected by food-restricting behaviors and/or medical complications.
   a. Activities may focus mainly on appearance, rather than on those that have meaning or purpose.
   b. Exercise activities previously done for fun (e.g., running, swimming, cycling) may now be done excessively without enjoyment to decrease weight.
5. Social participation (including family, community, and peer/friend) can be greatly impacted by the excessive use of food-restricting behaviors, the need to maintain secrecy about the behaviors, and feeling ashamed, guilty, embarrassed, and/or depressed about atypical and disturbed eating habits and patterns.

**D. Medical Management**

1. Individual psychotherapy.
2. Family counseling.
3. Behavioral and/or cognitive therapies.
4. The use of antidepressant medications may be used in anorexia nervosa, but they are more effective for individuals with bulimia.
5. Treatment of any of the resulting medical complications such as cardiac disturbances (hypotension, slow heart rate), reduced thyroid metabolism, osteoporosis, seizures, severe dehydration, electrolyte imbalances, irregular bowel movements, pancreatitis, peptic ulcers, gastric and/or esophageal inflammation and possible rupture,

tooth decay, etc., may also be necessary.

6. Treatment most often takes place in outpatient or day care programs.
7. Hospitalization may be necessary if the individual has medical difficulties, is suicidal, cannot care for him/her self, or needs to be removed from his/her environment.
8. Behavioral programs designed around a privileging system are often used.
   a. Consistency among staff is crucial for program effectiveness.

**E. Diagnostic-Specific Considerations for Occupational Therapy**

1. The building of trust is essential to effective intervention due to the secrecy, guilt, anger, resistance, and ego fragility often associated with the disorder and its stages of recovery.
2. The OT practitioner must be honest, supportive, and gently confrontal when indicated.
3. Evaluation and intervention must include the identification of the socio-emotional needs the eating disorder had fulfilled for the person so that health-promoting occupation-based alternatives can be explored and developed.
   a. Non-food related areas of interest and meaningful purposeful activities should be pursued to promote a reality-based body image and foster improved coping.
4. Education about nutritional food management and the development of healthy leisure time (i.e., does not involve excessive exercise) are key.
5. See sections XV and XVI in this chapter for additional evaluation and intervention guidelines.
6. Chapter 13 provides further information on general OT psychosocial evaluation and intervention approaches.

# X. Disruptive Behavior Disorders

**A. Diagnostic Criteria**

1. Oppositional defiant disorder.
   a. Negativistic, hostile, and defiant behaviors that result in functional impairment.
2. Conduct disorder.
   a. Disregard for the rights of others leading to aggression towards people and animals, destruction of property, deceitfulness, theft, or serious violation of rules.

**B. Onset, Prevalence and Prognosis**

1. Oppositional defiant disorder.
   a. Oppositional, negative behavior begins in early

childhood and may be seen in 1 to 16% of school-age children.

b. The course and prognosis depend on the severity of behaviors, the presence of other disorders, and the intactness of the family.

c. It is most likely to progress into a conduct disorder if aggression is prominent.

d. Lifetime prevalence of ODD is estimated to be 10.2% (males = 11.2%; females = 9.2%).

2. Conduct disorder.

a. It is estimated that 6 to 16% of boys and 2 to 9% of girls under the age of 18 have a conduct disorder.

b. Prognosis is related to the age of onset and the severity of symptoms and behavior.

(1) Severe conduct disorder is often associated with the development of other disorders and substance abuse later in life.

c. Assaultive behavior and parental criminality correlate highly with future incarceration.

**C. Impact on Function**

1. Children with disruptive behavior disorders have difficulty at school and with the formation of healthy social and familial relationships.

2. Difficulties within the family affect not only the child but all family members, impacting on their role performance.

**D. Medical Management**

1. Behavioral techniques are often the most effective forms of intervention with adolescents.

2. The identification and treatment of other disorders, (attention-deficit/hyperactivity disorder, learning disorders, substance use, depression, etc.) is important.

3. The use of medications such as antipsychotics, antidepressants, anxiolytics, and mood stabilizers may be helpful.

4. A consistent approach from all team members is essential.

**E. Diagnostic-Specific Considerations for Occupational Therapy**

1. Contributing disorders (attention deficit/hyperactivity disorder, mood disorders, learning disorders, etc.) and their effect on performance skills and areas of occupation must be evaluated and addressed in intervention.

2. The child's goals, stressors, and family and social relationships should be considered.

3. Skill development may improve emotional adjustment.

4. Behavioral approaches must be consistent throughout all programming.

5. The therapist should assist the parents, other family members, teachers, and other school personnel to understand the nature of the child's condition and to develop consistent strategies for behavior management.

6. See sections XV and XVI in this chapter for additional evaluation and intervention guidelines.

7. Chapter 13 provides further information on general OT psychosocial evaluation and intervention approaches and specific interventions to manage offensive, intrusive, and escalating behaviors.

## XI. Pervasive Developmental Disorders/ Autism Spectrum Disorders[3]

**A. Autism**

1. Etiology.

a. Organic brain pathology.

b. May or may not be seen with other disorders.

2. Onset, prevalence, and prognosis.

a. May occur from birth up to 3 years of age.

b. Occurs in 4 times as many boys than girls, and 1 in 110 live births.

c. The prognosis for functional independence is poor with 70% of children needing a supervised living setting (although the life expectancy is normal).

3. Diagnostic characteristics.

a. Presence of at least six items below, two or more from (1), and at least one from (2) and (3).

(1) Impaired social interaction and in most cases cognitive disabilities.

(a) Impaired nonverbal behaviors, e.g. infrequent/poor eye contact, impaired attachment behavior, anxiety with changes in typical routines.

(b) Difficulty relating to others and forming relationships at an age appropriate level.

(c) Lack of spontaneous social seeking behavioral interactions with others and awareness of others' bids for interactions (e.g. sharing, pointing).

(d) Lack of social reciprocation due to decreased ability to infer feelings and intentions of others.

(2) Difficulty with communication.

(a) Lack of initiation, reflection, develop-

---

[3]Jan Garbarini contributed this section on Pervasive Developmental Disorders

ment of spoken language or alternative means for communication.

    (b) If speech is developed, difficulty in initiating or engaging in conversation and lack of appropriate context.

    c) Stereotyped echolalia and/or use of indiscernible language.

    (d) Lack of spontaneous pretend, imitative or exploratory play.

  (3) Repetitive and stereotyped behaviors and movements in one or more of the following;

    (a) Ritualistic limited preoccupation of interest.

    (b) Rigid observance of nonfunctional routines or behavioral patterns.

    (c) Repetitive motor action (e.g., flapping and wiggling of fingers, head banging, rocking of the head or body).

    (d) Restrictive fixation on parts of a whole object (e.g., wheel of a toy car).

b. Prior to three years of age, delay or impairment in social interaction and/or language and/or play (symbolic or imaginative).

c. Not better described as Rett's syndrome or childhood disintegrative disorder.

d. Difficulty with sensory processing and perception of various sensory stimuli; difficulty in modulation of stimuli at various levels of the continuum, e.g. hyper- or hypo-responsiveness.

e. Common associated behaviors may include unanticipated mood swings, temper tantrums, lack of ability to focus, insomnia, and enuresis.

f. Deficits tend to be more severe in verbal sequencing and abstraction versus abilities in visuospatial and rote memory skills (e.g. calculation, musical abilities).

## B. Asperger's Disorder

1. Etiology is unknown; however, studies indicate a strong relation to autism. It is hypothesized to be due to genetic, metabolic, infectious, or perinatal causes.

2. Onset, prevalence, and prognosis.

  a. Little is known, and course and prognosis are variable.

  b. Those individuals with a normal IQ and high level social skills appear to have a good prognosis, although they tend to be socially uncomfortable and demonstrate illogical thinking.

3. Diagnostic characteristics.

  a. Difficulty with social interaction.

  b. Restricted interests and behaviors.

  c. Characterized by clumsiness.

  d. Delayed developmental motor milestones.

  e. Cognitive development is normal and persons with Asperger's have normal to superior intelligence.

  f. Differentiated from autism by adequate language and the level of social interaction and engagement in activities with others.

## C. Rett's Syndrome

1. Etiology is unknown; however, since deterioration occurs after a period of normal development, it is thought to be attributed to a genetic metabolic disorder.

2. Onset, prevalence, and prognosis.

  a. Occurs in girls, 1 in 10,000 girls.

  b. Motor and social skills are age appropriate from 6 months to 2 years of development when the onset of progressive encephalopathy develops.

  c. Deterioration occurs and is characterized by loss of purposeful hand movements, with development of stereotypical movements such as hand wringing and licking, biting, and slapping of fingers.

  d. Muscle tone becomes hypotonic, and then progresses to spasticity and then rigidity, resulting in ataxia and an uncoordinated and stiff gait.

  e. Breathing patterns become irregular, marked by hyperventilation, apnea, and holding of breath.

  f. Deterioration of language and social skills may plateau at a six month to one year developmental level.

  g. Regression in cognition and praxis.

  h. EEGs are abnormal and seizures common.

  i. Development of physical growth and head circumference plateau resulting in progressive encephalopathy.

  j. A child may live for over ten years following the onset.

3. Diagnostic characteristics and sequelae.

  a. Receptive and expressive communication skills and social skills deteriorate.

  b. Muscle wasting can make these children prone to scoliosis and eventually may necessitate the use of a wheelchair.

  c. Stereotypical movements of licking, biting, and slapping of the hands may result in deterioration of the integrity of the skin.

**D. Pervasive Developmental Disorder, Not Otherwise Specified**

1. Disorders that are similar with impairments seen in the above pervasive developmental disorders.
2. Impairments in social interaction, communication skills, stereotyped behavior, interests, and activities; however, cannot be classified as a pervasive developmental disorder as not all criteria are met.

**E. Medical Management**

1. Medications prescribed will depend on the presenting symptoms of a specific PDD.
   a. Seizure medications.
   b. Medication for muscle deterioration and/or complications due to abnormal tone.
   c. Medications to increase alertness.
   d. Medications to modulate behaviors.

**F. Diagnostic-Specific Considerations for Occupational Therapy**

1. Evaluate developmental and functional levels. See Chapter 5.
2. Develop sensorimotor, social interaction, vocational readiness, and community integration skills relevant to the child's level.
3. Provide sensory integrative intervention, if indicated. See Chapters 7 and 12.
4. If indicated, prescribe and train in technologically-based augmentive communication.
5. Provide adaptive and positioning equipment to facilitate function, e.g., the stereotypical movements of licking, biting and slapping of the hands in a child with Rett's Syndrome may require adaptations to maintain the integrity of the skin, such as dynamic elbow splints that inhibit a hand to mouth pattern by limiting full elbow flexion.
6. Collaborate with the family and interdisciplinary team to promote functional skills.
7. See sections XV and XVI in this chapter for additional evaluation and intervention guidelines.
8. Chapter 13 provides further information on general OT psychosocial evaluation and intervention approaches and specific interventions to manage behaviors.

# XII. Reactive Attachment Disorder (RAD) of Infancy or Early Childhood[4]

**A. Etiology**

1. Exact cause is unknown.
2. Early experiences with initial caregivers/pathogenic care may contribute to the disorder.

3. Indicators of pathogenic care.
   a. Persistent disregard of the child's basic emotional needs.
   b. Persistent disregard of the child's basic physical needs.
   c. Repeated changes of primary caregiver or a succession of caregivers prevents the establishment of stable, appropriate attachments.

**B. Onset, Prevalence, and Prognosis**

1. Onset begins before five years of age.
2. Exact prevalence or incidence of Reactive Attachment Disorder is unknown.
3. There is a high risk of prevalence for toddlers and children in foster care and orphanages and for children with frequently changing caregivers.
4. Prognosis: Unknown.

**C. Diagnostic Criteria**

1. There are two types of Reactive Attachment Disorder.
   a. Reactive Attachment Disorder, Inhibited type, characterized by:
      (1) Persistent failure to initiate or respond in a developmentally appropriate fashion to most social interactions.
      (2) Interactions are excessively inhibited, hypervigilant, or highly ambivalent and contradictory in nature.
   b. Reactive Attachment Disorder, Disinhibited Type, characterized by:
      (1) Indiscriminate sociability with inability to exhibit appropriate selective attachments.
      (2) Demonstrated by excessive familiarity with relative strangers or lack of selectivity.

**D. Impact on Function**

1. These children are frustrating to work with and difficult to parent.
2. They have a high need to be in control.
3. They frequently lie.
4. Affectionate and related with strangers.
5. Frequent episodes of hoarding or gorging on food without physical need.
6. Deny responsibility/project blame for their actions.

**E. Medical Management**

1. No one standard treatment for Reactive Attachment Disorder is apparent in the literature.
2. Interventions that may be efficacious:
   a. Nondirective play therapy.
   b. Sensory integrative therapy. See Chapter 12.
   c. Attachment therapy (somewhat controversial).
   d. Psychotherapy combined with psychoeducation.

[4] William Lambert contributed this section on reactive adjustment disorder.

**F. Diagnostic-Specific Considerations for Occupational Therapy**

1. Close and ongoing collaboration with the child's family facilitates successful outcomes.
2. Actively involve parents in treatment.
3. Assist children to form a more secure sense of self.
4. Limit the child's exposure to multiple caregivers.
5. Provide high levels of structure and consistency.
6. Goals need to be specific, realistic and attainable.
7. See sections XV and XVI in this chapter for additional evaluation and intervention guidelines.
8. Chapter 13 provides further information on general OT psychosocial evaluation and intervention approaches and specific interventions to manage behaviors.

# XIII. Attention-Deficit/Hyperactivity Disorders

**A. Etiology**

1. Unknown, however, there are suggested contributing factors.
   a. Genetic factors include higher occurrence in monozygotic twins than in dizygotic twins, and twice the occurrence in siblings of hyperactive children.
   b. Neurological factors include the possibility of minimal or subtle brain damage due to circulatory, toxic, metabolic, or mechanical effects during fetal or perinatal periods; and infection, inflammation, and/or trauma during early childhood.
   c. Neurochemical dysfunction related to neurotransmitters in the adrenergic and the dopaminergic systems.
   d. Psychosocial factors include stress, anxiety, or predisposing factors such as temperament.

**B. Subtypes of Attention-Deficit/Hyperactivity Disorder**

1. DSM-IV-TR delineates three subtypes.
   a. Predominantly inattentive type.
   b. Predominantly hyperactive-impulsive type.
   c. Combined type.

**C. Onset, Prevalence and Prognosis**

1. Symptoms are often noted during the toddler years, usually by the age of three.
   a. Caution is advised to not make a diagnosis in early childhood years
   b. Diagnosis is most often made during elementary school years when behavior interferes with adjustment to school.

2. Occurs in 5 to 8% of elementary school children.
   a. Incidence in boys to girls is a 3 to 1 ratio, most common in firstborn boys.
3. Partial remission may occur between the ages of 12 and 20, allowing for a productive adolescence and adulthood.
   a. Although hyperactivity may disappear, distractibility and impulsivity can persist.
4. Symptoms persist into adulthood in 60% of cases.

**D. Diagnostic Criteria**

1. The presence of six or more symptoms in the inattention domain, the hyperactivity-impulsivity domain, or both.
2. Symptoms in the inattention domain or hyperactivity-impulsivity domain that interfere with occupational activities are present for at least six months or more.
3. Symptoms of the inattention domain may include lack of attention to detail, poor listening, limited follow through of tasks, difficulty with organization, avoidance of tasks that require sustained attention, tendency to lose things, distractibility, and forgetfulness.
4. Symptoms of the hyperactivity domain may include fidgeting, inability to remain seated, inappropriate activity level for a given situation, difficulty with quiet sedentary activities, frequent movement, and excessive talking.
5. Symptoms of impulsivity include answering questions before they are fully stated, difficulty with turn taking, and interrupting the conversations or activities of others.
6. Visual-perceptual, auditory-perceptual, language, and/or cognitive problems may be present.
7. Some of the symptoms that result in impairment were evident before 7 years of age.
8. Symptoms that result in impairment are present in two settings, such as school, home, and/or work.
9. A detailed developmental history to confirm behavior patterns and the meeting of six or more symptoms of inattention or hyperactivity-impulsivity of the DSM-IV-TR diagnostic criteria.

**E. Impact on Function**

1. Infants are over-active, difficult to soothe when crying, and demonstrate poor sleeping habits.
2. Defensiveness to environmental stimuli, frequent irritability, aggressive behavior, emotional lability, and fluctuating and unpredictable performance.
3. Difficulty with delayed gratification in the school and home environment.

4. Deficits in academic and/or social functioning.
5. Deficits in perceptual motor tasks with disorders in reading, mathematics, written expression, and general coordination resulting.
6. Disorders of memory, thinking, speech, and hearing.
7. Depression secondary to frustration and difficulty with learning.
   a. This often leads to low self-esteem and conduct disorders.
8. Individuals with symptoms remaining in adolescence and adulthood are prone to antisocial personality disorders, and are at risk for substance-related disorders.

### F. Medical Management

1. Prescribed medications depend on presenting symptoms.
   a. Stimulants.
      (1) Most commonly used include dextroamphetamine (e.g., Dexedrine, Focalin) for children 3 years and older, and methylphenidate (e.g., Concerta, Ritalin, Adderall, Metadate) for children 6 years and older.
      (2) Side effects include loss of appetite, weight loss, loss of appetite, disturbed sleep patterns, and slow growth.
   b. Antidepressants.
      (1) Imipramine.
      (2 Used when stimulants are unable to be used.
      (3) Careful monitoring of cardiac functioning is required.
   c. Anxiolytics.
      (1) Clonidine. (Catapres).
      (2) Guanfacine (Tenex).
      (3) Require careful dosing and competent adults for administration.
         (a) Medications cannot be stopped suddenly because this could medically compromise the child.
2. Monitoring of medication and its impact on cognitive and psychosocial function, e.g., learning and self-esteem.
3. Psychotherapy, behavior modification, parent and individual counseling may be indicated.

### G. Diagnostic-Specific Considerations for Occupational Therapy

1. Behavior's impact on school, home, play/leisure, and social participation must be considered.
2. Environmental modifications and activity adaptations to structure the client's home environment can enhance function.
3. Environmental modifications and activity adaptations to structure the child's environment at school and the adult's environment at work can support more successful outcomes (e.g., the elimination of sensory distractors, the use of lists, datebooks, and/or texted reminders).
4. Training in social skills and self-management (i.e., the use of humor, personally initiated time-outs) can improve adaptive behaviors.
5. Interventions to promote sensory modulation are emphasized. See Chapter 12.
6. Consultation is provided to parents, family members, teachers, and employees regarding strategies for the provision of structure and expectations in a manner that fosters the person's psychosocial adaptation.
7. In school-based practice, ongoing collaboration with individualized education planning team members and parents is vital.
8. See sections XV and XVI in this chapter for additional evaluation and intervention guidelines.
9. Chapter 13 provides further information on general OT psychosocial evaluation and intervention approaches and specific interventions to manage problem behaviors

## XIV. Intellectual Disorders

### A. Etiology

1. Genetic conditions such as chromosomal abnormalities (e.g., Down syndrome, Fragile X Syndrome, Prader-Willi Syndrome, and Klinefelter's Syndrome).
2. Metabolic conditions such as phenylketonuria, hypothyroidism, and Tay-Sachs disease.
3. Prenatal infections such as rubella, toxoplasmosis, AIDS.
4. Maternal substance abuse.
5. Perinatal factors such as trauma and prematurity.
6. Acquired conditions including infections such as encephalitis, meningitis.
7. Head trauma sustained in motor vehicle accidents, falls, child abuse, etc.

### B. Diagnostic Classification and Functional Implications

1. In DSM-IV-TR, intellectual disorders are classified as mental retardation.
2. Based on the measurement of intelligence or IQ tests.
   a. Those individuals who score more than two

standard deviations below the norm or below an IQ of 70 are considered to have an intellectual disability.

3. IQ range of 55 to 69 indicates mild intellectual disability.
   a. Focus is placed on the individual acquiring social and vocational skills to function adequately.
   b. Minimal support is typically required.
   c. Additional intermittent support may be required in special circumstances.

4. IQ range of 40 to 54 indicates moderate intellectual disability.
   a. Focus is usually placed on the individual acquiring independence in routine daily skills and skills necessary to work in a sheltered workshop.
   b. Limited support and assistance may be required in specific occupational performance areas on a daily basis.
   c. Supervised living is required.

5. IQ range of 25 to 39 indicates severe intellectual disability.
   a. Focus is usually placed on the individual acquiring communication skills and some basic health habits.
   b. Assistance is required for performance of most tasks in all occupational performance areas on a daily basis.
   c. Supervised living is required.
   d. Significant impairments in motor functioning and physical development are typical.

6. IQ of 25 or below indicates profound intellectual disability.
   a. Assistance and ongoing supervision are required for basic survival skills.
   b. Significant impairments in motor functioning and physical development are typical.
   c. Supervised living is required.

7. Multiple disabilities such as hearing and other sensory impairments, seizures, and other neurological abnormalities may be associated with various syndromes (e.g. fetal alcohol syndrome).

## C. Impact on Development

1. The developmental impact of intellectual disabilities can vary greatly.
   a. The impact is greatest in children with severe and profound intellectual disabilities.

2. Cognitive development.
   a. Slower learning ability.
   b. Shorter attention span.
   c. Difficulty with problem-solving and critical thinking.
   d. Difficulty generalizing information and mastering abstract thinking.
   e. Increased distractibility.

3. Motor development.
   a. Slower development with the attainment of physical milestones occurring at a later age than typical.
   b. Uncoordinated appearance and movements.
   c. Low muscle tone.

4. Sensory development.
   a. Diminished sensory modulation abilities.
   b. Hyper- or hypo-sensitivity to all sensory stimuli.

5. Language development.
   a. Decreased ability in recalling and retrieving words secondary to cognitive deficits (e.g., inattention and impaired memory).
   b. Difficulty grasping and expressing concepts secondary to cognitive deficits (e.g., impaired abstract thinking).
   c. Difficulty with the motor aspects of creating language secondary to motor deficits (e.g., low tone).

6. Psychosocial development.
   a. Impaired ability to respond to social cues can result in a number of behavioral outcomes. These can include:
      (1) Excessive shyness.
      (2) Aggressiveness.
   b. Hyperactivity and distractibility can also impede psychosocial development.

## D. Medical Management

1. Dependent upon presenting symptoms and complications.
2. Psychological, hearing, and speech evaluations and interventions may be indicated.
3. Intermittent support may be required in special circumstances.

## E. Diagnostic-Specific Considerations for Occupational Therapy

1. Support and assistance may be required in specific occupational performance areas on a regular basis.
2. Development of community integration and social participation skills are a major focus.
3. Interdisciplinary team and family collaboration to promote independence in functional and social skills is emphasized.

4. Collaboration with educational team to contribute to a comprehensive educational program if individual is of school age is required.
5. See sections XV and XVI in this chapter for additional evaluation and intervention guidelines.
6. Chapter 13 provides further information on general OT psychosocial evaluation and intervention approaches.

# XV. Occupational Therapy Mental Health Evaluation

## A The Role of the OTA
1. The OTA contributes to the evaluation process.
2. The OTA can assist with the collection of data for the evaluation once service competency has been established.
3. The level of supervision required will be determined by the OTA's experience and established service competency.
4. The OTA cannot independently evaluate or interpret evaluation results.

## B. Evaluation Focus
1. Determination of values, interests, desired occupational roles, and self-determined goals.
2. Identification of cognitive, perceptual, and psychosocial strengths and skills and their ability to facilitate recovery.
3. Identification of cognitive, perceptual, and psychosocial deficits and limitations and their impact on function and life style.
4. Determination of functional problems associated with psychiatric symptoms (e.g., safety awareness and judgment).
5. Treatment history and ability and interest to engage in recovery.
6. Identification of coping skills, stressors, and environmental and social supports,
7. Chapter 13 provides further information on OT psychosocial evaluation approaches.

# XVI. Occupational Therapy Mental Health Intervention

## A The Role of the OTA
1. The OTA implements intervention with OT supervision.
2. The level of supervision required depends upon the OTA's experience and established service competency.
3. During the implementation of intervention, the OTA informs the supervising therapist of any change in the individual's status and any other relevant information that may affect treatment.

## B. Intervention Focus
1. The focus of intervention during periods of acute hospitalization includes:
   a. Management of all behaviors that threaten the safety and well being of the individual as well as that of others on the unit.
   b. Stabilization of behavior to enable engagement in intervention.
   c. Engagement in activities that are 'do-able' (e.g., brief and structured) to enable success and promote reality-based thinking.
      (1) Graded activities are designed to promote self-efficacy which can increase self-confidence, motivation, and participation in treatment.
   d. Engagement of the person in the treatment process.
   e. Development of relaxation and stress management skills to help decrease the incidence and severity of symptoms and facilitate recovery.
   f. Development of the skills needed to pursue desired occupational roles and attain self-determined goals.
   g. Engagement in activities to improve communication skills and self-expression.
   h. The gathering and sharing of ongoing assessment information with the treatment team.
      (1) The person's status typically changes drastically during the course of an acute hospitalization due to the stabilizing effects of psychotropic medications.
         (a) The input of OT practitioners about a patient's observed symptoms and functional behaviors is critical in assisting with the effective titration of psychotropic medications.
   i. Assistance with discharge planning to support recovery and a healthy life style.
2. The focus of intervention during periods of long term hospitalization include:
   a. Development and implementation of a plan for self-determined goal achievement.
   b. Provision of a normalizing environment that enables participation in meaningful and desired occupational roles.
   c. Engagement of the person in the treatment process.
   e. Provision of graded activities to develop the

skills needed for competence in ADL, IADL, social participation, leisure, school, and/or work.

f. Development of relaxation and stress management skills to help decrease the incidence and severity of symptoms and facilitate recovery.

g. Continuation of assessment to determine realistic and meaningful discharge goals.

h. Development of the skills and external supports needed to pursue desired post-discharge occupational roles, participate in the anticipated discharge environment, and attain self-determined discharge goals.

3. The focus of intervention in community settings.

a. Provision of services that facilitate recovery and assist in the maintenance of existing skills.

b. Assistance with the continued development of skills needed for community living, social participation and the pursuit of valued occupational roles.

c. Development of skills and supports to enable ongoing recovery (e.g., WRAP –Wellness and Recovery Action Plan, NAMI - National Alliance for the Mentally Ill).

d. Monitoring of the individual for changing clinical and social needs.

# References

American Academy of Child and Adolescent Psychiatry. (2009). *Facts for families: Children with oppositional defiant disorder.* Retrieved March 25, 2010 from http://www.aacap.org/galleries/FactsForFamilies/72_children_with_oppositional_defiant_disorder.pdf

American Psychiatric Association (2000). *Diagnostic and statistical manual of mental disorders (4th ed., text revision).* Washington, DC: Author.

American Psychiatric Association. (2000). *Quick reference to the diagnostic criteria from DSM-IV-TR.* Arlington, VA: Author.

Austism Speaks. (2010). *What is autism?* Retrieved March 25, 2010 from http://www.autismspeaks.org/whatisit/index.php

Ayd, F. J. (1995). *Lexicon of psychiatry, neurology, and the neurosciences.* Baltimore: William and Wilkins.

Bonder, B. (1991). *Psychopathology and function.* Thorofare, NJ: Slack.

Cara, E., & MacRae, A. (Eds.). (2005). *Psychosocial occupational therapy: A clinical practice, 2nd ed..* Clifton Park, NY: Thomson Delmar Learning.

Case-Smith, J. (Ed.). (2005). *Occupational therapy for children, 5th ed.* St. Louis, MO: Elsevier Mosby.

Cornell, C. & Hamrin, V. (2008). Clinical interventions for children with attachment problems. *Journal of Child and Adolescent Psychiatric Nursing, 21*(1), pp. 35-47.

Costa, D. (2009, June 29). Eating disorders: Occupational therapy's role. *OT Practice,* 13-16.

Cutler, J.L. and Marcus, E.R. (1999). *Psychiatry.* Philadelphia: W.B. Saunders.

Depression and Bipolar Support Alliance. (2009). *Bipolar statistics.* Retrieved March 25, 2010 from http://www.dbsalliance.org/site/PageServer?pagename=about_statistics_bipolar

Depression and Bipolar Support Alliance. (2009). *Statistics on depression.* Retrieved March 25, 2010 from http://www.dbsalliance.org/site/PageServer?pagename=about_statistics_depression

Fleming-Castaldy, R. (2009). Activities, human occupation, participation, and empowerment. In J. Hinojosa & M. L. Blount (Eds.). *The texture of life: Purposeful activities in occupational therapy, 3rd ed.,* (pp. 483- 521) Bethesda, MD: AOTA Press.

Glanzman, M.M. & Nathan J. Blum (2007) Attention deficits and hyperactivity. In M.L. Batshaw, L. Pellegrino, & N.J. Roizen (Ed.), *Children with disabilities* (6th ed., pp. 345-365). Baltimore, MD: Paul H. Brooks.

Hardy, L. (2007). Attachment theory and reactive attachment disorder: Theoretical perspectives and treatment implications. *Journal of Child & Adolescent Psychiatric Nursing 20*(1), pp.27-39.

Hyman, S.L. & Towbin, K.E. (2007). Autism spectrum disorders. In M.L. Batshaw, L. Pellegrino, & N.J. Roizen (Eds.), *Children with Disabilities* (6th ed., pp. 345-365). Baltimore, MD: Paul H. Brooks.

Kaplan, J.I., & Sadock, B.J. (2007). *Synopsis of psychiatry* (10th ed.). Philadelphia: Mosby.

Lenzenweger, M., Lane, M., Loranger, A., & Kessler, R. (2007). DSM-IV personality disorders in the National Comorbidity Survey Replication. *Biol Psychiatry, 62*(6), 553-64.

Livneh, H. & Antonak, R.F. (1997). *Psychosocial adaptation to chronic illness and disability.* Gaithersburg, MD: Aspen Publishers.

Merikangas, K., Akiskal, H., Angst, J., Greenberg, P., Hirschfeld, R., Petukhova, M., & Kessler, R. (2007). Lifetime and 12-month prevalence of bipolar spectrum disorder in the national comorbitity survey replication. *Archives of General Psychiatry, 64*(5), 543-552.

Myers, D.G. (1993). *Exploring psychology* (2nd ed.). New York: Worth.

Nock, M., Kazdin, A., Hiripi, E., & Kessler, R. (2007). Lifetime prevalence, correlates, and persistence of oppositional defiant disorder: Results from the National Comorbidity Survey Replication. *Journal of Child Psychology and Psychiatry, 48*(7), 703-713.

*Physicians desk reference* (53rd Ed.). (1999). Montvale, NY: Medical Economics.

Rett Syndrome Research Trust. (2008). *Prevalence of Rett and related disorders.* Retrieved March 25, 2010 from http://www.rsrt.org/about-Rett/prevelance-of-Rett-and-related-disorders.html

Right Health (2010). *Prevalence of autism.* Retrieved 3/8/2020 from: http://www.righthealth.Com.

Rogers, S. (2005) Common conditions that influence children's participation. In J. Case-Smith (Ed), *Occupational therapy for children* (5th ed., 160-215). St. Louis, MO: Elsevier Mosby.

Sheperis, C., Renfro-Michel, E. & Doggett, R. (2003). In-home treatment of reactive attachment disorder in a therapeutic foster care system: A case example. *Journal of Mental Health Counseling, 25*(1), pp.76-88.

Thomas, C.L. (Ed.). (1981). *Tabor's cyclopedic medical dictionary* (14th ed.). Philadelphia: F.A. Davis Company.

# CHAPTER 11

# BIOMECHANICAL APPROACHES: EVALUATION AND INTERVENTION

Colleen Maher • Rita P. Fleming-Castaldy

## I. Biomechanical Approach

### A. Overview

1. The biomechanical frame of reference is based on the works of Bird T. Baldwin (reconstruction model), Marjorie Taylor (orthopedic model), Dr. Sydney Licht, and William Dunton, Jr. (kinetic model).
2. The biomechanical approach focuses on the range of motion, strength, and endurance required to perform an occupation.
3. It is most commonly used to treat patients with lower motor neuron deficits and orthopedic problems.
4. The biomechanical approach is most effective when used in combination with other treatment approaches.
5. Settings that most commonly use the biomechanical approach.
   a. Hand clinics.
   b. Work programs.
   c. Physical medicine and rehabilitation (PM&R) departments.
   d. Ergonomic programs.

## II. Evaluation

### A. Role of the OTA

1. The OTA contributes to the evaluation process.
   a. The OTA can assist with the collection of data for the evaluation once service competency has been established.
   b. The level of supervision required will be determined by the OTA's experience, established service competency, and state regulations.
   c. The OTA cannot independently evaluate or interpret evaluation results.

### B. Range of Motion (ROM)

1. Measurement tool: goniometer consisting of an axis, stationary and movable arms.
2. Types of range of motion.
   a. Functional ROM: ROM needed to perform functional movements (e.g., reach to top of head, small of back, etc.).
   b. AROM: active ROM (contractile structures) movement produced by one's own muscle.
   c. PROM: passive ROM (noncontractile structures) movement produced by an external force.
   d. AAROM: active assistive ROM, movement produced by one's own muscles and assisted by an external force.
3. Recording measurements.
   a. Starting position/ending position (e.g., 0-150°).
   b. Do not use negatives.
   c. Within functional limits (WFL): ROM is functional.
   d. Within normal limits (WNL): ROM achieves normal ranges (e.g., shoulder flexion 0-180°).
4. Review bony landmarks and normal ranges. (Table 11-1).

## TABLE 11-1 - AVERAGE NORMAL ROM (180° METHOD)

| JOINT | ROM | ASSOCIATED GIRDLE MOTION |
|---|---|---|
| **CERVICAL SPINE** | | |
| Flexion | 0° to 45° | |
| Extension | 0° to 45° | |
| Lateral flexion | 0° to 45° | |
| Rotation | 0° to 60° | |
| **THORACIC AND LUMBAR SPINE** | | |
| Flexion | 0° to 80° | |
| Extension | 0° to 30° | |
| Lateral flexion | 0° to 40° | |
| Rotation | 0° to 45° | |
| **SHOULDER** | | |
| Flexion | 0° to 170° | Abduction, lateral tilt, slight elevation, slight upward rotation |
| Extension | 0° to 60° | Depression, adduction, upward tilt |
| Abduction | 0° to 170° | Upward rotation, elevation |
| Adduction | 0° | Depression, adduction, downward rotation |
| Horizontal abduction | 0° to 40° | Adduction, reduction of lateral tilt |
| Horizontal adduction | 0° to 130° | Abduction, lateral tilt |
| Internal rotation | | Abduction, lateral tilt |
| Arm in abduction | 0° to 70° | |
| Arm in adduction | 0° to 60° | |
| External rotation | | Adduction, reduction of lateral tilt |
| Arm in abduction | 0° to 90° | |
| Arm in adduction | 0° to 80° | |

## TABLE 11-1 - AVERAGE NORMAL ROM (180° METHOD) CONT.

| JOINT | ROM |
|---|---|
| **ELBOW** | |
| Flexion | 0° to 135°-150° |
| Extension | 0° |
| **FOREARM** | |
| Pronation | 0° to 80°-90° |
| Supination | 0° to 80°-90° |
| **WRIST** | |
| Flexion | 0° to 80° |
| Extension | 0° to 70° |
| Ulnar deviation (adduction) | 0° to 30° |
| Radial deviation (abduction) | 0° to 20° |
| **THUMB *** | |
| DIP flexion | 0° to 80°-90° |
| MP flexion | 0° to 50° |
| Adduction, radial and palmar | 0° |
| Palmar abduction | 0° to 50° |
| Radial abduction | 0° to 50° |
| Opposition | composite motion |
| **FINGERS *** | |
| MP flexion | 0° to 90° |
| MP hyperextension | 0° to 15°-45° |
| PIP flexion | 0° to 110° |
| DIP flexion | 0° to 80° |
| Abduction | 0° to 25° |
| **HIP** | |
| Flexion | 0° to 120° (bent knee) |
| Extension | 0° to 30° |
| Abduction | 0° to 40° |
| Adduction | 0° to 35° |
| Internal rotation | 0° to 45° |
| External rotation | 0° to 45° |
| **KNEE** | |
| Flexion | 0° to 145° |
| **ANKLE AND FOOT** | |
| Plantar flexion | 0° to 50° |
| Dorsiflexion | 0° to 15° |
| Inversion | 0° to 35° |
| Eversion | 0° to 20° |

*DIP, distal interphalangeal; MP, metacarpophalangeal; PIP, proximal interphalangeal

Data adapted from American Academy of Orthopaedic Surgeons: Joint motion: method of measuring and recording. Chicago, 1965, The Association; Esch D, Lepley M: Evaluation of joint motion: methods of measurement and recording, Minneapolis, 1974, University of Minnesota Press.

Pedretti, L.W. (1996). *Occupational therapy: Practice skills for physical dysfunction.* (4th ed., p. 84). St. Louis, MO: Mosby. Reprinted with permission.

C. **Muscle Strength**
1. Types of manual muscle tests (MMT).
   a. Break test is the most common MMT.
      (1) Test position: gravity eliminated (lessened) or against gravity.
      (2) Stabilization: usually proximal to the joint the muscle crosses over. Do not hold over the muscle belly being tested.
      (3) Resistance: applied in opposite direction of movement; should be gradual.
      (4) Muscle grades. (Table 11-2).

D. **Grip Strength**
1. Measurement tool: dynamometer.
2. Position of upper extremity: shoulder adducted to side, elbow flexed to 90° and forearm in neutral.
3. Types of grip strength tests.
   a. Dynamometer handle placed on position #2. The mean of three trials of each hand is compared to the norms.
   b. One trial in all five positions for each hand. A

bell curve is observed if the individual is applying maximal effort.

   c. Vigorometer or sphygmomanometer cuff should be used to evaluate the grip strength of a person with arthritis.

**E. Pinch Strength**

1. Measurement tool: pinch meter.
2. Position of upper extremity: shoulder adducted to side, elbow flexed to 90° and forearm in neutral.
3. Types of pinch strength test.
   a. Key or lateral pinch: thumb pulp to the lateral aspect of the index middle phalanx.
   b. Three jaw chuck: pulp of thumb to pulps of index and middle fingers.
   c. Tip to tip: thumb pulp to pulp of index finger.
4. Three trials on each hand are obtained for all pinch strengths. The mean of three trials on each hand is compared to the norms.

**F. Endurance/Activity Tolerance**

1. Count number of repetitions per unit of time.

---

### TABLE 11-2 -MUSCLE TESTING GRADING SYSTEM

| GRADE | DEFINITION | DESCRIPTION |
|---|---|---|
| 5 | Normal | The part moves throught full ROM against gravity and takes maximal resistance. |
| 4 | Good | The part moves throught full ROM against gravity and takes moderate resistance. |
| 4- | Good minus | The part moves throught full ROM against gravity and takes less than moderate resistance. |
| 3+ | Fair plus | The part moves through full ROM against gravity and takes minimal resistance before it breaks. |
| 3 | Fair | The part moves through full ROM against gravity and is unable to take any added resistance. |
| 3- | Fair minus | The part moves less than full range of motion against gravity. |
| 2+ | Poor | The part moves through full ROM in a gravity-eliminated plane with no added resistance. |
| 2- | Poor minus | The part moves less than full ROM in a gravity-eliminated plane. |
| 1 | Trace | Tension is palpated in the muscle or tendon, but no motion occurs at the joint. |
| 0 | Zero | No tension is palpted in the muscle or tendon. |

Radomski. M.V. & Trombly Latham , C.A. (2008). *Occupational therapy for physical dysfunction* 6th ed. Baltimore : Lippincott Williams and Wilkins. Reprinted with permission.

2. Determine percent of maximum heart rate.
3. Measure time until fatigue.

**G. Edema**

1. The body's initial response to injury.
   a. It is the transfer of exudate in which the fluid from the blood stream moves to the interstitial tissue.
   b. Edema can be localized or diffuse.
2. Types.
   a. Pitting - acute.
   b. Brawny - chronic.
3. Evaluation of circumference.
   a. Measurement tool: tape measure, recorded in centimeters.
   b. Compare extremities, document landmarks.
4. Evaluation of hand and arm mass.
   a. Measurement tool: volumeter, recorded in milliliters.
      (1) Significant change in edema would be more than 10 ml.
      (2) The only true objective tool.

**H. Sensation**

1. Demonstrate sensory test with vision; then occlude vision for actual testing.
2. Test uninvolved side first. Apply stimulus to volar and dorsal surfaces (exceptions will be noted).
3. Spinal cord injuries are tested proximal to distal following dermatomes.
4. Peripheral nerve injuries are tested distal to proximal.
5. Neurological disorders: assess for dermatome pattern.
6. Peripheral nerve injuries: assess for peripheral nerve involvement.
7. Types of sensory testing.
   a. Light touch: touch with cotton swab. Person responds "yes" or "touched" when touched. Scoring: + (intact), - (impaired), or 0 (absent).
   b. Localization: touch with cotton swab. Person responds "yes" when touched and then with vision points to area touched. Scoring +, -, 0.
   c. Pain: touch with paper clip. Person responds "sharp" or "dull". Scoring: S+, D+, D, S, S-, or D-.
   d. Temperature sensation: use test tubes or thermal kit. Person responds "hot" or "cold". Scoring: +, -, 0.
   e. Stereognosis: present with vision occluded and ask for recognition by touch of common objects. Scoring: number of correct objects.
      (1) A second set of identical common objects

should be used for individuals with expressive aphasia.

f. Two point discrimination: use disk-criminator or caliper. Person responds to the number of points he/she feels, i.e., one or two.

g. Proprioception: position sense.
   (1) The OTA positions involved extremity.
   (2) Person duplicates position with contralateral extremity.

h. Kinesthesia: movement sense.
   (1) The OTA moves segment.
   (2) Person responds up or down.

## I. Coordination/Dexterity

1. Commercial assessment tools are used to evaluate dexterity.
   a. NBCOT publications do not provide any information about whether the examination includes or does not include these published instruments.
   b. See Table 11-3 for commonly used assessments.

## III. Intervention

### A. Role of the OTA

1. The OTA implements intervention with OT supervision.
2. The level of supervision required depends upon the OTA's experience and established service competency.
3. During the implementation of intervention, the OTA informs the supervising OT of any change in the individual's status and any other relevant information that may affect treatment.

### B. Increasing Range of Motion

1. Passive ROM and passive stretching.
   a. PROM is moving the joint to the desired range using an external force.
      (1) PROM can be performed by the therapist gently moving the extremity to the desired range or when resistance is felt.
   b. Passive stretching is PROM with overpressure.
   c. A careful review of the physician's orders is paramount to distinguish the type of passive exercise being requested.
   d. Heat prior to PROM and passive stretching increases extensibility.
   e. Joint mobilization requires special training and the establishment of service competence.
      (1) More effective if performed before passive ROM and passive stretching.
   f. Manual passive stretching within individual's tolerance.
   g. Contract/relax and hold/relax also increase ROM.
   h. Instruction in home exercises. Stress the importance of home exercises to facilitate change in tissue length.
      (1) Post surgical patients performing self PROM must clearly understand the concept of passive ROM before including it as part of their home exercise program.
   i. Splinting: dynamic and serial splinting.
   j. Exercise equipment: continuous passive movement (CPM), pulleys, etc.

2. Active ROM.
   a. Differential tendon gliding exercises: differentiates tendon movement and increases tendon excursion. See Figure 11-1.
   b. Blocking exercises: used to isolate individual joint motion. Instruct the client to hold the end range position for 3-5 seconds.
   c. Preparatory interventions: wall walking, AROM, table glides, cane exercises, etc.
      (1) Consider place and hold exercises when PROM is greater than AROM: assist

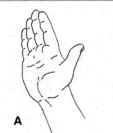 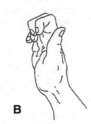 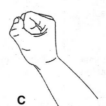 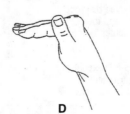 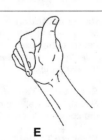

A                  B                  C                  D                  E

**Figure 11-1** Tendon Gliding Exercises: The five positions: **A**. Straight. **B**. Hook. **C**. Fist. **D**. Tabletop. **E**. Straight fist. Reprinted with permission. This figure was published in the *Journal of Hand Therapy, 11*. Rozmaryn, L. M., Dovelle, S., Rothman, E. R., Gorman, K., Olvey, K. M., & Bartko, J. J. Nerve and tendon gliding exercises and the conservative management of carpal tunnel syndrome. 171-179. Copyright Elsevier. 1998.

## TABLE 11-3 - DEXTERITY ASSESSMENTS

| NAME OF ASSESSMENT TOOL, AUTHOR AND PUBLICATION DATE | STANDARDIZED | VALIDITY/RELIABILITY | SETTING USED | AREAS ASSESSED | AGE GROUP |
|---|---|---|---|---|---|
| **Jebsen-Taylor Hand Function Test** Asses a broad range of hand functions used in daily activities. A seven-part test that uses common items such as paper clips, cans, pencils, etc. | Yes | Reliable | Seated requires adequate lighting | Writing page turning lifting small/large objects, simulated feeding | Ages 2-=94 |
| **Manipulative Aptitude Test** Measures hand/arm/finger dexterity and speed through sorting and assembling. | Yes | Valid and reliable | Seated at a table or desk | Dexterity, manipulatie aptitude, dominant hand | Ages 13+ |
| **Minnesota Rate of Manipulation** Assesses unilateral and bilateral manual dexterity along with eye-hand coordination. Provides information on standing tolerance, sustained neck flexion, weight bearing, and repetitive reach. | Yes | Valid and reliable | Table and chair | Manual dexterity turning, displacing | Ages 13+ |
| **Nine Hole Pet** Client places nine dowels in nine holes while being timed. | Yes | Valid and reliable | Table and chair | Finger dexterity turning, displacing | Ages 20+ |
| **O'Connor Finger Dexterity** Requires hand placement of 3 pins per hole. | Yes | | Table and chair | Predictor of rapid manipulation | Ages 13+ |
| **O'Connor Tweezer Dexterity Test** Measures the speed with which a client can pick up pins with a tweezer, one at time, and place the pin into a small hole. | Yes | | ´ Table and chair | Finger dexterity, fine motor coordination, speed, eye-hand coordination | Ages 13+ |
| **Pennsylvania Bi-manual Worksample** Requires hand placement of 3 pins per hole | Yes | Reliable | Table and chair | Finger dexterity of both hands, gross movement of both arms, eye-hand coordination | Ages 16+ |
| **Perdue Pegboard** Assembles gross movement of hands/ fingers/arms, as well as fingertip dexterity. | Yes | Valid and reliable | Table and chair | Gross movement of hands, fingers, and arms, fingertip dexterity | Ages 5+ |
| **Range of Motion** Measurement of the achievable distance between the flexed position and the extended position of a particular joint or muscle group. | Yes | Valid not 100% reliable | Table and chair | Gross movement of hands, fingers, and arms, fingertip dexterity | All ages |
| **Rosenbusch Test of Finger Dexterity** Measures the speed of inter-digital manipulation of each hand separately. | Yes | Valid and reliable | Table and chair | Manipulation of all parts of the hand | All ages |
| **Strength Testing** The strength of each muscle group is measured of each hand separately. | Yes | Valid, not 100% reliable | Comfortable for client, chair/mat | Biomechanical | All ages |

From Burns, A. (2010). Assessment tool grid. In K., Sladyk, Jacobs, K., & N., MacRae. (Eds.). *Occupational therapy essentials for clinical competence.* (534-535). Thorofare, NJ: Slack. Reprinted with permission.

extremity or hand to desired position and then slowly release. Ask the client to hold the position as you slowly release.

d. Purposeful activity: crafts, games, and sports. Incorporate individual's leisure interests.

e. Emphasize active use during purposeful and occupation based activities.

3. Precaution: myositis ossificans may result from overstretching (especially noted in elbow flexors).

## C. Increasing Strength

1. High resistance, low repetitions.
2. Type of contractions.
   a. Isometrics: contraction without movement.
      (1) Sometimes can produce more forceful contraction.
      (2) Isometrics are contraindicated for persons with hypertension and cardiovascular problems. They can increase blood pressure (BP) and heart rate (HR), so they should be avoided.
   b. Isotonic: contraction with movement; not concerned with length change.
   c. Eccentric = lengthening contraction.
   d. Concentric = shortening contraction.
3. Resistive exercises.
   a. Considered preparatory interventions. Common types include: progressive resistive exercises (PREs), hand grips, theraputty, theraband, and graded clothespins.
4. Improve strength using purposeful activities such as removing cans from a shelf or practice lifting pots.
5. Improve strength using occupation-based interventions such as grocery shopping and then preparing a meal.

## D. Increasing Endurance

1. Work at 50% of maximal resistance.
2. Increase repetitions, not resistance.
3. Use energy conservation methods.

## E. Edema Reduction Techniques

1. Elevation: extremity should be placed above the heart.
   a. This is contraindicated if the individual has circulation problems.
2. Retrograde massage assists the return of blood and lymphatic fluids to the venous system.
   a. Stroking is applied in centripetal direction.
   b. Massage should be performed with the extremity elevated.
3. Compression garments prevent re-accumulation of

fluids following retrograde massage.
   a. Common types.
      (1) Isotoner glove.
      (2) Tubigrip (stockinet with elastic).
      (3) Ace wraps.
      (4) Custom made compression garments.
      (5) Coban wrap (digit is wrapped distal to proximal).
         (a) Effective for decreasing edema in a digit.
         (b) Avoid too much tension.
         (c) The individual can exercise and use his/her hand for ADL and role activities while wearing Coban.
4. Cold packs: most effective when combined with elevation.
   a. Monitor vascular status.
5. Contrast bath.
   a. Move hand from warm (104-110°F) to cold (50-64°F) water.
   b. Begin in warm water (typically for 10 minutes), then transfer to cold water (typically for one minute), Then warm for typically 4 minutes. Continue this process. End in warm water.
   c. In the case of severe edema, some therapists suggest ending in cold water for one minute.
   d. Duration of this intervention can vary. The most common is 15 to 30 minutes.
      (1) Research on the efficacy of this approach is somewhat controversial, however, it is still a common method utilized in hand therapy settings.
6. Other edema techniques: string wrapping, ace bandage wraps and intermittent compression pump.
   a. These techniques are not as common.
7. Heat is commonly contraindicated. However, if the effects of heat are needed in a mild case of edema it could be cautiously used and combined with elevation.
8. Active exercise
9. Precautions/contraindications.
   a. Infection.
   b. Grafts or wounds.
   c. Vascular damage.
   d. Unstable fractures.
   e. Congestive heart failure (CHF).

## F. Scar Management

1. ROM: early mobilization programs are most effective.

2. Massage (circles and friction).
3. Scar pad with compression (Otoform, elastomers and topigel are the most common scar pads).
4. Splinting: to prevent contractures resulting from scar.
5. Edema control: especially in acute phase.

**G. Sensory Training**
1. Desensitization for hypersensitivity.
   a. If post-surgery, begin in periphery of the scar and as tolerated work over the scar.
   b. Massage.
   c. Textures.
   d. Vibration.
   e. Three phase desensitization kit.
   f. Fluidotherapy.
2. Sensory re-education.
   a. Same as number 1 above.
   b. Review safety precautions.
3. Compensation.
   a. Avoid use of hands where vision is occluded.
   b. Observe safety precautions.

**H. Improving Coordination**
1. Begin with gross motor activities and gradually grade up to fine motor activities.
2. Focus on accuracy and speed.

**I. Energy Conservation and Work Simplification Methods**
1. Plan short rest periods (5-10 minutes) during daily routine.
2. Schedule tasks for the day, week, and month to alternate and balance heavy and light work tasks.
3. Organize tasks; gather all necessary items and equipment before beginning task.
4. Avoid multiple trips to obtain items by using a utility cart, a bucket, walker bag, backpack, etc. to carry all items needed in one trip.
5. Eliminate tasks that are non-essential.
6. Delegate tasks that are beyond one's capacity.
7. Combine tasks to eliminate extraneous work.
8. Sit to work at a table or use a high stool for counter-top work.
9. Organize cabinets so that items are easy to reach and in convenient locations.
10. Use adaptive equipment (e.g., reachers) to avoid bending and stooping.
11. Use electrical appliances (e.g., mixers) to decrease personal effort.
12. Slide rather than lift heavy items.
13. Use lightweight equipment, tools and utensils.
14. Rest before fatigue sets in; intermittent rest during an activity is more effective than resting after exhaustion has occurred.

**J. Joint Protection Principles and Methods**
1. Maintain joint ROM by using maximal ROM during daily activities.
2. Maintain muscle strength by using maximal strength during daily activities.
3. Use the strongest and largest joint that is possible for task completion.
   a. Use knees and hips for lifting not the back.
   b. Push large items that need to be moved with a full body rather than pulling.
   c. Lift objects with both hands, palms pointed upward.
   d. Carry purses and bags on the forearm rather than wrist; most preferred is use of an ergonomically designed back pack.
4. Use each joint in its most stable and functional position.
   a. Stand directly in front of item to be reached for, opened or closed, rather than to the side.
   b. Keep wrists and fingers in proper alignment.
5. Avoid holding joints in one position or sustaining muscle contractions for extended periods of time.
   a. Use adaptive equipment to hold items for long periods of time (e.g., a book holder).
   b. Take breaks from extended activities.
6. Avoid positions of deformity and activities in the direction of deformity (e.g., ulnar drift).
   a. Perform movements in the direction opposite the potential deformity (e.g., opening a door with the right hand and closing it with the left hand to prevent ulnar drift).
   b. Use adaptive equipment that is ergonomically designed (e.g., tools and utensils with angled handles that eliminate deviations at the wrist).
7. Do not start an activity that cannot be immediately stopped if it requires capacities beyond existing capabilities.
8. Recognize that discomfort may be a reality of activity but that pain is a warning sign indicating that an activity should be modified or stopped.

**K. Body Mechanics Principles**
1. Do not move items that are too heavy; ask for assistance.
2. Slide or push an object along the surface rather than lift it, if possible.
3. Directly face the object about to be lifted. Do not face the direction in which the item is going to move.
4. Keep object close to the body during lifting and carrying.

5. Hold object centered at waist level.
6. Feet should be kept flat on the floor; balancing on toes should be avoided.
7. Maintain a firm and broad base of support. Maintain the body balanced over a wide stance.
8. Bend at the knees and hips, not at the waist.
9. Keep the back as straight as possible.
10. Breathe while lifting.
11. Lift by straightening legs; do not pull upward with arms and back.
12. Move smoothly; do not jerk.
13. Do not rotate the trunk. Pick up the object completely and then pivot the entire body.
14. Lower the body to the level of work.

**L. Splinting**
1. Types of splints.
   a. Static: has no resilient components and immobilizes a joint or part.
   b. Dynamic: includes a resilient component (elastic, rubber band, or spring) which the individual moves.
      (1) Designed to increase PROM or to augment AROM.
2. Purposes of splinting.
   a. Rest.
   b. Prevent deformities and contractures.
   c. Increase joint ROM.
   d. Protect bone, joint, and soft tissue.
   e. Increase functional use.
3. Hand splinting design standards.
   a. Maintain arches of the hand.
      (1) Proximal transverse arch.
      (2) Distal transverse arch.
      (3) Longitudinal arch.
   b. Do not impinge upon creases of the hand.
      (1) Distal and proximal palmar creases.
      (2) Distal and proximal wrist creases.
      (3) Thenar creases.
4. Mechanical principles of splinting.
   a. Decrease pressure: wide, long splint base is the most desirable. Round edges are needed.
   b. Use sling applied with a 90° angle of pull.
   c. Use low load to increase duration.
   d. Maintain three-point pressure versus circumference.
   e. Avoid the position of deformity.
      (1) Wrist flexion.
      (2) MCP hyperextension.
      (3) IP joints flexed.
      (4) Thumb adducted.
   f. Select the appropriate splinting position.

      (1) Functional position.
         (a) Wrist 20-30° extension.
         (b) MCPs 45° flexion.
         (c) IPs 20-30° flexion.
         (d) Thumb abducted.
      (2) Resting position (used for an inflammatory condition such as rheumatoid arthritis).
         (a) Wrist 10-20 extension.
         (b) MCPs 15-25 of flexion.
         (c) IPs in slight flexion.
         (d) Thumb palmarly abducted.
      (3) Safe position (following hand trauma). This position preserves the collateral ligaments.
         (a) Wrist 0-20° extension.
         (b) MCPs 70-90° flexion.
         (c) IPs in extension.
         (d) Thumb abducted and extended.
5. Precautions and education.
   a. Check individual's skin condition before and after making splint.
   b. Instruct splint wearer in procedures for splint maintenance and routine skin inspection and care.
      (1) Check skin when donning and doffing.
      (2) Provide wear and care instruction form.
   c. Ensure individual accepts and understands the purpose(s), function(s), and limitation(s) of the splint.
   d. Teach proper technique for donning and doffing splint.
   e. Provide functional training in use of splint in role activities (e.g., use of tenodesis splint to do schoolwork).
   f. Reevaluate individual's use of splint at periodic intervals.
6. OTA Role.
   a. Occupational therapist/OTA team must carefully assess for most appropriate splint.
   b. Occupational therapist must set splinting goals.
   c. Experienced OTAs can fabricate static splints and assist with dynamic splints upon establishment of service competency.
7. Splints for common diagnoses.
   a. Brachial plexus injury: flail arm splint.
   b. Radial nerve palsy: dynamic wrist, finger, and thumb extension splint.
   c. Spinal cord (C6-C7): tenodesis splint.
   d. Carpal tunnel syndrome: wrist splint positioned 0-15° extension.
   e. DeQuervain's: long thumb splint, includes wrist, IP joint free.
   f. CMC arthritis: hand based thumb splint.

g. Ulnar drift: ulnar drift splint.

h. Swan neck: silver rings or buttonhole splint.

i. Boutonniere: silver rings or dynamic PIP extension splint.

j. Arthritis: resting hand splint.

k. Flaccidity: resting splint.

l. Spasticity: spasticity splint or cone splint.

m. Muscle weakness (ALS, SCI, Guillain-Barré): balanced forearm orthosis (BFO), deltoid sling/suspension sling.

(1) Mounts to wheelchair.

(2) Individuals must have shoulder or trunk movement.

n. Burns to the axilla: airplane splint.

**M. Physical Agent Modalities (PAMs)**

1. Physical agent modalities (PAMs) can be used as facilitating procedures in preparation for purposeful activity.

a. PAMs are not an appropriate occupational therapy intervention if they are used in isolation of purposeful activity or occupation-based activities.

b PAMs are an appropriate occupational therapy intervention if they precede, support, and/or enable the individual's ability to perform purposeful activities and meaningful occupations.

c. PAMs are, therefore, preparatory OT intervention methods for they add to and complement the primary OT intervention methods of purposeful activity and occupation-based activities.

2. Types of PAMs.

a. Paraffin baths.

b. Hot packs.

c. Cold packs.

d. Fluidotherapy.

e. Whirlpool.

f. Contrast baths.

g. Ultrasound.

h. Electrical stimulation units.

(1) Functional electrical stimulation (FES).

(2) Neuromuscular electrical stimulation (NMES).

(3) Transcutaneous electrical nerve stimulator (TENS).

3. Benefits of superficial heat.

a. Relieves pain.

b. Increases tissue extensibility (increases ROM).

c. Assists with wound healing.

4. Benefits of cryotherapy.

a. Relieves pain.

b. Controls edema.

c. Decreases abnormal tone.

d. Facilitates muscle tone.

5. Benefits of electrical stimulation.

a. Relieves pain.

b. Stimulates and strengthens muscles.

c. Stimulates denervated muscle.

d. Decreases swelling

6. Benefits of ultrasound.

a. Relieves pain.

b. Decreases inflammation.

c. Increases tissue extensibility (increases ROM).

d. Decreases adhesions.

7. Benefit of contrast baths.

a. Reduces edema

8. Competent and ethical use of PAMs in occupational therapy.

a. PAMs should be used when they can benefit the individual's treatment program.

b. PAMs should be not be used when they will not benefit the individual's treatment program.

c. Indications, contraindications, and precautions for use of PAMs must be adhered to strictly.

(1) General contraindications for PAMs.

(a) Cancer.

(b) Pacemaker.

(c) Pregnancy.

(d) Cognitive impairment.

(e) Sensory impairment.

(f) Vascular impairment.

(g) Deep vein thrombophlebitis.

(h) Infection.

(i) Post surgery.

(2) Prior to using PAMs with an individual, diagnostic and age considerations must be carefully reviewed. For example, ultrasound is never used over growth plate.

d. Practitioner competence must be established for any and all PAMs used in OT intervention.

(1) The OTA can implement intervention with OT supervision.

(a) The level of supervision required depends upon the OTA's experience.

(2) During the implementation of intervention, the OTA informs the supervising therapist of any change in the individual's status and any other relevant information that may affect treatment.

# References

Amadottir, G. (1990). *The brain and behavior: Assessing cortical dysfunction through activities of daily living.* St. Louis, MO: Mosby.

American Occupational Therapy Association. (1995). *Standards of practice.* Bethesda, MD: Author.

American Society of Hand Therapists. (1992). *Clinical assessment recommendations.* (2nd ed.). Chicago: Author.

Bain, B. & Leger, D. (1997). *Assistive technology: An interdisciplinary approach.* Orlando, FL: Churchill Livingstone.

Bracciano, A.G. (2008). *Physical agent modaliites: Theory and application for the occupational therapist* (2nd ed.) Thorofare, NJ: SLACK Inc.

Cameron, M. (1999). *Physical agents in rehabilitation: From research to practice.* Orlando, FL: W.B. Saunders.

Clark, G., et al. (1993). *Hand rehabilitation: A practical guide.* Orlando, FL: Churchill Livingstone.

Clarkson, H.M. (2000). *Musculoskeletal assessment: Joint range of motion and manual muscles strength,* (2nd ed.), Philadelphia: Lippincott Williams and Wilkins.

Cooper, C. (2007). *Fundamentals of hand therapy: Clinical reasoning and treatment guidelines for common diagnoses of the upper extremity.* Philadelphia: Elsevier.

Gillen, G. & Burkhardt, A. (Eds.). (1998). *Stroke rehabilitation: A function-based approach.* St. Louis, MO: Mosby.

Greene, D.P. & Roberts, S.L. (2005). *Kinesiology: Movement in the context of activity* (2nd ed.), St Louis: Mosby.

Hopkins, H., & Smith, H. (1993). *Willard and Spackman's occupational therapy* (8th ed.) Philadelphia: Lippincott.

Hunter, J., Mackin, E. & Callahan, A. (1995). *Rehabilitation of the hand: Surgery and therapy* (4th ed.). St. Louis, MO: Mosby.

Katz, N. (1998). *Cognition and occupation in rehabilitation: Cognitive models for intervention in occupational therapy.* Bethesda, MD: American Occupational Therapy Association.

Kendall, F. (1995). *Muscle testing and function* (4th ed.). Baltimore, MD: Williams and Wilkins.

Malick, M., & Kasch, M. (1984). *Manual on management of specific hand problems.* Pittsburgh, PA: AREN Publications.

Michlovitz S.L. & Nolan T.P. (2005), *Modalities for therapeutic intervention,* (4th ed.), Philadelphia: F.A. Davis Company.

Neer, C. (1990). *Shoulder reconstruction.* Orlando, FL: W.B. Saunders.

Norkin, C.C. & White, D.J. (1995). *Measurement of joint range of motion.* (2nd ed.). Philadelphia: F.A. Davis.

*O'Connor Tweezer Dexterity Test.* (1986). Smith & Nephew Roylan, Inc. Menomonee Falls, WI 53051.

Okkema, K. (1993). *Cognition and occupation in rehabilitation: Cognitive models for intervention in occupational therapy.* Bethesda, MD: American Occupational Therapy Association.

Pedretti, L., Smith, R., Hammel, J., Rein, J., Anson, D., & McGuire, M.J. (1996). Use of adjunctive modalities in occupational therapy. In R.P. Cottrell (Ed.), *Perspectives on purposeful activity: Foundation and future of occupational therapy* (pp 451-458). Bethesda, MD: AOTA.

Pendleton, H. M. & Schultz-Krohn, W. (2006). *Pedretti's occupational therapy: Practice skills for physical dysfunction* (6th ed.). St. Louis: Mosby.

*Purdue Pegboard Procedure Manual.* Lafayette Instrument, PO Box 5729, Lafayette, IN 47903.

Radomski. M.V. & Trombly Latham, C.A. (2008). *Occupational therapy for physical dysfunction 6th ed.* Baltimore: Lippincott Williams and Wilkins.

Sladyk K., Jacobs, K. & MacRae, N. (2010). *Occupational therapy essentials for clinical competence.* Thorofare, NJ: Slack.

Sladyk K. & Ryan, S.E. (2001). *Ryan's occupational therapy assistant: Principles, practices, and techniques* (3rd ed.). Thorofare, NJ: Slack.

Unsworth, C. (1999). *Cognitive and perceptual dysfunction: A clinical reasoning approach.* Philadelphia: F.A. Davis.

Weiss, S. & Falkenstein, N. (2005). *Hand rehabilitation a quick reference guide and review.* 2nd ed, St. Louis: Elsevier Mosby.

# CHAPTER 12

# NEUROLOGICAL AND COGNITIVE-PERCEPTUAL APPROACHES: EVALUATION AND INTERVENTION

## Glen Gillen

## I. Neurological Frames of Reference Related to Motor Performance

### A. Contemporary Task-Oriented Approaches to Motor Control Training

1. General principles/assumptions.
   a. Contemporary approaches to motor control training are based on current research and knowledge of the motor behavior.
   b. Approaches reject assumptions of the reflex-hierarchical model of motor control and of the traditional neurophysiologic therapies.
   c. Remediation of performance components and environmental modifications to improve task performance is included.
   d. Based on a systems model of motor control.
      (1) Proposes that motor control is determined by interactive systems (motor, cultural, environmental, etc.), behavioral tasks, and adaptive/anticipatory mechanisms.
   e. Movement is controlled by the integration and interaction of multiple systems including environmental influences, sensorimotor factors, musculoskeletal factors, regulatory functions, and behavioral/emotional goals.
   f. The role of the structures responsible for motor control is to tune and prepare the motor system to respond to changing environmental and task demands.

   g. Interventions are also guided by the occupational therapist's or the OTA's understanding of motor learning principles.
   h. Control is not simply over muscle actions, but over the interactions of kinematic variables.
   i. Movement dysfunction following CNS damage reflects the system's best effort to accomplish task goals.

2. Principles of Carr and Shepherd's Motor Relearning Program (MRP).
   a. The person is an active participant whose goal is to relearn effective strategies for performing functional movement.
   b. Postural adjustments and limb movements are linked together in the learning process.
   c. Successful task relearning has occurred when activities are performed automatically and efficiently.
   d. The learning of skills does not follow a developmental sequence.
   e. Continued practice of compensatory strategies limits functional recovery.
   f. Intervention is not focused on learning specific movements but instead on learning general strategies for solving motor problems.
   g. Obstacles to efficient movement include loss of soft tissue extensibility, balance loss, fixation patterns due to postural insecurity, and muscle weakness.

h. Abnormal movement patterns are attributed to the repeated practice of compensatory movement strategies that become overlearned.
3. Principles of the Contemporary Task-Oriented Approach.
   a. Task performance emerges from the interaction of multiple systems including personal and performance contexts.
   b. An individual's behavioral changes reflect his/her attempts to compensate and to achieve functional goals.
   c. Individuals must practice with varied strategies to find optimal solutions for motor problems and develop skill in performance.
   d. Functional tasks help organize motor behavior.
   e. The practitioner must determine which control parameters or systems (personal, environmental, etc.) have positive or negative influences on motor behavior.
   f. Practice opportunities are provided that are appropriate to the person's stage of learning.
4. Principles of Motor Learning.
   a. Contemporary approaches to treating motor dysfunction incorporate principles of motor learning during interventions focused on remediating motor control in persons with CNS dysfunction.
   b. The ultimate goal of utilizing motor learning theory is the acquisition of functional skills that can be generalized to multiple situations and environments.
   c. Stages of motor learning.
      (1) Skill acquisition stage (cognitive stage) occurs during initial instruction and practice of a skill.
      (2) Skill retention stage (associated stage) involves "carry-over", as individuals are asked to demonstrate their newly acquired skill after initial practice.
      (3) Skill transfer stage (autonomous stage) involves the individual demonstrating the skill in a new context.
      (4) Refer to Table 12-1 for further description of these stages.
   d. Practice.
      (1) Random practice involves practice of several tasks that are presented in a random order encouraging reformulation of the solution to the presented motor problem.
      (2) Blocked practice involves repeated per-

formance of the same motor skill.
      (3) Variable conditions involve practice of skills in various contexts to improve transfer of learning and retention of skills.
      (4) Mental practice involves cognitive rehearsal of a skill without actually moving.
   e. Intrinsic feedback.
      (1) Information received by the learner as a result of performing the task.
      (2) Information is received from tactile, vestibular, and visual systems during and after the task.
   f. Extrinsic feedback.
      (1) Feedback provided from an outside source (i.e. the therapist or a mechanical device).
      (2) Includes knowledge of performance, which is verbal feedback about the process or performance itself.
      (3) Includes knowledge of results, which is the therapist's provision of feedback about the outcome or end product or results of the motor action.
   g. Factors/conditions that promote generalization of motor learning.
      (1) Capacity to generate intrinsic feedback.
      (2) High feedback regarding knowledge of performance.
      (3) Low extrinsic feedback regarding knowledge of results.
      (4) Practice conditions that are variable, random.
      (5) Whole task performance as opposed to breaking activities into contrived parts.
      (6) High contextual interference utilizes environmental conditions that increase the difficulty of learning such as noise distractions, crowded environments.
      (7) Practice in naturalistic settings, i.e. the setting in which the skill being taught will be utilized or an environment that closely resembles the one in which the skill will be performed.
   h. Refer to Table 12-1 for training strategies appropriate for each stage of motor learning.
5. The role of the OTA in intervention.
   a. The OTA implements intervention with OT supervision.
   b. The level of supervision required depends upon the OTA's experience and established service competency.

## TABLE 12-1
## MOTOR LEARNING STAGES AND TRAINING STRATEGIES

### COGNITIVE STAGE CHARACTERISTICS

- The learned develops an understanding of task; cognitive mapping assesses abilities, task demands; identifies stimuli, contacts memory; selects response; performs initial approximations of task; structures motor program; modifies initial responses
- "What to do" decision

### TRAINING STRATEGIES

- Highlight purpose of task in functionally relevant terms,
- Demonstrate ideal performance of task to establish a reference of correctness
- Have patients verbalize task components and requirements
- Point out similarities to other learned tasks
- Direct attention to critical task elements
- Select appropriate feedback
  - Emphasize intact sensory systems, intrinsic feedback systems.
  - Carefully pair extrinsic feedback with intrinsic feedback
  - High dependence on vision: have patient watch movement
  - Knowledge of Performance (KP): focus on errors as they become consistent; do not cue on large number of random errors
  - Knowledge of Results (KR): focus on success of movement outcome.
- Ask learner to evaluate performance, outcomes; identify problems, solutions
- Use reinforcements (praise) for correct performance, continuing motivation
- Organize feedback schedule
  - Feedback after every trial improves performance during early treatment
  - Variable feedback (summed, fading, bandwidth designs) increases depth of cognitive processing, improves retention; may decrease performance initially

- Organize initial practice
  - Stress controlled movement to minimize errors.
  - Provide adequate rest periods (distributed practice) if task is complex, long, or energy costly or if learner fatigues easily, has short attention, poor concentration
  - Use manual guidance to assist as appropriate
  - Break complex tasks down into component parts, teach both parts as integrated whole
  - Utilize bilateral transfer as appropriate
  - Use blocked (repeated) practice of same task to improve performance
  - Use variable practice (serial or random practice order) of related skills to increase depth of cognitive processing and retention; may decrease performance initially.
  - Use mental practice to improve performance and learning, reduce anxiety
- Assess, modify arousal levels as appropriate,
  - High or low arousal impairs performance and learning
  - Avoid stressors, mental fatigue
- Structure environment
  - Reduce extraneous environmental stimuli, distracters to ensure attention, concentration
  - Emphasize closed skills initially gradually progressing to open skills

### ASSOCIATED STAGE CHARACTERISTICS

- The learned practices movements, refines motor programs: spatial and temporal organization; decreases errors, extraneous movements
- Dependence on visual feedback decreases, increases for use of proprioceptive feedback; cognitive monitoring decreases
- "*How to do*" decisions

### TRAINING STRATEGIES

- Select appropriate feedback
  - Continue to provide KP, intervene when errors become consistent
  - Emphasize proprioceptive feedback, "feel of movement" to assist in establishing an internal reference of correctness
  - Continue to provide KR; stress relevance of functional outcomes
  - Assist learner to improve self evaluation, decision making skills
  - Facilitation techniques, guided movements may be counterproductive during this stage of learning

- Organize feedback schedule
  - Continue to provide feedback for continuing motivation; encourage patient to self-assess achievements
  - Avoid excessive augmented feedback
  - Focus on use of variable feedback (summed, fading, bandwidth) designs to improve retention
- Organize practice
  - Encourage consistency of performance
  - Focus on variable practice order (serial or random) of related skills to improve retention
- Structure environment
  - Progress toward open, changing environment.
  - Prepare the learner for home, community, work environments

### TABLE 12-1
## MOTOR LEARNING STAGES AND TRAINING STRATEGIES CONTINUED

**AUTONOMOUS STAGE CHARACTERISTICS**

- The learner practices movements, continues to refine motor responses, spatial and temporal highly organized, movements are largely error-free, minimal level of cognitive monitoring
- *"How to succeed"* decision

**TRAINING STRATEGIES**

- Assesses need for conscious attention, automaticity of movements
- Select appropriate feedback
  - Learner demonstrates appropriate self evaluation, decision-making skills
  - Provide occasional feedback (KP, KR) when errors evident

- Organize practice
  - Stress consistency of performance in variable environments, variations of tasks (open skills)
  - High levels of practice (massed practice) are appropriate
- Structure environment
  - Vary environments to challenge learner
  - Ready the learner for home, community, work environments.
- Focus on competitive aspects of skills as appropriate, e.g., wheelchair sports.

O'Sullivan, S. & Schmitz, T. (2007). *Physical rehabilitation* (5th ed.). Philadelphia: F.A. Davis Company. Reprinted with permission.

---

   c. During the implementation of intervention, the OTA informs the supervising therapist of any change in the individual's status and any other relevant information that may affect treatment.

**B. Review of Neurophysiologic ("Traditional") Frames of Reference**

1. Also known as sensorimotor or traditional approaches.
2. Utilized for persons with central nervous system dysfunction.
3. Approaches developed in the 1940s and 1950s based on the understanding of nervous system pathology at that time.
   a. Many of the assumptions upon which these approaches were based are questionable when a contemporary view of motor control is considered.
4. Treatment foundations.
   a. Application by the therapist of controlled sensory input to influence motor responses (i.e., a reflex model of control).
   b. Utilization of "facilitation" and "inhibition" techniques to improve motor performance.
   c. The assumption that controlled movement is preceded by stereotypic reflex responses.
   d. The assumption that sensory input regulates motor output and sensation is necessary for movement to take place.
   e. The assumption that normal movements are governed by hierarchical centralized motor programs that determine muscle activation patterns.
      (1) The cerebral cortex controls the middle levels (basal ganglia, brainstem, etc.) which in turn control the spinal cord.

   f. The assumption that damage to higher control centers release lower level or primitive reflexes and movement patterns from inhibition.
   g. The assumption that when basic movements and postures are normalized, skilled movement would occur automatically.
   h. The assumption that "integration" of lower level spinal and brainstem reflexes occurs by eliciting higher level righting and equilibrium responses.

**C. Margaret Rood's Approach**

1. Principles/assumptions.
   a. Utilization of controlled sensory stimulation.
      (1) Specific techniques are used to provide sensory input to the nervous system to evoke a reflex-based muscular response.
   b. Utilization of developmental sequences.
      (1) Individuals are placed in various developmental postures that evoke particular muscular responses.
   c. Utilization of activity to demand a purposeful response.
      (1) Purposeful activities are provided so that the person can actively utilize the evoked movement pattern in the context of a task.
   d. Normalization of tone and muscular responses are achieved via controlled sensory stimulation.
      (1) Sensory stimulation can elicit desired movement patterns.
   e. Sensorimotor control is developmentally based.
      (1) Treatment must begin at the person's current level and progress sequentially.
      (2) Treatment is based on a developmental

sequence.

f. Muscular responses of the agonists, antagonists, and synergists are believed to be reflexively programmed according to a purpose or plan.

   (1) Purposeful activity is chosen to subcortically elicit desired movement patterns.

g. Repetition/practice is necessary for motor learning.

2. Rood proposed four sequential phases of motor control.

   a. Reciprocal inhibition/innervation.

      (1) An early mobility pattern that is primarily a reflex governed by spinal and supraspinal centers.

   b. Co-contraction.

      (1) Defined as a simultaneous contraction of the agonist and antagonist that provides stability in a static pattern.

      (2) Utilized to hold a position or object for a long duration.

   c. Heavy work.

      (1) Also termed "mobility superimposed on stability".

      (2) In these patterns, proximal muscles contract and move and the distal segments are fixed.

   d. Skill.

      (1) Considered the highest level of control and combines stability and mobility.

      (2) These patterns consist of a stabilized proximal segment while the distal segments move in space.

3. Rood described a sequence of motor development termed "ontogenic motor patterns" that includes eight different patterns in sequence.

   a. Supine withdrawal.

      (1) A position of total flexion while in the supine position.

      (2) The arms cross the chest, the legs flex and abduct.

      (3) Utilized to gain trunk stability and elicit flexion responses.

   b. Rollover.

      (1) The arm and leg on the same side flex as the trunk rotates.

      (2) Utilized to elicit lateral trunk responses as well as for persons who are dominated by tonic reflexes.

   c. Prone extension.

      (1) The person lies prone with upper trunk and head extension.

      (2) The shoulders abduct, extend, and externally rotate, while the hips and knees extend off the support surface.

      (3) The pattern results in an isometric contraction of the extensors and abductors.

   d. Neck cocontraction.

      (1) The individual is lying prone and encouraged to lift the head into extension against gravity.

      (2) Utilized to develop head control.

   e. Prone on elbows.

      (1) A pattern of trunk extension utilized to inhibit tonic neck reflexes as well as provide trunk and proximal limb stability.

   f. Quadruped.

      (1) The person assumes an "on all fours" position to develop limb and trunk cocontraction patterns.

   g. Standing.

      (1) Standing is at first static followed by active weight shifting.

   h. Walking.

      (1) Gait patterns are integrated into functional activities.

4. The role of the OTA in intervention.

   a. The OTA implements intervention with OT supervision.

   b. The level of supervision required depends upon the OTA's experience and established service competency.

   c. During the implementation of intervention, the OTA informs the supervising therapist of any change in the individual's status and any other relevant information that may affect treatment.

5. Intervention methods /techniques.

   a. Utilize controlled sensory input (cutaneous, thermal, olfactory, gustatory, auditory, and/or visual) to evoke desired motor responses.

   b. Apply facilitation techniques to stimulate or maintain control of a muscle group.

   c. Apply inhibition techniques to quiet/relax/dampen overactive muscle groups.

   d. Engage the individual in activities appropriate to the developmental patterns in an effort to master each level and progress to more difficult patterns/activities.

   e. Utilize general facilitory and/or inhibitory stimuli to influence the person's central state (i.e., to increase arousal level or calm a disorganized state).

**D. Neurodevelopmental Treatment (NDT)/the Bobath Technique**

1. Principles/assumptions.
   a. Normalization of postural and limb tone.
   b. Normalization of movement patterns.
   c. Integration of both sides of the body.
   d. Establishment of the ability to weight bear and weight shift through the limbs.
   e. Establishment of normal righting and equilibrium patterns.
   f. Utilization of specific "handling" techniques to promote normal movement.
   g. Inhibition of primitive reflexes.
   h. Avoidance of movements and activities that increase tone.
   i. Inhibition of abnormal postural and limb movements.
   j. Development of normal patterns of posture and movement.
   k. Re-establishment of symmetry of the sides of the body to increase functional use.
   l. Improvement of the quality of movement and performance of the involved side.
   m. Normalization of tone is prerequisite to normal movement.
      (1) Tone abnormalities include flaccidity (low tone) or spasticity (high tone).
   n. Associated reactions (nonfunctional and involuntary changes in the uninvolved limb position and tone) should be avoided.
   o. Postural reactions are considered the basis for control of movement.
      (1) These reactions include righting, equilibrium, and protective responses.
   p. Loss of postural control results in overuse of the sound side and limits functional movements.
   q. The stereotypical patterns of the trunk and limbs observed in persons with CNS dysfunction are viewed as abnormal patterns of motor coordination.
   r. Focus is on improving the quality of movement.
2. The role of the OTA in intervention.
   a. The OTA implements intervention with OT supervision.
   b. The level of supervision required depends upon the OTA's experience and established service competency.
   c. During the implementation of intervention, the OTA informs the supervising therapist of any

change in the individual's status and any other relevant information that may affect treatment.
3. Interventions methods/techniques.
   a. Handling is the hallmark of NDT. The therapist's hands are utilized to attain intervention goals.
   b. Utilize "key points of control" when handling to control quality of movement response.
   c. Utilize inhibition techniques to decrease synergistic movement, hypertonicity, and asymmetrical posture.
   d. Utilize specific techniques to "normalize tone".
   e. Establish the ability to weight shift symmetrically in various postures in all directions.
   f. Retrain activities of daily living and mobility skills integrating both sides of the body while limiting abnormal responses (associated reactions, etc.).
   g. Utilize bilateral movement patterns to integrate both sides of the body into function.

**E. Proprioceptive Neuromuscular Facilitation (PNF)**

1. Principles/assumptions.
   a. The response of the neuromuscular mechanisms can be hastened through stimulation of the proprioceptors.
      (1) Utilized for neurologic and orthopedic populations throughout the lifespan.
   b. Techniques are superimposed on patterns of movement and posture, focusing on sensory stimulation from manual contacts, visual cues, and verbal commands.
   c. Normal motor development proceeds in a cervicocaudal and proximodistal direction.
   d. Early motor behavior is dominated by reflex activity.
      (1) Mature motor behavior is supported or reinforced by postural reflexes that are integrated throughout the lifespan.
   e. Early motor behavior is characterized by spontaneous movement, which oscillates between extremes of flexion and extension.
      (1) These movements are rhythmic and reversing in character.
   f. Developing motor behavior is expressed in an orderly sequence of total patterns of movement and posture.
   g. In development, there are shifts between flexor and extensor dominance.
   h. Normal motor development has an orderly sequence of total patterns of movement and

postures.

   i. Locomotion depends on reciprocal contraction of flexors and extensors.

   j. The maintenance of posture requires continual adjustment for nuances of imbalance.

   k. Frequency of stimulation and repetitive activity are used to promote and retain motor learning, and to develop strength and endurance.

   l. Goal directed activities coupled with techniques of facilitation are used to hasten learning of total patterns of walking and self-care activities.

   m. Goal directed activity is made up of reversing movements.

   n. Normal movement and posture depend upon "synergism" and balanced interaction of antagonists.

2. The role of the OTA in intervention.

   a. The OTA implements intervention with OT supervision.

   b. The level of supervision required depends upon the OTA's experience and established service competency.

   c. During the implementation of intervention, the OTA informs the supervising therapist of any change in the individual's status and any other relevant information that may affect treatment.

3. Intervention methods/techniques.

   a. Diagonal patterns or mass movement patterns are utilized during functional activities.

     (1) Patterns are chosen in an effort to remediate missing components.

     (2) For each body segment two pairs of diagonals exist. (Table 12-2).

     (3) Flexion or extension is the major component.

     (4) All patterns cross midline and encourage rotary components to movement. (Figures 12-1 and 12-2).

     (5) Combinations are utilized.

   b. Assisted diagonal patterns using techniques of "chop" and "lift".

   c. Total patterns of movement during treatment utilize a developmental approach.

   d. PNF techniques are superimposed on postures and movement patterns.

**F. Brunnstrom's Movement Therapy**

1. Principles/assumptions.

   a. The reader should note that the below principles/assumptions are not reflective of current understanding of the motor system. They are included as historical reference only for some test questions may reflect this historical perspective.

   b. In normal development, spinal cord and brain stem reflexes become modified and their components rearranged into purposeful movement through the influence of higher centers.

   c. The damaged central nervous system has undergone a "reverse evolution" and regresses to a phylogenetically older pattern of movement that includes the limb synergies and primitive reflexes.

   d. Reflexes and primitive movements are used to facilitate recovery of voluntary movement post-stroke.

   e. Proprioceptive and exteroceptive stimuli are used to facilitate desired movement as well as tonal changes.

   f. Newly produced movements must be practiced and learned.

   g. Treatment progresses developmentally from

**TABLE 12-2**
**PATTERN ANALYSIS OF DIAGONAL PATTERNS**

| | |
|---|---|
| **D1 Flexion (UE)** | Scapula: Abducted and upwardly rotated.<br>Shoulder: Flexed, adducted, externally rotated.<br>Elbow: Slightly flexed.<br>Forearm: Supinated.<br>Wrist: Flexed towards radial side.<br>Fingers: Flexed, adducted.<br>Thumb: Flexed, adducted. |
| **D1 Extension (UE)** | Scapula: Adducted, downwardly rotated.<br>Shoulder: Extended, abducted, internally rotated.<br>Elbow: Extended.<br>Forearm: Pronated.<br>Wrist: Extended toward ulnar side.<br>Fingers: Extended, abducted.<br>Thumb: Extended, abducted. |
| **D2 Flexion (UE)** | Scapula: Adducted and upwardly rotated.<br>Shoulder: Flexed, abducted, externally rotated.<br>Elbow: Extended.<br>Forearm: Supinated.<br>Wrist: Extended toward radial side.<br>Fingers: Extended, abducted.<br>Thumb: Extended, abducted. |
| **D2 Extension (UE)** | Scapula: Abducted and downwardly rotated.<br>Shoulder: Extended, adducted, internally rotated.<br>Elbow: Towards flexion.<br>Forearm: Pronated.<br>Wrist: Flexed toward ulnar side.<br>Fingers: Flexed, adducted.<br>Thumb: Flexed, abducted, opposed. |

reflex to voluntary to purposeful.

h. Movement is elicited by use of associated reactions and tactile stimulation.

i. Reversal of movement is stressed.

j. Emphasis is placed on the person's ability to overcome movement dominated by flexor or extensor synergies.

k. Recovery follows an ontogenic process.
   (1) Proximal to distal.
   (2) Flexion before extension.
   (3) Reflex movement before controlled/volitional movement.

2. Brunnstrom identified six stages of motor recovery following the onset of hemiplegia that the individual progresses through in a stereotypical fashion.

   a. Flaccidity or no voluntary motion.

   b. Developing synergies. (Figures 12-3 and 12-4 and Table 12-2).

   c. Beginning voluntary movement within the synergy pathways.

   d. Initial movements that deviate from synergy.

e. Independence from the basic synergies.

f. Isolated, near normal movement with minimal spasticity.

3. The role of the OTA in intervention.

   a. The OTA implements intervention with OT supervision.

### TABLE 12-3 - BASIC MOVEMENT SYNERGIES

|  | FLEXION | EXTENSION |
|---|---|---|
| Shoulder Girdle | Elevation/retraction | Depression/protraction |
| Shoulder | Abduction/external rotation | Adduction/internal rotation |
| Elbow | Flexion | Extension |
| Forearm | Supination | Pronation |
| Hand | Variable (usually flexion) | Variable (usually flexion) |
| Hip | Flexion/abduction/external rotation | Extension/adduction/internal rotation |
| Knee | Flexion | Extension |
| Ankle | Dorsiflexion | Plantar flexion |
| Foot | Inversion | Inversion |

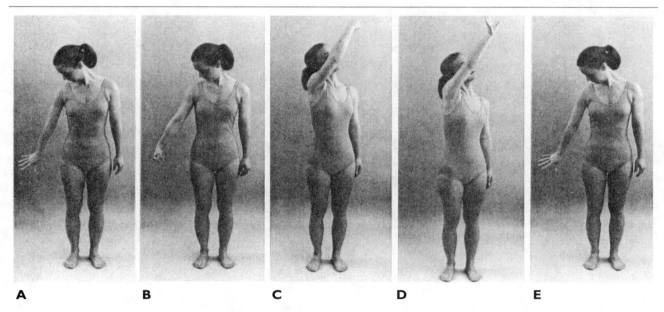

D1 flexion and D1 extension, elbows straight
Head and Neck: D flexion, R; D extension, L

**COMMANDS (left to right)**

A. "Ready! Look at your hand!"
B. "Close and turn your right hand toward your face!"
C. "Pull up and across!"

D. "Now open your hand!"
E. "And push down and away! And repeat! And again!"
(Speak the commands as you perform.)

**Figure 12-1**: Upper Extremities, Unilateral Patterns
From Voss, D.E. Ionta, M.K. & Myers, B.J. (1985). *P.N.F.: Patterns and techniques, p15*, Philadelphia, PA: J.B. Lippincott. Reprinted with permission.

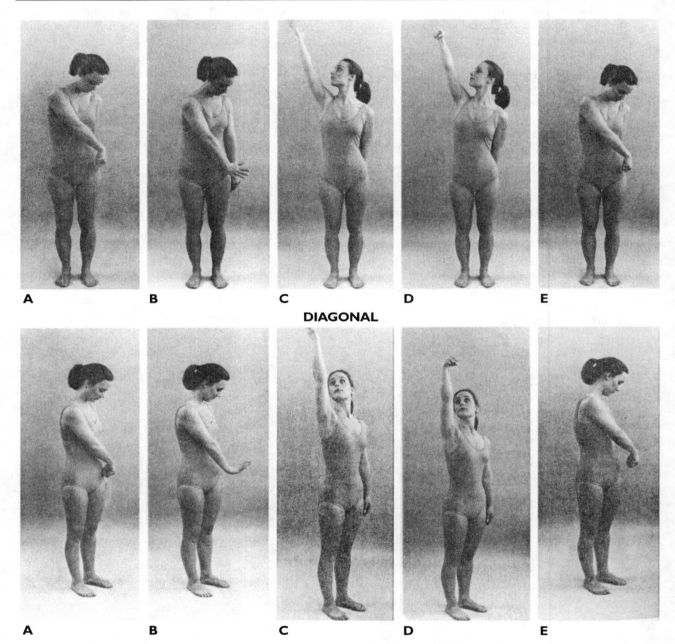

**DIAGONAL**

D2 flexion and D2 extension, elbows straight
Head and Neck: D extension, R; D flexion, L

## COMMANDS (left to right)

**A.** "Ready! Look at your hand!"

**B.** "Open and turn your right hand, thumb toward your face!"

**C.** "Lift up and out!"

**D.** "Now close your hand!"

**E.** "And pull down and across! And repeat! And again!"
(Speak the commands as you perform.)

**Figure 12-2**: Upper Extremities, Unilateral Patterns
From Voss, D.E. Ionta, M.K. & Myers, B.J. (1985). *P.N.F.: Patterns and techniques*, p14, Philadelphia, PA: J.B. Lippincott. Reprinted with permission.

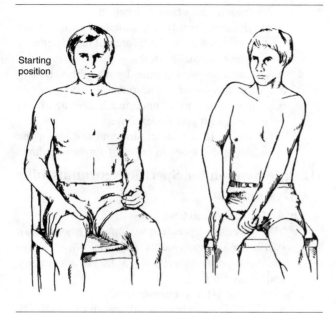

**Figure 12-3**: Extension synergy (Grade 4).
From Sawyer, K.A. & LaVigne, J.M. (1992) *Brunnstrom's movement therapy in hemiplegia: A neurophysiological approach* 2nd ed, p196. Philadelphia, P.A.: J.B. Lippincott. Reprinted with permission.

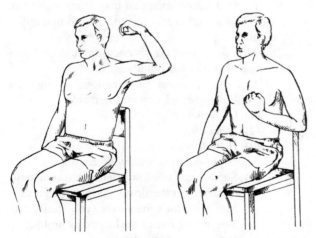

Alternate flexion pattern (shoulder hyperextension replaces abduction – external rotation)

**Figure 12-4**: Flexion synergy (Grade 4).
From Sawyer, K.A. & LaVigne, J.M. (1992) *Brunnstrom's movement therapy in hemiplegia: A neurophysiological approach* 2nd ed, p196. Philadelphia, P.A.: J.B. Lippincott. Reprinted with permission.

   b. The level of supervision required depends upon the OTA's experience and established service competency.
   c. During the implementation of intervention, the OTA informs the supervising therapist of any change in the individual's status and any other relevant information that may affect treatment.
4. Intervention methods/techniques.
   a. The reader should note that the below intervention techniques are rarely used, for they are not based on a current understanding of the motor system. They are included as historical reference only.
   b. Facilitate the individual's progress through the recovery stages that Brunnstrom identified.
   c. Recapitulate normal movement developmentally from a reflex base to voluntary control.
   d. Postural reflexes are utilized to change tone in specific muscles.
   e. Specific facilitory techniques are utilized.
   f. Movement demands progress from no muscle activity to movement within the synergy pathways to deviations out-of-synergy to normal movement.

## II. Evaluation of Motor Control Dysfunction

### A. The Role of the OTA in Evaluation
1. The OTA contributes to the evaluation process.
2. The OTA can assist with the collection of data for the evaluation once service competency has been established.
3. The level of supervision required will be determined by the OTA's experience and established service competency.
4. The OTA cannot independently evaluate or interpret evaluation results.

### B. Assessment for Components of Motor Control
1. Abnormal tone is evaluated by the elicitation of velocity-dependent stretch reflexes.
2. Reflex testing.
   a. Utilized to evaluate involuntary stereotyped responses to a particular stimulus.
   b. Responses develop during fetal life and persist through early infancy.
   c. Reflexes may be released after brain injury or not integrated during early development secondary to CNS pathology.
   d. Intensity and quality of the response in monitored.
   e. A response to stimulus is termed "positive" and no response to stimulus is "negative".

f. The therapist or the OTA notes the highest level of reflex control achieved.

g. The therapist or the OTA must be aware of the age range that is considered normal for each reflex. Refer to Chapter 5.

h. Treatment is planned to progress individual to an age-appropriate level of reflex hierarchy.

3. Qualitative descriptions of motor control.

a. Evaluation of motor control should include observations of the quality of movement during performance of functional tasks.

b. Examples of motor control issues resulting in observable poor quality of movement.

(1) Intention tremor is the worsening of action tremor as the limb approaches a target in space.

(2) Dysmetria is the undershooting (hypometria) or overshooting (hypermetria) of a target.

(3) Dyssynergia is a breakdown in movement resulting in joints being moved separately to reach a desired target as opposed to moving in a smooth trajectory; decomposition of movement.

(4) Dysdiadochokinesia is impaired ability to perform rapid alternating movements.

(5) Ataxia is loss of motor control including tremors, dysdiadochokinesia, dyssynergia, and visual nystagmus.

(6) Resting tremor is an involuntary tremor noted in resting postures.

(7) Rigidity is an increased resistance to passive movement throughout the range; may be "cogwheel" (alternative contraction/relaxation of muscles being stretched) or "leadpipe" (consistent contraction throughout range).

(8) Bradykinesia is an overall slowing of movement patterns.

(9) Akinesia is the inability to initiate movements.

(10) Athetosis is a dyskinetic condition that includes inadequate timing, force, and accuracy of movements in the trunk/limbs; movements are writhing and worm-like.

(11) Dystonia is an involuntary sustained distorted movement or posture involving contraction of groups of muscles.

(12) Chorea consists of involuntary movements of the face and extremities which are spas-modic and of short duration.

(13) Hemiballismus is a unilateral chorea characterized by violent, forceful movements of the proximal muscles.

4. Assessment for glenohumeral joint subluxation.

a. Allow the person's arm to dangle into gravity.

b. Palpate the space underneath the acromion process with your index finger.

c. Compare to the intact side and document the width of the space in terms of finger breadths.

## III. Intervention for Specific Neuromuscular Dysfunction

### A. Oral Motor Dysfunction

1. May result in speech impairments (dysarthria), swallowing impairments (dysphagia), or psychosocial stresses related to facial asymmetry and/or drooling.

2. Role of the OTA in intervention.

a. The OTA implements intervention with OT supervision.

b. The level of supervision required depends upon the OTA's experience and established service competency.

c. During the implementation of intervention, the OTA informs the supervising therapist of any change in the individual's status and any other relevant information that may affect treatment.

3. Direct intervention involves techniques that utilize a bolus.

a. Modification of consistency, amount, and pacing of solids and liquids.

b. Utilizing postural interventions to increase swallowing efficiency during meals.

(1) Chin tuck.

(2) Head tilt.

(3) Head turn.

c. Utilizing specific swallowing adaptations.

(1) Supraglottic swallow technique to voluntarily close/protect the airway during food intake.

(2) Mendelssohn's maneuver (voluntarily prolonging the rise of the larynx by prolonging tongue contraction).

4. Indirect intervention involves procedures that do not include use of a bolus.

a. Thermal (cold) stimulation provides sensory input to the inferior faucial arches via a chilled dental examination mirror to elicit a swallow reflex.

b. Reflex facilitation.

c. Strengthening, facilitation, and coordination of oral movements.

d. Airway adduction procedures.

e. Positioning to maintain the trunk/head/neck in correct postures.

5. Refer to Chapter 9 for further information on dysphagia and swallowing disorders.

**B. Orthotic/Splinting Interventions for Neuromotor Dysfunction**

1. The role of the OTA in intervention.

   a. The occupational therapist/OTA team must carefully assess for most appropriate splint.

   b. The occupational therapist must set splinting goals.

   c. Experienced OTAs can fabricate static splints and assist with dynamic splints upon establishment of service competency.

2. Orthoses may be utilized in the population with neuromuscular dysfunction to meet the following goals.

   a. Prevent/correct deformity via prolonged stretch and proper alignment.

   b. Control spasticity by aligning joints and providing prolonged stretch to spastic muscles.

   c. Prevent/decrease/accommodate contractures of the joint or soft tissue.

   d. Correct biomechanical malalignment by external force.

   e. Position the hand in a functional posture to promote engagement in activities.

   f. Compensate for weakness to allow intact muscle groups to function.

   g. Provide proximal support.

   h. Support a painful joint.

   i. Promote distal mobility.

   j. Enhance a specific activity, e.g., fabrication of a typing or writing splint or utilization of a cock-up splint for feeding.

   k. Immobilize joints and soft tissues to promote healing.

   l. Prevent or reduce scarring via prolonged pressure and appropriate stretch.

3. Splint classification.

   a. Static (no moving parts) splints are utilized for external support, prevention of motion, stretching of contractures, aligning joints for healing, resting joints, or reducing pain.

   b. Dynamic (moving parts are included) splints have a resilient component (elastic bands or spring) and are utilized to increase passive motion, assist weak motions, or substitute for lost motion.

   c. Serial splints are utilized to achieve a slow, progressive increase in motion by progressive remolding.

4. Types of inhibitory/tone normalizing orthoses.

   a. Based on the neurophysiologic frames of reference.

   b. Bobath finger spreader (abduction splint).

      (1) Based on Bobath's principle of reflex inhibiting patterns.

      (2) This soft splint positions the digits and thumb in abduction in an effort to reduce tone.

   c. Rood cone.

      (1) Based on Rood's inhibitory principles of sustained deep pressure.

      (2) This cone-shaped splint is utilized to reduce flexor spasticity in the hand.

   d. Orthokinetic splints.

      (1) This type of splint utilizes tactile input (e.g., via elastic bandages) to facilitate and/or inhibit appropriate muscle groups.

   e. Spasticity reduction splint.

      (1) This splint places the spastic distal extremity on submaximal stretch to reduce spasticity.

5. Types of supportive orthoses.

   a. Overhead suspension sling.

      (1) This orthotic device incorporates an arm support that is supported by a sling and suspended by an overhead rod.

      (2) Persons presenting with proximal weakness (amyotrophic lateral sclerosis, Guillain-Barré syndrome, muscular dystrophy) with muscle grades in the 1/5 to 3/5 range are appropriate candidates.

   b. Balanced forearm orthoses (mobile arm supports or ball-bearing forearm orthoses).

      (1) Consists of an arm trough, proximal and distal arms, and a support bracket.

      (2) Allows a patient with weak proximal musculature to utilize available control of the trunk and shoulder to engage in functional tasks.

   c. Shoulder slings.

      (1) Utilized to support a flaccid arm after neurologic insult for short and controlled periods of time.

      (2) Long term use may be detrimental in terms of soft-tissue contracture, edema, and the development of pain syndromes.

   d. Supports may be utilized on a wheelchair to

position a flaccid arm (e.g., lapboards, arm troughs, etc.).

6. Hand/wrist based splints may be dorsal or volar.
   a. Cock-up splints.
      (1) Supports the wrist in 10-20 degrees of extension to prevent contracture.
      (2) Allows the digits to function (e.g., to support flaccid wrist).
   b. Resting hand splint.
      (1) Utilized for persons who need to have their wrist, digits, and thumb supported in a functional position for prolonged periods (i.e., when developing contracture of the long flexors).
   c. Opponens splints.
      (1) May be short or long.
      (2) Designed to support the thumb in a position of abduction and opposition.
      (3) Utilized during functional activities to compensate for weakness patterns.
7. Splinting considerations.
   a. Wearing schedules must be prescribed to enhance the function of the splint.
      (1) Splints that are utilized to decrease spasticity or reverse contractures require longer wearing times.
   b. Splints must be monitored for pressure over bony prominences.
   c. Donning/doffing procedures should be reviewed with individuals and caretakers and be documented.
   d. The appropriate material must be chosen by the inclusion of necessary characteristics including resistance to stretch, memory, conformability/drape, rigidity/flexibility, and self-adherence.
   e. Refer to Chapter 11 for additional splinting information.

## IV. Sensory Integration Frame of Reference and Intervention[1]

### A. Overview
1. A sensory integrative approach to views the neural organization of sensory information for an adaptive response.
2. The sensory integration frame of reference was developed by Jean A. Ayres.

### B. Principles/Assumptions
1. Plasticity (structural changes) of the central nervous system allows for modification of the central nervous system (CNS).

2. Sensory integration occurs in a developmental sequential manner.
3. Higher cortical processing functions are dependent on adequate processing and organization of sensory stimuli by lower brain centers.
4. Adequate modulation of sensory stimuli must occur for an adaptive response to occur.
   a. Sensory stimuli can be either facilitory or inhibitory, and each sensory system influences other sensory systems.
5. Adaptive responses facilitate the integration of sensory stimuli.
6. Individuals seek out sensorimotor experiences that have an organizing effect.

### C. Intervention
1. Role of the OTA.
   a. The OTA implements intervention with OT supervision.
   b. The level of supervision required depends upon the OTA's experience and established service competency.
   c. During the implementation of intervention, the OTA informs the supervising therapist of any change in the individual's status and any other relevant information that may affect treatment.
2. Intervention follows the general principles of SI theory.
   a. Control sensory input to improve sensory processing, facilitate sensory integration, and elicit an adaptive response.
      (1) Grade for type and rate of movement, and for the amount of resistance while adhering to the precautions.
         (a) Firm pressure and resistance is less threatening than light touch.
         (b) Linear movement is less threatening than angular.
         (c) Slow movement is less threatening than rapid movement.
   b. Create an environment to facilitate active participation.
   c. Ensure registration of meaningful sensory input to obtain an adaptive response.
   d. The quality of input and the type of activities used will vary depending on the child's needs and the situational context.
   e. Balance structure and freedom, tapping into the child's inner drive to obtain neural organization.
   f. Gradually introduce activities requiring more mature and complex patterns of behaviors.

[1]Jan G. Garbarini contributed to this section on the sensory integration frame of reference.

g. Promote organized adaptive responses to enhance a child's general behavioral organization, including socialization.

3. Follow intervention principles for specific sensory processing deficits.
   a. Tactile.
      (1) Tactile modulation for tactile defensiveness and hypersensitivity/overresponsivity, and hyposensitivity/underresponsivity and sensory-seeking.
         (a) Self-applied stimuli are more tolerable than passive application of tactile stimuli (e.g., play using shaving crème, pretend dress-up play).
         (b) Provide deep touch/firm pressure where the child can see the source of the stimuli, which tends to be more tolerable versus light touch stimuli that tends to be aversive especially to the face, abdomen, and palmar surfaces of the extremities.
         (c) Provide controlled sensory activities that simultaneously provide tactile and vestibular-proprioceptive information.
         (d) Begin with slow linear movements and deep touch-pressure.
         (e) Apply tactile stimuli in the direction of hair growth which is less aversive.
         (f) Follow tactile stimuli with joint compression.
         (g) Monitor and adjust stimuli that seem to influence modulation of stimuli (e.g., lighting, sound, etc.).
         (h) Be alert and assess the child's behavioral responses up to a few hours following treatment when negative impacts may still be demonstrated.
         (i) Tactile defensiveness and sensory-seeking can be reduced if the treatment approach is effective.
      (2) Tactile discrimination.
         (a) Provide deep touch pressure to the hands as well as the body.
         (b) Deficits in tactile discrimination are rarely seen in isolation, and somatodyspraxia is typically seen; therefore, treatment for tactile discrimination is usually performed simultaneously when providing treatment for deficits in motor planning.
         (c) Provide graded activities requiring tactile discrimination activities using a mixture of textures and items (e.g., rice, sand).
   b. Proprioception.
      (1) Deficits in modulation demonstrated by hypersensitivity/overresponsivity.
         (a) Provide firm touch, pressure, joint compression or traction.
         (b) Provide resistance to active movement to help the child learn the appropriate amount of force to perform tasks.
         (c) Provide activities in various body positions combining vestibular proprioceptive information (e.g., yoga).
         (d) Provide slow linear movement, resistance, and deep pressure.
         (e) Use adaptive techniques (e.g., weighted vests).
      (2) Discrimination deficits.
         (a) Provide treatment as noted above.
         (b) Provide activities requiring the child to demonstrate the ability to grade the force or efforts of movement.
   c. Vestibular.
      (1) Deficits in modulation of vestibular input include hyposensitivity/underresponsivity, hypersensitivity/overresponsivity (aversion response), and gravitational insecurity (fear response).
         (a) Grade for type and rate of movement, and for the amount of resistance.
            • Precautions must be observed.
         (b) Slowly introduce linear movement with touch pressure in prone and provide resistance to active movements, especially for gravitational insecurity.
         (c) Use linear vestibular stimuli to increase awareness of spatial orientation (otolith organ).
         (d) Provide rapid rotary and angular movements with frequent starts/stops and acceleration/deceleration to increase ability to distinguish the pace of movement (semicircular canals).

4. Special advanced training and knowledge of the effects of various sensory stimuli is required.
   a. An occupational therapy assistant must be well aware of precautions for movements, as their impact may not be apparent for several hours.
   b. Continually ask the child how he/she is feeling,

and observe for signs involving the autonomic nervous system such as pupil dilation, sweaty palms, changes in the rate of respiration.

5. Provide compensatory skill development (e.g., environmental adaptations, hand writing supports).

6. Use group treatment to develop the social interaction skills needed for adaptive functional behavior in a classroom, in peer groups, and/or afterschool programs.

7. Consult with and/or educate teachers and parents.

8. Share intervention strategies for specific sensory processing deficits.

# V. Cognitive-Perceptual Approaches

## A. Overview of Cognitive-Perceptual Terminology and Symptoms

1. Perception.
   a. The integration/interpretation of sensory impressions received from the environment into psychologically meaningful information.

2. Cognition.
   a. The ability of the brain to process, store, retrieve, and manipulate information. It involves the skills of understanding and knowing, the ability to judge and make decisions, and an overall environmental awareness.

3. Cognitive-perceptual deficits.
   a. Occur as a result of multiple pathologies including CVA, TBI, neoplasms, acquired diseases, psychiatric disorders, etc.

4. Functional impairments.
   a. Impaired alertness or arousal.
      (1) The person has a decreased response to environmental stimuli.
   b. Astereognosis, also known as tactile agnosia.
      (1) The inability to recognize objects, forms, shapes, and sizes by touch alone.
      (2) A failure of tactile recognition although sensory testing (tactile and proprioceptive) is intact.
   c. Impaired attention.
      (1) An inability to attend to or focus on specific stimuli.
      (2) May result in distraction by irrelevant stimuli.
      (3) Includes difficulty with sustained attention and selective attention.
   d. Ideational apraxia.
      (1) A breakdown in the knowledge of what is to be done or how to perform.
      (2) A lack of knowledge regarding object use.
      (3) The neuronal model about the concept of how to perform is lost although the sensorimotor system may be intact.
   e. Motor apraxia/ideomotor apraxia.
      (1) Loss of access to kinesthetic memory so that purposeful movement cannot be achieved because of ineffective motor planning although sensation, movement, and coordination are intact.
   f. Long term memory loss.
      (1) Lack of storage, consolidation, and retention of information that has passed through working memory.
      (2) Includes the inability to retrieve this information.
   g. Short term memory loss.
      (1) Lack of registration and temporary storing of information received by various sensory modalities.
      (2) Includes the loss of working memory.
   h. Impaired organization/sequencing.
      (1) The inability to organize thoughts with activity steps properly sequenced.
   i. Right-left indiscrimination.
      (1) Inability to discriminate between the right and left sides of the body or to apply the concepts of right and left to the environment.
   j. Body scheme disorders.
      (1) Loss of awareness of body parts, as well as the relationship of the body parts to each other and objects.
      (2) Includes body neglect and somatoagnosia.
   k. Spatial relations impairment.
      (1) Difficulty relating objects to each other or to the self secondary to a loss of spatial concepts (up/down, front/back, under/over, etc.).
   l. Somatoagnosia.
      (1) A body scheme disorder that results in diminished awareness of body structure, and a failure to recognize body parts as one's own.
   m. Topographical disorientation.
      (1) Difficulty finding one's way in space secondary to memory dysfunction or an inability to interpret sensory stimuli.
   n. Unilateral body neglect.
      (1) Failure to respond to or report unilateral

stimulus presented to the body side contralateral to the lesion.

o. Unilateral spatial neglect.
   (1) Inattention to, or neglect of, stimuli presented in the extrapersonal space contralateral to the lesion.
   (2) May occur independently of visual deficits.
p. Figure/ground dysfunction.
   (1) An inability to distinguish foreground from background.
q. Anosognosia.
   (1) An unawareness of motor deficit.
   (2) May be related to a lack of insight regarding disabilities.
r. Perseveration.
   (1) The continuation or repetition of a motor act or task.
s. Acalculia.
   (1) The inability to perform calculations.
t. Alexia.
   (1) The inability to read.
u. Agraphia.
   (1) The inability to write.
v. Impaired problem solving.
   (1) The inability to manipulate a fund of knowledge and apply this information to new or unfamiliar situations.
w. Disorientation.
   (1) Lack of knowledge of person, place, and time.
x. Anomia.
   (1) Loss of the ability to name objects or retrieve names of people.
y. Broca's aphasia.
   (1) Loss of expressive language indicated by a loss of speech production.
z. Wernicke's aphasia.
   (1) A deficit in auditory comprehension that affects semantic speech performance, manifested in paraphasia or nonsensical syllables.

5. Visual foundation skills.
a. These skills must be evaluated to differentiate perceptual dysfunction and visual system deficits.
   (1) Visual acuity.
      (a) The clarity of vision both near and far.
   (2) Visual fields.
      (a) The available vision to the right, left, superior, and inferior.
      (b) An example of field loss is homonymous hemianopsia (the left temporal field and right nasal field are affected).
   (3) Oculomotor function.
      (a) Control of eye movements.
   (4) Scanning.
      (a) Ability to systematically observe and locate items in the environment.

B. **Cognitive-Perceptual Evaluation**
1. Role of the OTA.
   a. The OTA contributes to the evaluation process.
   b. The OTA can assist with the collection of data for the evaluation once service competency has been established.
   c. The level of supervision required will be determined by the OTA's experience and established service competency.
   d. The OTA cannot independently evaluate or interpret evaluation results.

C. **Cognitive-Perceptual Intervention**
1. Role of the OTA.
   a. The OTA implements intervention with OT supervision.
   b. The level of supervision required depends upon the OTA's experience and established service competency.
   c. During the implementation of intervention, the OTA informs the supervising therapist of any change in the individual's status and any other relevant information that may affect treatment.
2. Remedial/restorative/transfer of training approach.
   a. Focuses on restoration of components to increase skill.
   b. Deficit specific.
   c. Targets cause of symptoms.
   d. Emphasizes performance components.
   e. Assumes improvements in performance components will result in increased skill.
   f. Assumes the cerebral cortex is malleable and can reorganize.
   g. Utilizes tabletop and computer activities such as memory drills, block designs, parquetry, etc. as treatment modalities.
3. Compensatory/adaptive/functional approach.
   a. Involves repetitive practice of functional tasks.
   b. Emphasizes modification.
   c. Activity choice driven by tasks the person needs, or wants, to perform.
   d. Emphasizes intact skill training.
   e. Treats symptoms, not the cause.
   f. Utilizes techniques of environmental adapta-

tion and compensatory strategies.

g. Treatment is task specific.

h. Utilizes functional tasks (BADL, IADL, work, and leisure tasks) that the individual desires, or is required, to perform at discharge as the basis of treatment.

4. Information processing approach.

a. Provides information on how the individual approaches the task.

b. Investigates how performance changes with cueing.

c. Standardized cues are given to determine their effect on performance.

d. Cues or feedback are utilized to draw attention to relevant features of the task.

e. Investigative questions are used to provide insight to the underlying deficits.

5. Dynamic interactional approach.

a. Emphasizes transfer of information from one situation to the next.

b. Utilizes varying treatment environments.

c. Practice of a targeted strategy with varied tasks and situations (multicontextual).

d. Emphasizes metacognitive skills (self-awareness of strengths and deficits) as basis of learning and generalization of learning.

e. Transfer of learning must be taught from one situation to the next and does not occur automatically.

f. Transfer of learning occurs through a graded series of tasks that decrease in similarity (e.g., training scanning strategies for a person with a visual neglect to find items in a refrigerator to a less similar task such as scanning to cross the street).

g. The person's processing abilities and self-monitoring techniques are used to facilitate learning for different tasks or environments.

h. The therapist or OTA utilizes awareness questioning ("How do you know this is right?") to help the individual detect errors, estimate task difficulty, and predict outcomes.

6. The quadraphonic approach.

a. Based on remediation.

b. Based on information processing theory and teaching/learning theory.

c. Micro-perspective includes evaluation of management of performance component subskills such as attention, memory, motor planning, postural control, and problem solving.

d. Macro-perspective evaluation includes the use of narratives, interview, real-life occupations (shopping, cooking, etc.).

e. Makes use of several theories.

(1) Information processing.

(2) Teaching/learning evaluation.

(3) Neurodevelopmental evaluation.

(4) Biomechanical evaluation.

7. Neurofunctional approach.

a. Based on learning theory.

b. Specifically used for individuals with acquired neurological impairments.

c. Focuses on retraining real world skills rather than cognitive-perceptual processes.

d. Utilizes an overall adaptive approach but incorporates some remediation components.

e. Treatment is focused on training specific functional skills in true contexts.

8. Cognitive disabilities model.

a. Originally developed for use with individuals who have psychosocial dysfunction, currently also being utilized with persons with neurologic dysfunction and dementia.

b Describes cognitive function on a continuum from level 1 (profoundly impaired) to level 6 (normal).

c. Each level describes the extent of a person's disability and difficulty in performing occupations.

d. After the person's level has been established, routine tasks are presented that the person can perform or that have been adapted so that he/she can perform them.

e. Focus is placed on adaptive approaches and strengthening residual abilities.

9. General intervention strategies for specific deficits.

a. Intervention strategies for impaired alertness or arousal.

(1) Increase environmental stimuli.

(2) Use gross motor activities.

(3) Increase sensory stimuli.

b. Intervention strategies for motor/ideomotor apraxia.

(1) Utilize general verbal cues as opposed to specific.

(2) Decrease manipulation demands.

(3) Provide hand over hand tactile-kinesthetic input.

(4) Utilize visual cues.

c. Intervention strategies for ideational apraxia.

(1) Provide step by step instructions.

(2) Use hand over hand guiding techniques.

(3) Provide opportunities for motor planning and motor execution.

d. Intervention strategies for perseveration.

(1) Bring perseveration to a conscious level and train the person to inhibit the behavior.

(2) Redirect attention.

(3) Engage the individual in tasks that require repetitive action.

f. Intervention strategies for spatial neglect.

(1) Provide graded scanning activities.

(2) Grade activities from simple to complex.

(3) Use anchoring techniques to compensate.

(4) Utilize manipulative tasks in conjunction with scanning activities.

(5) Use external cues (e.g., colored markers and written directions).

g. Intervention strategies for body neglect.

(1) Provide bilateral activities.

(2) Guide the affected side through the activity.

(3) Increase sensory stimulation to the affected side.

h. Intervention strategies for aphasia.

(1) Decrease external auditory stimuli.

(2) Give the individual increased response time.

(3) Use visual cues and gestures.

(4) Use concise sentences.

(5) Investigate the use of augmentative communication devices.

i. Intervention strategies for sequencing and organization deficits.

(1) Use external cues (e.g., written directions, daily planners).

(2) Grade tasks that are increasingly complex in terms of number of steps required.

j. Intervention strategies for spatial relations dysfunction.

(1) Utilize activities that challenge underlying spatial skills.

(2) Utilize tasks that require discrimination of right/left.

k. Intervention strategies for memory loss.

(1) Use rehearsal strategies.

(2) "Chunk" information.

(3) Utilize memory aids (alarm watches, timers, etc.).

(4) Utilize "temporal tags", focusing on when the event to be remembered occurred.

# References

Bundy, A.C., Shelly, L.J., Fisher, A.C., & Murray, E.A. (2002). *Sensory integration: Theory and practice. 2nd ed.* Philadelphia: F.A. Davis.

Gillen, G., (2009). *Cognitive and perceptual rehabilitation: Optimizing function.* St. Louis, MO: Elsevier/Mosby.

Gillen, G., & Burkhardt, A. (Eds.). (2004). *Stroke rehabilitation: A function-based approach, ed. 2.* St. Louis, MO: Elsevier/Mosby.

Gutman, S. A., & Schonfeld, A. B. (2003). *Screening adult neurologic populations: A step-by-step instruction manual.* Bethesda, MD: American Occupational Therapy Association.

Katz, N. (2004). *Cognition and occupation across the lifespan: Models for intervention in occupational therapy.* Bethesda, MD: American Occupational Therapy Association.

Lane, S. J. (2002). Structure and function of the sensory systems. In A.C. Bundy, S.J. Lane, & E.A. Murray (Eds.), *Sensory integration: Theory and practice, 2nd ed.* (pp. 35-70). Philadelphia: F.A. Davis.

Lane, S.J. (2002). Sensory modulation. In A.C. Bundy, S.J. Lane, & E.A. Murray, (Eds.), *Sensory integration: Theory and Practice, 2nd ed.* (pp. 101-122). Philadelphia: F.A. Davis.

Miller, L. J. (2007). *Sensational kids hope and help for children with sensory processing disorder (SPD).* New York: G.P. Putnam's Sons.

Parham, L., D. & Mailoux, Z. (2005). Sensory integration. In J. Case-Smith (Ed.), *Occupational therapy for children, 5th ed.* (pp. 356-409). St. Louis, MO: Elsevier Mosby.

Schultz-Krohn, W. & Pendleton, H. (Eds.) (2006). *Occupational therapy: Practice skills for physical dysfunction, 6th ed.* St. Louis, MO: Elsevier Mosby.

Shaf, R. & Lane, S. (2009). Neuroscience foundations of vestibular, proprioceptive, and tactile sensory strategies. *OT Practice,* 14(22), CE1-CE8.

Shumway-Cook, A. & Woollacott, MH. (2001). Motor control: *Theory and practical applications, 2nd ed.* Baltimore: Lippincott Williams and Wilkins.

Vining-Radomski, M. & Trombly-Latham, C.A. (2007). *Occupational therapy for physical dysfunction* (6th ed.). Baltimore: Williams & Wilkins.

# CHAPTER 13

# PSYCHOSOCIAL APPROACHES: EVALUATION AND INTERVENTION

### Janice L. Romeo • Rita P. Fleming-Castaldy

## I. Psychosocial Frames of Reference[1]

### A. Overview

1. To the best of our knowledge, the NBCOT examination does not ask specific questions about frames of reference or models of practice except for Allen's Cognitive Disabilities model.
   a. Evaluation and intervention methods based on Allen's approach may be directly tested because this model is viewed as providing a classification system for cognitive deficits.
2. Information about other major frames of reference and models of practice is provided because it can be helpful in answering exam items that require clinical reasoning in the analysis of case scenarios.

### B. Model of Human Occupation (MOHO)

1. Developed by Gary Kielhofner, based on the Occupational Behavior model of Mary Reilly.
2. Principles.
   a. "Occupation is dynamic and context-dependent." (Kielhofner, 2004, p. 151)
   b. Personal occupational choices and engagement in occupation shape the individual.
   c. Three elements are inherent to humans.
      (1) Volition includes thoughts and feelings that motivate people to act and is comprised of personal causation, values, and interests.
      (2) Habituation includes organized, recurrent patterns of behavior and is comprised of roles and habits.
      (3) Performance capacity includes the physical and mental skills needed for performance and the subjective experience of engaging in occupation.
   d. The environment impacts on the individual through the opportunities, demands, resources, and constraints it provides.
      (1) The environment is divided into physical and social components.
      (2) Each component is influenced by the culture(s) in which it takes place.
   e. Evaluation focuses on exploring the individual's occupational history, goals, volition, habits, and occupational performance.
   f. Intervention focuses on occupational engagement and includes activities that are purposeful, relevant and meaningful to people and their social context.

### C. Life-Style Performance Model

1. Developed by Gail Fidler.
2. Principles.
   a. The Life-Style Performance Model seeks to identify and describe the nature and critical "doing" elements of an environment that support and foster achievement of a satisfying, productive life-style.

[1]Acknowledgment: William Lambert, MA, OTL, Lecturer in Occupational Therapy, The University of Scranton, Scranton PA critically reviewed this chapter and provided helpful input to ensure the accuracy and currency of the chapter's content.

b.  It proposes a method for looking at the match between that environment and the individual's needs.

c.  Four hypotheses are proposed.

(1)  "Mastery and competence in those activities that are valued and given priority in one's society or social group have greater meaning in defining one's social efficacy than competence in activities that carry less social significance.

(2)  "A total activity and each of its elements have symbolic as well as reality-based meanings that notably affect individual experiences and motivation.

(3)  "Mastery and competence are more readily achieved, and the sense of personal pleasure and intrinsic gratification is more intense, in those activities that are most closely matched to one's neurobiology and psychological structure.

(4)  "Competence and achievement are most readily seen and verified in the end-product or outcome of an activity; thus the ability to do, to overcome, and to achieve becomes obvious to self and others." (Fidler, 1996, pp. 115-116).

d.  Performance and quality of life can be enhanced by an environment that provides for ten fundamental human needs.

(1)  Autonomy: self-determination.

(2)  Individuality: self-differentiation.

(3)  Affiliation: evidence of belonging.

(4)  Volition: the having of alternatives.

(5)  Consensual validation: acknowledgment of achievement and verification of perspectives.

(6)  Predictability: discernment and evaluation of cause and effect.

(7)  Self-efficacy: evidence of competence.

(8)  Adventure: exploration of the new and unknown.

(9)  Accommodation: freedom from physical or mental harm and compensation for limitations.

(10) Reflection: contemplation of events and the meaning of things.

e.  Performance is measured in the quality of functioning in four domains.

(1)  Self-care and maintenance.

(2)  Intrinsic gratification.

(3)  Service to others.

(4)  Reciprocal relationships.

3.  Evaluation focuses on obtaining an activity history and a life-style performance profile related to the four skill domains. Environmental factors are explored.

4.  Intervention.

a.  Addresses five main questions that identify the focus of intervention.

(1)  What does the person need to be able to do?

(2)  What is the person able to do?

(3)  What is the person unable to do?

(4)  What interventions are needed, and in what order?

(5)  What are the characteristics and patterns of activity and of the environment that will enhance the person's quality of life?

b.  Any interventions or activities that promote performance in the four domains are acceptable.

**D. Occupational Adaptation**

1.  Developed by Janette Schkade and Sally Schultz.

2.  Principles.

a.  Occupational adaptation is concerned with the processes that the individual goes through to adapt to his/her environment.

b.  It consists of three elements: the person, the occupational environment, and the interaction between the two.

(1)  The person element consists of the sensorimotor, cognitive, and psychosocial components of the individual.

(2)  The occupation environment is viewed as the physical, social, and cultural systems within which work, play/leisure, and self-maintenance take place.

(3)  The outcome of the interaction between the person and the environment is referred to as the occupational response.

c.  The occupational adaptation model makes two basic assumptions.

(1)  "Occupation provides the means by which humans adapt to changing needs and conditions, and the desire to participate in occupation is the intrinsic motivational force leading to adaptation.

(2)  "Occupational adaptation is a normative process that is most pronounced in periods of transition, both large and small. The greater the adaptive transitional needs, the

greater the importance of the occupational adaptation process, and the greater the likelihood that the process will be disrupted." (Schkade & Shultz, 1992, pp. 829-830).

3. Evaluation focuses on occupational environment, role expectation, and the individual's potential for adaptation and the best means for adaptation to occur.

4. Intervention focuses on increasing the skills needed for occupational adaptation. It addresses both the individual and the environment.

## E. Role Acquisition

1. Developed by Ann Mosey.

2. Principles.

   a. Intervention is focused on the acquisition of the specific skills an individual needs in order to function in his/her environment.

   b. The individual employs task and social skills to meet the demands of personally desired and necessary roles.

   c. Performance is addressed through function/dysfunction continuums in seven categories.

      (1) Task skills.

      (2) Interpersonal skills.

      (3) Family interaction.

      (4) Activities of daily living.

      (5) School.

      (6) Work.

      (7) Play/leisure/recreation.

   d. Temporal adaptation addresses the individual's temporal orientation and ability to organize his/her use of time in a need-satisfying manner.

3. Evaluation focuses on gathering data indicative of function/ dysfunction in the above categories.

4. Intervention.

   a. The principles of learning are used to promote skill development.

   b. General postulates for change are provided to guide the treatment process.

      (1) Long-term goals are set based on the person's expected environment.

      (2) Initially, task and interpersonal skills can be taught separately or they can be taught within the context of the learning of social roles.

      (3) An adequate repertoire of behavior is acquired through activities that elicit the desired behavior, are interesting to the client, include socializing, and apply the

principles of learning. See Chapter 3.

      (4) Intrapsychic content is shared matter-of-factly with the client, and reality testing is provided.

      (5) The OT practitioner must know very specifically what kind of behavior he/she wishes to promote or enhance.

   c. Specific postulates are provided for each of the continuums.

   d. Any treatment activities or strategies that employ the teaching-learning principles are acceptable.

## F. Cognitive Disabilities

1. Developed by Claudia Allen.

2. Principles.

   a. Based on the stages of cognitive development as described by Piaget and the neurobiological sciences.

   b. Cognitive ability is determined by biological factors and the potential for improvement is dictated by those factors.

   c. Once the maximum level has been achieved, compensations must be made biologically, psychologically, or environmentally.

   d. Cognitive performance is placed on a continuum divided into six levels that are further divided into modes.

      (1) Automatic Actions, Level I, is characterized by automatic motor responses and changes in the autonomic nervous system. Conscious response to the external environment is minimal.

      (2) Postural Actions, Level II, is characterized by movement that is associated with comfort. There is some awareness of large objects in the environment, and the individual may assist the caregiver with simple tasks.

      (3) Manual Actions, Level III, begins with the use of the hands to manipulate objects. The individual may be able to perform a limited number of tasks with long-term repetitive training.

      (4) Goal Directed Actions, Level IV, is characterized by the ability to carry simple tasks through to completion. The individual relies heavily on visual cues. He/she may be able to perform established routines but cannot cope with unexpected events.

      (5) Exploratory Actions, Level V, is character-

ized by overt trial and error problem solving. New learning occurs. This may be the usual level of functioning for 20% of the population.

    (6) Planned Actions, Level VI, is characterized by the absence of disability. The person can think of hypothetical situations and do mental trial-and-error problem solving.

3. Evaluation.

  a. Focus is on identifying the individual's current cognitive abilities and their implications for performance, independence, and the need for assistance. The potential for improvement is also considered.

  b. Observation during functional tasks is emphasized.

  c. Several evaluation tools have been developed to assist with the identification of the individual's cognitive level.

    (1) The Allen Cognitive Levels Leather Lacing Task is a structured task that allows the therapist to observe the individual performing three increasingly complex stitches and make determinations about that person's cognitive skill level. Guidelines are available for designing other tasks that will also elicit the component skills of each level.

    (2) The Routine Task Inventory gathers data about the individual's ADL performance from an informed caregiver.

    (3) The Cognitive Performance Test was designed to assess the functional performance of individuals with Alzheimer's disease. The focus is on the identification of the effects that particular deficits have on the performance of ADL.

4. Intervention.

  a. Activities are used to elicit the individual's highest cognitive level.

  b. Therapy focuses on maintaining the individual's highest level of function.

  c. Environmental changes and activity adaptations are made to compensate for deficits and allow the greatest degree of independence.

  d. The OT practitioner works with the team to develop an appropriate discharge plan.

  e. The OT practitioner should meet with the family or other caregivers to develop understanding of the individual's abilities, deficits, and care needs.

## G. Psychodynamic/Psychoanalytic

1. An early OT frame of reference based on the work of S. Freud, A. Freud, Jung and Sullivan.

  a. Principle developers were Gail Fidler and Ann Mosey.

  b. Due to the advances in psychiatry, temporal and financial constraints, and the nature of the population served, these approaches are rarely used today.

  c. Proper use of this approach requires further training.

  d. Individuals may protect themselves from anxiety through the use of "defense mechanisms". Some are healthy; some are not.

  f. Understanding the function of defensive mechanisms is useful in therapeutic relationships.

  g. Defense mechanisms are grouped into a hierarchy according to the phases of maturity associated with them.

    (1) Narcissistic mechanisms.

      (a) Denial - the failure to acknowledge the existence of some aspect of reality that is apparent to others (e.g., an alcohol abuser is unable to acknowledge that his/her problems are a result of drinking).

      (b) Projection - attributing attributes or unacknowledged feelings, impulses or thoughts to others (e.g., someone who feels guilty attributes what others say as blaming them).

      (c) Splitting - rigid separating of positive and negative thoughts and of feelings (e.g., staff members may be seen as all good or all bad when variations of behavior are anxiety-provoking).

    (2) Immature mechanisms.

      (a) Passive-aggressive - aggression towards others which is indirectly or unassertively expressed (e.g., a patient is late for a treatment session when he/she is angry with the practitioner).

      (b) Regression - returning to an earlier stage of development to avoid the tension and conflict of the present one (e.g., an individual becomes needy and/or child-like during a period of stress or illness).

      (c) Somatization - the conversion of psychological symptoms into physical illness (e.g., a person who feels stuck in an unhappy marriage develops low back pain).

(3) Neurotic mechanisms.

(a) Rationalization - creating self-justifying explanations to hide the real reasons for one's own or another's behavior (e.g., a parent believes a lazy adult son is not working because the job market is poor).

(b) Repression - blocking from consciousness painful memories and anxiety-provoking thoughts (e.g., an adult child has no memory of being mistreated by a beloved parent).

(c) Displacement - redirecting an emotion or reaction from one object to a similar but less threatening one (e.g., a child gets angry with his/her parents and hits a younger sister).

(d) Reaction formation - the switching of unacceptable impulses into its opposite (e.g., hugging someone you would like to hit).

(4) Mature mechanisms.

(a) Humor - using comedy to express feelings and thoughts without provoking discomfort in self and others (e.g., making fun of yourself for coming inappropriately dressed for a specific function).

(b) Sublimation - redirecting energy from socially unacceptable impulses to socially acceptable activities (e.g., an angry individual channels that anger into aggressive sports play).

(c) Suppression - consciously or semi-consciously avoiding thinking about disturbing problems, thoughts or feelings (e.g., cleaning closets and drawers while waiting for the results of medical tests).

a. Projective and functional tasks are used to promote self-awareness and the identification of intrapsychic content.

## II. Psychosocial Assessment

### A. Role of the OTA

1. The OTA contributes to the evaluation process in collaboration with the occupational therapist.

a. The OTA can assist with the collection of data for the evaluation once service competency has been established.

b. The level of supervision required will be determined by the OTA's experience and established service competency.

c. The OTA cannot independently evaluate or interpret evaluation results.

### B. Areas Addressed in Assessment

1. Performance skills (i.e., cognitive, perceptual, psychological, and social) and their impact on performance in areas of occupation.

2. Client factors and physical conditions or limitations that impact functional behaviors and performance in areas of occupation.

3. The impact of the individual's social, cultural, spiritual, and physical contexts.

4. Identification of the roles and behaviors that are required of the individual either by society or for the achievement of his/her desired self-determined goals.

5. Precautions and safety issues such as suicidal and/or aggressive behavior.

6. History of behavior patterns.

7. Individual's goals, values, interests, and attitudes.

### C. Assessment Methods

1. Interviews - structured and unstructured.
   a. Occupational profile.
2. Standardized tests.
3. Clinical observation and rating scales.
4. Questionnaires.
5. Self-report inventories.

## III. Psychosocial Intervention

### A. Role of the OTA

1. The OTA implements intervention with OT supervision.

2. The level of supervision required depends upon the OTA's experience and established competency.

3. During the implementation of intervention, the OTA informs the supervising OT of any change in the individual's status and any other relevant information that may affect treatment.

### B. General Treatment Considerations

1. One-to-one versus group intervention.
   a. Indicators for one-to-one intervention.
      (1) Refusal to attend groups.
      (2) Inability to tolerate group interaction.
      (3) Presence of behaviors that would be disruptive to the goals of the group.

(4) The issues that must be addressed are specific to that patient/client only.

b. Indicators for group intervention.

(1) More cost effective.

(2) Effective at assisting members to learn to live in social environments.

(3) Takes advantage of group dynamics and therapeutic milieu.

(a) Groups that are facilitated in a therapeutic manner by an OT practitioner are inherently curative.

(b) See Chapter 3 for a comprehensive review of therapeutic groups and Yalom's curative factors.

2. Factors that influence the effectiveness of treatment.

a. Skillful therapeutic use of self. See Chapter 3.

b. An understanding of the individual's cognitive abilities.

c. Exploration of the needs and wants of the individual.

d. The establishment of realistic goals.

e. Skill with activity analysis. See Chapter 3.

f. An understanding of the realities of the treatment conditions.

g. Prioritization of the most goal-directed use of the person's time.

3. The relationship of treatment activities to desired self-determined goals.

a. Initial treatment may need to focus on the performance skills needed for desired occupational performance.

b. Once basic skills are in place, treatment focuses on performance of functional activities specific to the individual.

(1) Activities that require the actual desired skills or behaviors, in their natural environment, are often the most effective (e.g., assisting the client to use a checking account to pay bills).

(2) Activities that simulate desired behaviors in clinical setting may be less effective (e.g., using kits that simulate checking materials).

(3) Activities that utilize the performance components of desired behaviors and rely on generalization may be the least effective (e.g., practicing arithmetic calculation).

## C. General Group Intervention

1. Taxonomy of groups as described by Anne Mosey.

a. Evaluation groups.

(1) Designed to gather information about the individual's task and group interaction skills that can be used to establish goals and plan treatment.

(2) The primary purpose is assessment. However, they are often therapeutic through process or content.

b. Task-oriented groups.

(1) The purpose is to assist the members in becoming aware of their needs, values, ideas, and feelings through the performance of a shared task.

c. Developmental groups.

(1) The purpose is to assist the members to acquire and develop group interaction skills.

(2) Developmental groups offer five levels of interaction.

(a) Parallel groups use individual tasks with minimal interaction required.

(b) Project groups consist of common, short-term activities requiring some interaction and cooperation.

(c) Egocentric cooperative groups require joint interaction on long-term tasks; however, completion of the task is not the focus. The members are beginning to express their needs and address those of others.

(d) Cooperative groups learn to work together cooperatively, not specifically to complete a task, but to enjoy each other's company and meet emotional needs.

(e) Mature groups are responsive to all members' needs and can carry out a variety of tasks. There is good balance between carrying out the task and meeting the needs of the members.

d. Thematic groups are designed for the learning of specific skills.

e. Topical groups focus on the discussion of activities and issues outside of the group that are current or anticipated.

f. Instrumental groups are concerned with meeting health needs and maintaining function.

g. See Chapter 3 for more detail.

2. The curative factors of groups as described by Irving Yalom.

a. Groups and group activities that are designed to facilitate these curative factors are most effective.

 b. See Chapter 3 for a complete descriptive listing.

3. Considerations in group planning.

 a. Member demographics including gender, age, culture, and ethnicity.

 b. Individual characteristics of members.

  (1) Cognitive level.

  (2) Functional skill level.

  (3) Individual goals.

  (4) Contraindications and safety issues.

 c. Logistical considerations.

  (1) Number of people in the group.

  (2) Length of sessions.

  (3) Number of sessions.

  (4) Space availability.

  (5) Environmental characteristics.

  (6) Budget and materials required.

  (7) Number of leaders.

  (8) Frame of reference.

  (9) Open group vs. closed group.

4. Elements of a group protocol.

 a. Title/name: reflect the purpose or goal of the group (e.g., Communication Skills Group), not the media used, (e.g., Crafts Group).

 b. Purpose: a brief statement of what the group hopes to accomplish (e.g., to improve the members' ability to effectively and appropriately communicate to others their needs and feelings and to enter into satisfying interpersonal relationships).

 c. Rationale: explains the value of this group to the members, and why it is important to offer this service to this population.

 d. Theoretical base/frame of reference: explains in brief and readily understandable terms the theory on which this intervention is based and the rationale for its use.

 e. Criteria for membership: explains who should/ should not be included in the group, and what will indicate when the member will no longer benefit from participation.

 f. Goals/anticipated outcomes: the expectations of what the members will be able to do as a result of having attended this group.

  (1) A list of "Patient/client will…" statements (e.g., patient will be able to initiate and sustain social interactions with peers).

 g. Methodology/format: explains how the group will be carried out.

  (1) Includes the format, scheduling, activities, materials, procedures, etc.

  (2) Includes the information another therapist or OTA would need to lead this group.

 h. Role of the leader: the tasks of the leader in preparing for and conducting the group.

  (1) Includes such things as supplying materials, designing activities, facilitating interaction, providing a safe environment, etc.

  (2) See Chapter 3 for further discussion of leadership roles and styles.

 i. Quality assurance: explains how the need for this intervention and its effectiveness will be monitored.

 j. The actual format used to write protocols varies from setting to setting.

5. Procedure for developing a group.

 a. Conduct a needs assessment to identify intervention needs. (See Chapter 4 for needs assessment procedures).

 b. Develop the protocol.

 c. Present the protocol to the treatment team or program administrators.

 d. Select potential members who would benefit from the group.

 e. Meet with each potential member to explain the purpose and circumstances of the group.

 f. Hold introductory sessions of the group and revise the protocol as needed.

6. Group member leadership roles. See Chapter 3.

7. Considerations in activity selection.

 a. Degree of structure (inherent or imposed).

 b. Type(s) and degree of instruction provided.

 c. Degree of new learning required.

 d. Complexity of the activity.

 e. Length of time for completion.

 f. Nature and degree of skill required for engagement and completion.

 g. Degree of challenge to the members' skills.

**D. Intervention Groups**

1. Directive groups as developed by Kathy Kaplan.

 a. These are highly structured groups designed to assist low functioning patients in developing basic skills.

 b. Each session is divided into five parts followed by a 15 minute review of the session by the leaders.

  (1) Part I consists of an orientation to the purpose and goals of the group (maximum of 5 minutes).

  (2) Part II involves a review of everyone's

name and the introduction of new members (5-10 minutes).

   (3) Part III consists of warm-up activities to make members comfortable and engage them in the group (5-10 minutes).

   (4) Part IV involves one or more activities designed to address the goals of the group and the needs of its members (10-20 minutes).

   (5) Part V includes activities designed to give meaning to the activities and closure to the group (10 minutes).

2. Mildred Ross' Five Stage groups.

  a. Expanded on the sensory integration work of Lorna Jean King which examined the sensory distortions, postural disturbances, and vestibular stimulating activities that were observed in individuals with chronic schizophrenia.

   (1) King proposed that using non-cortical, alerting, stimulating, and pleasurable activities (e.g., parachute games) would normalize movement patterns, increase strength and flexibility, and facilitate adaptive behaviors.

  b. Ross extended the use of sensorimotor approaches to other chronic populations including persons with intellectual disabilities, Alzheimer's disease, neurological impairment, etc.

  c. Stage I consists of orienting the members to the session and each other.

  d. Stage II uses a variety of vigorous gross motor activities designed to be stimulating and alerting.

  e. Stage III uses brief (30 minutes or less) activities that utilize perceptual-motor skills designed to be calming and to increase ability to focus.

  f. Stage IV includes activities to provide cognitive stimulation to promote organized thinking.

  g. Stage V consists of brief discussions to promote a sense of satisfaction and closure.

3. Modular groups.

  a. The focus of each session is rotated in a way that allows an individual to join the group at any time and still cover each topic (e.g., an Independent Living Skills group that addresses nutrition the first session, money management the second, transportation the third, etc. and then begins the cycle again with a session on

nutrition).

4. Psychoeducational groups.

  a. An intervention approach that uses a classroom format and the principles of learning to provide information to members and to teach skills.

  b. A teacher/student relationship exists.

  c. The use of homework assignments is encouraged to facilitate skill development and generalization of learning.

5. Basic task skills groups.

  a. Include intervention activities designed to develop the basic cognitive skills necessary for the completion of simple tasks.

6. Social interaction groups.

  a. Include interventions to develop communication skills, socially acceptable behavior, and interpersonal relationship skills.

  b. May be conducted in a modular and/or psychoeducational format.

7. ADL/IADL groups.

  a. Focus is on self-care and independent living skills such as cooking, money management, transportation, etc.

  b. May be conducted in a modular and/or psychoeducational format.

8. Community participation.

  a. Focuses on identification and use of resources.

  b. May be conducted in a modular and/or psychoeducational format.

9. Prevocational.

  a. Includes such topics as identification of skills, limitations, interests, work behaviors, and job hunting skills.

10. Leisure.

  a. May include identification of interests, development of activity specific skills, identification of resources, and recognition of the importance of healthy use of unstructured time.

11. Reminiscence.

  a. Activities are designed to review past life experiences to promote cognition and a sense of personal worth.

  b. Current memory is not necessary nor is it facilitated.

12. Sensory awareness.

  a. Includes activities to promote sensory functions and environmental awareness.

13. Self-awareness.

  a. Includes such activities as values clarification, awareness of personal assets, limitations, and behaviors; and the individual's impact on others.

14. Goal setting.
   a. Consists of activities designed to identify personal objectives and treatment goals and the steps to their achievement.

15. Coping skills.
   a. Focuses on identifying the problem-solving and stress-management techniques needed to cope with life stressors.

16. Discharge planning.
   a. Focuses on activities to problem-solve potential obstacles and identify resources for successful community reintegration.

**E. Managing Problem Behaviors**

1. Hallucinations.
   a. Create an environment free of distractions that trigger hallucinatory thoughts and interfere with reality-based activity.
   b. Use highly structured simple, concrete activities that hold the individual's attention.
   c. When the person appears to be focusing on a hallucinatory experience, attempt to redirect him/her to reality-based thinking and actions.

2. Delusions.
   a. Redirect the individual's thoughts to reality-based thinking and actions.
   b. Avoid discussions and other experiences that focus on and validate or reinforce delusional material.

3. Akathisia.
   a. Allow the person to move around as needed if it can be done without causing disruption to the goals of the group.
   b. Keep in mind that participation on many levels and in many forms can be beneficial to the individual.
   c. Whenever possible, select gross motor activities over fine motor or sedentary ones.

4. Offensive behavior (physical or verbal).
   a. Set limits and immediately address the behavior during a session.
   b. Reasons that the behavior is not acceptable should be clearly presented in a manner that is not confrontational or judgmental.
   c. The consequences of continued offensive behavior should be clearly communicated.
   d. It is required that staff protects all patients from the threat of harm or abuse by another patient. The needs of the entire unit and/or group membership must be kept in mind.

5. Lack of initiation/participation.
   a. Together with the individual, identify the reasons for lack of participation, e.g., lack of skill, irrelevance of activity, attention deficits, embarrassment, depression, etc.
   b. Motivational hints.
      (1) Individuals are more likely to participate in activities that address issues that are of interest or concern to them.
      (2) The more ownership people have of the activity, the more they will participate.
      (3) Success is motivating.
      (4) Fun is motivating.
      (5) Positive feedback and rewards are motivating.
      (6) Everyone has his/her own motivators. It is important to identify what they are.
      (7) Curiosity can be used to motivate.
      (8) Food is often motivating (as per Maslow's hierarchy of needs; see Chapter 5).
         (a) Using secondary reinforcers such as praise is usually preferable to using primary reinforcers such as food.

6. Manic or monopolizing behavior.
   a. Select or design highly structured activities that hold the individual's attention and require a shift of focus from patient to patient.
   b. Thank the individual for their participation and redirect attention to another group member.
   c. Refer to limit-setting discussed above.

7. Escalating behavior.
   a. Avoid what can be perceived as challenging behavior (e.g., eye contact, standing directly in front of the patient).
   b. Maintain a comfortable distance.
   c. Actively listen.
   d. Use a calm, but not patronizing, tone.
      (1) Speaking in a softer or lower tone than the individual is often effective in decreasing the volume and intensity of the escalating individual.
   e. Speak simply, clearly, and directly. Avoid miscommunication.
   f. Do not make or communicate value judgments about the individual's thoughts, feelings, or behaviors.
   g. Clearly present what you would like the person to do.
   h. Avoid positions where either you or the patient feels trapped.

i. Individuals most often calm in response to the above interventions. If an individual continues to escalate and is nonresponsive to interventions, additional steps are needed to ensure safety.
   (1) Remove other patients from the area.
   (2) Get or send for other staff.

8. The effects of Alzheimer's disease.
   a. Make eye contact and show that you are interested in the person.
      (1) Value and validate what is said by the person.
   b. Maintain a positive and friendly facial expression and tone of voice during all communications.
      (1) Do not give orders.
      (2) Use short, simple words and sentences.
      (3) Do not argue or criticize.
   c. Do not speak about the individual as if he/she was not there.
   d. Use non-verbal communication.
   e. Create a routine that uses familiar and enjoyable activities.
      (1) Use activities that demonstrate and promote personal interests and independence.
      (2) Do not introduce infantilizing activities.
      (3) Analyze and grade activities carefully.
      (4) Do not rush activities.
         (a) It is the process of engaging in an activity that is important; task completion is not needed.
   f. Note the effects of the time of day on behavior and activity performance.
   g. Attend to safety issues at all times.

# IV. Special Considerations in Psychosocial Evaluation and Intervention

## A. Domestic Abuse

1. Facts and figures.
   a. Ninety percent of abuse is committed by men against women.
   b. Four million women are victims of domestic violence each year.
   c. Four women are killed every day by domestic violence.
   d. Seventy percent of men who abuse their partners also abuse their children.
   e. Children who witness domestic violence are 74% more likely to commit assaults against others.
   f. Fifty percent of homeless women and children are homeless because of violence at home.
   g. Many incidents involve alcohol and/or drug use.
   h. Domestic abuse knows no boundaries. It occurs regardless of socioeconomic factors, race, culture, ethnicity, religion, or age.

2. Definition and types.
   a. Definitions vary greatly from state to state.
   b. Definitions involve violence or abuse that is used to control another member of the household.
   c. Domestic abuse can take one or more forms.
      (1) Physical abuse: hitting, kicking, punching, slapping, choking, and/or burning.
      (2) Emotional abuse: criticizing, humiliating, playing mind games, abusing or killing pets, withholding affection, isolating, and/or dominating.
      (3) Economic abuse: making the other ask for money, giving an allowance, and/or preventing the other from taking a job.
      (4) Intimidation and coercion: making the other afraid, breaking things, displaying weapons, threatening to leave or report the other for something, and/or making the other do something illegal.
      (5) Using children: making the other feel guilty about the children, using the children to relay messages, using visitation to harass the other, and/or threatening to take the children away.
      (6) Stalking: following, having followed, invading home and privacy, and/or creating fear of immediate harm.
      (7) Sexual abuse: performing and/or requiring the other to perform unwanted sexual activities through force, threats, or intimidation.
   d. Patterns of abuse.
      (1) Impulsive abuse, during which the abuser has sudden attacks of rage, which may be regular or random.
      (2) Premeditated abuse, during which the abuser is cool and calculating.

3. Signs of physical abuse.
   a. Bruises at different stages of healing or in unusual places.
   b. Burns suggestive of specific objects.
   c. Lacerations to the face or genitals.
   d. Orthopedic injuries that are inconsistent with the explanations.

e. Internal injuries of the head and organs.

f. Head and facial injuries suggestive of hitting, shaking, or pulling.

g. Reluctance to talk about injuries.

h. Abuser not wanting to leave victim alone with others.

4. Reasons for failure to report or leave an abusive relationship.

  a. Economic pressure.

  b. Religious beliefs.

  c. Feeling of love for abuser.

  d. Believing the abuse is deserved.

  e. Viewing abuse as normal due to exposure to abuse/violence as a child.

  f. Fear of increasing abuse.

  g. Fear of retaliation.

  h. Belief things will change.

  i. Concern for children.

  j. Nowhere to go.

  k. Lack of support systems.

5. Role of OT practitioners.

  a. Refer to domestic shelters/safe houses. The National Hotline is 800-799-7233.

  b. Develop a trusting relationship.

  c. Provide information about treatment and support programs.

  d. Provide treatment for physical and emotional injuries and to develop independent living skills.

  e. Inform supervisor and or other treatment staff.

  f. Mandatory reporting is required in some states, but laws vary.

  g. Areas to discuss with person who has been/is being abused.

    (1) Stress and safety.

    (2) Fear and abuse.

    (3) Family, friends, and support network.

    (4) Emergency plan.

**B. Child Abuse**

1. See Section X in Chapter 5.

**C. Elder Abuse**

1. See Section XI J in Chapter 5.

**D. Patient/Client Abuse**

1. See Section I D in Chapter 3.

**E. Psychological Reaction to Disability**

1. Several factors influence the individual's reaction to disability.

  a. Permanency of the disability.

  b. Sudden vs. chronic onset.

  c. Appraisal of life experiences.

  d. Spiritual beliefs.

  e. Support systems.

  f. Cultural factors.

2. Adjustment.

  a. Active participation in social, vocational, and avocational pursuits.

  b. Successful negotiation of the physical environment.

  c. Awareness of remaining strengths and assets as well as functional limitations.

3. Phases of adjustment.

  a. Shock.

    (1) Initial reaction to a sudden physical or psychological trauma.

    (2) Characterized by emotional numbness, depersonalization, and reduced speech and mobility.

  b. Anxiety.

    (1) A panic-stricken reaction to awareness of the seriousness of the situation.

    (2) Characterized by restlessness, confusion, racing thoughts and psychological symptoms associated with anxiety.

  c. Denial.

    (1) Retreat from the realization of the seriousness and implications of the situation.

    (2) Characterized by minimization, negation, aloofness, and unrealistic expectations.

  d. Depression.

    (1) Bereavement for the associated losses as the realities of those losses are identified.

    (2) Characterized by hopelessness, helplessness, isolation, and decreased self-esteem.

  e. Internalized anger.

    (1) Resentment and bitterness directed towards self.

    (2) Characterized by blaming of self for the event, the extent of the loss, or the failure to recover.

  f. Externalized anger.

    (1) An attempt to retaliate for the imposed losses, directed against those associated with the onset or rehabilitation of the situation.

    (2) Characterized by aggression, antagonism, demanding and critical attitudes, and passive-aggressive behavior.

  g. Acknowledgement.

    (1) The first step towards acceptance of the situation.

(2) Characterized by acceptance of a new self-concept and the identification of values and goals.

h. Adjustment.

(1) An emotional acceptance of the situation and reintegration into identified roles.

(2) Characterized by a positive sense of self and potentialities, and achievement of meaningful goals.

4. OT intervention.

a. Identification of what the individual is able to do with emphasis on personal accomplishments.

b. Assistance to the individual in his/her assumption of an active role in shaping his/her life.

c. Reduction of limitations through changes in the physical and social environment.

d. Development of the skills necessary to participate in valued activities and meaningful occupations.

F. **Suicide.**

1. Facts and Figures

a. In the United States, suicide is a major social justice crisis and health care concern. The below facts and figures are provided to highlight the need for OTAs to be vigilant about the potential of suicide during all interactions with all clients and family members, regardless of age. These statistics will not be on the NBCOT examination.

b. In the United States, suicide is a leading cause of death. In 2006, it was seventh for males, sixteenth for females, and third for young people ages 15 to 24.

c. It is estimated that there are 12 to 25 nonfatal suicide attempts for every suicide death.

d. The attempts of men and the elderly are more likely to be more fatal than those of women and youth.

(1) The suicide rate for men is more than 4 times that of women due to men using firearms at a higher rate than women.

(2) The elderly commit suicide at twice the rate of younger adults due to the losses associated with age.

e. The suicide rate is increasing in children and adolescents.

f. Single individuals who were never married commit suicide at twice the rate of those who are or were married.

2. Identification of risk.

a. A member of the treatment team (usually physician) will ask the individual about suicidal thinking.

b. It is important to identify the degree of risk.

(1) The person is usually asked, if he/she was to try to hurt him/herself, how he/she would do it.

(2) The degree of detail given indicates the seriousness of intent.

(3) The potential for the plan to succeed also indicates the degree of risk.

(4) The preparation of a will and/or expression of concern for the effect of suicide on family members indicate the seriousness of intent.

c. Risk factors for suicide

(1) Previous attempt or fantasized suicide.

(2) Anxiety, depression, exhaustion, pervasive pessimism or hopelessness.

(3) Resignation after agitated depression.

(4) Availability of means of suicide; i.e., firearms in the home.

(5) Verbalized suicidal ideation.

(6) Proximal life crisis, such as mourning, pending surgery, divorce.

(7) Family history of suicide, exposure to suicide of others.

(8) Family violence, including physical or sexual abuse

(9) Clinically diagnosed depression or other mental disorder.

(10) Alcohol and other substance abuse.

(11) Incarceration

3. OT intervention.

a. Identification of the motivation behind the suicidal intention and the identification of alternatives.

b. Development of problem solving skills and stress management techniques to increase the individual's ability to manage life stressors.

c. Identification of positive goals and interests to increase motivation for recovery.

d. Identification of positive personal attributes and support systems to increase hopefulness.

(1) This may be facilitated by a review of past successes.

e. Activities that produce successful outcomes, especially those with a visible end-product, promote positive thinking.

f. Activities designed for the expression and validation of feelings.

  g.  Moderate physical activity elevates mood.

  h.  Development of skills that increase functional performance.

## G. Adjustment to Death and Dying

1.  Stages of the individual's response as described by Elizabeth Kubler-Ross.

  a.  Denial.

   (1)  A coping strategy that allows the individual to refuse to accept or address the reality of his/her illness (e.g., "There must have been a mistake with the x-rays").

   (2)  Denial may lead the individual to see many health professionals, hoping to find the one who will give a different prognosis.

   (3)  Denial may be a response to the denial or discomfort experienced by others.

   (4)  Denial will end when the individual is psychologically prepared to face the reality of the situation.

   (5)  OT intervention includes allowing the person to ask questions and discuss the situation at his/her own pace.

  b.  Anger.

   (1)  The individual becomes angry as he/she accepts the reality of impending death (e.g., "Get out of here. You don't know what it's like.").

   (2)  This anger may be projected onto anyone who is seen as healthy or in a better position.

   (3)  Rages, outbursts, and hurtful behavior must be identified for the purposes they serve.

   (4)  OT intervention allows the individual to vent anger while identifying its source and developing more effective coping strategies.

  c.  Bargaining.

   (1)  In an attempt to gain control, the individual may bargain with doctors, caretakers or God (e.g., "Just let me go to my son's graduation and then I'll be okay with this.").

   (2)  Bargains are an attempt to buy time.

   (3)  Bargains are often associated with guilt related to things not done or promises not kept.

   (4)  The individual should not be expected to keep to these bargains.

   (5)  OT intervention involves responding honestly to questions.

  d.  Depression.

   (1)  As the individual acknowledges impending death, he/she begins to identify the feelings of loss and become depressed.

   (2)  The tendency is to say good-byes to all but a few and isolate oneself as thoughts and feelings turn inward.

   (3)  Physical contact or just being together replaces conversation.

   (4)  OT intervention assists in providing physical and psychological comfort for both the individual and his/her loved ones.

  e.  Acceptance.

   (1)  As the individual recognizes impending death, he/she begins to make plans and think about the future for self and family.

   (2)  It may be a time of peace without fear or despair.

   (3)  As time goes on, the need to communicate diminishes.

   (4)  OT intervention is to provide ongoing support to the individual and family.

2.  General considerations.

  a.  People vary in the way they go through each stage.

  b.  They may stop at any stage (e.g., some may stay in denial as their preferred coping strategy).

  c.  The needs of loved ones must be considered as they are likely going through stages similar to the dying individual.

  d.  Occupational therapy practitioners should assist the individual in coping with each stage without pushing for progression into the next stage.

3.  Occupational therapy intervention throughout each stage.

  a.  Assist the individual in maintaining as much control and independence as possible.

  b.  Respond honestly and at the appropriate depth to questions.

  c.  Assist the individual in developing coping skills.

  d.  Encourage positive life review and support the legacies the individual leaves.

   (1)  Gifts and mementos can be made or selected for significant others.

  e.  Assist the individual in pursuing interests and maintaining meaningful roles.

  f.  Actively listen.

  g.  Incorporate family and friends into the treatment process.

h. While being realistic, the OT practitioner should not deprive the individual of hope.

# References

Allen, C.K., Earhart, C.A., & Blue, T. (1992). *Occupational therapy treatment goals for the physically and cognitively disabled.* Rockville, MD: American Occupational Therapy Association.

American Occupational Therapy Association. (2008). Occupational therapy practice framework: Domain and process, 2nd edition. *American Journal of Occupational Therapy, 62,* 625-688.

Alzheimer's Association. (2003). www.alz.com

Artemis Center for Alternatives to Domestic Violence (2001). *The facts.* Available:www.artemiscenter.org/facts.

Bruce, M. & Borg, B. (2002). *Psychosocial frames of reference: Core for occupation-based practice, 3rd ed.* Thorofare, NJ: Slack.

Cole, M.B. (2005). *Group dynamics in occupational therapy: The thoretical basis and practice application of group dynamics, 3rd ed.* Thorofare, NJ: Slack.

Domestic Abuse. (2001). *Metro Nashville Police Department.* Available: www.telalink.net/~police/abuse/symptoms.htm.

Early, M. (2009). *Mental health techniques and concepts for the occupational therapy assistant.* Philadelphia: Lippincott Williams and Wilkins.

Fidler, G.S. (1996). Life-style performance: From profile to conceptual model. In R.P. Cottrell (Ed), *Perspectives on purposeful activity: Foundation and future of occupational therapy* (pp. 113-121). Bethesda, MD: American Occupational Therapy Association.

Fleming-Castaldy, R. (2009). Activities, human occupation, participation, and empowerment. In J. Hinojosa & M. L. Blount (Eds.). *The texture of life: Purposeful activities in occupational therapy,* 3rd ed. (pp. 483- 521) Bethesda, MD: AOTA Press.

Greenward, B. (2001). *Death and dying.* Available: www.uic.edu/orgs/convening/deathdyi.htm.

Helfrich, C. A. (2000). Domestic violence: Implications and guidelines for occupational therapy practitioners. In R.P. Cottrell (Ed.), *Proactive approaches in psychosocial occupational therapy* (pp. 309-316). Thorofare, NJ: Slack.

Hemphill, B.J. (Ed.) (1988). *Mental health assessment in occupational therapy.* Thorofare, NJ: Slack.

Hopkins, H. & Smith, H. (Eds.). (2003). *Willard and Spackman's occupational therapy (10th ed.).* Philadelphia: J.B. Lippincott.

Hussey, S.; Sabonis-Chafee, B.; & O'Brien, J. (2007). *Introduction to occupational therapy, (3rd ed.).* St. Louis, MO: Elsevier Mosby.

Kielhofner, G. (2004). *Conceptual foundations of occupational therapy (3rd ed.)* Philadelphia: F.A. Davis.

Miller, P.J., & Walker, K.F. (Eds.) (1993). *Perspectives on theory for the practice of occupational therapy.* Gaithersburg, MD: Aspen Publishers.

Mosey, A.C. (1996). *Psychosocial components of occupational therapy.* New York: Raven Press.

National Institute of Mental Health (NIMH). (2009). *Suicide in the U.S.: Statistics and prevention.* Retrieved February 24, 2010, from http://www.nimh.nih.gov/health/publications/suicide-in-the-us-statistics-and-prevention/index.shtml#factors

Schkade, J.K., & Schultz, S. (1999). Occupational adaptation: Toward a holistic approach for contemporary practice, part 1, *American Journal of Occupational Therapy 46,* 829-837.

Schkade, J.K., & Schultz, S. (1999). Occupational adaptation: Toward a holistic approach for contemporary practice, part 2, *American Journal of Occupational Therapy 46,* 917-925.

# CHAPTER 14

# EVALUATION AND INTERVENTION FOR PERFORMANCE IN AREAS OF OCCUPATION

Rita P. Fleming-Castaldy

## I. Occupational Performance

### A. Definition

1. The engagement in, and completion of activities of daily living, work and productive activities, and play/leisure activities.

### B. Areas of Occupation

1. Activities of daily living (ADL) are often delineated into basic and instrumental tasks.
   a. Basic ADL (BADL) includes self-care tasks such as grooming, oral hygiene, bathing/showering, toilet hygiene, dressing, and eating. This is also termed "personal" activities of daily living (PADL).
   b. Instrumental ADL (IADL) includes home management tasks such as shopping, money management and meal preparation and community mobility.
2. Work includes competitive employment for pay and other productive activities that make a societal contribution, such as volunteer work.
3. Education includes activities needed to participate in a learning environment and fulfill the role of student.
4. Play/leisure includes discretionary activities done for pleasure, diversion, and entertainment.
5. Social participation includes activities engaged in as a member of a community, family, and/or peer/friend group.

6. Refer to Appendix 1 for a complete listing of areas of occupational performance as defined in AOTA's Practice Framework.

## II. Evaluation of Occupational Performance

### A. Overall Guidelines

1. The OTA contributes to the evaluation process by collecting data and sharing observations.
   a. Service competency must be established to ensure data will be collected effectively and safely.
   b. The level of supervision needed for the collection of evaluation data by the OTA will depend upon the OTA's experience and established service competence.
   c. The OTA cannot independently evaluate occupational performance.
2. The focus of OT evaluation must be the individual's ability to perform meaningful occupations that are needed and desired by the individual.
3. Assessments should follow a "top down" progression of considering the person's occupations first, rather than a "bottoms up" approach which focuses on performance components/skills.
   a. The first step in the evaluation process is obtaining "an understanding of the client's occupational history and experiences, patterns of daily living, interests, values, and needs"

(AOTA, 2008, p.646).

b. The desired outcome of evaluation is the identification of the person's occupational performance concerns and difficulties and the establishment of the individual's priorities for performance in areas of occupation.

c. In the OT Practice Framework, this determination is called the occupational profile.

4. After the completion of a person's occupational profile, the person's client factors, performance skills, patterns, and contexts, and activity demands are assessed to identify specific strengths and limitations that impact on desired and needed occupational performance.

a. All of the factors that may influence performance in areas of occupation are considered during screening.

(1) Based on the results of screening, aspects that are determined to warrant further evaluation are specifically assessed.

b. In certain practice settings (e.g., acute care with a 3 day length of stay) and in certain clinical situations (e.g., there are major concerns for a client's safety) this determination of underlying problems may take precedence over the determination of an occupational profile.

c. To determine these capabilities, the evaluation process should include observation of the person's actual performance of an activity in context.

(1) If it is pragmatically not possible during the evaluation process for the person to perform the activity in its natural context, an environment that closely simulates the natural one should be provided for the assessment (e.g., an ADL apartment on a rehabilitation unit to simulate the person's home).

d. In the OT Practice Framework, this part of the evaluation process is called an analysis of occupational performance.

5. Occupational performance assessment tools include interviews, checklists, task performance, rating scales, and standardized instruments.

**B. Evaluation of BADL and IADL**

1. Occupational performance assessment tools typically delineate activities of daily living (ADL) into basic and instrumental tasks.

a. Basic ADL (BADL) includes self-care tasks such as grooming, oral hygiene, bathing/showering, toilet hygiene, dressing, and eating. This is also termed personal ADL (PADL).

b. Instrumental ADL (IADL) includes home management tasks such as shopping, money management and meal preparation; and community mobility.

2. Many assessment tools used to measure occupational performance provide a determination of the person's level of functional performance (Table 14-1).

3. Interpretation of BADL and IADL assessments to determine a person's functional capabilities and ability to live independently are made by the occupational therapist.

a. The OTA contributes to this determination process.

b. Due to the self-report and/or simulated nature of certain items and the limited number of

---

### TABLE 14-1
### SCALES TO MEASURE FUNCTIONAL PERFORMANCE

**TOTAL ASSISTANCE:**
The need for 100% assistance by one or more persons to perform all physical activities and/or cognitive assistance to elicit a functional response to an external stimulation.

**MAXIMUM ASSISTANCE:**
The need for 75% assistance by one person to physically perform any part of a functional activity and/or cognitive assistance to perform gross motor actions in response to direction.

**MODERATE ASSISTANCE:**
The need for 50% assistance by one person to perform physical activities or provide cognitive assistance to sustain/complete simple, repetitive activities safely.

**MINIMUM ASSISTANCE:**
The need for 25% assistance by one person for physical activities and/or periodic, cognitive assistance to perform functional activities safely.

**STANDBY ASSISTANCE:**
The need for supervision by one person for the patient to perform new activity procedures that were adapted by the therapist for safe and effective performance. A patient requires standby assistance when errors and the need for safety precautions are not always anticipated by the patient.

**INDEPENDENT STATUS:**
No physical or cognitive assistance is required to perform functional activities. Patients at this level are able to implement the selected courses of action, consider potential errors, and anticipate safety hazards in familiar and new situations.

Adapted from Health Care Financing Administration. (1996). *Medicare intermediary manual, Publication 13, Section 3906.4.* Washington, DC: U.S. Government Printing Office, 21-21.

items tested in many evaluation tools, interpretations must be made cautiously.

**C. Sexual Expression/Activity Evaluation**

1. The ADL skill of sexual expression/activity is typically not included on commonly used ADL assessments and it does not have a published OT assessment available for clinical use.

2. The OT practitioner should assess this ADL during routine screenings and interviews, as appropriate.

3. The OTA contributes to the assessment of this ADL in collaboration with the OT supervisor.

   a. The aims of this process are to:

   (1) Determine if sexual expression/activity is valued.

   (2) Identify potential obstacles for the attainment and maintenance of safe, satisfying sexual expression/activity.

   (a) Pathophysiological changes related to disease, disability, and/or the aging process.

   (b) Psychological and/or cognitive changes related to disease, disability and/or the aging process.

   • Judgment, impulse control, and decision-making skills must be assessed to ensure safety.

   (c) Limited partner availability due to social demographics and/or sociocultural attitudes.

   (3) Determine if a person's knowledge of his/her sexuality is adequate and appropriate for his/her age, developmental level, expected roles, and environmental contexts.

4. If an individual is reticent about discussing his/her sexuality during the OT evaluation, the practitioner must respect and accept this preference.

   a. Sexual concerns that are unexpressed during initial OT sessions are often brought forth during later sessions as a therapeutic relationship develops between the individual and his/her OT practitioner.

   b. Sessions focused on intimate self-care issues frequently precipitate questions regarding sexuality.

   c. An atmosphere of continuing permission to discuss sexual expression should be maintained throughout the person's engagement in OT.

5. The potential realities of sexual abuse, assault, and exploitation must be considered during the evaluation of all individuals regardless of age.

   a. OT practitioners are required by practice acts, protective legislation, and our professional code of ethics to report any suspected incidents of child, adult, or elder abuse, exploitation, or assault to the appropriate agency and/or local law enforcement.

**D. Family Participation and Parenting/Childcare Evaluation**

1. There are no specific OT published assessments that deal exclusively with family interaction.

   a. Many commonly used assessments include family interaction (e.g., the Role Checklist).

2. The OT practitioner should assess this occupational performance during routine screenings and interviews.

3. The OTA contributes to the assessment of this occupational performance in collaboration with the OT supervisor.

   a. The aims of this process are to:

   (1) Determine past, current, and anticipated roles, responsibilities, and expectations of family members.

   (2) Determine parent(s)' ability to care for child's physical needs.

   (3) Determine parent(s)' ability to care for child's emotional needs.

   (4) Determine parent(s)' knowledge of child's developmental level and its corresponding play and communication level.

   (5) Identify potential obstacles for the attainment and maintenance of satisfying family interaction.

   b. If the family and the OT practitioner do not share a common language, interpreters must be used to ensure the validity of information obtained.

   c. The sociocultural background, values, and dynamics of the family must be considered during the evaluation process.

   d. Individuals who live in shared residential settings such as nursing homes, group homes, and assisted living facilities and their families should receive intervention to assist with role transitions.

   (1) Fellow residents and staff in these settings, often assume the roles of surrogate family members.

**E. Play/Leisure Evaluation**

1. The OTA contributes to the assessment of this occupational performance during routine screen-

ings and interviews, in collaboration with the OT supervisor.

a. The OTA may administer specific play/leisure assessments as determined by service competency.

(1) Assessment tools for play and leisure include interviews, checklists, task performance, rating scales, and standardized instruments.

b. The aims of this process are to:

(1) Determine the individual's perception of the meaning of leisure and the extent the individual participates in leisure activities.

(2) Identify motivational and situational issues that influence leisure (e.g., perceived barriers to leisure and knowledge of leisure opportunities).

(3) Determine a child's or adolescent's developmental level and the adequacy of his/her play environments.

(4) Identify ways leisure or play activities can be modified to better meet individual needs.

c. If the family and the OT practitioner do not share a common language, interpreters must be used to ensure the validity of information obtained.

## F. Work Evaluation

1. Prevocational Assessment Process

a. The OTA contributes to this process with OT supervision. The aims of this process are to:

(1) Screen to identify deficits in occupational performance areas, client factors, and/or performance skills that could impact on work abilities and potential.

(2) Determine if the individual is interested in prevocational assessment and intervention.

(3) Gather relevant work, educational, social and medical history information.

(4) Identify prevocational interests through the use of interest inventories and/or structured interviews.

(5) Assess current level of work-related skills. (Table 14-2 for a listing of essential behavior skills).

(6) Conduct structured observations of an individual performing work tasks or work samples in a prevocational group or vocational rehabilitation workshop or during a job simulation.

(7) Administer standardized work assessments.

- Aptitude tests to determine individual's strengths and weaknesses in a variety of areas such as verbal and numerical abilities.

- Behavioral and personality tests to determine personality characteristics, attitudes, motivators, and intra- and inter-personal strengths.

- Manual dexterity tests to determine motor coordination skills such as speed and accuracy in performing motor tasks.

(8) Determine if the individual can return to past employment.

(a) Identify existing abilities and supports.

(b) Identify existing limitations and barriers.

(c) Determine the need for a job analysis.

(d) Identify needed reasonable accommodations.

(9) Determine if pre-vocational and/or vocational training is indicated.

(10) Refer to Table 14-3 for an overview of the prevocational assessment process.

2. Work assessment.

a. The OTA contributes to this process with OT supervision.

b. If service competency is established the OTA may collect data under the supervision of the occupational therapist in the following areas:

(1) Initial screening and prevocational assessment as described above.

(2) Functional capacity evaluation (FCE) which evaluates an individual's capabilities in relation to one of several dimensions.

(a) The physical demands of a job which is often termed a physical capacity evaluation to assess the physical demands of a job according to the descriptions provided in the Dictionary of Occupational Titles (DOT), (e.g., the Smith Physical Capacity Evaluation).

(b) The critical demands of a specific job.

(c) The critical demands of an occupational group.

(d) The demands of competitive employment.

(3) Work capacity evaluation using real or simulated work activities to assess an individual's ability to return to work (e.g., Valpar Work Samples or BTE).

(4) Job site analysis to evaluate its expectations, supports, ergonomics, essential functions of the job, the marginal functions of the job and the potential reasonable accommodations in accordance with ADA.

   c. See Table 14-4 for assessment guidelines for determining the general ergonomic risks of work tasks.

   d. See Table 14-5 for assessment guidelines for determining the ergonomic risks of computer work.

   e. Refer to Chapter 4 for ADA information.

## III. Intervention for Occupational Performance Deficits

### A. Overview

1. The OTA implements intervention with OT supervision.
2. Intervention should follow a "top down" progression of considering the person's occupation first rather than a "bottoms up" approach which focuses initially and/or solely on performance components/skills.

   a. The impact of performance skill deficits and

## TABLE 14-2 - WORK BEHAVIOR SKILLS

| PHYSICAL TOLERANCE & DEMANDS | SENSORY/PERCEPTION | MOTOR |
|---|---|---|
| • Work pace/rhythm<br>• Standing tolerance<br>• Sitting tolerance<br>• Endurance<br>• Performance with repetition<br>• Muscle strength<br>• Walking<br>• Lifting<br>• Carrying<br>• Pushing<br>• Pulling<br>• Climbing | • Color discrimination<br>• Form perception<br>• Size discrimination<br>• Spatial relationship<br>• Ability to follow visual instruction<br>• Texture discrimination<br>• Digital discrimination<br>• Figure-ground<br>• Form constancy<br>• Visual closure<br>• Parts-to-whole<br>• Shape discrimination<br>• Kinesthesia | • Finger dexterity<br>• Manual dexterity<br>• Coordination:<br>  – eye-hand<br>  – eye-hand-foot<br>  – fine motor<br>  – gross motor<br>  – bimanual<br>  – bilateral<br>• Use of hand tools<br>• ROM:<br>  – stooping<br>  – kneeling<br>  – crouching<br>  – crawling<br>  – reaching<br>• Balancing |

| DAILY LIVING SKILLS | COGNITION | AFFECTIVE |
|---|---|---|
| • Self care:<br>  – personal hygiene<br>  – grooming<br>  – dressing<br>  – eating/feeding<br>  – object manipulation<br>• Mobility<br>  – transfers<br>  – travel (mode of)<br>  – transportation<br>• Communication<br>  – with peers<br>  – with supervisor<br>  – writing<br>  – dialing phone<br>  – talking on phone<br>  – typing | • Numerical ability<br>• Measuring ability<br>• Safety consciousness<br>• Care in handling work and tools<br>• Work quality<br>• Accuracy<br>• Neatness<br>• Attention span<br>• Planning/organization<br>• Ability to follow:<br>  – verbal instruction<br>  – written instruction<br>• Retention of instruction<br>• Work judgment<br>• Ability to learn new task<br>• Orientation | • Attendance<br>• Punctuality<br>• Response to:<br>  – praise<br>  – criticism<br>  – assistance<br>  – frustrating situation<br>• Relationship with<br>  – evaluator<br>  – co-worker<br>• Work flexibility<br>• Attitude toward work<br>• Behavior in structured setting<br>• Ability to work independently<br>• Initiative<br><br>(In psychiatry you would also observe for additional pathological behavior.) |

• Wayne County Community College, Occupational Therapy Assistant Program

client factors on occupational performance is considered after the establishment of individual's desired occupational outcome.

b. Specific interventions to remediate, alleviate, and/or compensate for the effects of performance component/skill deficits on occupational performance are often required.

---

### TABLE 14-3 - OCCUPATIONAL THERAPY PREVOCATIONAL ASSESSMENT PROCESS

**GATHER BACKGROUND INFORMATION**

1. Work history, education, and training background
2. Current medications and their side effects
3. History of mental and physical illnesses
4. Factors/stressors influencing symptomatology

**DETERMINE CONSUMER WORK INTERESTS AND SUPPORT SYSTEMS**

1. Available emotional support persons
2. Cultural/familial influences affecting employment
3. Skills needed for most recent employment
   a. Is that job still available?
   b. Will employer rehire?
   c. Are skills still in place?
   d. Does patient want to return to the job?

**RETURN TO MOST RECENT EMPLOYMENT**

1. Identify job stressors
2. Identify accommodations needed to stay employed
3. Identify strategies needed to be practiced to return to work (e.g., relaxation techniques, medication management, cognitive therapy, etc.)
4. Which employment opportunities are considered desired by consumer?
   a. Which skills are needed for identified employment?
   b. What training is needed?
   c. Is a job analysis needed?

**ASSESS SKILL LEVEL FOR EMPLOYMENT OPPORTUNITY**

1. Determine assessments directly relating to employment tasks
   a. Work tolerance screening
   b. Functional capacity evaluation
   c. Simulated job try-out
   d. Work samples
   e. Standardized assessments for specific job tasks
2. Consider a work behavior assessment
3. Determine job interview skills

**ASSESS FOR REASONABLE ACCOMMODATIONS**

Reprinted with permission from Hemphill-Pearson, B. (1999). *Assessments in Occupational Therapy Mental Health: An Integrative Approach.* Thorofare, NJ: SLACK Incorporated.

---

c. The focus of remediation interventions for performance component/skill deficits must be related to the individual's ability to perform meaningful occupations that are needed and desired by the individual.

3. Interventions for deficits that cannot be remediated should include recommendations for adaptive strategies and/or adaptive equipment that compensate for the deficits and ease occupational performance.

a. Strategies that can be generalized to different situations are particularly helpful (e.g., principles of energy conservation).

b. Multiple factors should be considered when recommending adaptive strategies. See Table 14-6.

   (1) These factors are also relevant to consider when selecting adaptive equipment.

c. Training in adaptive strategies and/or equipment used to enhance self-care performance must consider the person's privacy.

B. **Self-Care Intervention**

1. Determine with the OT supervisor whether the self-care activity should be modified to enable individual performance, performance with external assistance, or eliminated.

a. Activities that are valued, meaningful, and enjoyable to the person and related to desired role performance should be modified for individual performance, with appropriate supports provided as needed (e.g., brushing one's hair using an adapted brush to maintain one's appearance at school/work).

b. Activities that are difficult to perform and/or are not enjoyable should be eliminated or performed with the assistance of others (e.g., dressing requires a great deal of exertion that can exhaust an individual; fasteners can be modified or eliminated, physical assistance can facilitate task).

2. Recommend adaptive strategies for self-care task performance. (Table 14-6).

3. Provide adaptive equipment to compensate for functional impairments during self-care activity performance.

a. Toileting and toilet hygiene equipment.

   (1) Grab bars and/or toilet safety frame.

   (2) Bedside (3 in 1) commode or raised toilet seat.

   (3) Bowel training device, bladder control devices.

# TABLE 14-4 – GENERAL ERGONOMIC RISK ANALYSIS CHECKLIST

Check the box if your answer is "yes" to the question. A "yes" response indicates that an ergonomic risk factor that requires further analysis may be present.

## MANUAL MATERIAL HANDLING

❑ Is there lifting of loads, tools, or parts?

❑ Is there lowering of loads, tools, or parts?

❑ Is there overhead reaching for loads, tools, or parts?

❑ Is there bending at the waist to handle loads, tools, or parts?

❑ Is there twisting at the waist to handle loads, tools or parts?

## PHYSICAL ENERGY DEMANDS

❑ Do tools and parts weight more than 10 lbs?

❑ Is reaching greater than 20 inches?

❑ Is bending, stooping, or squatting a primary task activity?

❑ Is lifting or lowering loads a primary task activity?

❑ Is walking or carrying loads a primary task activity?

❑ Is stair or ladder climbing with loads a primary task activity?

❑ Is pushing or pulling loads a primary task activity?

❑ Is reaching overhead a primary task activity?

❑ Do any of the above tasks require five or more complete work cycles to be done within a minute?

❑ Do workers complain that rest breaks and fatigue allowances are insufficient?

## OTHER MUSCULOSKELETAL DEMANDS

❑ Do manual jobs require frequent, repetitive motions?

❑ Do work postures require frequent bending of the neck, shoulder, elbow, wrist, or finger joints?

❑ For seated work, do reaches for tools and materials exceed 15 inches from the worker's position?

❑ Is the worker unable to change his or her position often?

❑ Does the work involve forceful, quick, or sudden motions?

❑ Does the work involve shock or rapid buildup of forces?

❑ Is finger-pinch gripping used?

❑ Do job postures involve sustained muscle contraction of any limb?

## COMPUTER WORKSTATION

❑ Do operators use computer workstations for more than 4 hours a day?

❑ Are there complaints of discomfort from those working at these stations?

❑ Is the chair or desk nonadjustable?

❑ Is the display monitor, keyboard, or document holder nonadjustable?

❑ Does lighting cause glare or make the monitor screen hard to read?

❑ Is the room temperature too hot or too cold?

❑ Is there irritating vibration or noise?

## ENVIRONMENT

❑ Is the temperature too hot or too cold?

❑ Are the worker's hands exposed to temperatures less than 70° F?

❑ Is the workplace poorly lit?

❑ Is there glare?

❑ Is there excessive noise that is annoying, distracting, or producing hearing loss?

❑ Is there upper extremity or whole body vibration?

❑ Is air circulation too high or too low?

## GENERAL WORKPLACE

❑ Are walkways uneven, slippery, or obstructed?

❑ Is housekeeping poor?

❑ Is there inadequate clearance or accessibility for performing tasks?

❑ Are stairs cluttered or lacking railings?

❑ Is proper footwear worn?

## TOOLS

❑ Is the handle too small or too large?

❑ Does the handle shape cause the operator to bend the wrist in order to use the tool?

❑ Is the tool hard to access?

❑ Does the tool weigh more than 9 pounds?

❑ Does the tool vibrate excessively?

❑ Does the tool cause excessive kickback to the operator?

❑ Does the tool become too hot or too cold?

## GLOVES

❑ Do the gloves require the worker to use more force when performing job tasks?

❑ Do the gloves provide inadequate protection?

❑ Do the gloves present a hazard of catch points on the tool or in the workplace?

## ADMINISTRATION

❑ Is there little worker control over the work process?

❑ Is the task highly repetitive and monotonous?

❑ Does the job involve critical tasks with high accountability and little or no tolerance for error?

❑ Are work hours and breaks poorly organized?

General ergonomic risk analysis checklist. (From Cohen AL, et al: *Elements of ergonomics programs; a primer based on workplace evaluations of musculoskeletal disorders,* Washington DC, 1997, US Government Printing Office.)

## TABLE 14-5 – RISK ANALYSIS CHECKLIST FOR COMPUTER-USER WORKSTATIONS

"No" responses indicate potential problem areas which should receive further investigation.

1. Does the workstation ensure proper worker posture, such as

   - horizontal thighs? ❑ Yes ❑ No
   - vertical lower legs? ❑ Yes ❑ No
   - feet flat on floor or footrest? ❑ Yes ❑ No
   - neutral wrists? ❑ Yes ❑ No

2. Does the chair

   - adjust easily? ❑ Yes ❑ No
   - have a padded seat with a rounded front? ❑ Yes ❑ No
   - have an adjustable backrest? ❑ Yes ❑ No
   - provide lumbar support? ❑ Yes ❑ No
   - have casters? ❑ Yes ❑ No

3. Are the height and tilt of the work surface on which the keyboard is located adjustable? ❑ Yes ❑ No

4. Is the keyboard detachable? ❑ Yes ❑ No

5. Do keying actions require minimal force? ❑ Yes ❑ No

6. Is there an adjustable document holder? ❑ Yes ❑ No

7. Are arm rests provided where needed? ❑ Yes ❑ No

8. Are glare and reflections avoided? ❑ Yes ❑ No

9. Does the monitor have brightness and contrast controls? ❑ Yes ❑ No

10. Do the operators judge the distance between eyes and work to be satisfactory for their viewing needs? ❑ Yes ❑ No

11. Is there sufficient space for knees and feet? ❑ Yes ❑ No

12. Can the workstation be used for either right- or left-handed activity? ❑ Yes ❑ No

13. Are adequate rest breaks provided for task demands ❑ Yes ❑ No

14. Are high stroke rates avoided by

   - job rotation? ❑ Yes ❑ No
   - self-pacing? ❑ Yes ❑ No
   - adjusting the job to the skill of the worker? ❑ Yes ❑ No

15. Are employees trained in

   - proper postures? ❑ Yes ❑ No
   - proper work methods? ❑ Yes ❑ No
   - when and how to adjust their workstations? ❑ Yes ❑ No
   - how to seek assistance for their concerns? ❑ Yes ❑ No

Risk analysis checklist for computer-user workstations. (From Cohen AL, et al: *Elements of ergonomics programs; a primer based on workplace evaluations of musculoskeletal disorders,* Washington DC, 1997, US Government Printing Office.)

    (4) Skin inspection mirror.

    (5) Toilet paper holder.

  b. Grooming/oral hygiene adaptive equipment.

    (1) Universal cuff to hold toothbrush, razor, comb, and/or brush.

    (2) Built-up, angled, or long-handled brushes and/or razors.

    (3) Blow dryer, nail clipper, nail polish holders.

    (4) Faucet turners.

    (5) Electric toothbrush, floss holders, water pik, denture brush.

  c. Bathing/showering.

    (1) Grab bars and non-skid mat.

    (2) Tub transfer bench/shower bench.

    (3) Shower or commode chair.

    (4) Handheld shower.

    (5) Anti-scald valves and/or faucets.

    (6) Built-up, angled, and/or long-handled bath sponge or bath mitt.

    (7) Soap on a rope, soap dish with suction cup.

    (8) Storage units.

  d. Dressing.

    (1) Reachers, dressing sticks/hooks, and pants dressing poles.

    (2) Built-up, angled, or long-handled shoe horn.

    (3) Pull-on clothing, Velcro-type and/or front opening closures for clothing.

    (4) Elastic shoelaces, slip on shoes.

---

### TABLE 14-6 - FACTORS TO CONSIDER WHEN RECOMMENDING ADAPTIVE STRATEGIES

- What is important to the individual about the task?

- Is the strategy viewed as compatible with the particular social context?

- Does the strategy enhance the individual's sense of personal control?

- Does the strategy minimize the effort?

- Does the strategy interfere with social opportunities or diminish the presentation of self?

- Is the recommended strategy temporally realistic given the context?

- Does the strategy provide for safety?

---

From Self-care management for adults with movement disorders by M. McCraig. In C. Christiansen (Ed.). *Ways of living: Self-care strategies for special needs* (p. 261). Copyright 1994 by American Occupational Therapy Association. Reprinted with permission.

    (5) Button hook, zipper pull and zipper loop or ring.

    (6) Sock/stocking aid.

  e. Feeding/eating.

    (1) Adapted nipples and bottles for infants.

    (2) Scoop dish or plate guards.

    (3) Non-slip placemat or dycem.

    (4) Built-up, angled, weighted or long-handled utensils, swivel utensils.

    (5) Rocker knife and/or spork.

    (6) Adapted cups, i.e., weighted, two handled, nosey cup, travel mugs.

    (7) Longhandled or angled straws.

    (8) See Chapter 5 Section VI.A.2 for information on interventions to facilitate development of oral-motor control and feeding skills.

  f. Medication management.

    (1) Easy open, non-child-proof medication bottles.

    (2) Pill organizers, medication minders.

  g. Refer to Table 14-7 for spinal cord injury levels and self-care abilities.

4. Recognize the multiple dimensions of a person with a disability and the complexities of many disorders. For example, Friedreich's ataxia is characterized by tremors that may indicate the need for weighted utensils, but muscle strength is also limited so these utensils may be too heavy for functional use.

5. Train in safe use of adaptive equipment and assistive technology.

6. Practice to attain proficiency in activity performance at appropriate times and in real environments (e.g., brush teeth in the bathroom in the morning).

7. Provide cues and assistance as needed.

  a. Verbal reminders and prompts.

  b. Nonverbal gestures, written directions, physical prompt to initiate.

  c. Physical hand over hand assistance through complete activity movement.

  d. Visual supervision to ensure safety with minimal or no verbal or nonverbal cues.

8. Use thematic and topical groups to develop needed skills (e.g., grooming group, medication management).

9. Teach principles and methods of energy conservation, work simplification, joint protection, and proper body mechanics. Refer to Chapter 11.

10. Educate and train caregivers to provide needed

cues, physical assistance, and/or supervision.

    a. Teach organizational strategies (e.g., place clothing in proper sequence for dressing).

    b. Teach activity analysis, gradation, simplification, and adaptation skills (e.g., provide multiple small meals to decrease the amount of attention required to eat for a person with Alzheimer's disease).

11. Educate the individual with disabilities on personal care attendant training.

## TABLE 14-7 - SCI LEVELS AND SELF-CARE ABILITIES

| C1-C3 | Totally dependent in self-care but can instruct others in preferences for care. Can chew and swallow. |
|---|---|
| C4 | Totally dependent in self-care but can instruct others in preferences for care. Can drink from a glass with a long straw. |
| C5 | 1. Feeding requires assistance with setup. Equipment used may include: <br>• Suspension sling or mobile arm support. <br>• Dorsal wrist splint with universal cuff. <br>• Dycem to prevent slippage of plate. <br>• Scoop dish or plate guard. <br>• Angled utensils. <br>2. Dressing requires minimal to moderate assistance with upper body dressing. Dependent with lower body dressing. <br>3. Bathing requires moderate to minimal assistance. <br>4. Grooming requires assistance with setup; however, with splint and universal cuff can be independent with brushing teeth and combing hair. Independent using electric shaver that fits around the hand. |
| C6 | 1 Feeding: Independent using adaptive equipment. <br>• Universal cuff or tenodesis splint. <br>• Rocker knife. <br>• Cup with large handles. <br>2. Dressing: Independent in lower body dressing performed while in bed. Requires maximal assistance with socks and shoes. Independent with upper body dressing using button hook and zipper pull. <br>3. Bathing: Minimal assistance using tub bench and sliding board transfer. <br>4. Grooming: Independent using tenodesis grasp or splint. |
| C7 | 1. Feeding: Independent. <br>2. Dressing: Independent, but may need button hook. <br>3. Bathing: Same as C6 but performs depression transfers. <br>4. Grooming: Same as C6. |
| C8-T1 | Self Care: Independent <br>Performs depressions transfers. Can transfer from wheelchair to floor and back to chair with standby assist. |
| T6 to L4 | Independent in all self-care. |

    a. Practice methods for directing self-care in the personally desired and acceptable manner.

    b. Provide assertiveness and personal advocacy training.

12. Modify the environment to maximize performance and ensure safety. Refer to Chapter 15.

## C. Sexual Expression/Activity Intervention

1. Occupational therapy intervention is provided to enable satisfying, safe sexual expression/activity regardless of disability, disease, or advanced age.

2. Myths about the sexuality of the aged and individuals with disability or disease processes must be confronted and debunked.

3. Myths include:

    a. They are asexual and have less interest in sexual expression than younger and/or healthier persons.

    b. They are physically unattractive and not desirable as a sexual partner and will be a burden to their partners.

    c. They inherently have poor judgment and cannot make appropriate decisions about their sexuality.

    d. Intercourse with mutual orgasm is the desired and primary means to express oneself sexually.

      (1) Intimate behaviors, such as mutual stimulation, cuddling, oral sex, and/or caressing are not adequate sexual activity.

      (2) Self-stimulation/masturbation is not an appropriate means of sexual expression.

    e. Individuals who live in shared residential settings such as nursing homes, group homes, and assisted living facilities are asexual.

      (1) They should be segregated according to gender.

      (2) Privacy for the individual is not essential and does not need to be respected.

    f. Individuals with disabilities and/or elders who desire and/or engage in sexual activity are oversexed and inappropriate.

4. OT practitioners should use the PLISSIT model as a guide for appropriate interventions.

    a. P = permission which requires the practitioner to create an atmosphere which gives the individual permission to raise concerns about his/her sexuality and sexual activity(ies).

      (1) Incorporating sexuality into the OT initial and ongoing evaluation in a matter-of-fact manner is an effective method.

      (2) An OT practitioner who is not comfortable with creating a permissive atmosphere for

the discussion of sexuality due to personal, social, cultural, and/or religious reasons must honestly acknowledge this fact to the client and refer him/her immediately to a team member who is comfortable with addressing the individual's concerns.

    (3) It is the team's responsibility to ensure that at least one team member is comfortable with evaluating and intervening with individuals with sexual expression concerns.

    (4) Supervision and continuing professional development activities should be pursued by all to develop this needed comfort.

b. LI = limited information that is provided by the OT practitioner to ensure that the individual has accurate knowledge about his/her sexual abilities and potentials.

    (1) Facts are shared (e.g., there is sex after disability), and myths are dispelled (see prior section).

c. SS = specific suggestions that are provided by the OT practitioner to facilitate the individual's pursuit of satisfying sexual expression, either alone or with a partner.

    (1) The individual's (and partner's) goals for sexual expression and activity are identified and strategies for achieving goals are explored.

    (2) Principles of activity analysis, gradation, modification, and simplification are used to facilitate goal attainment.

    (3) Nonmedical methods to manage pain and stiffness (e.g., warm baths) are provided.

    (4) Positioning alternatives and adaptive equipment to facilitate desired sexual expression are suggested.

    (5) Energy conservation methods (e.g., timing sex for when one has the most energy and use of sexual positions that require less energy expenditures) are suggested to those with limited endurance.

    (6) Catheter care, hygiene concerns, and skin care are addressed.

    (7) Referrals to a physician for medical management of pain, impotence or other sexual dysfunctions, and hormonal treatment.

d. IT = intensive therapy which is indicated when the individual requires intervention for long-standing relationship problems and/or enduring sexual problems.

    (1) These problems are often due to difficulties beyond the onset or presence of a disability.

    (2) Specialized training is required to provide intensive therapy so a referral to the appropriate professional (e.g., marriage counselor, sex therapist) is indicated.

5. Methods of intervention can include one-on-one counseling sessions, therapeutic groups, and/or dissemination of printed materials.

6. Interventions for individuals with cognitive impairments (e.g., poor impulse control, limited judgment) are essential to ensure safety and to protect the individual from sexual abuse, assault, and/or exploitation.

a. Assertiveness training to increase understanding of the right, and develop the ability, to set limits.

b. Training and practice in physical self-protection techniques.

c. Role playing to simulate potential scenarios which can challenge the individual's sexual judgment.

d. Sex education (e.g. menstrual cycle information, prevention of sexually transmitted diseases).

e. Caregiver and family education.

    (1) Socially inappropriate sexual activity is often difficult for families to understand (e.g., an elder with Alzheimer's disease begins to disrobe in the living room).

        (a) Recognizing that this behavior is indicative of an underlying disease process is important.

        (b) Providing strategies for effectively managing undesirable behaviors is main OT focus (e.g., eliminate clothing fasteners in the front, divert the person's attention to an activity of interest).

## D. Home Management Intervention

1. Determine with the OT supervisor the home management expectations and demands of the individual's current and expected environment.

a. Supportive living environments can range in expectations from requiring that a resident only clean his/her room (e.g., in a group home) to complete management of a home with minimal supervision (e.g., a supported apartment).

b. Independent living environments can also have a range of expectations and demands (e.g., only wife does the budget, only husband cooks).

2. Determine with the OT supervisor and the individual whether the home management activity should be modified to enable independent performance, performance with external assistance, or eliminated.
   a. Activities that are valued, meaningful and enjoyable to the person and related to desired role performance should be modified for individual performance, with appropriate supports provided as needed (e.g., preparing after-school snacks for children).
   b. Activities that are difficult to perform and/or are not enjoyable should be eliminated or performed with the assistance of others (e.g., cleaning a refrigerator can be delegated to another person, or a self-cleaning oven can eliminate a task).
3. Recommend adaptive strategies for home management task performance. (Table 14-6).
4. Provide adaptive equipment to compensate for functional impairments during home management activity performance.
   a. Cleaning.
      (1) Suction bottom bottle and glass brushes.
      (2) Reachers.
      (3) Aerosol can holders.
      (4) Built up, angled, or long-handled sponges, dusters, brooms, mops, dustpans.
      (5) Front-loading washers and dryers.
      (6) Electronic dishwasher, self-cleaning oven, automatic defrosting refrigerator.
   b. Cooking.
      (1) Faucet and knob turners.
      (2) Anti-scald faucets and/or valves.
      (3) Jar openers, bowl holders, and saucepan stabilizers.
      (4) Nonskid pad, placemat, or dycem.
      (5) Cutting board with a stabilizing nail and built-up edges.
      (6) Built-up or angled utensils and rocker knives.
      (7) Adapted timers.
      (8) Electric can opener.
      (9) Lightweight pots, pans, dishware.
      (10) Automatic hot water dispenser and/or hot-pots.
      (11) Strap loops to open refrigerator, cabinet, and oven doors.
      (12) Reachers and step stools.
      (13) Utility cart.
      (14) High kitchen stool.

5. Train in safe use of adaptive equipment and assistive technology.
6. Teach principles and methods of energy conservation, work simplification, joint protection, and proper body mechanics. Refer to Chapter 11.
7. Provide cues and assistance as needed.
   a. Verbal reminders and prompts.
   b. Nonverbal gestures, written directions, physical prompt to initiate.
   c. Physical hand over hand assistance through complete activity movement.
   d. Visual supervision to ensure safety with minimal or no verbal or nonverbal cues.
8. Practice to attain proficiency in activity performance at appropriate times and in real environments (e.g., cooking a meal in a kitchen at lunchtime).
9. Recognize and respect personal, sociocultural, and socioeconomic differences (e.g., standards of cleanliness, dietary restrictions and preferences).
   a. Use equipment that is socioeconomically appropriate (e.g., do not use an oven to teach meal preparation if someone only uses a hot plate).
10. Use thematic and topical groups to develop needed skills (e.g., cooking group, money management group).
11. Modify environment to maximize performance and ensure safety. Refer to Chapter 15.
12. Educate and train caregivers to provide needed cues, physical assistance, and/or supervision.
13. Refer to relevant social service programs (e.g., food stamps, home energy assistance program [HEAP]).
14. Refer to the appropriate supportive living environment if independent living is not attainable (e.g., group home, halfway house, supported apartment).

**E. Family Participation Intervention**
1. Collaborate with family on identifying desired goals.
   a. Provide interpreters, if necessary.
2. Determine with the OT supervisor and the individual whether the family activity should be modified to enable independent performance, performance with external assistance, or eliminated.
   a. Activities that are valued, meaningful, and enjoyable to the person and related to desired role performance should be modified for individual performance, with appropriate supports provided as needed (e.g., reading a bedtime

story to children).

   b. Activities that are difficult to perform and/or are not safe should be eliminated or performed with the assistance of others (e.g., bathing a toddler).

3. Methods of intervention can include one-on-one counseling sessions, therapeutic groups, and/or dissemination of printed materials.

4. Design interventions using activities that are meaningful to the individual's role within the family.

5. Use topical and thematic groups to develop effective family interaction skills.

   a. Role play to simulate potential scenarios which can challenge the individual's family skills (e.g., assertiveness training, anger management).

   b. Practice effective family communication.

   c. Teach principles and methods of energy conservation, work simplification, joint protection, and proper body mechanics for family activities. Refer to Chapter 11.

   d. Develop parenting skills, as needed.

     (1) Teach how to care for a child's physical needs and physically practice parenting tasks (e.g., placing child into a front pack using proper body mechanics).

     (2) Instruct parent about normal developmental roles and tasks to ensure expectations of child/children are realistic.

6. Recommend adaptive strategies for home management task performance that are related that to family participation and/or parenting (e.g., preparation of child's bag lunch for school). See Table 14-6.

7. Provide adaptive equipment to compensate for functional impairments during parenting tasks.

   a. Adapted drop-side crib, raised and/or adjustable height crib mattress, child-resistant one-handed crib wall release mechanism.

   b. Foam rubber bathing pads for sink, portable plastic tub and/or reclining infant seat placed in tub.

   c. Changing tables at proper height with safety straps and touch fasteners.

   d. Pillow to support breast feeding (which physically is the easiest method to feed an infant).

   e. Light weight and/or angled bottles.

   f. One handed swing away release tray on high chair with safety strap.

   g. Food warmer tray.

   h. Pullover clothes, velcro fasteners for bibs, diaper covers, clothing.

   i. Infant carriers.

8. Baby furniture and equipment should be tested and used on a trial basis to ensure it matches the parent's capabilities.

9. The family's socioeconomic status and cost of recommendations must be considered (e.g., premeasured formula and disposable diapers are convenient, energy saving, and expensive options).

10. Recognize and respect personal, sociocultural, and socioeconomic differences within families.

11. Teach the child/children of a parent with a disability self-reliance at a young age.

   a. Arrange tasks so they are accessible to a child (e.g. storage for dishes and glasses next to dishwasher, not in a high cabinet).

   b. Delegate tasks that are achievable for child's/children's developmental level (e.g., even a young child can move clothes from a front-loading washer to a front-loading dryer).

12. Modify the environment to maximize parenting task performance and ensure safety of the parent and child. Refer to Chapter 15.

13. Refer family members to support groups, local and national organizations.

14. Provide caregiver/family education in verbal and written formats in family's language of choice.

15. Be aware of signs of family neglect or abuse.

   a. OT practitioners are required by practice acts, protective legislation, and our professional code of ethics to report any suspected incidents of child, adult, or elder abuse, assault, or exploitation to the appropriate agency and local law enforcement.

**F. Play/Leisure Intervention**

1. Recognize that the acquisition of a disability often results in increased leisure time due to loss of roles.

   a. Provide support for losses, refer to support group.

   b. Renew or adapt old interests.

2. Leisure activities that are valued, meaningful, and enjoyable to the person should be adapted, modified, and/or simplified to facilitate satisfying engagement.

3. Provide assistive technology and adaptive equipment to compensate for functional impairments during leisure activity performance.

   a. Universal cuff.

b. Card holders.

c. Book holders and page turners.

d. Writing orthosis, typing aids, weighted pens.

e. Environmental control unit (ECU) to activate electronic equipment (e.g., CD players, TVs).

f. Adapted computer, keyboard guards, voice-activated computer.

g. Headsticks, mouthsticks.

h. Speaker phones.

i. Use switches to activate toys that a child with a disability cannot operate by conventional means.

j. Refer to Table 14-8 for a description of SCI levels and play/leisure abilities.

4. Plan with the OT supervisor play interventions that consider developmental issues and the child's developmental level.

a. Provide opportunities for culturally relevant solitary play and environmental mastery.

b. Facilitate active participation in cause and effect learning.

c. Provide opportunities for play with siblings and/or peers.

d. Provide toys that are safe, durable, and colorful.

e. Provide toys and activities that are visually and auditorally stimulating.

5. Use thematic and topical groups to develop needed skills (e.g., a parenting play group, a retirement planning group).

6. Teach principles and methods of energy conservation, work simplification, joint protection, and proper body mechanics. Refer to Chapter 11.

7. Refer to relevant community and national resources (e.g. senior centers, free concerts, parks, Compeer, Special Olympics).

8. Explore and present internet and web-based opportunities for play and leisure participation (e.g., social networking, chat rooms, gaming sites).

**G. Work Intervention**

1. Evaluate the work site and adapt the environment and job tasks to enable the individual to perform essential job functions. See Table 14-1 and Table 14-2.

a. Determine with the OT supervisor the person's feasibility to return to work.

2. Provide assistive devices, adaptive strategies, and equipment to compensate for functional impairments during work activity performance. See Table 14-6.

a. Adapted computers.

b. Typing aids.

c. Universal cuff.

d. Teach principles and methods of energy conservation and work simplification. Refer to Chapter 11.

3. Practice, modify, and instruct in work activities.

4. Provide conditioning exercises and activities.

5. Educate about work safety and injury prevention.

a. Teach principles and methods of joint protection and proper body mechanics. Refer to Chapter 11.

6. Educate employer regarding reasonable accommodations to enable performance of essential job functions. See Table 14-9 and Chapter 15.

7. Collaborate with employee assistance programs to obtain additional needed services (e.g., substance abuse counseling).

8. Educate family.

9. Explore alternatives to competitive work if it is not an attainable goal (e.g., volunteer work) and/or if the person is retiring.

10. Use thematic and topical groups to develop needed skills.

a. Task skills to enable successful completion of work tasks.

b. Social skills to facilitate appropriate interactions with coworkers and employer.

c. Work behaviors to ensure a successful work experience. See Table 14-2.

---

### TABLE 14-8 - SCI LEVELS AND PLAY/LEISURE ABILITIES

| | |
|---|---|
| C1-C4 | Can play computer games and access the Internet and e-mail using a mouthstick, head pointer or voice activation. Can read using a mouthstick, head pointer or electronic page turner to turn pages. Can paint with a mouthstick or head pointer. Can control radios, TVs and other electronic devices through use of a mouthstick, head pointer or voice activated environmental control unit. |
| C5 | Can independently play computer games, access the Internet and e-mail, use a speakerphone and ECU, turn pages for reading, play board games and do some crafts using a splint, universal cuff and typing splint. |
| C6 and C7 | Can hold a phone, typing stick and pen using a tenodesis grasp. Can independently use computer using a tenodesis grasp or universal cuff to hold a typing stick. Can play board games and some wheelchair sports. Can do some crafts. |
| C8 - T1 | Can do the same activities as C7 but performance is easier due to good functional use of both upper extremities. |

# TABLE 14-9 - REASONABLE ACCOMMODATIONS FOR RECURRENT FUNCTIONAL PROBLEMS AMONG PERSONS WITH PSYCHIATRIC DISORDERS

## PERSONAL SELF-EFFICACY

- Reinforce or coach appropriate behaviors.
- Test for job skills on the job and avoid self-report of abilities.
- Place in job where there is a model to follow or imitate.
- Teach self-advocacy skills.
- Provide successful job experiences. Use positive feedback.
- Begin with close supervision and then cut back slowly as skills are maintained.
- Maintain similarity or consistency in work tasks.
- Encourage positive self-talk and eliminate negative self-talk.

## DURATION OF CONCENTRATION[1]

- Put each work request in writing and leave in "to do" box to avoid interruptions.
- Provide ongoing consultation, mediation, problem solving and conflict resolution.
- Provide good working conditions, such as adequate light, smoke-free environment, and reduced noise.
- Provide directive commands on a regular basis.

## SCREENING OUT ENVIRONMENTAL STIMULI[1]

- Place in a separate office.
- Provide opaque room dividers between workstations.
- Allow person to work after hours or when others are not around.
- Ensure that workstation facilitates work production and organization.

## MAINTAINING STAMINA THROUGHOUT THE WORKDAY[1]

- Provide additional breaks or shortened workday.
- Allow an extended day to allow for breaks or rest periods.
- Avoid work during lunch, such as answering the phone; use of an answering machine instead.
- Distribute tasks throughout the day according to energy level.
- Job share with another employee.
- Develop work simplification techniques, such as collect all copying to be done at one time or use a wheeled cart to move supplies.
- Have a liberal leave policy for health problems, flexible hours, and back-up coverage.
- Individualize work agreements.
- Verify employees' efficacy regarding their ability to sustain effort or persist with a task.
- Teach on-the-job relaxation and stress-reduction techniques.

## MANAGING TIME PRESSURE AND DEADLINES[1]

- Maintain structure through a daily time and task schedule using hourly goals.
- Provide positive reinforcement when tasks are completed within the expected time lines.
- Arrange a separate work area to reduce noise and interruptions.
- Screen out unnecessary business.

## INITIATING INTERPERSONAL CONTACT[1]

- Purposely plan orientation to meet and work alongside co-workers.
- Allow sufficient time to make good, unhurried contacts.
- Make contacts during work, break, and even lunch times, adjusting the conversation to the situation.
- When standing, instead of facing each other, try standing at a 90° angle to each other.
- Allow the person to work at home.
- Have an advocate to advise and support the person.
- Communicate honestly.
- Plan supervision times and maintain them.
- Develop tolerance for and helpful responses to unusual behaviors.
- Provide awareness and advocacy training for all workers.

## TABLE 14-9 - REASONABLE ACCOMMODATIONS FOR RECURRENT FUNCTIONAL PROBLEMS AMONG PERSONS WITH PSYCHIATRIC DISORDERS CONT.

### FOCUSING ON MULTIPLE TASKS SIMULTANEOUSLY[1]

- Eliminate the number of simultaneous tasks.
- Redistribute tasks among employees with the same responsibilities, so each can do more of one type of job task than a lot of different tasks.
- Establish priorities for task completion.
- Arrange for all work tasks to be put in writing with due dates or times.

### RESPONDING TO NEGATIVE FEEDBACK[1]

- Have employee prepare own work appraisal to compare with supervisor's.
- Work together to establish methods employee can use to change negative behavior.
- Provide positive reinforcement for observed behavioral change.
- Provide on-site crisis intervention and counseling services to develop self-esteem, provide emotional support, and promote comfort with accommodations.
- Establish guidelines for feedback.

### SYMPTOMS SECONDARY TO PRESCRIBED PSYCHOTROPIC MEDICATIONS[1]

- Provide release time to see psychiatrist or primary physician.
- Encourage employee to work with physician to establish a time schedule to take medications that are conducive to work responsibilities.
- Provide release time or changes in job tasks that match condition.

[1]From: Mancuso (1990).

11. Provide pre-retirement planning to ease transition from competitive employment.

12. Provide follow-up care, as needed (e.g., counseling, work support group, psychosocial clubhouse).

13. Refer to state offices for vocational and educational services for individuals with disabilities for further education and/or vocational training.

14. Specific work program characteristics.
    a. Work hardening program characteristics.
       (1) An interdisciplinary approach is used.
       (2) Real or simulated work activities are used.
       (3) A transition between acute care and return to work is provided.
       (4) The issues of productivity, safety, physical tolerance, and worker behaviors are addressed.
       (5) CARF accreditation is required.
    b. Work conditioning programs.
       (1) One discipline is the provider of services.
       (2) Real or simulated work activities are used.
       (3) A transition between acute care and return to work is provided.
       (4) Flexibility, strength, movement, and endurance are addressed.
       (5) Accreditation is not a requirement.
    c. Ergonomic program characteristics.
       (1) Prevention is the main focus to fit the work place to the human body.
       (2) Types of programs.
           (a) Ergonomic survey.
           (b) Specific job site analysis.
           (c) Manager and employee training.
           (d) Educational seminars.
           (e) Exercise and stretching programs.
    d. Vocational (sheltered) workshops, supported employment programs, transitional employment programs (TEP).
       (1) A multidisciplinary or interdisciplinary approach is used.
       (2) Real work activities are used.
           (a) Participants are paid at a piece-work rate in vocational (sheltered) workshops.
           (b) Participants are paid at the prevailing competitive wage for positions in TEP and supported employment programs.
       (3) Participants are considered as employees with supports provided as needed.

(a) Job coaches are used.

(b) Reasonable accommodations are provided. See Table 14-9.

(4) A transition between program participation and competitive employment is provided according to participant's functional level.

(5) Vocational (sheltered) workshops and supported employment can be the final and permanent employment goal for an individual.

(6) Accreditation is not a requirement.

(a) Vocational (sheltered) workshops, TEPs, and supported employment programs are usually part of an accredited hospital system or a major agency (e.g., ARC).

15. Interventions for the most common work related injuries.

a. Cumulative trauma such as carpal tunnel syndrome and low back pain.

(1) Avoid static positions, repetition, awkward postures, forceful exertions, and vibration.

(2) Design workplace and work station to be ergonomically correct to prevent further trauma.

b. Psychosocial and cognitive deficits.

(1) Engage person in program suitable to functional vocational abilities (e.g., vocational workshop, supportive employment).

(2) Table 14-6.

16. Discharge criteria from work programs.

a. Individual exhibits limited potential for improvement.

b. Individual has declined services.

c. Individual is non-compliant with the program.

d. Individual has met program goals.

e. Individual has returned to work.

# References

Allen, C.K., Earhart, C.A., & Blue, T. (1992). *Occupational therapy treatment goals for the physically and cognitively disabled.* Bethesda, MD: American Occupational Therapy Association.

American Occupational Therapy Association. (2008). Occupational therapy practice framework: Domain and process, 2nd edition. *American Journal of Occupational Therapy, 62,* 625-688

American Occupational Therapy Association. (2006). *Reference manual of the official documents of the American Occupational Therapy Association* (11th ed.). Bethesda, MD: Author.

American Occupational Therapy Association. (2005). Standards of practice for occupational therapy. *American Journal of Occupational Therapy, 59,* 663-665.

Asher, I.E. (2007). *An annotated index of occupational therapy evaluation tools.* (3rd ed.). Bethesda, MD: American Occupational Therapy Association.

Asrael, W. (1993). The PLISSIT model of sexuality counseling and education. In R.P. Cottrell (Ed.). *Psychosocial occupational therapy: Proactive approaches* (pp. 451-452). Bethesda, MD: American Occupational Therapy.

Backman, C. (1994). Assessment of self-care skills. In C. Christiansen (Ed.). *Ways of living: Self-care strategies for special needs* (pp. 51-75). Bethesda, MD: American Occupational Therapy Association.

Case-Smith, J. (Ed.). (2005). *Occupational therapy for children* (5th ed.). St. Louis, MO: Elsevier Mosby.

Christiansen, C. (1994). *Ways of living: Self-care strategies for special needs.* Bethesda, MD: American Occupational Therapy Association.

Clifton, D. (2004, December). *Workers' Comp: A plethora of opportunities. Rehab Management, 32,* 34-36.

Crist, P.A., & Stoffel, V.C. (1996). The Americans with Disabilities Act of 1990 and employees with mental impairments: Personal efficacy and the environment. In R. P. Cottrell (Ed.). *Perspectives on purposeful activity: Foundation and future of occupational therapy.* (pp. 217-228). Bethesda, MD: American Occupational Therapy Association.

Gutman, S., Mortera, M. Hinojosa, J., & Kramer, P. (2007). The Issue Is--Revision of the Occupational Therapy Practice Framework. *American Journal of Occupational Therapy,* 61,119-126.

Hinojosa, J., & Kramer, P., & Crist, P. (Eds.) (2005). *Evaluation: Obtaining and interpreting data* (2nd ed.). Bethesda, MD: American Occupational Therapy Association.

Holm, M.B., Rogers, J.C. & James, A.B. (1998). Treatment of occupational performance areas. In M.E. Neistadt and E.B. Crepeau (Eds.). *Willard and Spackman's occupational therapy* (9th ed., pp. 323-390). Philadelphia, PA: Lippincott.

Hopkins, H. & Smith, H. (Eds.). (2003). *Willard and Spackman's occupational therapy* (10th ed.). Philadelphia: J.B. Lippincott.

Hussey, S.; Sabonis-Chafee, B.; & O'Brien, J. (2007). *Introduction to occupational therapy,* (3rd ed.). St. Louis, MO: Elsevier Mosby.

Larson, K., Stevens-Ratchford, R.G., Pedretti, L., & Crabtree, J. (1996). *ROTE: The role of occupational therapy with the elderly* (2nd ed.). Bethesda, MD: American Occupational Therapy Association.

McHugh Pendleton, H. & Schultz-Krohn, W. (Eds.), *Pedretti's occupational therapy: Practice skills for physical dysfunction* (6th ed.). St. Louis, MO: Mosby

Mosey, A. (1996). *Psychosocial components of occupational therapy.* Philadelphia: Lippincott-Raven.

Moyers, P. & Dale, L. (2007). *The guide to occupational therapy practice.* Bethesda, MD: American Occupational Therapy Association.

Spencer, E. (1998). Functional restoration: Preliminary concepts and planning. In H. Hopkins and H. Smith (Eds.). *Willard and Spackman's occupational therapy* (7th ed., pp.435-460). Philadelphia: Lippincott.

Trombly, C. (1995). *Occupational therapy for physical dysfunction* (4th ed.). Hagerstown, MD: Williams and Wilkins.

# CHAPTER 15

# MASTERY OF THE ENVIRONMENT: EVALUATION AND INTERVENTION

Colleen Ann DeRitis • Rita P. Fleming-Castaldy

## I. General Environmental Considerations

### A. Definition and Major Concepts

1. The environment is "the aggregate of phenomena that surrounds the individual and influences his (her) development and existence" (Mosey, 1996, p. 171).
2. The environment in which a person lives, and the exposure to various settings, influences his or her development and adaptation.
3. The environment can facilitate growth because it allows for adaptation and problem solving strategies to be developed.
4. Conversely, the environment can hinder development and adaptation if it is impoverished or hostile.
5. A person's abilities, skills, limitations, problems, activities, and/or occupations cannot be fully understood without considerations of his/her current and expected environment.
6. Physical/non-human environment.
   a. Everything that is non-human (i.e., buildings, objects, tools, devices, animals, trees).
7. Sensory environment.
   a. Visual: lighting, colors, clutter (i.e., posters all over a wall).
   b. Auditory: loudness of radios, loudspeakers, classroom noise.
   c. Tactile: room temperature, seating textures.

d. Olfactory: pleasant or offensive odors.
   e. Gustatory: pleasant or offensive tastes.
8. Social-cultural/ human environment.
   a. Social roles: "an organized pattern of behavior that is characteristic and expected of the occupant of a defined position in a social system" (Mosey, 1996, p. 64). For example, a student, a parent, a worker.
   b. Social network: "the web of voluntary relationships that make up an individual's social environment" (Mosey, 1996, p. 184).
   c. Cultural aspects: "the social structures, values, norms, and expectations that are accepted and shared by a group of people" (Mosey, 1996, p. 172).
   d. Psychological aspects: environmental characteristics that can affect mood and stress level (e.g., a calming, comfortable, cheerful environment versus a chaotic, uncomfortable, depressing setting).
9. The AOTA practice framework has expanded the description of environment beyond the physical and social environment to include the concept of context. In the AOTA practice framework, context "refers to a variety of interrelated conditions that are within and surrounding the client. These interrelated contexts often are less tangible than physical and social environments but nonetheless exert a strong

influence on performance" (AOTA 2008, p. 642).

a. Contexts include cultural, personal, temporal, and virtual.

   (1) The "cultural context includes customs, beliefs, activity patterns, behavior standards, and expectations accepted by the society of which the client is a member (AOTA 2008, p. 642).

   (2) The "personal context refers to demographic features of the individual such as age, gender, socioeconomic status, and educational level that are not part of a health condition (AOTA 2008, p. 642).

   (3) The "temporal context includes stages of life, time of year, time of day and duration rhythm of activity, or history" (AOTA 2008, p. 645).

   (4) The virtual context refers to the "environment in which communication occurs by means of airways or computers and an absence of physical contact" (AOTA 2008, p. 645); for example, email, video-conferencing, web-based social networking.

B. **Legislation Related to the Environment**

1. Americans with Disabilities Act (ADA): a civil rights law aimed at allowing full participation in society for people with disabilities.

   a. Several sections mandate accessible environments for persons with disabilities.

   b. Included are policies dealing with public service, employment, and public accommodations.

2. Omnibus Budget Reconciliation Act (OBRA): mandates that restraints cannot be used without proper justification, agreement, and documentation.

3. Individuals with Disabilities Education Act (IDEA): mandates that children with disabilities receive education in the least restrictive and most natural environment.

   a. Inclusive models are to be used to enable the child to be taught in a regular classroom.

   b. Education must prepare a child for independent living and employment environments.

4. The role of OT practitioners in environmental assessment and modification has increased with the implementation of the ADA, OBRA, and IDEA (See Chapter 4 for specific information on the ADA, OBRA, and IDEA).

C. **The Role of OT Practitioners**

1. OT practitioners should be familiar with all aspects of a person's environment – living, vocational, and leisure – whether it takes place in a hospital, nursing home, school, or home.

2. OT practitioners can advocate for and design environments that use principles of universal design to meet the physical, sensory, sociocultural, and psychological needs of the individual.

   a. See Table 15-1.

3. OT practitioners can help to identify settings and approaches to implement the ADA, OBRA, and IDEA.

4. OT practitioners can advocate for ADA, OBRA, and IDEA compliance to enable individuals to function as independently – and with the least restriction – as possible, in their environment.

D. **The Role of the Team**

1. OT practitioners are often part of an interdisciplinary team that determines the needs and abilities of an individual with a disability in a specific environment.

2. Basis for team construction.

   a. The facility in which the individual with a disability presently resides and/or participates.

   b. The individual's needs and his or her abilities/functional status.

   c. Geographical location.

   d. Funding available to the individual with a disability (i.e., third party payers and/ or state offices for individuals with disabilities).

   e. Support available from caregivers.

3. The team should always include the consumer and caregivers.

4. Professional team members may belong to the Rehabilitation Engineers Society of North America (RESNA) and/or National Registry of Rehabilitation Technology Suppliers (NRRTS).

   a. Both professional organizations help to develop standards and measuring tools to ensure proper design, fabrication, prescription, and delivery of rehabilitation technology.

5. Potential professional team members.

   a. Physicians, to authorize and assess services and purchases.

   b. Occupational therapists and occupational therapy assistants (See section I.C.).

   c. Physical therapists, to assess mobility difficulties an individual may encounter in the environment.

   d. Speech language pathologists, to assess and recommend augmentative communication aids.

   e. Rehabilitation engineers, to design equipment

## TABLE 15-1 – PRINCIPLES OF UNIVERSAL DESIGN

### PRINCIPLE 1

**Equitable Use:** The design is useful and marketable to people with diverse abilities.

**Guidelines:**

**1a.** Provide the same means of use for all users; identical whenever possible; equivalent when not.

**1b.** Avoid segregating or stigmatizing any users.

**1c.** Provisions for privacy, security, and safety should be equally available to all users.

**1d.** Make the design appealing to all users.

### PRINCIPLE 2

**Flexibility in Use:** The design accommodates a wide range of individual preferences and abilities.

**Guidelines:**

**2a.** Provide choice in methods of use.

**2b.** Accommodate right- or left-handed access and use.

**2c.** Facilitate the user's accuracy and precision.

**2d.** Provide adaptability to the user's pace.

### PRINCIPLE 3

**Simple and Intuitive Use:** Use of the design is easy to understand, regardless of the user's experience, knowledge, language skills, or current concentration level.

**Guidelines:**

**3a.** Eliminate unnecessary complexity.

**3b.** Be consistent with user expectations and intuition.

**3c.** Accommodate a wide range of literacy and language skills.

**3d.** Arrange information consistent with its importance

**3e.** Provide effective prompting and feedback during and after task completion.

### PRINCIPLE 4

**Perceptible Information:** The design communicates necessary information effectively to the user, regardless of ambient conditions or the user's sensory abilities.

**Guidelines:**

**4a.** Use different modes (pictorial, verbal, tactile) for redundant presentation of essential information.

**4b.** Provide adequate contrast between essential information and its surroundings.

**4c.** Maximize "legibility" of essential information.

**4d.** Differentiate elements in ways that can be described (i.e., make it easy to give instructions or directions).

**4e.** Provide compatibility with a variety of techniques or devices used by people with sensory limitations.

### PRINCIPLE 5

**Tolerance for Error:** The design minimizes hazards and the adverse consequences of accidental or unintended actions.

**Guidelines:**

**5a.** Arrange elements to minimize hazards and errors: most used elements, most accessible; hazardous elements eliminated, isolated, or shielded.

**5b.** Provide warnings of hazards and errors.

**5c.** Provide fail-safe features.

**5d.** Discourage unconscious action in tasks that require vigilance.

### PRINCIPLE 6

**Low Physical Effort:** The design can be used efficiently and comfortably and with a minimum of fatigue.

**Guidelines:**

**6a.** Allow user to maintain a neutral body position.

**6b.** Use reasonable operating forces.

**6c.** Minimize repetitive actions.

**6d.** Minimize sustained physical effort.

### PRINCIPLE 7

**Size and Space for Approach and Use:** Appropriate size and space is provided for approach, reach, manipulation, and use regardless of user's body size, posture, or mobility.

**Guidelines:**

**7a.** Provide a clear line of sight to important elements for any seated or standing user.

**7b.** Make reach to all components comfortable for any seated or standing user.

**7c.** Accommodate variations in hand and grip size.

**7d.** Provide adequate space for the use of assistive devices or personal assistance.

From C. Christiansen and K. Matuska. (Eds.). (2004). *Ways of living: Adaptive strategies for special needs,* 3rd edition (p. 428). Bethesda, MD: American Occupational Therapy Association. Reprinted with permission.

and to assist with modifications of adaptive equipment.

f. Computer experts, to assist with the design and provision of efficient technology.

g. Rehabilitation counselors, to assess and advise on vocational issues.

h. Social workers, to assist in obtaining funding.

i. Psychologists, to assist with adjustment disorders, if indicated.

j. Nurses, to ensure carry-over of medical care and medication regimes prescribed by the doctor.

k. Teachers, for children in the school system, to help carry over any modifications within the classroom setting.

l. Driver trainers, for those who may require driving adaptations.

m. Vendors, to provide items requested by therapists and required for the individual to function.

n. Third party payers or their respective case managers, to approve and/or provide funding for the individual's needed environmental modifications.

### E. Purposes of Environmental Evaluation and Intervention

1. Identify and prioritize the needs, goals, desires, and problem areas of an individual with a disability within his/her environments.

2. Establish the individual's abilities regarding everyday functional activities within his/her environment.

3. Assess functional use of devices being considered for a particular individual to facilitate mastery of the environment.

4. Identify a device's availability, safety, and cost.

5. Determine a device's location and frequency of use.

6. Determine funding and financial resources for equipment and/or modifications.

   a. It is of questionable ethics and not in the best interest of the individual with a disability to show him or her a device or order top of the line equipment that is not covered by his or her insurance, if he/she does not have the financial resources to self-pay.

7. Determine environmental constraints.

   a. For example, an individual may be living in a four flight walk-up apartment and have to leave a device locked up in a lobby, opening it up to the risk of vandalism or theft.

8. Assess if the individual with a disability and the device will allow for re-evaluation.

9. Ensure the device will allow for possible modifications, if upon reassessment of the individual a change in status is found.

## II. Overall Environmental Evaluation

### A. Evaluation of Performance Skills and Client Factors

1. The role of the OTA.

   a. The OTA contributes to the evaluation process in collaboration with the OT supervisor.

      (1) Supervision is required.

      (2) The level of supervision required will be determined by the OTA's experience and established service competence.

   b. Service competency must be established.

   c. The OTA cannot independently evaluate or interpret evaluation results.

2. Performance skills and client factors are essential to assess when conducting an environmental evaluation, for they are the fundamental abilities that allow a person to function in his or her environment.

3. Upon establishment of service competency, the OTA can collect data in the following areas:

   a. Sensory skills (e.g., tactile to assess sensation to determine if there is an impairment with discrimination that could influence safety in the manipulation of devices).

   b. Visual perceptual processing skills (e.g., Minnesota Rate of Manipulation Test, a standardized test to assess visual motor perception to assess for potential difficulties with computer use).

   c. Musculoskeletal skills (e.g., range of motion, strength, and endurance, to assess if the person will be able to physically use the devices to optimal capability).

   d. Neuromuscular skills (e.g., tone, coordination, to assess the person's ability to utilize all limbs rhythmically in mobility and environmental manipulation).

   e. Cognitive skills (e.g., following directions and judgment, to assess if a person is aware of limitations and able to follow and recall directions regarding operation of assistive technology and wheelchairs) and the safe use of devices.

   f. Psychosocial skills (e.g., social support, to

assess if an individual with a disability can ask for assistance and obtain needed information from the right person).

**B. Contextual Evaluation**
1. The OTA contributes to the evaluation process with OT supervision.
2. Areas targeted for evaluation include:
   a. Physical considerations.
      (1) Arrangement of furniture.
      (2) Accessibility of items needed for desired activities and for safe use.
      (3) Ease of use.
      (4) Housing/workplace design.
      (5) Neighborhood characteristics.
         (a) Availability and use of transportation.
         (b) Overall accessibility.
   b. Sociocultural considerations.
      (1) The individual's social network: the relationships between the individual with the disability and others.
      (2) Social roles: expectations for role performance of the individual with a disability and others.
      (3) Opportunities for socialization.
      (4) Sociocultural norms, values, and expectations for independent function.
      (5) Community resources available.

# III. Home Evaluation

**A. General Considerations**
1. OTAs can perform home assessments and make adaptations, modifications, and recommendations to the anticipated dwelling to increase safe, independent functioning with OT supervision.
2. If an individual with a disability is to be discharged to home from a facility, the on-site home evaluation should be done before the discharge date.
3. The person's current status (abilities and limitations) will drive the need for modification.

**B. Overall Characteristics of the Home**
1. Type of dwelling: private house, one-family, two-family, apartment, walk-up, elevator access.
2. Protection from weather/environmental changes.
3. Presence and use of a driveway.
4. Level of the dwelling in which the person lives.
5. Entrance to the dwelling: wheelchair access, ramp, level entrance, stairs.
6. Number of entrances that are accessible to the individual.

   a. Some apartment buildings allow residents to use delivery entrance because it has a ramp.
7. Steps: the number present outside dwelling, inside the dwelling, to the laundry room, and to the mailbox.
8. Railings: the location and number of railings when outside and facing the entrance door; the presence of secure railings for interior stairways.
   a. Interior railings should be mounted 1½" from the wall to ease grasp.
   b. Exterior railings should be waist high for those who walk; 34" – 38" depending on person's height.
   c. Railings should be 1½" – 2" in diameter with non-skid surfaces.
9. Door sills: identify where they are present, i.e., entrance to dwelling, bedroom doors, bathroom doors, kitchen doorway.
10. Elevators: width of elevator doorway, type of manual operation.
11. Hallways: width of hallway entrance.
12. Doorways: width of entrance door(s); measure from open door to frame; not frame to frame.
13. Doorways: direction of opening for entrance door(s) and any other doors throughout dwelling which must be opened.
    a. Space to accommodate door swing must be available.
       (1) A minimum of 18" is needed for those using walkers.
       (2) A minimum of 26" is needed for those using wheelchairs.
14. Type(s) of door handles: lever handles are more functional than round knobs.
15. Identification of objects which may be obstructing doorways and/or pathways.
16. Presence of pets: they can become obstacles and/or safety concerns to those with low vision, balance problems, and those who require assistive devices.
17. Carpeting: location and type, i.e., wall to wall, throw rugs, and height of pile.
18. Electrical cords: placed out of flow of traffic, in good condition or frayed, overloaded or under rugs/carpeting.
19. Presence of a firm chair in the dwelling and its height.
20. Light switches: accessibility from various levels (standing and chair).
21. Telephones: number of phones, their location,

cordless phone availability, type of phones (push button or rotary), emergency numbers by telephone.

22. Presence of working smoke detectors.
23. Presence of space heaters or wood burning equipment.
24. Presence of an emergency call system and an emergency exit plan.

**C. Bedroom Considerations**
1. Bed: size of bed, height from floor to top mattress, type of mattress and bed, wheeled frame or not, position of bed (against the wall or freestanding).
2. Side of the bed from which the individual with a disability enters/exits.
3. Ability to change bed location, if needed.
4. Accessibility of clothes and dresser drawers.
5. Sufficient room available for a bedside commode, if needed.

**D. Bathroom Considerations**
1. Number of bathrooms in the home.
2. Location of bathroom(s) relative to the bedroom, living room, kitchen, and other living spaces important to the individual.
3. Width of the bathroom doorway.
4. Type of bathing the individual with a disability performs (i.e., bath, shower, sponge bath) previously and currently.
5. Type of shower/tub: separate stall, glass door tub with shower, curtain-enclosed tub with shower, old fashioned claw-legged tub.
6. Presence and location of grab bars for toilet and bath/shower (the soap dish and towel bar are not grab bars).
   a. If home is rental, landlord's agreement to allow grab bars to be installed if needed.
7. Height of tub, sink, and toilet.
8. Presence of a non-skid mat or skid-free surface in the shower/tub.
9. Presence of a throw rug outside of shower.
10. Availability of a hand-held shower.
11. Presence of anti-scald valves and/or faucets.
12. Location of toilet paper holder.

**E. Kitchen Considerations**
1. Location of meal preparation devices that the individual uses most frequently (i.e., oven, microwave, stove).
2. Presence of a countertop area between the stove and sink, between the stove and refrigerator.
3. Accessibility of food, pots, pans, dishes, and preparation materials.

4. Direction of opening for refrigerator, cabinetry, and/or pantry doors.
5. Presence of a charged fire extinguisher.
6. Presence of anti-scald valves and/or faucets.

# IV. Fall Prevention and Management
## A. Falls Etiology, Prevalence, and Prognosis
1. The unintentional loss of balance causing one to make unexpected contact with ground of floor.
2. Falls and fall injury are a major public health concern for the elderly. The facts and figures that follow are provided to highlight the need for OT practitioners to be active in the prevention of falls. These statistics will not be on the NBCOT examination.
   a. Between 30 and 50% of persons over the age of 65 fall each year. Note: Percentages may be greater because data is based only upon reported falls.
   b. Twenty-four percent of falls result in severe soft tissue injury and fractures.
   c. Falls are the sixth leading cause of death for the elderly. 12% of all deaths for persons aged 65 or older are caused by falls.
   d. Falls are a factor in 40% of admissions to nursing homes.
   e. Women are more at risk for falls than men, due to their increased incidence of osteoporosis; 20% of men aged 65-74 fall, whereas 42% of women of the same age fall.
   f. Within six months of a fall, more than $2/3$ of the elderly who have fallen will fall again.
3. Results of falls.
   a. Fractures: Most common fracture sites are the pelvis, hip, femur, vertebrae, and humerus head.
   b. Increased caution and fear of falling.
   c. Loss of confidence to function independently.
   d. Decreased engagement in activity and restriction of activities which can result in severe physical deconditioning and deterioration, contributing to the likelihood of reoccurrence.
   e. Increased risk of recurrent falls.

## B. Evaluation of Risk Factors for Falls
1. The OTA contributes to the evaluation process with OT supervision.
   a. Upon establishment of service competency, the OTA can collect data about the intrinsic and extrinsic factors that contribute to falls.
2. Intrinsic factors requiring evaluation.

a. Age related changes in sensory system resulting in reduced sensory capacity.
   (1) Vision.
       (a) Presbyopia (decreased acuity).
       (b) Reduced night vision means that vision in low light situations is also reduced.
       (c) Impaired depth perception.
   (2) Vestibular.
       (a) Vertigo.
       (b) Postural sway combined with vision problems results in a compound risk.

b. Age related changes in the neuromuscular system.
   (1) Decreased number of neurons results in decreased reaction or response time.
   (2) Decreased number of muscle fibers leads to decreased lower extremity strength and endurance.
   (3) Two manifestations of the combination of the above factors include difficulties in rising from a chair and maintaining gait speed.

c. Comorbidity and pathological states including congestive heart failure, arrhythmias, hypotension, cerebrovascular disease, Parkinson's disease, arteriosclerosis and atherosclerosis, diabetes mellitus.

d. Medication side effects and/or polypharmacy.

e. Delirium and/or dementia.

f. Anxiety and/or depression.

g. Cognitive deficits, decreased attention span, distractibility, impaired judgment.

h. Prior history of falls within past year.

i. Fear of falling can lead to decreased mobility and progressive deconditioning, which increase the risk of subsequent falls.

3. Extrinsic factors requiring evaluation: Safety hazards within the environment that predispose one to slip and fall.
   a. General.
      (1) Floors: slippery or uneven, presence of throw rugs.
      (2) Toys or other clutter left on floors or stairs.
      (3) Pets under foot.
      (4) High pile carpets.
      (5) Low lying furniture.
      (6) Stairs, excessive steepness, lack of or loose handrails.
      (7) Improper footwear.
      (8) Poor lighting or glare.
      (9) Poor thresholds.
      (10) Extension cords.
      (11) Use of furniture or other unstable objects for support.
      (12) Improper transfer techniques.
      (13) Problems with adaptive equipment, lack of needed equipment, or excessive equipment.
   b. Bathroom.
      (1) No grab bars.
      (2) Utilization of unstable soap dish or towel bar for support.
      (3) Toilet seat too low.
      (4) Wet floor surfaces.
      (5) Utilization of wet sink surface for support.
      (6) Loose rug on floor.
   c. Kitchen.
      (1) Low cabinet doors open.
      (2) Step stool without handles.
      (3) Chairs pulled out.
      (4) Wet floor surfaces.
      (5) Loose rug on floor.
   d. Bedroom.
      (1) Bed too high or too low.
      (2) Movement of bed.
      (3) Reaching into closets.
   e. Living room.
      (1) Wires and/or clutter across floor.
      (2) Chairs too high or too low.
      (3) High pile or loose rugs.
      (4) Poor lighting.

## C. Interventions to Prevent Falls

1. Intervention is based upon the determination of the individual's functional problems and the causative factors of falls as identified in evaluation.

2. The OTA implements intervention with OT supervision to:
   a. Eliminate or minimize all fall risk factors; stabilize disease states, manage medication.
   b. Improve functional mobility.
      (1) Active or resistive muscle strengthening exercises with weights and general conditioning exercises (GCE) to improve or maintain flexibility, strength, endurance, and coordination.
      (2) PROM stretching as indicated to increase joint ROM.
      (3) Specific coordination training.
      (4) Neuromuscular reeducation training.
      (5) Balance training.
          (a) Sit and stand positions.

(b) Static and dynamic.

(c) Turning, walking, stairs.

(6) Transfer training.

(7) Bed mobility training.

(8) Wheelchair safety training.

(9) Referral to physical therapy for gait/ambulation training.

c. Provide sensory compensation strategies.

d. Modify activities of daily living for safety.

(1) Order appropriate adaptive devices and train in safe use (i.e., reachers, long shoe horn, stocking/sock aid, leg lifter, dressing stick, walker baskets, etc.).

(2) Allow adequate time for activities; instruct in gradual position changes.

e. Teach energy conservation techniques.

f. Communicate with family and caregivers.

g. Modify environment to reduce falls and instability; use environmental checklist.

(1) Ensure adequate lighting.

(2) Use contrasting colors to delineate hazardous areas.

(3) Simplify environment, reduce clutter.

(4) Firmly attach carpet.

(5) Stairs.

(a) Securely fasten handrails on both sides of stairs.

(b) Provide light switches at top and bottom.

(c) Install non-skid secure surface.

(6) Bathrooms.

(a) Install grab bars located in and out of tubs and shower and near toilets.

(b) Provide nonskid mats and nightlights.

(c) Use elevated toilet seat.

(7) Bedrooms.

(a) Install night lights or light switch within reach of bed.

(b) Place telephones in an easy to reach position near bed.

(c) Replace existing mattress with one either thinner or thicker to lower or to raise bed height as needed.

(d) Arrange furniture to ease maneuvering.

(8) Living areas.

(a) Ensure couches and chairs are at proper height to get in and out of easily.

(b) Remove clutter and loose electrical cords.

(c) Arrange furniture for easy maneuverability.

(9) Kitchen and closet shelves.

(a) Store items on reachable shelves (between person's eye and hip level).

(10) Outdoors.

(a) Fix cracked pavement or steps.

(b) Install stable outside handrail.

h. Provide specific safety guidelines for the individual to follow.

(1) Ask for assistance to transfer or ambulate. (Do not stand up alone; do not walk to the bathroom or kitchen alone, etc.).

(2) Utilize prescribed assistive device(s) to ambulate, especially on any uneven or unfamiliar ground. Keep assistive device near at all times.

(3) Use prescribed adaptive equipment.

(4) Stand in place before beginning to walk to avoid dizziness from change in position and to regain balance.

(5) Do not bend forward.

(6) Wear supportive rubber-soled or low heeled shoes.

(7) Avoid wearing smooth-soled slippers or only socks, which makes it easier to slip.

10. Provide psychological support and specific interventions to deal with the fear of falling.

a. Acknowledge the validity of the individual's concerns.

b. Initiate discussions about risk factors and encourage active problem solving.

c. Modify activities to be safe and achievable to build confidence.

d. Provide activities to maintain physical conditioning to decrease risk of fear becoming a reality.

e. Develop a contingency plan to use in the event of a fall to maintain safety.

11. Complete appropriate referrals.

a. Refer to physician for medical check-up, assessment of polymedication.

b. Refer to optometrist/vision specialist for vision assessment.

**D. Interventions for Occurrence of Falls**

1. Check for fall injury.

a. Hip fracture: complaints of pain in hip, especially on palpation; external rotation of leg; inability to bear weight on leg; changes in gait or weight bearing status.

b. Head injury: loss of consciousness, mental confusion.

c. Spinal cord injury: loss of sensation or voluntary movement.

d. Cuts, bruises, painful swelling.

2. Check for dizziness that may have preceded the fall.

3. Provide reassurance.

4. Provide first aid, call emergency services if necessary.

5. Do not attempt to lift the individual alone, get help.

6. Solicit witnesses of fall event.

7. Document the incident as per setting's established procedures.

8. Refer the individual to a fall prevention intervention program to prevent reoccurrences.

# V. Modifications for Sensorimotor Deficits

## A. Architectural Barriers

1. Architectural features in the home and the community that make negotiation of space difficult or impossible (e.g., steps, narrow doors) or require modifications to allow accessibility.

2. Modifications should be made according to the International Code Council, Inc., Falls Church, Virginia.

3. Wheelchair dimensions and accessibility needs.

   a. Average wheelchair width is 24"-26" rim to rim.

(1) Some doorways and room spaces may be too narrow, limiting clear mobility.

(2) The minimal clearance width for doorways and halls: 32" doorway width minimum, with ideal being 36".

   (a) An additional 26" is needed beside the door to allow for door swing.

   (b) Doorways can be widened or removed if necessary.

   • Removing doorstops can add 3/4" in width.

   • Replacing existing hinges with offset hinges can add 1½" – 2" in width.

   (c) Doorway saddles can be removed and the floor patched, or a wedge can be placed in front of the saddle, or a thin rubber mat can be placed over the saddle.

(3) Hallways should be 36" wide (Figure 15-1.).

   b. Average wheelchair length is 42"-43" (Figure 15-2)

(1) Adequate turning spaces are needed. (Figure 15-3.)

(2) A 360 degree wheelchair turning space requires a clearance space of 60" x 60". (Figure 15-3.)

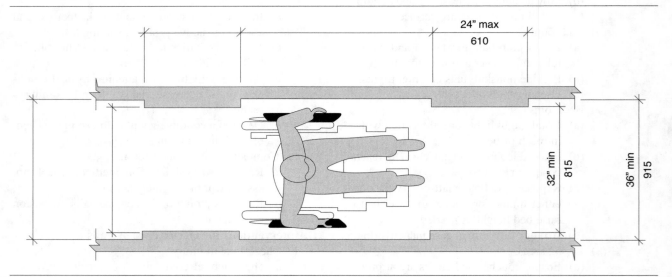

**Figure 15-1** Minimum clear width for doorways and halls. A minimum of 32" of doorway width is required; the ideal is 36". Hallways should be a minimum of 36" wide to provide sufficient clearance for wheelchair passage and allow the user to propel the chair without scraping the hands.

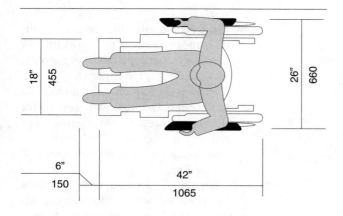

**Figure 15-2** Dimensions of standard adult manual wheelchair. Width 24 to 26" from rim to rim. Length: 42 to 43". Height to push handles from floor: 36". Height to seat from floor: 19 to 19.5 " (excluding cushion). Height to armrest from floor: 29 to 30". Note: Footrests may extend farther for very large people.

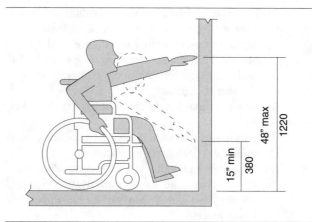

**Figure 15-4** Forward reach. The maximal height an individual can reach from a seated position is 48". Height should be at least 15" to prevent the wheelchair from tipping forward.

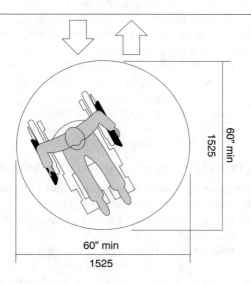

**Figure 15-3** 360° wheelchair turning space. A 360° turn requires a clear space of 60" by 60". This space enables the individual to turn without scraping the feet or maneuvering multiple times to accomplish a full turn.

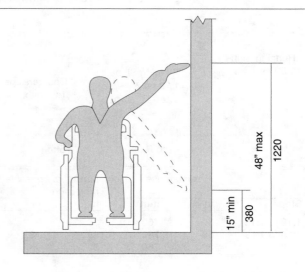

**Figure 15-5** Side reach. The maximal height for reaching from the side position without an obstruction is 48". If an obstruction such as a countertop or shelf is present the maximal height for side reach is 46".

c. The maximal height the individual can reach forward from sitting is 48" and at least 15" is needed to prevent tipping. (Figure 15-4.)

d. Maximal height for reaching sideways is 54" and when an obstruction is present is 46". (Figure 15-5.)

e. The maximal height for countertops should be 31".

f. Parking spaces should have an adjacent 4' aisle to allow wheelchairs to maneuver.

g. Pathways and walkways should be 48" wide.

h. Ramps should be a minimum of 36" wide and should have a non-skid surface on upper and lower levels.

(1) The ratio of slope to rise is 1:12 (for every 1" of vertical rise, 12" of ramp is required). (Figure 15-6.)

(2) Railings should be between 29" and 36" high depending on person's arm reach. 32" is average.

(3) Curbs on ramps should be at least 4" high.

(4) Level platforms must be included in the ramp design.

(a) If the ramp is excessively long, 4'x4' landing(s) are required to allow for rest.

(b) If the person using the ramp has limited upper extremity strength or decreased cardiopulmonary capacity, 4'x4' landing(s) are required.

(c) If there is a sharp turn in the direction of the ramp, landing(s) are required for turning space. A 90 degree turn requires a minimum 4'x4' landing; a 180 degree turn requires a minimum 4' x8' landing.

(5) If the ramp leads to a door, there must be a 5'x5' platform before the door that extends at least 12" (18" is preferred) along the side of the door to allow for door swing without backing up.

i. Electric porch lifts and stair lifts are alternatives to ramps.

## B. Funding for Environmental Modifications

1. State One-Stop Centers, Vocational and Educational Services for Individuals with Disabilities (VESID), Offices for Vocational Rehabilitation (OVRs), and Divisions of Vocational Rehabilitation (DVRs) will pay for home and work modifications, if the modifications enable a person to go to work or school.

2. Private companies will fund modifications to ensure ADA compliance.

3. Private insurance, Medicare, Medicaid and Workmen's Compensation will possibly reimburse for certain devices/adaptations.

4. Centers for Independent Living and disability rights organizations may fund modifications to enable full community participation.

# VI. Wheelchair Prescription and Assessment

## A. Purposes of Wheelchair Seating and Positioning

1. Promote comfort during upright ADL.

2. Promote functional posture by provision of appropriate back and leg supports.

3. Provide physiological maintenance and tissue protection through prevention of shearing.

4. Promote sensory readiness through provision of proper eye and head position.

5. Facilitate upper limb function which occurs with proper trunk support.

6. Promote social acceptance by allowing eye contact.

7. To decrease progression of deformity through customized seating as needed.

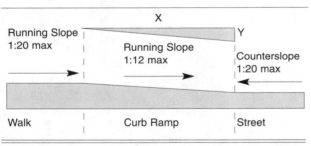

| | Maximum rise | | Maximum horizontal projection | |
|---|---|---|---|---|
| Slope | in | mm | ft | m |
| 1:12 to 1:15 | 30 | 760 | 30 | 9 |
| 1:16 to 1:19 | 30 | 760 | 40 | 12 |
| 1:20 | 30 | 760 | 50 | 15 |

**Figure 15-6** Slope and rise of ramps. This diagram provides the components of a single ramp run and a sample of ramp dimensions. The slope ratio is an important consideration when designing a ramp; slope creates hazardous wheelchair propulsion conditions if it is too steep.

8. Decrease pain through provision of proper support to all limbs.
9. Facilitate mobility with what means the person with a disability has available.
10. Increase self-esteem through provision of a wheelchair which meets the person's needs and facilitates mastery of the environment.

**B. General Assessment and Prescription Considerations**

1. The OTA contributes to the evaluation process with OT supervision to:
   a. Assess the ability of the wheelchair to interact/interface with other assistive devices.
   b. Determine the individual's medical status, including prognosis (is condition temporary, stable, or progressive?) and functional level/needs.
2. Collaborate with the consumer, caregiver(s), and interdisciplinary team members as identified in Section I.D. of this chapter.

**C. Specific Assessments for Wheelchair Prescription**

1. Upon establishment of service competency, the OTA can collect data in the following areas:
   a. Client factor and performance skill assessments.
      (1) Sensory (e.g., sensory loss places the person at risk for the development of decubiti, therefore necessitating a special seat cushion).
      (2) Neuromuscular (e.g., the individual's sitting posture can require application of seating and positioning knowledge. Poor trunk control requires postural supports).
      (3) Musculoskeletal (e.g., physical limitations, such as a compromised respiratory status, may impede mobility, requiring a powered wheelchair prescription). Hip precautions may require a cushion to raise seat height.
      (4) Cognition (e.g., deficits in cognitive function may impede ability to operate powered devices).
      (5) Psychosocial (e.g., the availability of social supports to assist with transporting and transferring to the wheelchair).
   b. Personal assessment.
      (1) Age and developmental status.
      (2) Medical history, current medical status, and weight.
      (3) Education and work history.
      (4) Leisure interests and pursuits (e.g., a spe-

cial sports chair can enable the individual to pursue past or new interests).
      (5) Daily routines and habits.
      (6) Goals and desired occupations.
      (7) Socioeconomic status, financial assets and limitations.
   c. Contextual assessments.
      (1) Physical environment.
         (a) Areas of travel and wheelchair use.
         (b) Surfaces and terrains that will be traveled on indoors (e.g., floor surfaces) and outdoors (e.g., sidewalks).
      (2) Building characteristics of school, work, leisure, and/or worship.
         (a) Entrance accessibility.
         (b) Doorways.
         (c) Hallways.
         (d) Restrooms.
         (e) Workspace design.
         (f) Parking.
         (g) Other specifics as described in the home evaluation section of this chapter.
   d. Wheelchair characteristics considered in assessment.
      (1) Transportability/portability.
      (2) Ride quality.
      (3) Wheelchair types available.
         (a) Control mechanism (e.g., type of brakes used, use of anti-tippers).
         (b) Features (e.g., use of lap tray, cushion, backpack to hold personal items and/or medical equipment, racing model for more athletic individuals).
         (c) Propulsion method (e.g., one arm drive, use of hand rim projections, motorized, use of lower extremities to propel).
   e. Developmental considerations in assessment.
      (1) Transportability to, from, and in school.
      (2) Allowance for adjustment when growth changes are experienced.
      (3) Allowance for use of other adaptive equipment (i.e., computer, augmentative communication).
      (4) Facilitation of social acceptance.

**D. Wheelchair Components**

1. Armrests.
   a. Fixed: minimal benefit but may be seen in older wheelchairs and/or in rentals.
   b. Detached: helpful for transfers.

c. Height adjustable: allows for ease in transfers and better support of a lap tray.

d. Desk arms: allow for moving closer to work surfaces.

e. Full arms: allow for holding of a lap tray and possibly ease transfers.

f. Wraparound, space saver arm rests: reduces the overall width of the chair by one inch.

2. Leg rests.

a. Fixed: minimal benefit but may be seen in older wheelchairs and/or in rentals.

b. Swing-away: allows feet to be placed on the floor to prepare for transfers and for a front approach to wheelchair.

c. Detachable: allows for a safe path for transfers.

d. Elevating: allows for edema control and reduction.

3. Footplates.

a. Fixed: minimal benefit but may be seen in older wheelchairs and/or in rentals.

b. Swing-away: allows feet to reach floor.

c. Heel loops: prevent feet from slipping off footrest in a posterior direction.

d. Ankle straps: prevent slipping off footrest.

4. Tires.

a. Pneumatic: air-filled, requires maintenance, more cushioned ride, shock absorbent.

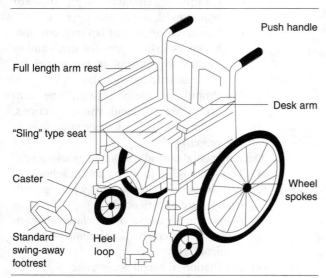

**Figure 15-7** Basic style of wheelchair frame.

Salemo, C. (1998). Seating and wheeled mobility prescription. In G. Gillen and A. Burkhardt (Eds). *Stroke rehabilitation: A function based approach* (page 443). St. Louis: Mosby-Year Book, Inc. Reprinted with permission.

b. Semi-pneumatic: airless foam inserts, less maintenance, good cushioning.

c. Solid-core rubber: minimal maintenance, tires are mounted on spoked or molded wheels.

5. Casters.

a. Smaller ones facilitate maneuverability.

b. Pneumatic and semi-pneumatic types available, but solid-core are best for indoors and smooth surfaces.

c. Caster locks can be added for increased stability during transfers.

6. Frame.

a. Fixed: minimal benefit but may be seen in older wheelchairs or sports chairs.

b. Folding: eases storage and facilitates mobility in community as it can fold to fit in car or van.

c. Weight: ultra-light, active-duty lightweight, lightweight, standard and heavy duty frame construction is available.

(1) The lighter the weight of the chair generally, the greater the ease of use.

(2) The demands of the individual's expected and desired activities must be considered.

7. Additional attachments.

a. Anti-tippers to prevent wheelchair from tipping backward or forward.

(1) Can get caught on doorsills and curbs.

b. Seatbelts for safety during mobility and functional activities.

(1) Attach at hip level not waist level.

(2) Extend across hips and into lap at 45-degree angle.

c. Harnesses to position a person lacking sufficient trunk control.

d. Arm troughs to position and support a flaccid upper extremity and prevent edema through elevation.

e. Lapboards can serve the same purpose as an arm trough, but are also beneficial as a working "table top" surface.

f. Head supports allow for improved eye contact, improved communication, and feeding assistance, as the head is kept in a neutral position.

g. Mobile arm supports allow for use of an upper extremity with proximal weakness to engage in feeding and other activities.

h. Brake extensions allow a person with limited range in one upper extremity to independently manipulate the wheelchair's brakes.

i. Handrim projections ease independent propulsion in persons with weak handgrip.

    (1) These increase the width of the chair and can decrease mobility through narrow doors and/or narrow spaces.

  j. Hillholder devices allow the wheelchair to move forward but automatically brake when the chair goes backward.

    (1) Useful for individuals unable to ascend a long ramp or hill without a rest.

  k. Seating and positioning systems (see Section VII for details).

## E. Wheelchair Measurement and Considerations

1. General.

  a. The size of a wheelchair should be proportional to the person. See Section VI.G for bariatric considerations.

    (1) Standard-sized chairs should be matched to a person whenever possible due to the increased expense of customized chairs.

    (2) Refer to Table 15-2.

  b. Measure on a firm surface, but also observe in a variety of positions to account for tonal influences on posture.

  c. The cushion that will be selected for the individual needs to be considered.

2. Seat width.

  a. Measure the widest point across the hips and thighs to allow for maximal seating space and comfort, and then add 2".

  b. This allows for clearance on the sides to prevent friction/rubbing and to allow the individual to wear heavier material clothing without being cumbersome.

  c. The bariatric client with a pear-shape will have increased gluteal femoral weight distribution.

    (1) Measurement should consider the widest

## TABLE 15-2
## STANDARD DIMENSIONS FOR WHEELCHAIRS

| CHAIR STYLE | SEAT WIDTH | SEAT DEPTH | SEAT HEIGHT |
|---|---|---|---|
| Adult | 18″ | 16″ | 20″ |
| Narrow Adult | 16″ | 16″ | 20″ |
| Slim Adult | 14″ | 16″ | 20″ |
| Hemi/low Seat | | | 17.5″ |
| Junior | 16″ | 16″ | 18.5″ |
| Child | 14″ | 11.5″ | 18.75″ |
| Tiny Tot | 12″ | 11.5″ | 19.5″ |

portion of the seated position (e.g., at the forward edge of the seated position).

    (2) Also consider room for weightshifting maneuvers for pressure relief, and possible use of lift devices.

3. Seat depth.

  a. Measure both lower extremities (LEs) and take the greatest length; measure from the posterior portion of the buttocks to the popliteal fossa and then subtract 2" from this measurement.

  b. This prevents rubbing and potential decubiti to posterior knee region, while also allowing maximal leg swing.

4. Back height.

  a. Measurement is based on the need for postural stability, upper extremity (UE) movements, and potential for independent wheelchair propulsion.

  b. Take measurement from seat surface (including the cushion) upward to one of the following depending on trunk control, activity level, strength, and size of person with disability.

    (1) Mid-back under scapula: 1"-2" below.

    (2) Mid-scapula or axilla.

    (3) Top of the shoulder.

  c. Lower back height can increase functional mobility as in sports chairs.

    (1) Lower back height can increase back strain.

  d. Higher back height may be needed if poor trunk stability.

    (1) If back height of chair is extended, potential problems must be recognized.

      (a) Added back height may prevent the individual from locking onto the push handle for stabilization and/or weight shifting.

      (b) Added back height may increase difficulty of fitting chair into car or van.

5. Seat height.

  a. Knees and ankles should be positioned at 90 degrees; measure from distal thigh to heel.

  b. Footrests should have 2" clearance from the floor, so cushion selected will affect this measurement.

  c. Standard height: 20".

  d. Hemi-height: 17.5".

  e. Super-low: 14.5".

6. Armrest height.

  a. Shoulders should be neutral; arms hanging at the sides; elbow flexed to 90 degrees.

b. Measure under each elbow to cushioned seating surface.

c. Armrests that are too low will encourage leaning forward.

d. Armrests that are too high will cause shoulder elevation.

F. Types of Wheelchairs

1. Refer to Table 15-3 for descriptions of general types of wheelchairs and indications/contraindications for use.

2. Specialized wheelchairs.

a. Reclining back: indicated for individuals who are unable to independently maintain an upright sitting position.

b. Tilt in space: indicated for pressure relief or for an individual with severe extensor spasms that may throw him or her out of the chair; entire seat and back tilt back to maintain a normal seat to back angle.

c. One arm-drive, hemi-chair, amputee frame, and powered chairs as outlined in Table 15-3.

d. Recreational: designed with large thick inner tube type tires and large front casters for all terrain use including sand, mud, snow, and off-road surfaces.

e Sports: specially designed for racing, cycling, basketball, and other competitive sports.

(1) Typically ultra lightweight with a solid frame, low seat, low back, seat that accommodates a tucked position, leg straps, slanted drive wheels, small push rims.

f. Stander: designed to enable a person to independently change seat height and/or elevate to a standing position.

g. Stair-climbing: designed to navigate stairs while balancing on two wheels using sensors and gyroscopes.

h. Bariatric wheelchair: heavy-duty, extra-wide wheelchair designed to assist mobility for individuals who are obese.

G. Bariatric Considerations for Wheelchair Prescription[1]

1. Wheelchair users who are obese must be prescribed wheelchairs that are rated for their obesity category.

a. Selection based on patient characteristics, safe-

## TABLE 15-3

| ATTENDANT PROPELLED | MANUAL WHEELCHAIR | POWERED MOBILITY |
|---|---|---|
| **Description** | **Description** | **Description** |
| • Pushed by another | • Rigid or folding frames | • Usually add-on unit to allow for manual use |
| • Usually is manual wheelchair | • Various frames and weights | • Scooter |
| | • Lightweight chair: 25-40 pounds | • Battery operated: |
| | • Standard: >50 pounds without seating | – deep cycle lead acid |
| | | – wet cell |
| | • Amputee frame: weight is more towards front axle | – sealed cell |
| | • Hemi-chair: use non-affected upper extremity and/or lower extremity | • Method of operation: |
| | • One-arm drive | – micro-switch |
| | • Gurneys: for prone position | – proportional joystick |
| | | – sip and puff |
| | | – sensing system |
| | | – body part to be used |
| **Indications/Benefits** | **Indications/Benefits** | **Indications/Benefits** |
| • Brief or chronic disability | • May independently propel | • Cannot use hands or feet |
| • Transport in the community | • May use quick release wheels (easier for cars) | • Energy expenditure limitations |
| • Used for extended periods of time | | • Arthritic upper extremities |
| • When powered mobility cannot be used | | • Prone to repetitive stress injury |
| • Fit and comfort considered for all involved | | • Neuromuscular injury: to prevent associated reactions |
| | | • Can change seat height or tilt |
| **Limitations** | **Limitations** | **Limitations** |
| • Dependent on another person | • Standard weight is heavy when considering adding seating system | • Large and heavy to transport |
| | | • May need to use lifts |

Based upon Dietz, J. and Dudgeon, B. (1995).

[1]This section and the section on bariatric considerations for wheelchair measurement (E.2.c) were contributed by Susan O'Sullivan.

ty, and function.

2. The bariatric client has a center of body mass that is positioned several inches forward in comparison with the non-obese person.
   a. In order to ensure wheelchair stability, the rear axle is displaced forward in comparison with the standard wheelchair.
      (1) This forward position allows for a more efficient arm push (full arm stroke with less wrist extension).
3. Bariatric wheelchair can be ordered with special adaptations.
   a. Hard tires versus pneumatic tires for increased durability.
   b. Adjustable backrest to accommodate excessive posterior bulk.
   c. Reclining wheelchair to accommodate excessive anterior bulk, cardiorespiratory compromise (e.g., orthostatic hypotension).
   d. Power application attached to a heavy duty wheelchair to accommodate excessive fatigue.

### H. Wheelchair Training

1. Assess cognition to determine the individual's ability to learn mobility.
2. Instruct in proper sitting posture.
3. Instruct in pressure relief (i.e., push ups, weight shifts leaning to one side, then the other).
4. Instruct in the purpose and use of additional devices used with the wheelchair (i.e., cushion, lap board).
5. Provide time schedule for weight shifts and use of devices.
6. Instruct in wheelchair propulsion (e.g., manual, joystick, head control, sip and puff).
   a. Use of wheelchair gloves to ease propulsion and protect hands.
   b. Compensation techniques (e.g., use of feet to assist for propulsion when upper extremity is affected).
7. Instruct in safety concerns when operating a mobility device.
   a. Need to set/release brakes.
   b. Use of swing-away leg rests and removable armrests with transferring.
   c. Caution when using powered wheelchair.
   d. Safe ways to fall from a wheelchair and to return to wheelchair from the ground.
8. Instruct in how to manipulate basic parts of the wheelchair.
9. Instruct in how to maneuver wheelchair through-

out the community.
   a. Practice in natural environments is essential.
      (1) Ascend and descend inclines.
      (2) Negotiate lips and curbs; how to "pop a wheelie".
      (3) Negotiate obstacles.
10. Instruct in basic maintenance of wheelchair parts.
11. Developmental considerations.
    a. Teach children early to foster independence with wheelchair mobility in their environment.
    b. Discourage use of strollers that prevent child from independent propulsion.

## VII. Seating and Positioning Systems

### A. Definition

1. "The primary unit that influences body posture and prepares the individual for functional control" (Johann, 1998, p. 438).

### B. Goals

1. Provide stability, control, and comfort.
2. Promote proximal stability.
3. Decrease the risk of muscle contracture, deformity, and decubiti.
4. Increase sitting tolerance and energy level.
5. Increase function as proper seating will allow for use of upper extremities in ADL.
6. Allow for pressure relief and support.
7. Allow for proper positioning and correct alignment of trunk and extremities.

### C. Assessment Considerations

1. It is crucial to distinguish between flexible deformity (i.e., where the OT practitioner can manually correct the position), and fixed abnormal postures and deformities (i.e., where changes cannot occur).
2. The pelvis should be evaluated first, and then LEs, trunk, UEs, head and neck, and feet as stability is required prior to mobility and proximal control allows for better distal function.

### D. Basic Styles of Seating

1. Linear.
   a. Flat, non-contoured.
   b. Custom or factory-ordered.
   c. Firm, rigid seating.
   d. Good for active individuals, those who perform independent transfers and/or those with minimal musculoskeletal involvement.
2. Contoured and/or custom-contoured.
   a. Ergonomically supports the individual.
   b. Provides excellent support.

c. Enhances postural alignment.

d. Decreases abnormal posturing.

e. Provides pressure relief.

f. May be difficult for independent transfers if decreased UE muscle strength.

g. Good for individuals with moderate to severe central nervous system dysfunction or neurological disease.

**E. Major Styles and Accessories of Seating Systems**

1. Solid wood insert prevents hammock effect, provides solid base of support.

2. Solid seat prevents hammock effect, provides stable base of support; easy to remove, can lower seat to floor height.

3. Lumbar back support helps to give proper lumbar curve.

4. Foam cushion (of various densities) can enhance sitting posture and comfort.

5. Contoured foam cushion enhances pelvic and LE alignment.

6. Pressure relief cushions.

   a. Fluid.

      (1) Facilitates pelvic and LE alignment.

      (2) Provides pressure relief without changing support.

      (3) Good for individuals who need increased stability.

   b. Air.

      (1) Minimal postural support offered.

      (2) Provides pressure relief.

      (3) Good trunk control is needed.

7. Wedge cushions or antithrust seats have a front that is higher than the back to prevent the individual from sliding out of their seat.

8. Pelvic guides inserted on the interior sides of the wheelchair at hip level keep hips stable.

9. Lateral supports extend up the side of the chair to just below person's armpits to provide trunk support.

**F. Pediatric Seating and Positioning Systems**

1. Purposes.

   a. Allow for contractures and deformities.

   b. Allow for function at home and in school setting.

   c. Facilitate eye contact and parent/teacher/sibling/peer interactions.

   d. General positioning goals as previously stated.

2. Types.

   a. Usually custom molded created systems.

   b. Standers provide weight bearing experience

which maintains hips, knees, ankles and trunk in optimal position, facilitate formation of acetabulum and long bone development, and aid in bowel and bladder function.

   (1) Prone standers decrease effect of tonic labyrinthine reflex (TLR.)

   (2) Supine standers provide more support posteriorly.

   c. Sidelyers decrease effects of TLR and put hands in visual field.

   d. Triwall construction for infants and toddlers.

   e. Abductor pads at hips to decrease scissoring extensor pattern.

# VIII. Mobility and Mobility Aids

## A. Overview

1. Functional mobility involves "moving from one position or place to another (during performance of everyday activities), such as in-bed mobility, wheelchair mobility, and transfers (e.g., wheelchair, bed, car, tub, toilet, tub/shower, chair, floor). Includes functional ambulation and transporting objects" (AOTA, 2008, p. 631).

2. Functional mobility is prerequisite to perform self-care, work/school and leisure tasks and activities.

3. Evaluation includes a full client factor and performance skill assessment to determine potential ability to perform mobility (including sensation, perceptual, neuromuscular, musculoskeletal, cognitive, and psychosocial areas).

## B. Functional Mobility Aids

1. Ambulation aids.

   a. Orthotic devices (sometimes referred to as braces) are used to prevent contractures and provide stability to joints involved.

      (1) AFO: ankle-foot orthosis.

      (2) KAFO: knee-ankle-foot orthosis.

      (3) HKAFO: hip-knee-ankle-foot orthosis.

   b. Canes.

      (1) Straight: one leg.

      (2) Wide based quad cane (WBQC): one shaft is connected to a four-pronged base to increase stability when a person is not able to balance on a straight cane.

      (3) Narrow based quad cane (NBQC): same premise as WBQC, but prongs are situated closer together for a client who may not require as much support.

   c. Walkers.

      (1) Standard: requires the person to have fair

balance and the ability to lift device with upper extremities to advance.

(2) Hemi-walker: for those who do not have the ability to use two hands.

(3) Side-stepper: a walker situated on a non-affected side of a person.

(4) Rolling walker: for those who cannot lift a standard walker due to upper extremity weakness or impaired balance.

(5) Walker bags, trays and baskets to assist in transporting personal items.

d. Crutches.

(1) Standard: situated in person's axillary region to allow ambulation.

(2) Platform: forearms are neutral and are supported and hands are in neutral position.

(3) Lofstrand: proximal arm has closure around it instead of support in axillary region.

e. Slings provide support to upper extremity which may have fractured and prevent poor handling of flaccid upper extremity.

2. Wheelchairs and wheelchair training: see information previously provided in this chapter.

3. Scooters provide mobility to those who are not able to ambulate for distances.

4. Sliding boards allow independent transfers from different surfaces for those who are not able to stand-pivot.

5. Upper extremity mobility aids for task performance.

6. Bariatric considerations.

a. Selection of mobility aides are based on specific patient needs (patient safety, gait pattern, fatigue) and weight capacity.

b. Typical gait changes include greater hip abduction and hip rotation, less knee flexion, difficulty rotating from side-to-side with increased girth.

c. Extra wide walkers are used to assist ambulation and changes in elevation (e.g., sit-to-stand).

d. Heavy duty, extra wide walkers are used to assist ambulation.

**C. Bed Mobility**

1. Rolling, bridging, sidelying, supine, and sitting.

2. Some diagnoses require special positioning in bed to:

a. Maintain alignment of vulnerable joints.

b. Provide variation in postures.

c. Decrease the effect of pathological reflex

activity.

d. Provide variations in ranges of motion.

e. Provide stretch to muscles prone to contracture.

f. Increase comfort.

g. Include supine as well as right and left side positioning.

3. Specific mobility/positioning techniques.

a. Status-post total hip replacement.

(1) May not be permitted to roll on the non-operated side. This may result in internal rotation of the operated hip, which may cause dislocation.

(2) May require use of abductor pillow between lower extremities to prevent adduction of the operated hip.

b. Status-post CVA.

(1) May need education regarding proper positioning of upper extremity to increase awareness, minimize pain, decrease swelling, and promote normalization of tone.

(2) May also require use of pillows between knees while in sidelying to increase comfort and promote proper positioning.

c. Status-post amputation of the lower extremity.

(1) May require training regarding use of pillows to prevent edema in the lower extremity.

(2) May also need training on how to provide passive stretching to residual limb while in bed to prevent shortening or contracture, which would make prosthetic training difficult and painful.

4. Bed mobility aids.

a. Hospital beds, usually with bedrails and elevating head and foot surfaces.

b. Trapeze frame attached to bed.

c. Hoyer lift/trans-aid: a hammock device that is attached to either hydraulic or manual lift systems to transfer individuals who are dependent.

d. Bedpans and urinals to decrease need to leave bed.

# IX. Transfers

## A. Purpose

1. To move from one surface to another safely and effectively.

## B. Transfer Considerations

1. Assess and identify an individual's assets and deficits, especially cognitive and physical abilities.

2. The OTA should be aware of his or her own limitations to avoid personal or consumer injury.

3. Use of proper body mechanics should be strictly enforced.
   a. Use broad base of support.
   b. The OTA must know where his/her center of gravity is at all times.
   c. Individual to be transferred should be lifted with the OT practitioner using his/her lower extremities to lift and not his/her back.
4. Perform wheelchair transfers safely.
   a. Clear areas involved in transfers of any clutter.
   b. Ask for help or standby assist if questioning ability to transfer safely.
   c. Use transfer belts if needed.
   d. Stabilize/lock brakes.
   e. Swing away leg rests and flip up footplates.
   f. Remove armrest if individual is unable to assist, is too heavy to bring to a standing position, or if the individual has a weight bearing precaution.
5. Allow for variability of individuals and environment.
   a. Adjust transfer methods according to individual's strengths and limitations regarding performance component/skills and client factors.
   b. Be aware of different floor/ground surfaces.
   c. Be aware of the increased risk of personal injury when transferring a bariatric client.
      (1) Use good body mechanics, obtain adequate assistance during transfers, and use mechanical lifts.
6. Train in transfers to and from a variety of different surfaces (i.e., bed, wheelchair, chair, toilet, tub, and/or car).

## C. Transfer Types

1. Stand-pivot: individual stands and turns to transfer surface.
2. Pop-over or seated sitting: a full stand position is not required and is used for those with decreased endurance and/or weight bearing precautions.
3. Sliding board for those who are not able to stand to transfer (i.e., individuals with spinal cord injuries or amputations).
   a. Board is placed under individual's gluteal region during a weight shift, while the other end of board is placed on surface being transferred to.
   b. Individual then uses upper extremities to push buttocks up and "slide" over to transfer surface.
   c. If the individual uses a tenodesis grasp or splint for functional activities, the person should weightbear on clenched fists with wrists extended.
4. Dependent: caregiver is required to fully perform the transfer.
5. Mechanical lift: use of Hoyer lift or trans-aid.
6. Use of adaptive or mobility devices.
   a. Bed transfer aids.
      (1) Trapeze.
      (2) Bedrail.
   b. Bath transfer aids.
      (1) Grab bars.
      (2) Active-aid commode, a commode with small wheels to allow transfer to bathroom and shower stall when otherwise not possible.
      (3) Bedside or 3-in-1 commode.
      (4) Ambulatory devices (i.e., canes, walkers).
      (5) Wheelchairs (i.e., removable arms, swing arms, leg rests).
7. Chair lifts: chairs with power control to allow elevation from surface for individuals who may otherwise not be able to transfer independently.

# X. Assistive Technology/Electronic Aids to Daily Living (EADLs)

## A. Assistive Technology Devices (ATDs)

1. Definition: "...any piece of equipment or product... used to increase, maintain, improve functional capabilities of individuals with disabilities..." (Bain, 1998, p. 466).
2. An expansion of adaptive equipment.
3. Assistive devices for the environment may be considered "high tech" or "low tech".
   a. High tech: costly devices that may require custom ordering and may require specific training to use (e.g., environmental control units [ECUs], augmentative communication devices, computers).
   b. Low tech: inexpensive household and/or catalog items that are readily available for use, (e.g., jar opener, shoehorn, sock aid).
   c. Some components of high tech devices (e.g., ECUs) can be fabricated in a cost-effective manner using inexpensive commercially available micro-switch technology (e.g., simple switches to turn on and off lights, appliances and other electronic equipment).

## B. Electronic Aids to Daily Living (EADLs)

1. Definition: EADLs were formerly known as environmental control units (ECUs) and are a "...means to purposefully manipulate and interact

with the environment by alternately accessing one or more electrical devices via switch, voice activation, remote control, computer interface..." (Bain, 1998, p. 469).

2. Purposes.
   a. Maximize functional ability and independence in home, school, work, and other environments.
   b. Allow energy conservation during home management and work tasks.

3. Uses.
   a. Turn on/off lights and appliances, open and close doors/drapes.
   b. Allow use of phones and machinery.
   c. Summon assistance. (Bain, 1998).

4. Considerations in device selection.
   a. Input method: selection requires knowledge of the distance of throughput/transmission.
   b. Output method.
   c. Portability.
   d. Safety.
   e. Reliability.
   f. Durability.
   g. Assembly ease.
   h. Operation ease.
   i. Maintenance schedule.
   j. Current and future affordability.

5. Types of EADL technology.
   a. Phones: large number pads, automatic dialing phones, speaker-phones, amplifiers.
   b. Monitoring systems allow for communication between areas.
   c. Personal emergency response system (PERS): enables a client to summon help by the push of a button.
   d. Electronically controlled door openers and closers.
   e. Computers enable individuals with disabilities to more fully participate in social, leisure, work and productive activities.
      (1) Facilitate performance of multiple functional tasks (e.g., turning on and off household items, banking, shopping).
      (2) Allow for communication and socialization through e-mail and Internet support groups.
      (3) Provide the means for productive work via tele-commuting.
      (4) Have alternative access modes that can compensate for a diversity of disabilities. Adaptations can include:
         (a) Eye gaze for individuals with severe mobility impairments (e.g., individuals with amyotrophic lateral sclerosis).
         (b) Programmable keyboards that allow for customized overlays (e.g., enlarged letters and numbers for persons with low vision; graphics and symbols for individuals with cognitive impairments).
         (c) Expanded keyboards that provide large keys for persons with limited motor accuracy and control (e.g., individuals with ataxia).
         (d) Contracted keyboards that provide smaller keys in a constrained space for persons with limited range of motion and functional motor control (e.g., individuals with arthritis).
         (e) Light-touch keyboard activation systems for persons with decreased strength and/or mobility (e.g., individuals with muscular dystrophy).
         (f) Delayed touch keyboard activation systems for persons with poor motor control (e.g., individuals with athetoid movements).
         (g) Chorded keyboards that consist of a few keys which generate standard characters by pressing various combinations of keys for persons with one-handed use (e.g., individuals with hemiplegia).
   f. Augmentative alternative communication: methods of communication that do not require speech. Need to consider:
      (1) Speed at which message is conveyed.
      (2) Portability: easy to use in a variety of environmental settings.
      (3) Accessibility: ability of individual to independently operate.
      (4) Dependability: quality, durability and warranty/service record.
      (5) Independence of user.
      (6) Vocabulary flexibility.
      (7) Time for repairs and maintenance.
      (8) Types range from simple communication boards or albums with a limited number of pictures to complex portable computer systems with extensive language capacity.

**C. Evaluation and Intervention**
   1. The role of the OTA in evaluation,

a. The OTA contributes to the evaluation process.

b. The OTA can assist with the collection of data for the evaluation once service competency has been established.

c. The level of supervision required will be determined by the OTA's experience and established service competence.

d. The OTA cannot independently evaluate or interpret evaluation results.

2. The OTA collaborates with the OT supervisor to:

a. Identify tasks an individual with a disability wants to accomplish.

b. Assess the individual's abilities and deficits, including client factors and performance skills.

(1) Stability of positioning and seating must be assessed as this will affect the person's ability to use devices.

(2) The anatomic site at which the person demonstrates purposeful controlled movement must be determined as this will influence a device's control site (e.g., device activated by shoulder, head, elbow, hand, tongue, or eye movements).

c. Determine the environments in which a device will be used and when it will be used.

d. Identify assistive technology devices.

(1) Consider input method; how the device will be activated (e.g., infrared, sonic, electric, or radio frequency switches).

(2) Consider the processing method; how the device will process the information from the input method.

(3) Consider the output method; results are needed (response from input occurs).

(4) Consider the feedback method; ensures the device is being used in the right way (could be auditory, visual, or proprioceptive).

e. Document recommended ATD(s)/EADLs selected and the rationale for each item for reimbursement justification.

4. The role of the OTA in intervention.

a. The OTA implements intervention with OT supervision.

b. The level of supervision required depends upon the OTA's experience and established service competence.

c. During the implementation of intervention, the OTA informs the supervising occupational therapist of any change in the individual's status and any other relevant information that may affect treatment.

5. Intervention principles.

a. Select and use several devices on a trial basis to determine what serve the individual's needs best.

b. Determine the specific device, after reviewing and incorporating all of the team members' information.

c. Keep devices as simple as possible.

d. If device is stationary, ensure that it is positioned to enable ease of access.

e. Provide multiple training sessions.

6. Re-evaluation guidelines.

a. Assess for change in status of the individual with a disability.

b. Determine efficiency and efficacy of use of assistive devices.

c. Check parts of the device for durability.

**D. Additional Considerations for ATDs and EADLs**

1. The appliances and electrical cords to be used with ATDs and EADLs must be determined.

2. Charging instructions must be followed, as some have strict schedules.

3. The individual's telephone answering machine should be evaluated to see if it permits ATDs/EADLs to be attached.

4. The computer abilities of an individual with a disability should be determined.

5. Surge protectors must be used to avoid blown circuits.

6. Back-up systems for electrical high-tech devices should be established.

7. Instruction must be provided to the individual to ensure carry-over when an OT practitioner is not present.

8. Warranty information should be obtained and the consumer educated about these terms and conditions.

**E. Funding for ATDs and EADLs**

1. State One Stop Centers, Vocational and Educational Services for Individuals with Disabilities (VESID), Offices for Vocational Rehabilitation (OVRs), and Divisions of Vocational Rehabilitation (DVRs) will pay for ATDs and EADLs, if they enable a person to go to work or school.

2. Private companies will fund ATDs and EADLs to ensure ADA compliance.

3. Private insurance, Medicare, Medicaid and Workmen's Compensation will possibly reimburse for certain devices.

4. Centers for Independent Living and disability rights organizations may fund ATDs and EADLs to enable full community participation.

## XI. Driver Rehabilitation

### A. Overview

1. Driving is an instrumental activity of living.
2. Purposes.
   a. Provide mobility within one's community.
   b. Allow for autonomy for self-directed activity pursuit.
   c. Enable engagement in life roles including vocational, avocational, social, and familial role activities.
3. Physical, cognitive, psychiatric, and developmental disabilities can affect the ability to drive safely and effectively.
4. Driver rehabilitation requires extensive on-the-road training and behind the wheel driving in a diversity of driving environments.
5. Knowledge of general state driving regulations and statutes specifically related to individuals with disabilities must be acquired prior to initiating a driver rehabilitation program.
   a. An OT practitioner who performs on-the-road driver training must become a state licensed driving instructor.
6. OT practitioners who practice driver rehabilitation should become certified driving rehabilitation specialists.

### B. Evaluation of Driver Ability

1. The OTA can contribute to the evaluation process with OT supervision.
2. Upon establishment of service competency the OTA can participate in the clinical screening of performance skills, prerequisite abilities, and client factors.
   a. Visual-perceptual: intact acuity, night vision, contrast sensitivity, peripheral field, scanning, spatial relations, and depth perception are needed to access essential visual input and to accurately interpret the driving environment.
      (1) Color recognition is not a state mandated requirement as color blindness can be readily compensated for while driving.
   b. Cognitive-perceptual: intact orientation, alertness, memory, ability to shift attention, problem solving, response time, topographical orientation, sign recognition, and knowledge of 'rules of the road' are required to drive safely

and appropriately for different driving conditions, and to anticipate the actions of other drivers on the road and the consequences of one's own actions.
   c. Motor: adequate range of motion, strength, endurance, and response time are needed for basic vehicle control including accurate steering to remain in lane and make turns, and for smooth acceleration and braking.
   d. Psychosocial: the presence of impulsive and/or agitated behaviors, and/or psychiatric symptoms such as, suicidal intentions, delusions, and hallucinations can affect an individual's ability to drive safely.
   e. Side-effects of medications can affect motor performance, alertness, attention, judgment, and reaction time.
   f. Past driving experiences (which can range from none, to poor, to competent) can influence the individual's potential to drive with a disability.
   g. OTAs with OT supervision can perform clinical screenings for all of the above factors that can affect driving without additional specialized training.
      (1) If screening identifies areas requiring further evaluation, the occupational therapist should refer the individual to a driving rehabilitation specialist.
3. On-the-road evaluation: there are two levels of driving that must be considered when evaluating a person's abilities when he/she are behind the wheel and actually driving.
   a. Operation: the ability to steer, brake, and turn.
   b. Tactical: the ability to respond to changes in road conditions and traffic/driving risks.
   c. The ergonomics of driving should also be assessed to increase safety and prevent discomfort. Considerations include:
      (1) Seat position in relation to visibility of car's endpoints.
      (2) Positioning of seatbelt and shoulder restraint.
      (3) Access to foot pedals and/or steering column controls.
      (4) Airbag clearance of 12 inches between the person and the steering wheel in case of airbag deployment.
   d. The person's ability to manage automotive emergencies and obtain assistance should also

be assessed.

e. An OT practitioner who performs on-the-road evaluations must become a state licensed driving instructor.

(1) State regulations will determine OTA eligibility.

**C. Intervention**

1. Adaptive driving equipment can be prescribed for individuals with specific limitations.

a. Hand controls can replace accelerators and brake foot pedals.

b. Steering knobs for one-handed steering control can include a:

(1) Standard round spinning knob for a person with one intact upper extremity.

(2) Ring to accommodate a prosthesis.

(3) Tri-pin or cuff to accommodate absent or weak grasp.

c. Pedal extensions can be added if feet do not reach standard foot pedals.

d. Zero effort or reduced effort steering can accommodate for decreased range, strength, and endurance.

e. Steering wheel positioning adjustments can place the steering wheel in atypical positions to allow for access.

2. If, and when, a person is determined to be unsafe or unable to drive, alternatives to maintain community mobility must be explored and implemented.

a. Support must be provided to the individual to deal with this loss and its ramifications on the person's daily life.

**D. Funding for Driver Rehabilitation**

1. State Vocational and Educational Services for Individuals with Disabilities (VESID), Offices for Vocational Rehabilitation (OVRs), and Divisions of Vocational Rehabilitation (DVRs) will pay for driver rehabilitation if it will enable a person to go to work or school.

2. Private insurance, Medicare, Medicaid, and Worker's Compensation will possibly reimburse for certain driver rehabilitation devices/adaptations.

# XI. Environmental Modifications for Cognitive and Sensory Deficits

**A. General Interventions**

1. The environment needs to be familiar, consistent, and predictable.

a. Provide structure in the environment to increase orientation to time, place, person, and situation.

b. Remove clutter to decrease extraneous stimuli when an individual is easily distracted or has limited vision.

c. Provide visual reminders or tactile cues to decrease confusion, increase awareness, and facilitate independence (e.g., written directions, Braille labels).

d. Keep things in the same place for consistency and ease.

2. Use contrasting colors to discriminate background from foreground or figures from background.

3. Use restraint reduction techniques if a person is confused, agitated, and/or a wanderer.

4. Educate consumer, caregiver, and family.

a. Train caregivers for persons with memory and/or sensory impairments on effective communication techniques.

b. Facilitate carry-over of intervention techniques in the modified environment.

c. Increase awareness of potential resources available to the individual and his/her families.

d. Increase awareness of his/her rights to access these resources.

5. Monitor changes and adjustment after a disability to assess carry-over of information.

6. Make home modifications to ensure safety as needed.

a. Remove potential hazards such as cleaning solutions, medications, sharp objects, matches, stove knobs, and firearms if a person is confused or forgetful.

b. Follow modifications identified earlier in this chapter for the prevention of falls.

c. See Chapter 5 for additional modifications for sensory loss.

7. Provide a personal emergency system and train in its use.

**B. Restraint Reduction**

1. The OTA contributes to the assessment of behaviors that result in agitation, restlessness, and/or wandering with OT supervision. Areas to assess include:

a. Pain, physical discomfort.

b. Hunger, thirst, need for toileting.

c. Loneliness, fear.

d. Boredom.

e. Unfamiliar environment.

2. The OTA implements intervention with OT supervision to address contributing factors/correct

underlying problems. Interventions include:

a. Referral to physician for medical evaluation/pain management.

b. Proper positioning.

c. Provision of snacks, unbreakable water bottles, or other appropriate safe source of nourishment and hydration.

d. Adequate and client-directed toileting routine.

e. Active listening, attention to underlying feelings and expressed concerns to promote trust.

f. Family, peer, and/or pastoral visits.

g. Animal-assisted or pet therapy.

h. Social and leisure activities.

i. Exercise and/or other outlets for restless, anxious behavior.

j. Night-time activities.

k. Eliminate loudspeaker and other extraneous noise, provide soothing background music.

l. Inclusion of familiar and favorite objects in person's living space to personalize it.

m. Provide a structured home-like environment with a set routine to promote sense of safety and security.

3. The OTA implements interventions with OT supervision to address agitation and/or wandering incidents. Interventions include:

a. Approach from person's front at his/her eye level.

b. Communicate calmly with the use of simple statements/instructions.

c. Distract with an activity or topic of interest to the person.

d. Re-direct back to desired location.

e. Engage in an activity of interest or diversion.

f. Camouflage doors, exits, and elevators with full-length mirrors, stop or no-crossing signs, wallpaper, vertical blinds.

g. Put tape on floors or planters to mark end of hall.

h. Install locks or Velcro doors.

i. Use door alarms, personal alarms or monitoring devices.

j. Make contained areas interesting and safe.

k. Rearrange furniture to deter wandering.

l. Provide a variety of comfortable seating and furniture including broad-based rockers and footstools.

# References

American Occupational Therapy Association. (2008). Occupational therapy practice framework: Domain and process, 2nd edition. *American Journal of Occupational Therapy, 62,* 625-688.

American Occupational Therapy Association

American National Standards Institute. (1992). *Accessible and usable buildings and facilities.* New York: Author.

Bain, B. (1997). Evaluation. In B. Bain & D. Leger (Eds.), *Assistive technology: An interdisciplinary approach* (pp. 17-27). New York: Churchill Livingstone.

Bain, B. (1998). Assistive technology. In G. Gillen & A. Burkhardt (Eds.), *Stroke rehabilitation: A function based approach* (pp. 465-478). St. Louis, MO: Mosby.

Bain, B., Dooley, K. & Leger, D. (1997). Assistive technology: An interdisciplinary approach. In B. Bain & D. Leger (Eds.), *Assistive technology: An interdisciplinary approach* (pp. 1-7). New York, NY: Churchill Livingstone.

Bolding, D., Adler, C., Tipton-Burton, M., & Lillie, S. (2007). Mobility. In In H. McHugh Pendleton & W. Schultz-Krohn (Eds.), *Pedretti's occupational therapy: Practice skills for physical dysfunction,* 6th ed. (pp. 195-247.). St. Louis, MO: Mosby.

Case-Smith, J. (Ed.), (2005). *Occupational therapy for children* (5th ed.). St. Louis, MO: Elsevier Mosby.

Cuccurullo, S.J. (2004) *Physical Medicine and Rehabilitation Board Review.* Retrieved from http://www.ncbi.nlm.nih.gov/books/bv.fcgi?index ed=google&rid=physmedrehab.section.13884.

Deitz, J. & Dudgeon, B. (2008). Wheelchair selection process. In C. A. Trombly (Ed.), *Occupational therapy for physical dysfunction,* 6th ed. (pp. 487-509.). Baltimore: Williams & Wilkins.

Deitz, J. & Dudgeon, B. (1995). Wheelchair selection process. In C. A. Trombly (Ed.), *Occupational therapy for physical dysfunction* pp. 599-609). (4th ed.). Baltimore: Williams & Wilkins.

Foti, D. & Kanazawa, L (2006). Activities of daily living. In H. McHugh Pendleton & W. Schultz-Krohn (Eds.), *Pedretti's occupational therapy: Practice skills for physical dysfunction,* 6th ed. (pp. 146-194.). St. Louis, MO: Mosby.

Gourley, M. (2002, March 25). Driver rehabilitation. *OT Practice,* 15-20.

Hopkins, H. & Smith, H. (Eds.). (2003). *Willard and Spackman's occupational therapy* (10th ed.). Philadelphia: J.B. Lippincott.

Johann, C. (1998). Seating and wheeled mobility prescription. In G. Gillen & A. Burkhardt (Eds.), *Stroke rehabilitation: A function based approach* (pp. 437-451). St. Louis, MO: Mosby.

Kane, L. & Buckley, K. (1998). Functional mobility. In G. Gillen & A. Burkhardt (Eds.), *Stroke rehabilitation: A function based approach* (pp. 305-242). St. Louis, MO: Mosby.

Lange, M.L. (2001, July 2). Alternative keyboards. *OT Practice,* 19-20.

Lange, M.L. (2001, Aug. 6). EADLs and aging clients. *OT Practice,* 16-18.

Lange, M.L. (2001, Aug. 6). EADLs in the school setting. *OT Practice,* 17-18.

Larson, K., Stevens-Ratchford, Pedretti, L., & Crabtree, J. (1996). ROTE: T*he role of occupational therapy with the elderly* (2nd ed.). Bethesda, MD: American Occupational Therapy Association.

Mosey, A.C. (1996). *Psychosocial components of occupational therapy.* New York: Raven Press.

Moyers, P. & Dale, L. (2007). *The guide to occupational therapy practice.* Bethesda, MD: American Occupational Therapy Association.

O'Toole, M. (Ed.). (1997). *Miller-Keane encyclopedia and dictionary of medicine, nursing, and allied health* (6th ed.). Philadelphia: W. B. Saunders.

Pedretti, L. (1990). Activities of daily living. In L. Pedretti & B. Zoltan (Eds.), *Occupational therapy: Practice skills for physical dysfunction* pp. 230-271. (3rd ed.). St. Louis, MO: Mosby.

Peterson, E.W., & Murphy, S. (2002). Fear of falling: Part II - Assessment and intervention. *Home and Community Health Special Interest Section Quarterly,* 9(1), 1, 2, 4.

Salerno, C. (1998). Home evaluation and modification. In G. Gillen & A. Burkhardt (Eds.), *Stroke rehabilitation: A function based approach* (pp. 452-464). St. Louis, MO: Mosby.

Spencer, E. (1998). Functional restoration: Preliminary concepts and planning. In H. Hopkins & H. Smith (Eds.), *Willard and Spackman's occupational therapy* (7th ed., pp. 435-460). Philadelphia: J.B. Lippincott Company.

Stav, W. & Kaebel, M. (2002, October). On the road again. *Rehab Management.* 26-27.

Walls, B.S. (1999, December 6). A dangerous secret: I had a fall. *OT Practice,* 12-16.

West Virginia Research and Training Center. (1990). ADA - *The Americans with Disabilities Act of 1990 PL 101-336, Volume I - The Law.* Dunbar, WV: Author.

Wheatley, C.J. (2001, July 16). Shifting into drive: Evaluating potential drivers with disabilities. *OT Practice,* 12-15.

# EPILOGUE

# PROFESSIONAL DEVELOPMENT AFTER INITIAL CERTIFICATION

## Rita P. Fleming-Castaldy

Successfully passing the NBCOT occupational therapy assistant examination results in national certification as a certified occupational therapy assistant (COTA®) and marks the beginning of a rewarding and fulfilling professional career. This concept of beginning is a critical one for the reader to embrace. While the pursuit of the goal to become an occupational therapy assistant may end with NBCOT certification, it is at this point that the life-long process of being a professional has just begun.

> Being a member of a profession requires an ongoing commitment to the attainment and maintenance of excellence. Competent practitioners value this pursuit of excellence and are personally responsible for this professional development.... The benefits of a life-long commitment to one's professional development are numerous. Increased personal pride and satisfaction in one's work; improved health care services for consumers and their families; enhanced professional image among policy makers, reimbursers, administrators, and the multidisciplinary team; and the prevention of burnout and professional stagnation are all viable outcomes of the continual pursuit of professional excellence (Cottrell, 2000, p.465).

Numerous professional development resources are available to facilitate growth from entry-level novice to master practitioner. Clinical supervision, peer support, networking, professional associations, mentorships, self-study, inservices, workshops, conferences, and post-professional education can all be used to attain and maintain professional mastery and excellence. The advent of the technological era has increased the availability and decreased the cost of many professional development activities through the use of e-mail, social networking, chat rooms, and distance learning. I strongly urge the reader to take advantage of both high-tech (e.g., video conferencing) and low-tech (e.g., brainstorming with a colleague over a practice dilemma) learning opportunities early and often in his/her professional life. I also highly recommend that each reader become an active member in his/her state association (and/or the local district in a large state). This action will immediately provide the reader with a network of OT practitioners who are proactive forces for professional advancement and role models for excellence. See Appendix 3 for State Association contact information.

As Yerxa (1985) noted, an authentic professional is one who recognizes his/her responsibility to be a life-long student. I wish the reader well at the beginning of this journey, the journey to learn and pursue an authentic occupational therapy career. I can think of no better way to practice or live.

# References

American Occupational Therapy Association Continuing Competency Task Force (1999). *Professional development for continuing competency*. Bethesda, MD: AOTA.

Cottrell, R.P. (2000). Professional development: The attainment, maintenance and promotion of excellence. In R.P. Cottrell (Ed.), *Proactive approaches in psychosocial occupational therapy* (pp. 465-468). Thorofare, NJ: Slack.

Yerxa, E. (1985). Authentic occupational therapy. *In a professional legacy: The Eleanor Clark Slagle lectures in occupational therapy* (pp.155-175). Bethesda, MD: American Occupational Therapy Association.

# APPENDIX 1

# THE PRACTICE FRAMEWORK

## AREAS OF OCCUPATION

Various kinds of life activities in which people, populations, or organizations engage, including ADL, IADL, rest and sleep, education, work, play, leisure, and social participation.

**ACTIVITIES OF DAILY LIVING (ADL)**—activities that are oriented toward taking care of one's own body (adapted from Rogers & Holm, 1994, pp. 181-202). ADL also is referred to as *basic activities of daily living (BADLs) and personal activities of daily living (PADLs).* These activities are "fundamental to living in a social world; they enable basic survival and well-being" (Christiansen & Hammecker, 2001, pl 156).

- **Bathing, showering**—Obtaining and using supplies; soaping, rinsing, and drying body parts; maintaining bathing position; and transferring to and from bathing positions.
- **Bowel and bladder management**—Includes completing intentional control of bowel movements and urinary bladder and, if necessary, using equipment or agents for bladder control (Uniform Data System for Medical Rehabilitation, 1996, pp. III-20, III-24).
- **Dressing**—Selecting clothing and accessories appropriate to time of day, weather, and occasion; obtaining clothing from storage area; dressing and undressing in a sequential fashion; fastening and adjusting clothing and shoes; and applying and removing personal devices, prostheses, or orthoses.
- **Eating**—"The ability to keep and manipulate food or fluid in the mouth and swallow it; *eating* and *swallowing* are often used interchangeably" (AOTA, 2007b).
- **Feeding**—"The process of setting up, arranging, and bringing food [or fluid] from the plate or cup to the mouth; sometimes called self-feeding" (AOTA, 2007b).
- **Functional mobility**—Moving from one position or place to another [during performance of everyday activities], such as in-bed mobility, wheelchair mobility, and transfers (e.g., wheelchair, bed, car, tub, toilet, tub/shower, chair, floor). Includes functional ambulation and transporting objects.
- **Personal device care**—Using, cleaning, and maintaining personal care items, such as hearing aids, contact lenses, glasses, orthotics, prosthetics, adaptive equipment, and contraceptive and sexual devices.
- **Personal hygiene and grooming**—Obtaining and using supplies; removing body hair (e.g., use of razors, tweezers, lotions); applying and removing cosmetics; washing, drying, combing, styling, brushing, and trimming hair; caring for nails (hands and feet); caring for skin, ears, eyes, and nose; applying deodorant; cleaning mouth; brushing and flossing teeth; or removing, cleaning, and reinserting dental orthotics and prosthetics.
- **Sexual activity**—Engagement in activities that result in sexual satisfaction.
- **Toilet hygiene**—Obtaining and using supplies; clothing management; maintaining toileting position; transferring to and from toileting position; cleaning body; and caring for menstrual and continence needs (including catheters, colostomies, and suppository management).

**INSTRUMENTAL ACTIVITIES OF DAILY LIVING (IADLs)**—Activities to support daily life within the home and community that often require more complex interactions than self-care used in ADL.

- **Care of others (including selecting and supervising caregivers)**—Arranging, supervising, or providing the care for others.
- **Care of pets**—Arranging, supervising, or providing the care for pets and service animals.
- **Child rearing**—Providing the care and supervision to support the developmental needs of a child.
- **Communication management**—Sending, receiving, and interpreting information using a variety of systems and equipment, including writing tools, telephones, typewriters, audiovisual recorders, computers, communication boards, call lights, emergency systems, Braille writers, telecommunication devices for the deaf, augmentative communication systems, and personal digital assistants.
- **Community mobility**—Moving around in the community and using public or private transportation, such as driving, walking, bicycling, or accessing and riding in buses, taxi cabs, or other transportation systems.
- **Financial management**—Using fiscal resources, including alternate methods of financial transaction and planning and using finances with long-term and short-term goals.
- **Health management and maintenance**—Developing, managing, and maintaining routines for health and wellness promotion, such as physical fitness, nutrition, decreasing health risk behaviors, and medication routines.
- **Home establishment and management**—Obtaining and maintaining personal and household possessions and environment (e.g., home, yard, garden, appliances, vehicles), including maintaining and repairing personal possessions (clothing and household items) and knowing how to seek help or whom to contact.
- **Meal preparation and cleanup**—Planning, preparing, and serving well-balanced, nutritional meals and cleaning up food and utensils after meals.
- **Religious observance**— Participation in religion, "an organized system of beliefs, practices, rituals, and symbols designed to facilitate closeness to the sacred or transcendent" (Moreira-Almeida & Koenig, 2006, p. 844).
- **Safety and emergency maintenance**—Knowing and performing preventive procedures to maintain a safe environment as well as recognizing sudden, unexpected hazardous situations and initialing emergency action to reduce the threat to health and safety.
- **Shopping**—Preparing shopping lists (grocery and other); selecting, purchasing, and transporting items; selecting method of payment; and completing money transactions.

**REST AND SLEEP**—Includes activities related to obtaining restorative rest and sleep that supports healthy active engagement in other areas of occupation.

- **Rest**—Quiet and effortless actions that interrupt physical and mental activity resulting in a relaxed state (Nurit & Michel, 2003, p. 227). Includes identifying the need to relax; reducing involvement in taxing physical, mental or social activities; and engaging in relaxation or other endeavors that restore energy, calm, and renewed interest in engagement.
- **Sleep**—A series of activities resulting in going to sleep, staying asleep, and ensuring health and safety through participation in sleep involving engagement with the physical and social environments.
- **Sleep preparation**—(1) Engaging in routines that prepare the self for a comfortable rest, such as grooming and undressing, reading or listening to music to fall asleep, saying goodnight to others, and meditation or prayers; determining the time of day and length of time desired for sleeping or the time needed to wake; and establishing sleep patterns that support growth and health (patterns are often personally and culturally determined). (2) Preparing the physical environment for periods of unconsciousness, such as making the bed or space on which to sleep; ensuring warmth/coolness and protection; setting an alarm clock; securing the home, such as locking doors or closing windows or curtains; and turning off electronics or lights.
- **Sleep participation**—Taking care of personal need for sleep such as cessation of activities to ensure onset of sleep, napping, dreaming, sustaining a sleep state without disruption, and nighttime care of toileting needs or hydration. Negotiating the needs and requirements of others within the social environment, interacting with those sharing the sleep space such as children or partners, providing nighttime care giving such as breastfeeding, and monitoring the comfort and safety of others such as the family while sleeping.

**EDUCATION**—Includes activities needed for learning and participating in the environment.
- **Formal educational participation**—Including the categories of academic (e.g., math, reading, working on a degree), nonacademic (e.g., recess, lunchroom, hallway), extracurricular (e.g., sports, band, cheerleading, dances), and vocational (pre-vocational and vocational) participation.
- **Informal personal educational needs or interests exploration (beyond formal education)**—Identifying topics and methods for obtaining topic-related information or skills
- **Informal personal education participation**—Participating in classes, programs, and activities that provide instruction/training in identified areas of interest.

**WORK**—Includes activities needed for engaging in remunerative employment or volunteer activities (Mosey, 1996, p. 341).
- **Employment interests and pursuits**—Identifying and selecting work opportunities based on assets, limitations, likes, and dislikes relative to work (adapted from Mosey, 1996 p. 342).
- **Employment seeking and acquisition**—Identifying and recruiting for job opportunities; completing, submitting, and reviewing appropriate application materials; preparing for interviews; participating in interviews and following up afterward; discussing job benefits; and finalizing negotiations.
- **Job performance**—Job performance including work skills and patterns; time management; relationships with co-workers, managers, and customers; creation, production, and distribution of products and services; initiation, sustainment, and completion of work; and compliance with work norms and procedures.
- **Retirement preparation and adjustment**—Determining aptitudes, developing interests and skills, and selecting appropriate avocational pursuits.
- **Volunteer exploration**—Determining community causes, organizations, or opportunities for unpaid "work" in relationship to personal skills, interests, location, and time available.
- **Volunteer participation**—Performing unpaid "work" activities for the benefit of identified selected causes, organizations, or facilities.

**PLAY**—"Any spontaneous or organized activity that provides enjoyment, entertainment, amusement, or diversion" (Parham & Fazio, 1997, p. 252).
- **Play exploration**—Identifying appropriate play activities, which can include exploration play, practice play, pretend play, games with rules, constructive play, and symbolic play (adapted from Bergen, 1986, pp. 64-65).
- **Play participation**—Participating in play; maintaining a balance of play with other areas of occupation; and obtaining, using, and maintaining toys, equipment, and supplies appropriately.

**LEISURE**—"A nonobligatory activity that is intrinsically motivated and engaged in during discretionary item, that is, time not committed to obligatory occupations such as work, self-care, or sleep" (Parham & Fazio, 1997, p. 250).
- **Leisure exploration**—identifying interests, skills opportunities, and appropriate leisure activities.
- **Leisure participation**—Planning and participating in appropriate leisure activities; maintaining a balance of leisure activities with other areas of occupation; and obtaining, using, and maintaining equipment and supplies as appropriate.

**SOCIAL PARTICIPATION**—"Organized patterns of behavior that are characteristic and expected of an individual or a given position within a social system" (Mosey, 1996, p. 340).
- **Community**—Engaging in activities that result in successful interaction at the community level (i.e., neighborhood, organizations, work, school).
- **Family**—Engaging in "[activities that result in] successful interaction in specific required and/or desired familial roles" (Mosey, 1996, p. 340).
- **Peer, friend**—Engaging in activities at different levels of intimacy, including engaging in desired sexual activity.

*Note.* Some of the terms used in this table are from, or adapted from, the rescinded *Uniform Terminology for Occupational Therapy*—Third Edition (AOTA, 1994, pp. 1047-1054).

# CLIENT FACTORS

Client factors include (1) values, beliefs, and spirituality; (2) body functions; and (3) body structures that reside within the client and may affect performance in areas of occupation.

## VALUES, BELIEFS, AND SPIRITUALITY

| CATEGORY AND DEFINITION | EXAMPLES |
|---|---|
| **Values:** Principles, standards, or qualities considered worthwhile or desirable by the client who holds them. | **Person**<br>1. Honesty with self and with others<br>2. Personal religious convictions<br>3. Commitment to family.<br>**Organization**<br>1. Obligation to serve the community<br>2. Fairness.<br>**Population**<br>1. Freedom of speech<br>2. Equal opportunities for all<br>3. Tolerance toward others. |
| **Beliefs:** Cognitive content held as true. | **Person**<br>1. He or she is powerless to influence others<br>2. Hard work pays off.<br>**Organization**<br>1. Profits are more important than people<br>2. Achieving the mission of providing service can effect positive change in the world.<br>**Population**<br>1. People can influence government by voting<br>2. Accessibility is a right, not a privilege. |
| **Spiritual:** The "personal quest for understanding answers to ultimate questions about life, about meaning, and the sacred" (Moyers & Dale, 2007, p, 28). | **Person**<br>1. Daily search for purpose and meaning in one's life<br>2. Guiding actions from a sense of value beyond the personal acquisition of wealth or fame.<br>**Organization and Population**<br>(see "Person" examples related to individuals within an organization and population). |

**BODY FUNCTIONS:** "[T]he physiological functions of body systems (including psychological functions)" (WHO, 2001, p. 10). The "Body Functions" section of the table below is organized according to the classifications of the International Classification of Functioning, Disability, and Health (ICF) classifications. For fuller descriptions and definitions, refer to WHO (2001).

| CATEGORIES | BODY FUNCTIONS COMMONLY CONSIDERED BY OCCUPATIONAL THERAPY PRACTITIONERS (Not intended to be all-inclusive list) |
|---|---|
| **Mental functions** (affective, cognitive, perceptual)<br>■ **Specific mental functions**<br> • Higher-level cognitive<br><br> • Attention<br> • Memory<br> • Perception | **Specific mental functions**<br>Judgement, concept formation, metacognition, cognitive flexibility, insight, attention, awareness<br>Sustained, selective, and divided attention<br>Short-term, long-term, and working memory<br>Discrimination of sensations (e.g., auditory, tactile, visual, olfactory, gusfatory, vestibular-proprioception), including multi-sensory processing, sensory memory, spatial, and temporal relationships (Calvert, Spence, & Stein, 2004) |

| CATEGORIES | BODY FUNCTIONS COMMONLY CONSIDERED BY OCCUPATIONAL THERAPY PRACTITIONERS (Not intended to be all-inclusive list) |
|---|---|
| **Mental functions** (affective, cognitive, perceptual) (continued)<br>■ **Specific mental functions**<br> • Thought<br><br> • Mental functions of sequencing complex movement<br> • Emotional<br> • Experience of self and time | **Specific mental functions**<br>Recognition, categorization, generalization, awareness of reality, logical/coherent thought, and appropriate thought content<br>Execution of learned movement patterns<br>Coping and behavioral regulation (Scheil, Cohn, & Crepeau, 2008)<br>Body image, self-concept, self-esteem |
| ■ **Global mental functions**<br> • Consciousness<br> • Orientation<br> • Temperament of personality<br> • Energy and drive<br> • Sleep (physiological process) | **Global mental functions**<br>Level of arousal, level of consciousness<br>Orentation to person, place, time, self, and others<br>Emotional stablity<br>Motivation, impulse control, and appetite |
| **Sensory functions and pain**<br> • Seeing and related functions, including visual acuity, visual stability, visual field functions<br><br> • Hearing functions<br><br> • Vestibular functions<br> • Taste functions<br> • Smell functions<br> • Proprioceptive functions<br> • Touch functions<br><br> • Pain (e.g., diffuse, dull, sharp, phantom)<br> • Temperature and pressure | **Sensory functions and pain**<br>Detection/registration, modulation, and integration of sensations form the body and environment<br>Visual awareness of environment at various distances<br>Tolerance of ambient sounds; awareness of location and distance of sounds such as an approaching car<br>Sensation of securely moving against gravity<br>Association of taste<br>Association of smell<br>Awareness of body position and space<br>Comfort with the feeling of being touched by others or touching various textures such as food<br>Localizing pain<br>Thermal awareness |
| **Neuromusculoskeletal and movement-related functions**<br>■ **Functions of joints and bones**<br> • Joint mobility<br> • Joint stability<br><br><br> • Muscle power<br> • Muscle tone<br> • Muscle endurance<br> • Involuntary movements reactions | **Neuromusculoskeletal and movement-related functions**<br><br>Joint range of motion<br>Postural alignment (this refers to the physiological stability of the joint related to its structural integrity as compared to the motor skill of aligning the body while moving in relation to task objects)<br>Strength<br>Degree of muscle tone (e.g., flaccidity, spasticity, fluctuation)<br>Endurance<br>Stretch, asymmetrical tonic neck, symmetrical tonic neck<br>Righting and supporting<br>Eye-hand/foot coordination, bilateral integration, crossing the midline, fine- and gross-motor control, and oculomotor (e.g., saccades, pursuits, accommodation, binocularity)<br>Walking patterns and impairment such as asymmetric gait, stiff gait. (Note: Gait patterns are considered in relation to how they affect ability to engage in occupations in daily life activities.) |

| CATEGORIES | BODY FUNCTIONS COMMONLY CONSIDERED BY OCCUPATIONAL THERAPY PRACTITIONERS (Not intended to be all-inclusive list) |
|---|---|
| **Cardiovascular, hematological, immunological, and respiratory system function** | **Cardiovascular, hematological, immunological, and respiratory system function** |
| • Cardiovascular system function | Blood pressure functions (hypertension, hypotension, postural hypotension), and heart rate |
| • Hematological and immunological system function<br>• Respiratory system function | (Note: Occupational therapy practitioners have knowledge of these body functions and understand broadly the interaction that occurs between these functions to support health and participation in life through engagement in occupation. Some therapists may specialize in evaluating and intervening with a specific function as it is related to supporting performance and engagement in occupations and activities targeted for intervention.) |
| • Additional functions and sensations of the cardiovascular and respiratory systems | Rate, rhythm, and depth of respiration<br>Physical endurance, aerobic capacity, stamina, and fatigability |
| **Voice and speech functions**<br>• Voice functions<br>• Fluency and rhythm<br>• Alternative vocalization functions<br>**Digestive, metabolic, and endocrine system function**<br>• Digestive system function<br>• Metabolic system and endocrine system function<br>**Genitourinary and reproductive functions**<br>• Urinary functions<br>• Genital and reproductive functions | (Note: Occupational therapy practitioners have knowledge of these body functions and understand broadly the interaction that occurs between these functions to support health and participation in life through engagement in occupation. Some therapists may specialize in evaluating and intervening with a specific functions, such as incontinence and pelvic floor disorders, as it is related to supporting performance and engagement in occupations and activities targeted for intervention.) |
| **Skin and related-structure functions**<br>• Skin functions<br>• Hair and nail functions | **Skin and related-structure functions**<br>Protective functions of the skin—presence or absence of wounds, cuts, or abrasions<br>Repair function of the skin—wound healing<br>(Note: Occupational therapy practitioners have knowledge of these body functions and understand broadly the interaction that occurs between these functions to support health and participation in life through engagement in occupation. Some therapists may specialize in evaluating and intervening with a specific function, as it is related to supporting performance and engagement in occupations and activities targeted for intervention.) |

**BODY STRUCTURES:** "*Body structures* are "anatomical parts of the body, such as organs, limbs, and their components [that support body function]" (WHO, 2001, p. 10). The "Body Structures" section of the table below is organized according to the ICF classifications. For fuller descriptions and definitions, refer to WHO (2001).

| CATEGORIES | BODY FUNCTIONS COMMONLY CONSIDERED BY OCCUPATIONAL THERAPY PRACTITIONERS (Not intended to be all-inclusive list) |
|---|---|
| Structure of the nervous system | (Note: Occupational therapy practitioners have knowledge of these body functions and understand broadly the interaction that occurs between these functions to support health and participation in life through engagement in occupation. Some therapists may specialize in evaluating and intervening with a specific function, as it is related to supporting performance and engagement in occupations and activities targeted for intervention.) |
| Eyes, ear, and related structures | |
| Structures involved in voice and speech | |
| Structures of the cardiovascular, immunological, and respiratory systems | |
| Structures related to the digestive, metabolic, and endocrine systems | |
| Structures related to the genitourinary and reproductive systems | |
| Structures related to movement | |
| Skin and related structures | |

*Note.* Some data adapted from the ICF (WHO, 2001).

From Occupational therapy practice framework: Domain and process, 2nd edition. (pp. 634-638).  Copyright by the American Occupational Therapy Association, Inc. Reprinted with permission.

# PERFORMANCE SKILLS

Performance skills are the abilities clients demonstrate in the actions they perform.

| SKILL | DEFINITION | EXAMPLES |
|-------|------------|----------|
| **Motor and praxis skills** | *Motor:* actions or behaviors a client uses to move and physically interact with tasks, objects, contexts, and environments (adapted from Fisher, 2006). Includes planning, sequencing, and executing new and novel movements.<br><br>*Praxis*: Skilled purposeful movements (Heilman & Rothl, 1993). Ability to carry out sequential motor acts as part of an overall plan rather than individual acts (Liepmann 1920). Ability to carry our learned motor activity, including following through on a verbal command, visual-spatial construction, ocular and oral-motor skills, imitation of a person or an object, and sequencing actions (Ayres, 1985; Filey, 2001). Organization of temporal sequences of actions within the spatial context, which form meaningful occupations (Blanche & Parham, 2002). | • *Bending and reaching* for a toy or tool in a storage bin<br>• *Pacing* tempo of movements to clean the room<br>• *Coordinating* the body movements to complete a job task<br>• *Maintaining balance* while walking on an uneven surface or while showering<br>• *Anticipating or adjusting posture and body position* in response to environmental circumstances, such as obstacles<br>• *Manipulating keys* or lock to open the door. |
| **Sensory-perceptual skills** | Actions or behaviors a client uses to locate, identify, and respond to sensations and to select, interpret, associate, organize, and remember sensory events based on discriminating experiences through a variety of sensations that include visual, auditory, proprioceptive, tactile, olfactory, gustatory, and vestibular. | • *Positioning the body* in the exact location of a safe jump<br>• *Hearing and locating* the voice of your child in a crowd<br>• *Visually* determining the correct size of a storage container for leftover soup<br>• *Locating* keys by touch from many objects in a pocket or purse (i.e., stereognosis)<br>• *Timing the appropriate moment* to cross the street safely by determining one's own position and speed relative to the speed of traffic<br>• *Discerning* distinct flavors within foods or beverages |
| **Emotional regulation skills** | Actions or behaviors a client uses to identify, manage, and express feelings while engaging in activities or interacting with others | • *Responding* to the feelings of others by acknowledgement or showing support<br>• *Persisting* in a task despite frustrations<br>• *Controlling* anger toward others and reducing aggressive acts<br>• *Recovering* from a hurt or disappointment without lashing out at others |

**PERFORMANCE SKILLS CONTINUED**

| SKILL | DEFINITION | EXAMPLES |
|---|---|---|
| **Cognitive skills** | Actions or behaviors a client uses to plan and manage the performance of an activity | • *Judging* the importance or appropriateness of clothes for the circumstance<br>• *Selecting* tools and supplies needed to clean the bathroom<br>• *Sequencing* tasks needed for a school project<br>• *Organizing* activities within the time required to meet a deadline<br>• *Prioritizing* steps and *identifying* solutions to access transportation<br>• *Creating* different activities with friends that are fun, novel, and enjoyable<br>• *Multitasking*—doing more than one thing at a time, necessary for tasks such as work, driving, and household management |
| **Communication and social skills** | Actions or behaviors a person uses to comminicate and interact with others in an interactive environment (Fisher, 2006) | • *Looking* where someone else is pointing or gazing<br>• *Gesturing* to emphasize intentions<br>• *Maintaining* acceptable physical space during conversation<br>• *Initating and answering* questions with relevant information<br>• *Taking turns* during an interchange with another person verbally and physically<br>• *Acknowledging* another peron's perspective during an interchange |

From Occupational therapy practice framework: Domain and process, 2nd edition. (pp. 640-641). Copyright by the American Occupational Therapy Association, Inc. Reprinted with permission.

# APPENDIX 2

## SELECTED PREFIXES AND SUFFIXES

A working knowledge of the components of medical terminology can often help decipher the meaning of an unknown word. This can assist in question analysis and the selection of the best answer. Remember Latin is not a dying language, it is alive and well in the language of health care. This Appendix does not list all medical terms that may be on the examination, but it does provide many foundational components of medical terminology. For a complete and exhaustive presentation of medical terminology the reader is referred to this Appendix's reference.

a-. . . . . . . . . . without
ab-. . . . . . . . . away from
abdomin/o. . . . abdomen
acous/o . . . . . . hearing
acr/o . . . . . . . . extremity or topmost
-acusis. . . . . . . hearing condition
ad-. . . . . . . . . . .to, toward, or near
aden/o. . . . . . . gland
adip/o . . . . . . . fat
adren/o . . . . . . adrenal gland
aer/o . . . . . . . . air or gas
-algia. . . . . . . . pain
alveol/o. . . . . . alveolus (air sac)
ambi- . . . . . . . both
an-. . . . . . . . . . without
angi/o . . . . . . . vessel
ankyl/o . . . . . . crooked or stiff
ante- . . . . . . . . before
anti- . . . . . . . . against or opposed to
-arche . . . . . . . beginning
arteri/o . . . . . . artery
arthr/o. . . . . . . joint
articul/o . . . . . joint
-ase . . . . . . . . . enzyme
-asthenia . . . . . weakness
ather/o. . . . . . . fat
-ation . . . . . . . process
audi/o . . . . . . . hearing
aur/i . . . . . . . . ear

bi-. . . . . . . . . . two or both
-blast. . . . . . . . germ or bud
blast/o. . . . . . . germ or bud
brachi/o. . . . . . arm
brady-. . . . . . . slow
bronch/o . . . . . bronchus (airway)
bucc/o. . . . . . . cheek
carcin/o. . . . . . cancer
cardi/o. . . . . . . heart
celi/o. . . . . . . . abdomen
cephal/o . . . . . head
cerebell/o . . . . cerebellum
 . . . . . . . . . . . . (little brain)
cerebr/o. . . . . . brain
cervic/o. . . . . . neck or cervix
chondr/o . . . . . cartilage
chrom/o . . . . . color
circum-. . . . . . around
con-. . . . . . . . . together or with
contra- . . . . . . against or opposed to
cost/o . . . . . . . rib
crani/o. . . . . . . skull
cutane/o . . . . . skin
cyan/o. . . . . . . blue
cyst/o . . . . . . . bladder or sac
dacry/o . . . . . . .tear
dactyl/o. . . . . . digit (finger or toe)
de-. . . . . . . . . . from, down, or not
derm/o . . . . . . skin

-desis . . . . . . . binding
dextr/o . . . . . . right, or on
 . . . . . . . . . . . . the right side
dia-. . . . . . . . . across or through
diaphor/o . . . . profuse sweat
dips/o . . . . . . . thirst
dis- . . . . . . . . . separate from or apart
-dynia . . . . . . . pain
dys-. . . . . . . . . painful, difficult, or
 . . . . . . . . . . . . faulty
ec- . . . . . . . . . . out or away
-ectasis . . . . . . expansion or dilation
ecto- . . . . . . . . outside
-ectomy. . . . . . excision (removal)
-emesis . . . . . . vomiting
-emia. . . . . . . . blood condition
en-. . . . . . . . . . within
encephal/o . . . brain
endo-. . . . . . . . within
epi- . . . . . . . . . upon
erythr/o. . . . . . red
esthesi/o . . . . . sensation
eu-. . . . . . . . . . good or normal
ex-. . . . . . . . . . out or away
exo-. . . . . . . . . outside
extra- . . . . . . . outside
fasci/o. . . . . . . fascia (a band)
fibr/o. . . . . . . . fiber
gangli/o. . . . . . ganglion (knot)

gastr/o . . . . . . stomach
-gen. . . . . . . . origin or production
glomerul/o . . . glomerulus
          (little ball)
gloss/o . . . . . . .tongue
glott/o . . . . . . . opening
gluc/o . . . . . . . sugar
glyc/o . . . . . . . sugar
gnos/o . . . . . . knowing
-gram . . . . . . record
-graph . . . . . . . instrument for
          recording
-graphy . . . . . . process of recording
hem/o . . . . . . . blood
hemat/o. . . . . . blood
hemi- . . . . . . . half
hepat/o . . . . . . liver
hepatic/o . . . . . liver
herni/o . . . . . . hernia
hidr/o . . . . . . . sweat
hist/o. . . . . . . . tissue
histi/o . . . . . . . tissue
hydr/o . . . . . . . water
hyper- . . . . . . . above or excessive
hypo- . . . . . . . below or deficient
-ia . . . . . . . . . . condition of
-iasis . . . . . . . . formation of or
          presence of
-iatrics. . . . . . . treatment
-iatry . . . . . . . . treatment
-icle. . . . . . . . . small
immun/o . . . . . safe
infra-. . . . . . . . below or under
inter-. . . . . . . . between
intra-. . . . . . . . within
-ism. . . . . . . . . condition of
iso- . . . . . . . . . equal, like
-itis . . . . . . . . . inflammation
-ium . . . . . . . . structure or tissue
kyph/o. . . . . . . humped
lacrim/o . . . . . tear
lapar/o . . . . . . . abdomen
lei/o. . . . . . . . . smooth
lip/o . . . . . . . . fat
lob/o . . . . . . . . lobe (a portion)
lord/o . . . . . . . bent
lumb/o . . . . . . . loin (lower back)
lymph/o . . . . . clear fluid
-lysis. . . . . . . . breaking down or
          dissolution
macr/o. . . . . . . large or long

-malacia . . . . . softening
meat/o. . . . . . . opening
-megaly. . . . . . enlargement
meso- . . . . . . . middle
meta-. . . . . . . . beyond, after, or
          change
-meter . . . . . . . instrument for
          measuring
-metry . . . . . . . process of measuring
micro-. . . . . . . small
mono-. . . . . . . one
morph/o . . . . . form
multi- . . . . . . . many
muscul/o. . . . . muscle
myel/o. . . . . . . bone marrow or
          spinal cord
myring/o . . . . . eardrum
narc/o . . . . . . . stupor
nas/o. . . . . . . . nose
nat/i. . . . . . . . . birth
necr/o . . . . . . . death
neo-. . . . . . . . . new
nephr/o . . . . . . kidney
neur/o . . . . . . . nerve
ocul/o . . . . . . . eye
-oid . . . . . . . . . resembling
-ole . . . . . . . . . small
olig/o . . . . . . . few or deficient
-oma . . . . . . . . tumor
ophthalm/o . . . eye
opt/o . . . . . . . . eye
or/o . . . . . . . . . mouth
orth/o . . . . . . . straight, normal, or
          correct
-osis . . . . . . . . condition or increase
oste/o . . . . . . . bone
ot/o . . . . . . . . . ear
pachy-. . . . . . . thick
pan-. . . . . . . . . all
para- . . . . . . . . alongside of or
          abnormal
-paresis . . . . . . slight paralysis
path/o . . . . . . . disease
pector/o. . . . . . chest
ped/o . . . . . . . . child or foot
pelv/i. . . . . . . . hip bone
pelv/o . . . . . . . hip bone
-penia . . . . . . . abnormal reduction
per- . . . . . . . . . through
peri- . . . . . . . . around
phag/o. . . . . . . eat or swallow

phas/o . . . . . . . speech
-phil . . . . . . . . attraction for
-philia . . . . . . . attraction for
phleb/o . . . . . . vein
phob/o. . . . . . . exaggerated fear or
          sensitivity
phon/o. . . . . . . voice or speech
phot/o . . . . . . . light
phren/o . . . . . . diaphragm
          (also mind)
plas/o . . . . . . . formation
-plasty. . . . . . . surgical repair or
          reconstruction
-plegia. . . . . . . paralysis
pleur/o . . . . . . pleura
-pnea. . . . . . . . breathing
pneum/o . . . . . air or lung
pod/o. . . . . . . . foot
-poiesis . . . . . . formation
poly-. . . . . . . . many
post- . . . . . . . . after or behind
pre-. . . . . . . . . before
presby/o . . . . . old age
pro-. . . . . . . . . before
-ptosis . . . . . . . falling or downward
          displacement
pulmon/o . . . . lung
quadr/i . . . . . . four
re-. . . . . . . . . . again or back
reticul/o . . . . . a net
retro-. . . . . . . . backward or behind
rhabd/o . . . . . . rod shaped or striated
          (skeletal)
-rrhage . . . . . . to burst forth
-rrhexis . . . . . . rupture
sarc/o . . . . . . . flesh
scler/o. . . . . . . hard or sclera
scoli/o. . . . . . . twisted
semi . . . . . . . . half
sinistr/o. . . . . . left, or on the left side
somat/o. . . . . . body
somn/o . . . . . . sleep
son/o. . . . . . . . sound
-spasm . . . . . . involuntary
          contraction
sphygm/o . . . . pulse
spin/o . . . . . . . spine (thorn)
spir/o. . . . . . . . breathing
spondyl/o . . . . vertebra
squam/o . . . . . scale
-stasis . . . . . . . stop or stand

steat/o . . . . . . . fat
sten/o . . . . . . . narrow
stere/o . . . . . . . three dimensional
                or solid
stern/o . . . . . . sternum (breastbone)
steth/o . . . . . . . chest
stomat/o . . . . . mouth
-stomy . . . . . . creation of an
                opening
sub- . . . . . . . . below or under
super- . . . . . . . above or excessive
supra- . . . . . . . above or excessive
sym- . . . . . . . . together or with
syn- . . . . . . . . . together or with
tachy- . . . . . . . fast
tax/o . . . . . . . . order or coordination
ten/o . . . . . . . . tendon (to stretch)
thorac/o . . . . . . chest
thromb/o . . . . . clot
-tomy . . . . . . . incision
ton/o . . . . . . . . tone or tension
top/o . . . . . . . . place
tox/o . . . . . . . . poison
trache/o . . . . . . trachea (windpipe)
trans- . . . . . . . . across or through
tri- . . . . . . . . . . three
-tripsy . . . . . . . crushing
troph/o . . . . . . nourishment or
                development
-ula, -ule . . . . . small
ultra- . . . . . . . . beyond or excessive
uni- . . . . . . . . . one
ur/o . . . . . . . . . urine
varic/o . . . . . . . swollen or twisted
                vein
vas/o . . . . . . . . vessel
vertebr/o . . . . . vertebra
vesic/o . . . . . . bladder or sac
xanth/o . . . . . . yellow
xer/o . . . . . . . . dry
-y . . . . . . . . . . condition or
                process of

# References

Willis, M.C. (1996). *Medical terminology: The language of healthcare*. Philadelphia: Williams & Wilkins.

# APPENDIX 3

# STATE OCCUPATIONAL THERAPY REGULATORY BOARD AND STATE OT ASSOCIATION CONTACT INFORMATION

## ALABAMA

**Type of Regulation:** Licensure

**Regulatory Authority Contact:**

Alabama State Board of Occupational Therapy
64 N. Union Street Suite 734
Montgomery, AL 36130-4510
Phone: 334-353-4466
Fax: 334-353-4465
Website: www.ot.alabama.gov

**State Association Contact:**

Alabama Occupational Therapy Association (ALOTA)
204 Wild Timber Parkway
Pelham, AL 35124
Website: www.alota.org

## ALASKA

**Type of Regulation:** Licensure

**Regulatory Authority Contact:**

Alaska State PT & OT Board
Division of Corporations, Business, & Professional Licensing
333 Willoughby Avenue, 9th Floor
Juneau, AK 99811
Phone: 907-465-2580
Fax: 907-465-2974
Website: http://www.commerce.state.ak.us/occ/pphy.htm

**State Association Contact:**

Alaska Occupational Therapy Association (AKOTA)
PMB 1616
3705 Arctic Blvd.

Anchorage, AK 99503
Phone: 907-336-7808
Website: http://www.akota.org

## ARIZONA

**Type of Regulation:** Licensure

**Regulatory Authority Contact:**

Arizona Board of Occupational Therapy Examiners
5060 North 19th Avenue Suite 216
Phoenix, AZ 85015
Phone: 602-589-8352
Fax: 602-589-8354
Website: http://www.occupationaltherapyboard.az.gov/

**State Association Contact:**

Arizona Occupational Therapy Association (ArizOTA)
P.O. Box 5214
Peoria, AZ 85385
Phone: 623-937-0920
Website: arizota.org

## ARKANSAS

**Type of Regulation:** Licensure

**Regulatory Authority Contact:**

Arkansas State Occupational Therapy Examining Committee
2100 Riverfront Drive Suite 200
Little Rock, AR 72202
Phone: 501-296-1802
Fax: 501-296-1972
Website: www.armedicalboard.org

**State Association Contact:**

Arkansas Occupational Therapy Association (AROTA)
P.O. Box 337
Bryant, AR 72089
Website: www.arota.org

## CALIFORNIA

**Type of Regulation:** Licensure—OT, Certification—**OTA**
**Regulatory Authority Contact:**

California Board of Occupational Therapy
444 North 3rd Street, Suite 410
Sacramento, CA 95814
Phone: 916-322-3394
Fax: 916-445-6167
Website: http://www.bot.ca.gov/

**State Association Contact:**

Occupational Therapy Association of California (OTAC)
P.O. Box 276567
Sacramento, CA 95827
Website: www.otaconline.org

## COLORADO

**Type of Regulation: Trademark Law** (Does not regulate OTAs)
**Regulatory Authority Contact:**

OT Association of Colorado
Post Office Box 18387
Boulder, CO 80308
Phone: 303-546-6822
Fax: 303-226-4499
Website: www.otacco.org

**State Association Contact:**

OT Association of Colorado
Post Office Box 18387
Boulder, CO 80308
Phone: 303-546-6822
Fax: 303-226-4499
Website: www.otacco.org

## CONNECTICUT

**Type of Regulation:** Licensure
**Regulatory Authority Contact:**

Department of Public Health Occupational Therapy Licensure
410 Capital Avenue Mail Stop # 12APP PO BOX 340308
Hartford, CT 06134
Phone: 860-509-7603
Fax: 860-509-8457
Website: http://www.ct-clic.com/trantype.asp?code=824

**State Association Contact:**

Connecticut Occupational Therapy Association (ConnOTA)
370 Prospect Street
Wethersfield, CT 06109
Phone: (860) 257-1371
Website: http://www.connota.org/

## DELAWARE

**Type of Regulation:** Licensure
**Regulatory Authority Contact:**

Department of Administrative Services Professional Regulation
861 Silver Lake Blvd. Suite 203
Dover, DE 19904
Phone: 302-744-4532
Fax: 302-739-2711
Website:http://www.professionallicensing.state.de.us/boards/occupationaltherapy/index.shtml

**State Association Contact:**

Delaware Occupational Therapy Association (DOTA)
P.O. Box 11726
Wilmington, DE 19850
Phone: (302) 456-1962
Website: http://www.dotaonline.org/

## DISTRICT OF COLUMBIA

**Type of Regulation:** Licensure
**Regulatory Authority Contact:**

District of Columbia Board of Occupational Therapy
Washington, DC 20005
Phone: 202-724-8739
Website:http://dchealth.dc.gov/prof_license/servies/boards_main_action.asp?strAppId=13

**District of Columbia Association Contact:**

330 13th Street, SE
Washington, District of Columbia 20003
Phone: 202-806-7614
Fax: 202-462-5248

## FLORIDA

**Type of Regulation:** Licensure
**Regulatory Authority Contact:**

Florida Board of Occupational Therapy Practice
4052 Bald Cypress Way, Bin # C05
Tallahassee, FL 32399
Phone: 850-245-4373
Fax: 850-414-6860
Website:http://www.doh.state.fl.us/mqa/occupational/index.html

**State Association Contact:**
Florida Occupational Therapy Association (FOTA)
P.O. Box 5606
Ft Lauderdale, FL   33310
Phone:  954-840-FOTA (3682)
Website: http://www.flota.org

## GEORGIA
**Type of Regulation:** Licensure
**Regulatory Authority Contact:**
Georgia State Board of Occupational Therapy
237 Coliseum Drive
Macon, GA 31217
Phone: 478-207-2440
Fax: 478-207-1633
Website: http://www.sos.state.ga.us/plb/ot
**State Association Contact:**
Georgia Occupational Therapy Association (GOTA)
1260 Winchester Parkway, Suite 205
Smyrna, GA 30080
Phone: 770-435-5910
Fax: 770-433-2907
Website: http://www.gaota.com

## HAWAII
**Type of Regulation:** Licensure (Does not regulate OTAs)
**Regulatory Authority Contact:**
Hawaii Professional & Vocational Licensing Division
DCCA/PVL-Occupational Therapist Program
PO Box 3469
Honolulu, HI 6801
Phone: 808-586-2701
Fax: 808-586-2689
Website: http://www.hawaii.gov/dcca/areas/pvl/
programs/occupational/
**State Association Contact:**
Occupational Therapy Association of Hawaii (OTAH)
1360 S.Beretania St, Suite 301
Honolulu, HI 96814
Phone: 808-544-3336
Website: http://www.otah-hawaii.com

## IDAHO
**Type of Regulation:** Licensure
**Regulatory Authority Contact:**
Idaho Occupational Therapy Board
Idaho State Board of Medicine, P O Box 83720
Boise, ID 83720-0058
Phone: 208-327-7000
Fax: 208-327-7005
Website: http://www.bom.state.id.us

**State Association Contact:**
Idaho Occupational Therapy Association (IOTA)
PO Box 7364
Boise, Idaho 83707
Phone: 208-388-4682
Website: http://www.id-ota.com/

## ILLINOIS
**Type of Regulation:** Licensure
**Regulatory Authority Contact:**
Illinois Occupational Therapy Board (ILOTA)
320 West Washington
Springfield, IL 62786
Phone: 217-782-8556
Fax: 217-782-7645
Email: mkim.scoh@illinois.gov
**State Association Contact:**
Illinois Occupational Therapy Association (ILOTA)
7234 West North Avenue Suite 409
Elmwood Park, IL 60707
Phone: 708-452-7640
Website: http://ilota.org

## INDIANA
**Type of Regulation:** Certification
**Regulatory Authority Contact:**
Indiana Occupational Therapy Committee
402 W. Washington St. Room W072
Indianapolis, IN 46204
Phone: 317-234-1999
Fax: 317-233-4236
Website: http://www.in.gov/hpb/boards/otc/
**State Association Contact:**
Indiana Occupational Therapy Association (IOTA)
PO Box 3494
Muncie, IN 47307
Phone: 866-653-7429
Fax: 765-381-0958
Website: http://www.inota.com

## IOWA
**Type of Regulation:** Licensure
**Regulatory Authority Contact:**
Iowa Board of PT and OT Examiners
Professional Licensure Office Lucas State Office
Bldg., 5th Floor 321 East 12th Street
Des Moines, IA 50319
Phone: 515-281-4401
Fax: 515-281-3121
Website: http://www.idph.state.ia.us/licensure/

**State Association Contact:**

Iowa Occupational Therapy Association (IOTA)

PO Box 57221

Des Moines, IA 50317

Phone: 515-266-4525

Fax: 515-266-4525

Website: http://www.iowaot.org

## KANSAS

**Type of Regulation:** Registration

**Regulatory Authority Contact:**

Kansas State Board of Healing Arts

235 South Topeka Blvd

Topeka, KS 66602

Phone: 785-296-7413

Fax: 785-296-0852

Website: http://www.ksbha.org/

**State Association Contact:**

Kansas Occupational Therapy Association (KOTA)

825 S. Kansas Avenue, Suite 500

Topeka, KS 66612

Phone: (785) 232-8044

Toll Free: (877) 904-0529

Fax: (785) 233-2206

Website: http://www.kotaonline.org/

## KENTUCKY

**Type of Regulation:** Licensure

**Regulatory Authority Contact:**

Kentucky Board of Licensure for Occupational

Therapy

911 Leawood Drive

Frankfort, KY 40601

Phone: 502-564-3296

Fax: 502-564-4818

Website: http://finance.ky.gov/ourcabinet/caboff/OAS/op/occupth/

**State Association Contact:**

Kentucky Occupational Therapy Association (KOTA)

P.O. Box 21502

Louisville, KY 40221

Phone: 1-888-987-KOTA (5682)

Website: http://www.kotaweb.org/

## LOUISIANA

**Type of Regulation:** Licensure

**Regulatory Authority Contact:**

Louisiana State Board of Medical Examiners

State Board of Medical Examiners P.O. Box 30250

630 Camp Street

New Orleans, LA 70190

Phone: 800-296-7549

Fax: 504-568-6880

Website: http://www.lsbme.louisiana.gov/

**State Association Contact:**

Louisiana Occupational Therapy Association (LOTA)

P.O. Box 14806

Baton Rouge, LA 70898

Phone: 225-291-4014

Website: http://www.lota.org/

## MAINE

**Type of Regulation:** Licensure

**Regulatory Authority Contact:**

Maine Board of Occupational Therapy Practice

Dept. of Prof.& Financial Regulation 35 State House Station

Augusta, ME 04333

Phone: 207-624-8626

Fax: (207) 624-8637

Website: http://www.state.me.us/pfr/olr/categories/cat28.htm

**State Association Contact:**

Maine Occupational Therapy Association (MEOTA)

c/o Kennebec Valley Community College

92 Western Ave

Fairfield, ME 04937

Phone: (207) 453-5172

Website: http://www.meota.org/

## MARYLAND

**Type of Regulation:** Licensure

**Regulatory Authority Contact:**

Maryland Board of Occupational Therapy Practice

Spring Grove Hospital Center Benjamin Rush

Bldg. 55 Wade Avenue-Tulip Drive

Baltimore, MD 21228

Phone: 410-402-8560

Fax: 410-402-8561

Website: http://mdotboard.org/

**State Association Contact:**

Maryland Occupational Therapy Association

P.O. Box 2742

Columbia, MD 21045-1742

Phone: 410-290-3283

Website: http://www.mdota.org/

## MASSACHUSETTS

**Type of Regulation:** Licensure

**Regulatory Authority Contact:**

Massachusetts Board of Registration Allied
Health Professions
Division of Professional Licensure Board
of Allied Health
239 Causeway Street, Suite 500
Boston, MA 02114
Phone: 617-727-3071
Fax: 617-727-2669
Website: http://www.state.ma.us/reg/boards/ah/

**State Association Contact:**

Massachusetts Occupational Therapy Association
(MAOTA)
57 Madison Road
Waltham, MA 02453-6718
Phone: 781-647-5556
Fax: 781-642-9742
Website: http://www.maot.org/

## MICHIGAN

**Type of Regulation:** Licensure
**Regulatory Authority Contact:**

Michigan Board of Occupational Therapy
Department of Community Health Bureau of
Health Professions P.O. Box 30670
Lansing, MI48909
Phone: 517-335-0918
Fax: 517-373-2179
Website: http://www.michigan.gov/mdch/0,1607,
7-132-27417_27529_27545---,00.html

**State Association Contact:**

Michigan Occupational Therapy Association (MiOTA)
124 W. Allegan, Suite 1900
Lansing, MI  48933
Phone: 517-267-3918
Fax: 517-484-4442
Website: http://www.mi-ota.com/

## MINNESOTA

**Type of Regulation:** Licensure
**Regulatory Authority Contact:**

Minnesota Department of Health OT/OTA Licensing
Advisory Council
MDH/HOP, OTP Licensing Advisory Council,
Post Office Box 64882
St. Paul, MN 55164
Phone: 651-282-5624
Fax: 651-282-3839
Website: http://www.health.state.mn.us/divs/hpsc/
hop/otp/index.html

**State Association Contact:**

Minnesota Occupational Therapy Association
(MOTA)
1000 Westgate Drive, Suite 252
St. Paul, MN 55114
Phone: 651-290-7498
Fax: 651-290-2266
Website: http://www.motafunctionfirst.org/

## MISSISSIPPI

**Type of Regulation:** Licensure
**Regulatory Authority Contact:**

Professional Licensure 143 Lefleur's Square
Jackson, MS 39211
Phone: 601-364-7360
Fax: 601-364-5057
Website: www.msdh.state.ms.us

**State Association Contact:**

Mississippi Occupational Therapy Association
(MSOTA)
PO Box 13706
Jackson, MS  39236
Phone: 601-956-4105
Fax: 601-956-4105
Website: http://www.angelfire.com/ms/msota/

## MISSOURI

**Type of Regulation:** Licensure
**Regulatory Authority Contact:**

Missouri State Board of Occupational Therapy
3605 Missouri Blvd P.O. Box 1335
Jefferson City, MO 65109
Phone: 573-751-0877
Fax: 573-526-3489
Website: http://pr.mo.gov/

**State Association Contact:**

Missouri Occupational Therapy Association (MOTA)
360 S. Missouri BLVD.
Jefferson City, MO 65102
Phone: 636-441-4146
Website: http://www.motamo.net/index.htm

## MONTANA

**Type of Regulation:** Licensure
**Regulatory Authority Contact:**

Montana Board of Occupational Therapy Practice
Department of Labor and Industry
PO Box 200513 301 South Park, 4th floor
Helena, MT 59620

Phone: 406-841-2385
Fax: 406-841-2305
Website: http://www.discoveringmontana.com/dli/otp
**State Association Contact:**
Montana Occupational Therapy Association (MOTA)
PO Box 1441
Ennis, MT 59729
Phone: 406-855-5894
Website: http://mtota.org/home.html

## NEBRASKA
**Type of Regulation:** Licensure
**Regulatory Authority Contact:**
Nebraska Board of Occupational Therapy Practice
Credentialing Division, Post Office Box 94986
Lincoln, NE 68509
Phone: 402-471-2299
Fax: 402-471-3577
Website: www.hhs.state.ne.us/crl/profindex1.htm
**State Association Contact:**
Nebraska Occupational Therapy Association (NOTA)
PO Box 31594
Omaha, NE 68131-0594
Website: http://www.notaonline.org/

## NEW HAMPSHIRE
**Type of Regulation:** Licensure
**Regulatory Authority Contact:**
Occupational Therapy Governing Board
2 Industrial Park Drive
Concord, NH 03301
Phone: 603-271-8389
Fax: 603-271-6702
Website: http://www.nh.gov/alliedhealth/boards/
occupationaltherapy/index.htm
**State Association Contact:**
New Hampshire Occupational Therapy Association
(NHOTA)
P.O. Box 4232
Concord, NH 03302-4232
Phone: 603-225-9290
Website: http://www.nhota.org/

## NEW JERSEY
**Type of Regulation:** Licensure
**Regulatory Authority Contact:**
NJ Occupational Therapy Advisory Council
PO Box 45037
Newark, NJ 08833
Phone: 973-504-6570
Fax: 973-648-3536

Website: www.state.nj.us/lps/ca/medical/
occuptherapy.htm
**State Association Contact:**
New Jersey Occupational Therapy Association
(NJOTA)
P.O. Box 401
Summit, NJ 07902
Phone: 1-888-80NJOTA.
Website: http://www.njota.org/

## NEW MEXICO
**Type of Regulation:** Licensure
**Regulatory Authority Contact:**
NM Board of Examiners for Occupational Therapy
2550 Cerrillos Rd
Santa Fe, NM 87505
Phone: 505-476-4827
Fax: 505-476-4645
Website: http://www.rld.state.nm.us/b&c/otb/
**State Association Contact:**
New Mexico Occupational Therapy Association
(NMOTA)
P.O. Box 3036
Albuquerque, NM 87190
Phone: 603-225-9290
Website: http://www.nmota.org/

## NEW YORK
**Type of Regulation:** Licensure—OT, Registration—OTA
**Regulatory Authority Contact:**
New York State Board for Occupational Therapy
Room 2W EB 89 Washington Ave
Albany, NY 12234
Phone: 518-474-3817
Fax: 518-486-4846
Website: http://www.op.nysed.gov/ot.htm
**State Association Contact:**
New York Occupational Therapy Association
(NYOTA)
119 Washington Avenue, 2nd floor
Albany, NY 12210
Phone: 518-462-3717
Fax: 518-432-5902
Website: http://www.nysota.org/

## NORTH CAROLINA
**Type of Regulation:** Licensure
**Regulatory Authority Contact:**
North Carolina Board of Occupational Therapy
Post Office Box 2280
Raleigh, NC 27602

Phone: 919-832-1380
Fax: 919-833-1059
Website: http://www.ncbot.org/
**State Association Contact:**
North Carolina Occupational Therapy Association
(NCOTA)
P.O. Box 20432
Raleigh, NC 27619
Phone: 919-785-9700
Fax: 919-771-0115
Website: http://www.ncota.org

## NORTH DAKOTA
**Type of Regulation:** Licensure
**Regulatory Authority Contact:**
North Dakota State Board of OT Practice
Post Office Box 4005, 2900 E Broadway #3
Bismarck, ND 58502-4005
Phone: 701-250-0847
Fax: 701-224-9824
Website: http://www.ndotboard.com
**State Association Contact:**
North Dakota Occupational Therapy Association
(NDOTA)
P.O. Box 14118
Grand Forks, ND 585208-4118-
Phone: 701-221-3758
Website: http://www.ndota.com

## OHIO
**Type of Regulation:** Licensure
**Regulatory Authority Contact:**
Ohio Occupational Therapy, Physical Therapy and
Athletic Trainers Board
77 South High Street, 16th Floor
Columbus, OH 43215
Phone: 614-466-3774
Fax: 614-995-0816
Website: www.otptat.ohio.gov
**State Association Contact:**
Ohio Occupational Therapy Association (OOTA)
P.O. Box 32252
Columbus, OH 43232
Phone: 614-920-9445
Fax: 614-920-0830
Website: http://www.oota.org/

## OKLAHOMA
**Type of Regulation:** Licensure
**Regulatory Authority Contact:**
Oklahoma State Board of Medical Licensure and
Supervision

PO Box 18256
Oklahoma City, OK 73154
Phone: 405-848-6841
Fax: 405-848-8240
Website: www.okmedicalboard.org
**State Association Contact:**
Oklahoma Occupational Therapy Association (OOTA)
PO Box 2602
Oklahoma City, OK 74101-2602
Phone: 918-231-1300
Website: http://www.okota.org/

## OREGON
**Type of Regulation:** Licensure
**Regulatory Authority Contact:**
Oregon Occupational Therapy Licensing Board
800 NE Oregon Street, Suite 407
Portland, OR 97232
Phone: 971-673-0198
Fax: 971-673-0226
Website: http://www.otlb.state.or.us
**State Association Contact:**
Occupational Therapy Association of Oregon (OTAO)
P.O. Box 7133
Aloha, OR 97007
Phone: 503-658-6384
Fax: 503-690-1819
Website: http://www.otao.com

## PENNSYLVANIA
**Type of Regulation:** Licensure
**Regulatory Authority Contact:**
Pennsylvania State Board of Occupational Therapy
Education and Licensure
Box 2649
Harrisburg, PA 17105
Phone: 717-783-1389 0
Fax: 717-787-7769
Website: http://www.dos.state.pa.us/therapy
**State Association Contact:**
Pennsylvania Occupational Therapy Association (POTA)
100 South 21st Street
Harrisburg, PA 17104
Phone: 1-800-UR1POTA
Website: http://www.pota.org/

## RHODE ISLAND
**Type of Regulation:** Licensure
**Regulatory Authority Contact:**
Rhode Island Board of Occupational Therapy Practice
Health Professions Regulation
Cannon Building 3 Capital Hill Room 104

Providence, RI 02908
Phone: 401-222-2828
Fax: 401-222-1272
Website: http://www.health.ri.gov/hsr/professions/
occ_therap.php

**State Association Contact:**

Rhode Island Occupational Therapy Association (RIOTA)
P.O. Box 8585
Warwick RI 02888-0599
Phone: 401-345-8356
Website: http://www.riota.org/

## SOUTH CAROLINA

**Type of Regulation:** Licensure

**Regulatory Authority Contact:**

South Carolina Board of Occupational Therapy
110 Centerview Drive PO Box 11329
Columbia, SC 29211
Phone: 803-896-4683
Fax: 803-896-4719
Website:
http://www.llr.state.sc.us/POL/OccupationalTherapy/

**State Association Contact:**

South Carolina Occupational Therapy Association
(SCOTA)
401 Pittsdowne Road
Columbia, SC 29210
Phone: 888-647-2682
Website: http://www.scota.net/

## SOUTH DAKOTA

**Type of Regulation:** Licensure

**Regulatory Authority Contact:**

South Dakota Occupational Therapy Committee
123 S. Main Ave. Ste 100
Sioux Falls, SD 57104
Phone: 605-367-7781
Fax: 605-367-7786
Website: http://www.state.sd.us/dcr/medical/ot.htm

**State Association Contact:**

South Dakota Occupational Therapy Association
(SDOTA)
PO Box 88732
Sioux Falls, SD 57109-8732
Phone: 605-335-5542
Website: http://www.sdota.org

## TENNESSEE

**Type of Regulation:** Licensure

**Regulatory Authority Contact:**

Tennessee Board of Occupational Therapy & Physical
Therapy Examiners

227 French Landing, Suite 300 Heritage Place Metro
Center
Nashville, TN 37243-
Phone: 800-778-4123 ext. 25161
Fax: 615-741-7698
Website: http://www2.state.tn.us/health/Boards/OPT/

**State Association Contact:**

Tennessee Occupational Therapy Association (TOTA)
P.O. Box 70
Spring Hill, Tennessee 37174
Phone: 931-487-9871
Fax: 931-487-9870
Website: http://www.tnota.org

## TEXAS

**Type of Regulation:** Licensure

**Regulatory Authority Contact:**

Texas Executive Council of PT & OT Examiners
333 Guadalupe Street #2-510
Austin, TX 78701
Phone: 512-305-6900
Fax: 512-305-6970
Website: http://www.ecptote.state.tx.us/ot/

**State Association Contact:**

Texas Occupational Therapy Association (TOTA)
P.O. Box 15576
Austin, Texas 78761-5576
Phone: 512-454-8682
Fax: 512-450-1777
Website: http://www.tota.org

## UTAH

**Type of Regulation:** Licensure

**Regulatory Authority Contact:**

Utah Occupational Therapy Board
P.O. Box 146741
Salt Lake city, UT 84114-6741
Phone: 801-530-6621
Fax: 801-530-6511
Website: www.dopl.utah.gov

**State Association Contact:**

Utah Occupational Therapy Association (TOTA)
P.O. Box 58412
Salt Lake City, Utah 84108-9998
Phone: 800-748-4063
Website: http://www.uotaonline.org/

## VERMONT

**Type of Regulation: Licensure** (Does not regulate OTAs)

**Regulatory Authority Contact:**

Vermont Occupational Therapy Advisors
26 Terrace Street, Drawer 09

Montpelier, VT 05609-1101
Phone: 802-828-2191
Fax: 802-828-2465
Website: http://www.vtprofessionals.org/opr1/o_therapists/

**State Association Contact:**

Vermont Occupational Therapy Association (VOTA)
PO Box 5567
Essex Junction, VT 05453-5567
Phone: 802-264-9671
Website: http://www.vtot.org/

## VIRGINIA

**Type of Regulation:** Licensure

**Regulatory Authority Contact:**

Virginia Advisory Board on Occupational Therapy
6603 W Broad Street, 5th Floor
Richmond, VA 23230-1712
Phone: 804-662-9073
Fax: 804-662-7281
Website: www.dhp.virginia.gov

**State Association Contact:**

Virginia Occupational Therapy Association (VOTA)
2231 Oak Bay Lane
Richmond, Virginia 23233
Phone: 804-754-4120
Fax: 804-754-0801
Website: http://www.vaota.org/

## WASHINGTON

**Type of Regulation: Licensure**

**Regulatory Authority Contact:**

Washington Occupational Therapy Practice Board
P.O. Box 47867
Olympia, WA 98504-7867
Phone: 360-236-4865
Fax: 360-664-9077
Website: www.doh.wa.gov

**State Association Contact:**

Washington Occupational Therapy Association (WOTA)
P.O. Box 731356
Puyallup WA 98373
Phone: 206.242.9862
Fax: 253.864.7992
Website: http://www.wota.org/

## WEST VIRGINIA

**Type of Regulation:** Licensure

**Regulatory Authority Contact:**

West Virginia Board of Occupational Therapy
WVBOT - 3041 University Ave. 2nd Fl., Ste 6 3041
University Avenue 2nd Floor, Suite 6
Morgantown, WV 26505
Phone: 304-285-3150
Fax: 304-285-3150
Website: http://www.wvbot.org/

**State Association Contact:**

West Virginia Occupational Therapy Association
(WVOTA)
1840 Oakridge Drive
Charleston, WV 25311
Website: http://www.wvota.org/Home.htm

## WISCONSIN

**Type of Regulation:** Licensure

**Regulatory Authority Contact:**

Bureau of Health Professions Department of Regulation
and Licensing
OT Affiliated Credentialing Board
PO Box 8935
Madison, WI 53708
Phone: 608-266-8098
Fax: 608-267-3816
Website: http://drl.wi.gov/prof/occt/def.htm

**State Association Contact:**

Wisconsin Occupational Therapy Association (WOTA)
122 E. Olin Ave., Suite 165
Madison, WI 53713
Phone: 608-287-1606
Fax: 608-287-1608
Website: http://www.wota.net/online/index.php

## WYOMING

**Type of Regulation:** Licensure

**Regulatory Authority Contact:**

Wyoming Board of Occupational Therapy
6101 Yellowstone Road Suite 510
Cheyenne, WY 82002
Phone: 307-777-7764
Fax: 307-777-3314
Website: http://www.ot.state.wy.us

**State Association Contact:**

Wyoming Occupational Therapy Association (WYOTA)
5423 Liberty Street
Cheyenne, WY 82001
Phone: 307-778-2568
Website: http://www.wyota.org/

# COMPUTER SIMULATED EXAMINATIONS

## Guidelines for Effective Use of the Computer-based Examinations

Complete each of the of the two examinations on this text's computer disc in a manner that will simulate the administration of your NBCOT examination; that is, during a four hour period with no additional time allotted for breaks. During the NBCOT examination, the exam clock keeps running and does not stop until you exit the exam. You can take a short (3-5 minutes) break, if needed, but do not add this time to your four hour simulated exam session.

Upon completing each computer-based examination, you will receive an analysis of your exam performance. This detailed analysis will identify all of the exam items that you answered incorrectly. Extensive rationales for correct and incorrect answers are provided in this text section. *DO NOT* read these rationales until after you have completed the exam in its computerized format. The analysis of your exam performance will also provide a breakdown of your areas of strengths and weaknesses according to the content categories and critical reasoning strategies listed below. After reviewing the rationales for the exam answers and the computerized analysis of your performance on the specific content areas, you should revise your study plan using this very specific information. To help you know what to study, the content categories are labeled in accordance with this text's chapter titles. You should also reflect on the feedback provided on your critical reasoning strategies. If you had difficulty with a specific area(s) of reasoning, review the self-assessment questions and the examination preparation guidelines provided in Table 5 in Chapter 2. After implementing your revised study plan and using effective exam preparation strategies, complete the second computer-based exam. Use your next exam performance analysis to further revise your study plan. Additional guidelines for effective examination preparation are provided in Chapter 2 of this text. It is important to understand that your performance on these practice exams is *not* indicative of your future performance on the NBCOT exam. The exam items on these practice tests are purposefully designed to assist you in developing, critiquing, and revising your study plan so that you are well prepared for NBCOT exam.

## Content Categories

**C1** Human Development and Aging
**C2** The Process of Occupational Therapy
**C3** Musculoskeletal System Disorders and Biomechanical Approaches
**C4** Neurological System and Cognitive-perceptual Disorders and Neurological and Cognitive-perceptual Approaches
**C5** Cardiopulmonary, Gastrointestinal, Renal-genitourinary, Immunological, Endocrine, and Integumentary System Disorders and Evaluation and Intervention Approaches
**C6** Psychiatric Disorders and Psychosocial Approaches
**C7** Evaluation and Intervention for Performance in Areas of Occupation
**C8** Evaluation and Intervention for Environmental Mastery
**C9** Professional Standards and Responsibilities

## Critical Reasoning Strategies

 Inductive Reasoning

 Inferential Reasoning

 Deductive Reasoning

 Evaluative Reasoning

 Analytical Reasoning

# *Examination A*

## A1  C9

An OTA leads a community integration group for individuals with mild intellectual disabilities who reside in a group home. During a travel training session, a member of the group slips while going up the stairs of a bus. The client quickly gets up, pays the fare, sits down, and jokingly states, "Good thing I bounce well". Which action should the OTA take after assessing that the person is not injured?

**Correct Answer: C. Continue with the planned activity and file an occurrence report upon return to the group home.**

**Incorrect Answers:**

A.  Cancel the planned activity and return to the group home to file an occurrence report.

B.  Ask the bus driver to radio for an ambulance to obtain a medical assessment to validate that the client was not injured.

D.  Continue with the activity and ask the client to report any development of symptoms related to the fall.

**Rationale:**

Upon determination that the client has not been injured there is no need to cancel the planned activity. It is standard policy to file a report about any incidents that involve clients but occurrence reports about minor events do not have to be done immediately. There is no information in the scenario provided to indicate a need to call an ambulance. Asking the client to report any symptoms related to the fall is appropriate, but it is not the most important action for the OTA to take. Proper documentation is a professional and legal requirement that must be met.

**Type of Reasoning: Evaluative**

This question requires a value judgment in a situation regarding safety, which is an evaluative reasoning skill. In this situation, the most prudent procedure should be followed given the individual's status, which is to continue with the planned activity and file an occurrence report upon return to the group home. Review guidelines for reporting occurrences if answered incorrectly.

## A2  C5

An adult is hospitalized and diagnosed with mild chronic obstructive pulmonary disease (COPD). During the discharge planning session, the person identifies a desire to exercise regularly. Which of the following should the OTA recommend the client pursue?

**Correct Answer: A. The hospital wellness program's yoga group.**

**Incorrect Answers:**

B.  Low-impact aerobics at a local gym.

C.  Weight-lifting under the direction of a personal trainer.

D.  Jogging with friends.

**Rationale:**

The yoga and stretching program put the least amount of pressure on the pulmonary and cardiovascular systems. Also, the program is monitored by hospital personnel. All of the other activities can stress the cardiovascular and pulmonary systems too much. Also, they are not monitored by health care professionals familiar with COPD.

**Type of Reasoning: Inferential**

One must consider the diagnosis and needs of the client in order to choose the best exercise program for the patient. For patients with COPD, a monitored exercise program with the least amount of pressure on the pulmonary and cardiovascular systems is best. Questions that ask for a best course of action or what will best consider a patient's needs often necessitate inferential reasoning skill. If answered incorrectly, review information on exercise guidelines for patients with COPD.

**A3  C2**

In a program for survivors of domestic violence which of the following would the OTA do when using a client-centered approach?

**Correct Answer: D. Paraphrase the consumers' statements about past difficulties to help clarify feelings.**

**Incorrect Answers:**

A.  Offer specific suggestions for more effectively dealing with confrontations.

B.  Respond to self-deprecating comments with positive feedback on personal characteristics.

C.  Reinforce only the consumers' neutral comments about themselves and their skills.

**Rationale:**

The focus of client-centered therapy is to be directed by the consumer. The goal is to encourage awareness of feelings and exploration of possible consequences of future actions. Offering suggestions is not a component of client-centered therapy. The OTA should use techniques to encourage the consumers to generate such suggestions. In the client-centered approach, the OTA should withhold judgment on self-deprecating comments. The best approach is to accept the consumer unconditionally. To foster self-esteem, the OTA does best to focus on the consumers' ability to discover positive feelings independent of what other people may say.

**Type of Reasoning: Inferential**

This question requires one to determine a best course of action based on the information provided, which is an inferential reasoning skill. For this situation, paraphrasing the consumer's statements about past difficulties making decisions to help clarify feelings is best. If answered incorrectly, review information on the therapeutic process for victims of domestic violence.

**A4  C6**

An OTA working on an acute psychiatric inpatient unit conducts a series of groups for clients newly admitted to the unit. Which group leadership style is most effective for the OTA to assume when leading these groups?

**Correct Answer: D. Directive.**

**Incorrect Answers:**

A.  Advisory.

B.  Facilitative.

C.  Laissez-faire.

**Rationale:**

Directive leadership involves the provision of structure, clear directions, and immediate and consistent feedback. These qualities are needed in a group whose members are acutely ill with psychiatric disorders. The other choices do not provide the structure or organization needed for individuals whose symptoms often include decreased attention span, distractibility, poor social skills and/or thought disorders.

**Type of Reasoning: Inductive**

Clinical knowledge and judgment are the most important skills needed for answering this question, which requires inductive reasoning skill. Knowledge of the leadership styles and the most effective style in leading groups of newly admitted clients is essential to arriving at a correct conclusion. In this case, the most effective style is directive leadership, which should be reviewed if answered incorrectly.

**A5  C4**

An OTA works with an eight year-old with pervasive developmental disabilities in order to improve self-care skills. In teaching the child to brush teeth, the OTA places the toothbrush in the child's hand and guides it to the mouth. To help the child learn to complete the activity the OTA uses the somatosensory system. Which of the following is most effective for the OTA to use next during intervention with this child?

**Correct Answer: B. Provide hand-over-hand assistance to brush the child's teeth.**

**Incorrect Answers:**

A.  Tell the child to brush up and down.

C.  Touch the child's hand to prompt hand-to-mouth movements.

D.  Instruct the child to follow a pictorial sequence card depicting tooth-brushing.

**Rationale:**

In providing hand-over-hand assistance, the OTA is using tactile, proprioceptive, and movement stimuli to cue the child. The somatosensory system is inclusive of these sensory systems. Providing auditory, tactile, or visual input does not provide sufficient input for the child to learn the task.

**Type of Reasoning: Inferential**

One must have knowledge of somatosensory interventions in children with pervasive developmental disabilities in order to choose the best intervention approach. This is an inferential reasoning skill where one must infer or draw conclusions about a best course of action. For this case, the OTA should next provide hand-over-hand assistant to brush the child's teeth. If answered incorrectly, review sensory system terminology and interventions using a somatosensory approach.

**A6  C8**

An individual with advanced Huntington's chorea is admitted to a skilled nursing facility. The resident weighs 280 pounds and cannot independently transfer. What is the best recommendation for the OTA to make to the resident's direct care staff to ensure a safe transfer?

**Correct Answer: A. A mechanical lift transfer.**

**Incorrect Answers:**

B.  A two-person lift transfer.

C.  A stand pivot transfer.

D.  An assisted sliding board transfer.

**Rationale:**

A mechanical lift transfer is the safest for both the resident and the staff. The other transfers require motor and cognitive abilities that are beyond the capacity of an individual with advanced Huntington's chorea. Huntington's chorea, an autosomal dominant neuromuscular disease, is characterized by choreiform movements, progressive intellectual deterioration, and psychiatric disturbances. The individual's movement disorder combined with potential confused and/or agitated behaviors requires the use of a mechanical lift for safe and efficient transfers.

**Type of Reasoning: Inductive**

This question requires one to determine the best recommendation for an individual, given an understanding of the diagnosis and limitations. This requires inductive reasoning skill, where clinical judgment is paramount to arriving at a correct conclusion. For this situation, the OTA should recommend a mechanical lift transfer for the safety of the resident and staff. If answered incorrectly, review guidelines for mechanical lift transfers and the information about the sequelae of Huntington's chorea. The integration of this knowledge is needed to determine the correct answer.

**A7  C4**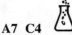

Two weeks after beginning kindergarten, a five year-old with myelomeningocele develops sudden onset of headaches, vomiting, irritability, and "sunken" appearance of eyes without signs of a fever. When the OTA reports the child's presenting symptoms, which condition should the OTA identify as a concern?

**Correct Answer: D. Shunt malfunction.**

**Incorrect Answers:**

A.  Stomach flu.

B.  Tethered cord.

C.  School anxiety.

**Rationale:**

These identified symptoms, along with seizures, are all symptoms of shunt malfunction. Shunt malfunction is a medical emergency. Stomach flu might be a possible reason for several of these symptoms, but given the clustering of the symptoms, the child should be checked for shunt malfunction. The signs of tethered cord include difficulties with bowel and bladder, gait disturbances, and/or foot deformities. A child may have a tendency to complain of stomach aches and other complaints to avoid school, if anxious. However, school anxiety would not include physical evidence of illness such as sunken eyes.

**Type of Reasoning: Analytical**

This question provides a group of symptoms and the test taker must determine the likely diagnosis. This requires analytical reasoning, where one must determine the precise meaning of the information presented. For this case, shunt malfunction is the most likely cause and should be reported. If answered incorrectly, review shunts for myelomeningocele and symptoms of malfunction.

**A8  C4**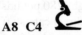

A client with a spinal cord injury and an OTA set a goal for the client to be independent in all aspects of bowel and bladder care, including skin inspection. Which of the following is the highest or most severe level of complete spinal cord injury the client can have to be able to achieve this goal?

**Correct Answer: A. C7-8.**

**Incorrect Answers:**

B.  C4-5.

C.  C5.

D.  C6.

**Rationale:**

These skills correspond to the C7-8 level. Individuals with SCIs at the other levels do not have the fine motor control to perform the skills independently.

**Type of Reasoning: Deductive**

This question requires factual recall of functional abilities according to spinal level lesions. Specifically, one must recall the expected outcomes of a patient with a complete C7-8 injury. Therefore a client with this level of injury could be expected to be independent in bowel and bladder care and skin inspection. Review functional outcomes of cervical level injuries if answered incorrectly, especially bowel and bladder care.

## A9  C2

The members of a clubhouse attain a level of cohesion which enables them to perform at a cooperative level. Two members disagree with the others on the details of a group project. How should the OTA leading this group respond to this conflict?

**Correct Answer: D. Encourage the members to explore alternative methods to resolve the conflict.**

**Incorrect Answers:**

A.  Clarify all viewpoints and facilitate the members in decision making.

B.  Listen to all viewpoints and suggest that members vote to determine the project details.

C.  Mediate only when the members have reached a deadlocked situation.

**Rationale:**

In a cooperative group, the OTA acts as an advisor. Group members are mutually responsible for giving feedback and meeting group needs. The OTA's interventions should facilitate group problem-solving rather direct the course of actions or decisions. Waiting until a group is deadlocked would not be beneficial to group cohesion.

**Type of Reasoning: Evaluative**

One must weigh the merits of the courses of action in order to arrive at a correct conclusion. This requires evaluative reasoning skill, where judgment based on values and principles is paramount to choosing the best solution. In this situation, where two members disagree in a cooperative level group, the OTA should encourage the members to explore alternative methods to resolve the conflict. Review the characteristics of cooperative groups and guidelines for group conflict resolution if answered incorrectly.

## A10  C3

After a work-related injury to the left index finger, an assembly line worker is fit with a buddy strap incorporating the index and middle fingers. In describing the primary purpose of the strap to the client, which of the following explanations is most accurate for the OTA to state?

**Correct Answer: A. "The strap provides passive ROM to the index finger".**

**Incorrect Answers:**

B.  "The strap reduces edema in the index finger".

C.  "The strap immobilizes the index finger".

D.  "The strap provides active ROM to the index finger".

**Rationale:**

The buddy strap provides passive ROM to the injured finger. The buddy strap can also help to improve a deformity that has been caused by immobilization due to injury, weakness, or casting. Elevation of the finger, retrograde massage, and contrast baths are techniques that help to reduce edema. Sometimes the strap on the finger can actually restrict circulation and increase edema. The strap mobilizes the finger and limits active ROM.

**Type of Reasoning: Inferential**

One must infer or draw conclusions about the possible effects of a buddy strap involving the middle or index finger. The benefit is typically passive ROM to the injured finger. In order to arrive at a correct conclusion, one must understand the indications for issuing a buddy strap, which should be reviewed if answered incorrectly.

346

## A11 C5

Several patients in a cardiovascular unit are referred to occupational therapy for rehabilitation in areas of occupation. Which diagnosis would be an inclusive criterion for participation in the home management activity group conducted in the department's simulated apartment?

**Correct Answer: A. Hypotension.**

**Incorrect Answers:**

B. Unstable angina.

C. Venous thrombosis.

D. Uncontrolled atrial arrhythmia.

**Rationale:**

Persons with hypotension can be included in a rehabilitation group that includes instrumental activities of daily living. Engagement in these activities would be contraindicated for patients with the other conditions. Unstable angina is a coronary insufficiency with risk for myocardial infarction or sudden death. The person's pain is difficult to control and it is present with low level activity or rest. Venous thrombosis and uncontrolled atrial arrhythmia must be monitored closely and persons with these diagnoses would be better candidates for OT services that are provided bedside.

**Type of Reasoning: Deductive**

This question requires the test taker to recall symptoms of cardiac dysfunction and guidelines for cardiac rehabilitation. Deductive reasoning skills are utilized, as one must recall factual information about indications and contraindications for cardiac rehabilitation programs associated with certain diagnoses. In this situation only patients with hypotension are allowed to engage in instrumental activities of daily living. If answered incorrectly, review cardiac rehabilitation guidelines, especially for patients with the identified symptoms.

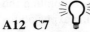

## A12 C7

An OTA is conducting a community transportation group with individuals attending a traumatic brain injury day treatment program in an urban area. Which should the group do first?

**Correct Answer: C. Determine a destination.**

**Incorrect Answers:**

A. Read a subway map.

B. Take a subway as a group.

D. Purchase a subway fare card.

**Rationale:**

The first step is to determine a desired destination. Map reading skills would be the next step in determining the subway route(s) to take to arrive at the desired destination. Purchasing a fare card and taking the subway as a group comes after planning a route.

**Type of Reasoning: Inferential**

One must infer or draw conclusions regarding the ideal first step in a functional task. After reviewing all of the possible choices, one must determine that one step must come before all the others in order to have a successful outcome. For this situation, determining a destination must come first in order for the remaining steps to be executed effectively. If answered incorrectly, review community transportation group guidelines.

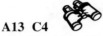

## A13 C4

A child with tactile defensiveness is receiving intervention from an OTA who uses a sensory integrative approach. Which method is most effective for the OTA to use when introducing tactile stimuli to the child?

**Correct Answer: A. Provide deep touch and firm pressure where the child can see the stimuli.**

**Incorrect Answers:**

B. Apply the stimuli in the direction opposite of hair growth with vision occluded.
C. Apply light touch across the face and abdomen with vision occluded.
D. Provide light brushing across the palmar surfaces of the extremities with the child watching.

**Rationale:**

Deep touch and firm pressure help to decrease tactile defensiveness. To decrease defensiveness, the child needs to see the stimuli. The self application of stimuli can also increase tolerance. Light touch, brushing across the face and abdomen, and application of stimuli in the direction opposite of hair growth are all aversive to a person with tactile defensiveness. Stimuli should be applied in the direction of hair growth for this is less aversive.

**Type of Reasoning: Inductive**

This question requires one to determine the most appropriate method for introducing tactile stimuli. This requires inductive reasoning skill, where clinical judgment is paramount to arriving at a correct conclusion. For this situation, the OTA should provide deep touch and firm pressure where the child can see the stimuli. If answered incorrectly, review tactile approaches for sensory integration intervention.

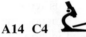

## A14 C4

An OTA uses the Rood approach to facilitate motor development. A pediatric client has mastered the neck co-contraction pattern. Which pattern is best for the OTA to implement next?

**Correct Answer: B. Prone on elbows.**

**Incorrect Answers:**

A. Quadruped.
C. Rollover.
D. Standing.

**Rationale:**

According to Rood there are eight different patterns which occur in the following sequence: (1) supine withdrawal, (2) rollover, (3) prone extension, (4) neck co-contraction, (5) prone on elbows, (6) quadruped, (7) standing, and (8) walking.

**Type of Reasoning: Deductive**

This question requires recall of guidelines and principles, which is factual knowledge. Deductive reasoning skills are utilized whenever one must recall facts and guidelines to solve novel problems. In this situation, after mastering neck co-contraction, the OTA should address prone on elbows. Review Rood theory and the development of motor patterns if answered incorrectly.

348

### A15 C4

The parents of a five year-old with attention deficit with hyperactivity disorder (ADHD) express difficulty managing the child's aggressive behavior towards older siblings. Which is the most effective strategy for the OTA to recommend to the parents?

**Correct Answer:  B. Redirect the child's energy into acceptable and safe play activities.**

**Incorrect Answers:**

A.  Allow the child to vent aggressive feelings on a stuffed animal or doll.

C.  Provide consistent punishment for aggressive behavior.

D.  Send the child to stay with a family member or close friend for an extended "time-out".

**Rationale:**

Redirecting the child's energy to activities can be an effective management of the child's aggressive behavior.  It would also be appropriate to have the parents observe and record the precipitants to these behaviors to determine potential environmental modifications.  This is not an option provided.  Allowing the child to vent aggression onto a stuffed animal or doll would not provide the structure the child needs to learn appropriate, safe behaviors.  Also, aggressive behaviors are not always coupled with aggressive feelings. Sometimes the hyperactivity of a child simply asserts itself in socially unacceptable ways, such as when a child pushes a sibling very hard in an effort to get the sibling to play "chase".  Punishing the child or removing the child from the family does not address the child's needs.  Taking punitive actions towards the child can increase feelings of resentment and promote a decrease in feelings of self-worth, which are typically already low in children with ADHD, which can fuel aggressive behavior.

**Type of Reasoning: Inductive**

This question requires one to determine the most appropriate recommendation for a child with ADHD. This requires inductive reasoning skill, where clinical judgment is paramount to arriving at a correct conclusion. For this situation, the OTA should recommend redirecting the child's energy into acceptable and safe play activities. If answered incorrectly, review treatment guidelines for children with ADHD, especially behavior management techniques.

### A16  C4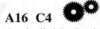

An individual with a spinal cord injury at the level of T-1 is practicing a stand pivot transfer in the OT department of a rehabilitation center. The patient complains of dizziness and nausea. Which action is most important for the OTA to take first?

**Correct Answer: C. Return the person to the wheelchair and immediately recline it.**

**Incorrect Answers:**

A.  Call for help according to facility procedures.

B.  Return the patient to the wheelchair for a five minute rest break.

D.  Return the patient to the wheelchair and transport the patient back to rest in bed.

**Rationale:**

Individuals with SCIs are at risk for orthostatic hypotension. Complaints of dizziness and nausea are indications of orthostatic hypotension and require an immediate response. Reclining the individual in his/her wheelchair will return blood pressure to a normal range. The other choices do not address the need for immediate remediation of this crisis.

**Type of Reasoning: Evaluative**

This question requires professional judgment based on knowledge of the symptoms and safety guidelines, which is an evaluative reasoning skill. Because the patient's symptoms indicate orthostatic hypotension, the OTA should return the person to the wheelchair and immediately recline it to relieve symptoms. Review care guidelines for orthostatic hypotension, especially in SCI if answered incorrectly.

## A17  C2

The members of a group are not working well together and show decreased levels of trust. Which action is most effective for the OTA to take to enhance the group's cohesiveness?

**Correct Answer: B. Verbally reinforce the goals and norms of the group.**

**Incorrect Answers:**

A.  Begin the group with inspirational phrases.

C.  Have each member write a journal about his/her perspectives about the group.

D.  Ask members to talk about what they do not like about the group.

**Rationale:**

The most effective choice is to verbally reinforce the goals and norms of the group. This helps to direct the focus of the members and to address difficulties in keeping that focus. Inspirational phrases can be helpful to instill a positive attitude but they do not address the need to develop group cohesion. Writing in a journal can help develop personal insights but it would not increase group cohesion. Asking for self-disclosure in a group with decreased levels of trust will decrease cohesion. Also, the topic of what members do not like about the group is not likely to facilitate trust, openness, and willingness to share.

**Type of Reasoning: Inferential**

One must determine which course of action will result in improved group cohesiveness. This requires inferential reasoning where one must draw conclusions about each course of action as achieving the ultimate purpose of group cohesion. In this case, verbally reinforcing the goals and purposes of the group will best enhance group cohesion. If answered incorrectly, review group facilitation techniques.

## A18  C3

A child with juvenile rheumatoid arthritis wears bilateral night resting splints with wrists in zero degrees of extension, MPs and IPs flexed, ulnar deviation of 10 degrees, and thumbs in opposition. The child complains of pain in wrists upon awakening. No redness is noted upon removing splints. ROM measurements show ulnar deviation of 5 degrees. Which action should the OTA take in response to this complaint and these observations?

**Correct Answer: A. Modify the splints at the wrist.**

**Incorrect Answers:**

B.  Pad the ulnar aspect on the inside of the splints.

C.  Discontinue the splints and monitor the status of pain for two weeks.

D.  Construct volar cock-up splints for use during the day.

**Rationale:**

The splints should be adjusted by use of heat to accommodate to the current position of ulnar deviation. Padding is frequently used to attempt to modify the position of a splint, but it does not correctly allow distribution of pressure. Discontinuing the splints will serve to increase deformities and pain. The child might benefit from day splints, but this does not address the issue of the night resting splints causing pain and being set at an incorrect angle for the child's ulnar deviation measurement.

**Type of Reasoning: Evaluative**

One must evaluate the symptoms provided and then determine a best course of action based upon this information. This utilizes evaluative reasoning skill, where the value of the information should guide one's thinking and action in clinical situations. For this case, the most appropriate action would be to modify the night splints at the wrist. If answered incorrectly, review splinting guidelines.

## A19 C8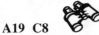

An adolescent with myelomeningocele (spina bifida) at the C8 level wants to access a new computerized play system. Which is the best adaptation for the OTA to recommend the adolescent use to access this system?

**Correct Answer: D. A joy stick control.**

**Incorrect Answers:**

A.  A chin switch.

B.  A tenodesis splint.

C.  A dorsal wrist splint with a universal cuff.

**Rationale:**

At the level of C-8, the teenager can independently use a joy stick control. A chin switch would be indicated for a C-3, C-4 level lesion; a tenodesis splint is indicated for a C-6 level lesion; and a dorsal splint with a universal cuff is indicated for a C-5 level lesion.

**Type of Reasoning: Inductive**

This question requires one to determine the best recommendation for a child with cervical spina bifida. This requires inductive reasoning skill, where clinical judgment and knowledge of the diagnosis, including functional abilities, are paramount to arriving at a correct conclusion. For this situation, the OT should recommend a joy stick control. If answered incorrectly, review the functional abilities associated with each spinal cord level, especially C8 level.

## A20 C8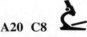

An individual is scheduled for a right hip total arthroplasty (THA). Following surgery, which is the most appropriate bed positioning intervention for the OTA to recommend?

**Correct Answer: B. Use of an abductor pillow between the lower extremities.**

**Incorrect Answers:**

A.  Sidelying with the lower extremities adducted.

C.  Use of a hospital bed to elevate the lower extremities to 90 degrees.

D.  Change of position from supine to prone every 2 hours.

**Rationale:**

An abductor pillow will prevent adduction of the operated hip, which is an important post-surgery precaution. Using a hospital bed to elevate the lower extremities to flex the hips to 90 degrees is contraindicated because a major hip precaution is not to flex beyond 90 degrees. Changing position from supine to prone requires rolling which can result in internal rotation of the hip. External rotation should be avoided if an anterolateral approach is used. This is contraindicated for it can result in dislocation.

**Type of Reasoning: Deductive**

One must recall the post-surgery guidelines for total hip replacement. This is factual knowledge, which is a deductive reasoning skill. In this situation, the only appropriate guideline listed is to use an abductor pillow between the legs. If answered incorrectly, review total hip precautions, especially bed positioning.

## A21 C4

An OTA works with an individual recovering from a traumatic brain injury in a rehabilitation hospital. The OTA uses a transfer of training approach to help the patient develop and carry out a daily schedule of activities upon the patient's return home. What is the most effective activity for the OTA to use during an intervention session with this client?

**Correct Answer: B. Organization of a list of daily activities.**

**Incorrect Answers:**

A. Preparation of a simple meal.

C. Composition of a shopping list.

D. Completion of an interest checklist.

**Rationale:**

A transfer of training approach is a remedial/restorative approach that focuses on restoration of components to increase skill. It is deficit specific and utilizes tabletop and computer activities as treatment modalities. According to this approach, the activity of organizing a list of daily activities will help with the ability to formulate a schedule in one's home environment. Preparing a meal, composing a shopping list, and completing an interest checklist are each discrete activities that would develop skills related to the performance of these activities, but they do not address the skills needed to schedule the multiple activities of a typical day.

**Type of Reasoning: Inductive**

This question requires the test taker to determine the most effective activity for a client with traumatic brain injury using a transfer of training approach. This is an inductive reasoning skill, as questions of this nature often ask one to utilize clinical judgment to determine therapeutic courses of action. For this case, the OTA should emphasize organization of a list of daily activities in treatment. Review transfer of training approach if answered incorrectly.

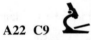

## A22  C9

An OTA observes a colleague using fluidotherapy on a patient with an insensate hand after being informed by the supervising therapist that this physical agent modality (PAM) is contraindicated for this specific case. The colleague justifies the use of this PAM based on the patient's request for the intervention. The OTA meets with the OT supervisor to express concern about the colleague's behavior. Which ethical principle does the OTA identify the colleague is violating?

**Correct Answer: B. Competence.**

**Incorrect Answers:**

A. Judgment.

C. Autonomy.

D. Justice.

**Rationale:**

Competence means practicing correctly. In this scenario, the colleague is incorrectly performing or administering the therapeutic activity. Judgment refers to decision-making skills in implementing services and is not an ethical principle of practice. Autonomy refers to having the patient involved in the decisions of therapy to reflect personal goals, values, and interests. Justice refers to complying with the laws of the profession as well as legality of local, state, and federal laws. While not practicing competently is a violation of state practice regulations and licensure laws, there is no law specifically against providing fluidotherapy for a person with an insensate hand.

**Type of Reasoning: Deductive**

One must recall the OT Code of Ethics and definitions for each principle in order to arrive at a correct conclusion. This requires deductive reasoning skill, where factual knowledge is paramount to choosing the correct solution. In this situation, the OTA is violating the principle of competence. Review the AOTA Code of Ethics and the principle of competence if answered incorrectly.

## A23  C6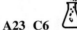

A person is recovering from a major cardiac infarct. During the initial OT session, the patient loudly and vigorously expresses plans to immediately resume a daily rigorous exercise routine. The OTA reports the individual's plan to the cardiac rehabilitation team and explains that the individual appears to be in which of the following disability adjustment stages?

**Correct Answer: B. Denial.**

**Incorrect Answers:**

A. Shock.

C. Acting out.

D. Acceptance.

**Rationale:**

During the psychosocial adjustment to disability/illness, denial is characterized by unrealistic expectations of recovery and minimizing one's difficulties. Shock is characterized by emotional numbness, depersonalization and reduced speech and mobility. Acceptance is reflected in the acknowledgement of the situation and the development of a new self-concept reflective of one's assets and potentialities. Acting out is a term used to describe behavior that challenges societal norms.

**Type of Reasoning: Analytical**

This question provides a description of a behavior and the test taker must draw conclusions about what the behavior indicates. This is an analytical reasoning skill, as questions of this nature often ask one to analyze descriptors and symptoms in order to determine a diagnosis or draw a conclusion. In this situation the behavior indicates denial. If answered incorrectly review disability adjustment guidelines.

## A24  C5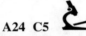

An OTA working on an acute cardiopulmonary rehabilitation unit collaborates with the occupational therapist to plan intervention for an individual who can complete activities in Stage II of cardiac recovery at a MET level of 1.4 -2.0. Which activities should the OTA recommend be included in this intervention plan?

**Correct Answer: A. Shaving and crafts.**

**Incorrect Answers:**

B. Self-feeding and reading.

C. Deep breathing exercises and table top games.

D. Showering and isometric exercises.

**Rationale:**

Shaving and crafts meet the 1.4-2.0 MET criteria of Stage II of cardiopulmonary recovery. Self-feeding, reading, deep breathing and table top games are at a 1.0-1.4 MET level and would be appropriate for an individual in Stage I. Showering is at the MET level of 2.0-3.0 and would be appropriate for an individual in Stage III of recovery. Isometrics are contraindicated during Stage II.

**Type of Reasoning: Deductive**

One must recall the guidelines for MET level activity for patients in stage II of cardiopulmonary recovery. This is factual knowledge, which is a deductive reasoning skill. For this situation, the patient is allowed to do shaving and crafts, which falls within the 1.4-2.0 MET range for stage II recovery. Review stage II recovery guidelines and MET level activity if answered incorrectly.

**A25  C2**

Several adolescents with behavior problems attend a school-based after-school program. They work at an egocentric-cooperative level in a group dealing with issues related to peer pressure. Which of the following would be most likely for the OTA to observe the participants doing in the group?

**Correct Answer: B. Focusing on the group tasks rather than the feelings of the participants.**

**Incorrect Answers:**

A.  Actively taking on roles such as energizer, coordinator, or opinion giver.

C.  Making decisions with minimal to no supervision from the group leader.

D.  Performing group skills consistent with the developmental level of 15 to 18 years of age.

**Rationale:**

The egocentric-cooperative group tends to focus on the tasks to be completed with little attention devoted to the feelings of the participants. At this level, members do not actively assume diverse group roles. A mature group would require little or no supervision and performs at the 15 to 18 year-old developmental level. An egocentric-cooperative group performs at the five to seven year developmental level.

**Type of Reasoning: Inferential**

One must recall the typical manifestations of clients who function at an egocentric-cooperative level in order to arrive at a correct conclusion. This requires one to determine what may be true for a group of clients, which is an inferential reasoning skill. For this situation, the group members are most likely to focus on the group tasks rather than the feelings of the participants. If answered incorrectly, review egocentric-cooperative level group guidelines and functional level of group participants.

**A26  C4**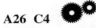

An OTA conducts an intervention session with a client recovering from a CVA to develop transfer skills. The client has a co-morbidity of epilepsy. As the client stands to complete a transfer from the wheelchair to the bed, the client reports feeling sensations that are indicative of an aura. Which is the best immediate action for the OTA to take in response to this situation?

**Correct Answer: D. Guide the person into a sidelying position on the bed.**

**Incorrect Answers:**

A. Provide reassurance and ask for guidance from the occupational therapist.

B. Return the client to a seated position in the wheelchair until the sensations pass.

C. End the session so the client can rest.

**Rationale:**

An aura is the brief warning stage before the tonic phase of an epileptic seizure. During an aura, changes in tactile, gustatory, olfactory, or other sensations are experienced (e.g., numbness, unexplained smells). After this brief stage, a tonic-clonic seizure will occur. The tonic phase includes a loss of consciousness, stiffening of the body, heavy and irregular breathing, drooling, skin pallor, and occasional bladder and bowel incontinence for a few seconds before the clonic phase begins. The clonic phase includes alternating rigidity and relaxation of muscles. Since a person could fall and harm him/herself during a seizure, the OTA must immediately ensure the client's safety. Therefore, the best action for the OTA to take is to place the person in sidelying on the bed. If there are bed rails these should be raised. This will prevent the client from falling or choking. Providing reassurance, having the client remain seated, and ending the session does not effectively deal with the immediate need to provide interventions for the impending seizure. The OTA does not need (nor should wait for) the input of the occupational therapist.

**Type of reasoning: Evaluative**

This question requires the test taker to weigh the merits of the four courses of action presented and then determine the action that most effectively addresses the needs of the client. This requires evaluative reasoning skill. For this situation, the OTA should guide the person into a side-lying position on the bed. Review first aid guidelines for clients with seizure disorders if answered incorrectly.

**A27 C4**

An OTA provides intervention for an individual with a swallowing disorder. To elicit a swallow reflex, the OTA provides sensory input to the inferior faucial arches. Which should the OTA use to provide this intervention?

**Correct Answer: C. A chilled dental examination mirror.**

**Incorrect Answers:**

A. A tongue depressor.
B. A moistened cotton swab.
D. A warmed metal teaspoon.

**Rationale:**

The use of cold stimulation to the inferior faucial arches via a chilled dental examination mirror will elicit a swallow reflex. The others will not.

**Type of Reasoning: Inferential**

One must determine the guidelines for eliciting a swallow reflex and then determine which of the listed devices is aligned with the stimulation of this reflex. This requires inferential reasoning skill. In this situation, a chilled dental examination mirror is ideal. If answered incorrectly, review elicitation of the swallow reflex.

**A28 C1**

A two year-old child receives home care early intervention services. The occupational therapy intervention plan includes a goal to develop the child's pincer grasp. Which is the most appropriate activity for the OTA to work on with the child during an intervention session?

**Correct Answer: A. Finger-feeding of O-shaped cereal.**

**Incorrect Answers:**

B. Picking up marbles.
C. Drawing with jumbo crayons.
D. Stacking one inch cubes.

**Rationale:**

Picking up O-shaped cereal to finger-feed will facilitate the use a pincer grasp. While picking up marbles also uses a pincer grasp, this activity presents a potential choking hazard, as two year-olds frequently put items they pick up into their mouths. Drawing with a jumbo crayon uses a gross grasp. Stacking cubes uses a radial digital grasp.

**Type of Reasoning: Inductive**

Clinical knowledge and judgment are the most important skills needed for answering this question, which requires inductive reasoning skill. Knowledge of the development of pincer grasp and effective strategies to facilitate it are essential to choosing the best solution. In this case, the OTA should recommend finger-feeding O-shaped cereal. Review the developmental sequence of grasp and the characteristics of different grasp patterns if answered incorrectly.

## A29 C1

A child with autism receives home care OT intervention services. The parent identifies a primary goal of developing the child's independent toileting skills. The child is completely dependent and the parent reports not attempting toilet training for several years. The OTA collaborates with the occupational therapist to establish the first intervention goal for the child. Which behavior should this goal address?

**Correct Answer: D. The child's ability to indicate when the diaper is wet or soiled.**

**Incorrect Answers:**

A. The child's ability to sit on the toilet with supervision.
B. The child's ability to verbally tell someone of the need to go to the bathroom.
C. The child's ability to non-verbally indicate the need to go to the bathroom.

**Rationale:**

The first toileting skill that must be developed is the child's recognition of being wet or soiled. This typically occurs at 12 months. Subsequent toileting skills such as sitting on the toilet with supervision and indicating the need to go to the bathroom can develop after this initial recognition of being wet or soiled.

**Type of Reasoning: Inferential**

One must have knowledge of the typical developmental sequence of toilet skills and toilet training guidelines in order to arrive at a correct conclusion. This is an inferential reasoning skill where knowledge of guidelines and judgment based on facts are utilized to reach conclusions. In this situation, the first intervention goal would be to have the child indicate when his/her diaper is wet or soiled. If answered incorrectly, review the typical developmental sequence of toilet skills and toilet training guidelines for children.

## A30 C3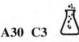

A client with arthritis of both hands has ulnar drift of MPs during finger extension and flexion and at rest. The person also has a lengthening of the central slips of the extensor digitorum communis tendons of the right index and middle fingers. Which of the following should the OTA report the person is exhibiting?

**Correct Answer: D. Boutonniere deformities.**

**Incorrect Answers:**

A. Swan-neck deformities.
B. Trigger-finger deformities.
C. MP palmar subluxation-dislocations.

**Rationale:**

A boutonniere deformity is caused by a lengthening or rupture of the extensor digitorum communis tendons and is expressed by DIP hyperextension and PIP flexion. A swan-neck deformity can result from the rupture of the lateral slips of the extensor digitorum communis or flexor digitorum superficialis tendon and results in DIP flexion and PIP hyperextension. A trigger-finger deformity results from a thickening of the flexor digitorum superficialis tendon at the flexor tunnel, also called a tendon sheath. The affected joint tends to stay open upon attempt to close or fist the hand. Synovitis of the MP joints can cause damage to the MP ligaments with palmar dislocation in conjunction with, or independent of, ulnar drift.

**Type of Reasoning: Analytical**

This question requires the test taker to determine the likely diagnosis from a set of symptoms, which is an analytical reasoning skill. For this situation, the symptoms indicate boutonniere deformities. If answered incorrectly, review characteristics of boutonniere deformity.

356

## A31 C9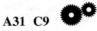

An OTA is hired to work in the occupational therapy department of an acute psychiatric unit. The OTA requests an orientation to hospital policies and procedures. Which is the most important focus for the OTA to learn the policies and procedures of during the initial orientation session?

**Correct Answer: A. Crisis intervention.**

**Incorrect Answers:**

B. Reimbursement.

C. Employee benefits.

D. Group program scheduling.

**Rationale:**

Crises can occur at any time in any acute facility. All employees must immediately learn the policies and procedures for dealing with crises to ensure the safety of patients and staff. Reimbursement issues and group program scheduling can be reviewed during regular supervisory sessions. These issues are not immediate concerns. Employee benefits are the responsibility of the personnel/human resources department.

**Type of Reasoning: Evaluative**

One must weigh the possible courses of action and then make a judgment about which focus is the most immediate need. This requires evaluative reasoning skill, which often requires one to make value judgments. For this case, the OTA should initially learn about the crisis intervention policies and procedures as they are the most critical to know in an acute psychiatric setting. The other policies and procedures are important but they are not immediate concerns. Review policies and procedures guidelines for acute psychiatric practice settings if answered incorrectly.

## A32 C1

An individual with bilateral lower extremity amputations and cataracts is newly admitted to a skilled nursing facility. The individual retains some residual vision. During intervention sessions, which is the most effective placement for the OTA to use when presenting materials to the person?

**Correct Answer: A. To the side of the person, with no direct lighting.**

**Incorrect Answers:**

B. Directly in front of the person, at eye level.

C. Directly in front of the person, at table top level.

D. To the side of the person, with a strong light shining.

**Rationale:**

An individual with cataracts loses central vision first; therefore, presenting evaluation materials directly in front of the person will be ineffective. Peripheral vision gradually decreases with cataracts, so presenting materials to the side will enable the person to use his/her residual vision. Individuals with cataracts have increased difficulty with glare, so indirect lighting is indicated.

**Type of Reasoning: Inferential**

One must have knowledge of cataracts and visual limitations in order to choose the best manner of presenting evaluation materials. This is an inferential reasoning skill where knowledge of the visual disorder and presenting deficits is pivotal to choosing the correct solution. For this situation, the OTA should present materials to the side of the person, with no direct lighting. If answered incorrectly, review the clinical presentation of cataracts and engagement in functional activities.

## A33  C4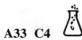

An adult who incurred a CVA has difficulty dealing with increasing amounts of stimuli. This is noted in all modalities. The OTA documents these observations. Which cognitive perceptual dysfunction should the OTA report the client is exhibiting?

**Correct Answer: D. Generalized attention deficit.**

**Incorrect Answers:**

A.  Inability to abstract.
B.  Poor organizational skills.
C.  Poor semantic memory.

**Rationale:**

Attention requires the ability to focus on a specific stimulus without being distracted by external or internal stimuli. The other options describe deficits with different manifestations. The ability to abstract requires the person to see relationships between concepts, ideas and events. Organization is the ability to structure thoughts and actions. Semantic memory is the general knowledge shared by groups of people, such as social norms.

**Type of Reasoning: Analytical**

This question provides a group of symptoms and the test taker must determine the cause. This requires analytical reasoning skill where one must analyze the symptoms in order to correctly determine a diagnosis. In this situation, the symptoms indicate generalized attention deficit. Review symptoms of generalized attention deficit disorder, especially related to CVA if answered incorrectly.

## A34  C4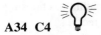

An adolescent with spinal muscle atrophy shows decreased trunk balance and strength during intervention sessions. Upper extremity strength and ROM appear unchanged. When discussing these observations with the occupational therapist, which is the best recommendation for the OTA to make?

**Correct Answer: A. A re-evaluation of the client be completed.**

**Incorrect Answers:**

B.  The client be referred to an orthotist for a soft spinal support.
C.  The client be measured for a power wheelchair.
D.  A trunk strengthening program be initiated with the client.

**Rationale:**

The most important action to take after noticing a change in the functional status of a person with a progressive condition is to re-evaluate. Based on the results of the evaluation, interventions can be planned. These interventions can include orthotics, powered mobility and/or a strengthening program; only the results of a re-evaluation can appropriately determine intervention needs. The occupational therapist would perform the re-evaluation.

**Type of Reasoning: Inferential**

One must determine the recommendation that would best provide address the adolescent's needs. Re-evaluation of the adolescent's capabilities and limitations is the best approach in order to determine if the decreases in trunk balance and strength will necessitate modifications to the treatment program. If answered incorrectly, review evaluation and treatment planning guidelines for patients with spinal muscle atrophy.

358

## A35 C8

The parent of a newborn infant has bilateral shoulder weakness and is referred to OT for training in energy conservation techniques for the performance of parenting and home management tasks. Which adaptation(s) is/are most effective for the OTA to recommend the parent use?

**Correct Answer: B. A steamer, steamer basket, and/or crock pot for meal preparation.**

**Incorrect Answers:**

A. A top-loading washer and dryer for clothing care.

C. A front pack carrier for holding the infant.

D. Cloth diapers and the use of a weekly diaper care service.

**Rationale:**

A steamer, steamer basket, and crock pot eliminate the need to move and lift heavy pans and pots; tasks which require intact bilateral upper extremity strength. A top-loading washer and dryer require more work than frontloading machines. The extra lifting required for top-loading appliances would be difficult with shoulder weakness. A front pack infant carrier has straps which cross the shoulders so this would be contraindicated in this case. The child's weight in the carrier could contribute to shoulder strain. While a weekly diaper service can provide clean diapers each week, cloth diapers require additional care (i.e., rinsing) which can consume the client's time and energy. Lifting the week's load of wet diapers to bring to the door and picking up the week's allotment of clean diapers can be difficult with shoulder weakness.

**Type of Reasoning: Inductive**

This question requires one to review all of the potential recommendations and determine which one is most aligned with conserving energy, given the patient's limitations. For this situation, use of a steamer, steamer basket or crock pot to prepare meals will best conserve energy. Inductive reasoning skills are utilized as clinical judgment is paramount to choosing the best solution. Review energy conservation strategies for home management tasks if answered incorrectly.

## A36 C8

An OTA provides home care services to an individual with advanced stages of dementia. The family caregiver expresses increased concern over the person's wandering behavior during late night and early morning hours. The caregiver expresses fear that the individual will leave the house while everyone is asleep. Which recommendation is best for the OTA to initially make to the caregiver in response to this potentially dangerous situation?

**Correct Answer: D. Use full-length mirrors or wallpaper to camouflage exit doorways.**

**Incorrect Answers:**

A. Consult with the home care case manager for an assessment for skilled nursing facility placement.

B. Use bed guard rails to ensure that the individual remains in bed at night.

C. Install a deadbolt lock on the individual's bedroom door.

**Rationale:**

Camouflaging the doorways is often an effective intervention to decrease wandering behavior in individuals with dementia or other cognitive deficits. One cannot open a door if one does not see a door. There are many additional intervention options to explore to decrease wandering prior to placing an individual in a SNF (e.g., the use of personal alarms, Velcro doors, and/or diversional activities, and/or the rearrangement of furniture). The use of bed guard rails can be dangerous as the individual may attempt to climb over the rails and fall. The installation of a dead bolt lock on the person's bedroom door is very dangerous for it can prevent timely rescue in the event of a fire or accident.

**Type of Reasoning: Inferential**

One must link the individual's diagnosis to an appropriate intervention approach that considers safety and functioning. This requires inferential reasoning, where one must draw conclusions about a course of action. In this case the OTA's best initial recommendation would be to try techniques that camouflage exit doorways. Review approaches to reduce wandering behavior in patients with dementia if answered incorrectly.

**A37 C1**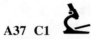

A four month-old with arthrogryposis remains in a position when placed and shows little spontaneous movement. The OTA implements intervention to work on rolling. Which positional changes should the OTA include in the intervention session?

**Correct Answer: B. Supine to side-lying.**

**Incorrect Answers:**

A. Prone to supine.
C. Prone to side-lying.
D. Supine to prone.

**Rationale:**

Developmentally, rolling from supine to side-lying starts at about two months. Rolling from prone to supine is the next stage that begins at about four months. The other options begin at about seven months.

**Type of Reasoning: Deductive**

One must recall the developmental guidelines in mobility for infants. This is factual knowledge, which is a deductive reasoning skill. Supine to side-lying is the first skill to develop, therefore the OTA should initiate mobility with this skill first. If answered incorrectly, review developmental milestones of infants for gross motor skills.

**A38 C4**

An OTA implements intervention using a contemporary neurorehabilitation approach by having a person with a neurological impairment practice an activity in different contexts. Which is the primary purpose of this approach?

**Correct Answer: A. To facilitate the generalization of learning.**

**Incorrect Answers:**

B. To make it more difficult to transfer learning.
C. To foster an unstructured approach to different situations.
D. To determine if the client is easily confused.

**Rationale:**

A major principle in contemporary approaches in neurorehabilitation is the use of multiple contexts to facilitate the generalization of learning. This generalization can then make it easier for an individual to transfer his/her learning to new situations which increases performance consistency, decreases confusion, and helps the person perform effectively in diverse situations.

**Type of Reasoning: Inferential**

One must have knowledge of neurorehabilitation and the benefits of practice in different contexts in order to draw a correct conclusion. This is an inferential reasoning skill where the test taker must infer information in order draw conclusions. In this situation practice in different contexts can facilitate the generalization of learning. Review contemporary neurorehabilitation practice theories and generalization of learning if answered incorrectly.

360

## A39 C1

An eight year-old with hypotonic cerebral palsy receives school-based occupational therapy to improve fine motor skills. The child holds a thick marker with a static tripod grasp and holds a No. 2 pencil with a gross grasp. The OTA collaborates with the occupational therapist to modify the intervention plan. The improvement of which grasp would be best to include in the revised occupational therapy intervention plan as a short-term goal?

**Correct Answer: B. Static tripod with a pencil.**

**Incorrect Answers:**

A. Dynamic tripod with the thick marker.

C. Lateral pinch with a thick marker.

D. Dynamic tripod with a pencil.

**Rationale:**

Developmentally, the best way to progressively grade the grasp is to work on static tripod with a thinner object before going to work on dynamic tripod. A lateral pinch is not an effective grasp for holding a thick marker.

**Type of Reasoning: Inductive**

This question requires one to determine the best modification to the treatment plan to reflect progress to the next developmental stage of grasp. This requires inductive reasoning skill, where clinical judgment is paramount to arriving at a correct conclusion. For this situation, a short-term goal of improving static tripod grasp with a pencil is the best modification to the treatment plan based on current ability. If answered incorrectly, review developmental patterns of hand grasp for writing.

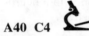

## A40 C4

A patient with a left CVA and resulting contralateral hemiplegia participates in occupational therapy. When documenting the patient's performance during an intervention session, which ability is most likely for the OTA to state is intact?

**Correct Answer: C. Spatial perception while in the ADL apartment.**

**Incorrect Answers:**

A. Temporal sequencing of a morning self-care routine.

B. Receptive language during a leisure planning group.

D. Motor planning during a Tai Chi group.

**Rationale:**

Difficulties in spatial perception are typically related to a right CVA. With a left CVA, these abilities would remain intact. The other options are all typically affected by a left CVA.

**Type of Reasoning: Deductive**

This question requires one to recall factual knowledge about expected symptoms of a patient with right CVA. This necessitates deductive reasoning skill, where recall of facts and previous knowledge are paramount to drawing the correct conclusion. For this case, spatial perception is most likely to be intact. If answered incorrectly, review symptoms of CVA, especially right CVA.

## A41  C1

An elder expresses concerns about the ability to perform daily tasks. The individual has somatosensory deficits consistent with the normal aging process. The OTA recommends adaptive equipment to assist with task performance. Which adaptive equipment should the OTA recommend the person use during meal preparation and feeding?

**Correct Answer: B. Utensils with wide textured grips.**

**Incorrect Answers:**

A. Utensils with narrow smooth grips.

C. A rocker knife.

D. Dycem pads.

**Rationale:**

Wide textured grips will provide augmented sensory feedback to the individual and will be easier to grip than narrow smooth handles. Somatosensory changes associated with aging include decreased tactile sensation, decreased proprioception, and increased pain thresholds. A rocker knife and dycem pads would not address these deficits. A rocker knife is suitable for one-handed cutting and dycem pads are used to provide stability to an object.

**Type of Reasoning: Inferential**

One must have knowledge of somatosensory deficits and the aging process in order to arrive at a correct conclusion. This is an inferential reasoning skill where knowledge of deficits and judgment based on facts are utilized to reach conclusions. For this situation, the OTA should recommend utensils with wide textured grips. If answered incorrectly, review somatosensory deficits in older adults and recommendations for adaptive equipment.

## A42  C5

An OTA works on feeding with a toddler who has a hyperactive gag reflex. What should the OTA do to decrease the gag reflex?

**Correct Answer: B. Walk a tongue depressor from the front of the tongue to its back.**

**Incorrect Answers:**

A. Have the child suck through straws of progressively longer lengths.

C. Quickly ice the child's throat laterally.

D. Have the child blow bubbles.

**Rationale:**

Walking a tongue depressor from the front of the tongue to the back can desensitize a hyperactive gag reflex. The other interventions do not address a hyperactive gag reflex. Sipping on a straw can increase the sucking reflex. Quick icing is a traditional Rood technique that theoretically stimulates a muscle group. Stimulating the neck muscles would not influence a gag reflex.

**Type of Reasoning: Inductive**

This question requires one to determine the best approach for decreasing a hyperactive gag reflex. This requires inductive reasoning skill, where clinical judgment is paramount to arriving at a correct conclusion. For this situation, the OTA should walk a tongue depressor from the front to the back of the tongue. If answered incorrectly, review treatment guidelines for a hyperactive gag reflex.

## A43 C1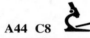

During an intervention session, an eight month-old child demonstrates a positive downward parachute reflex. Which is the most accurate statement for the OTA to include in the documentation of this observed behavior?

**Correct Answer: A. The child exhibits normal reflex development.**

**Incorrect Answers:**

B. The child exhibits a developmental delay.

C. The child's protective extension downward reflex needs to be evaluated by the occupational therapist.

D. The child's standing tilting reflex needs to be evaluated by the occupational therapist.

**Rationale:**

A downward parachute reflex is normal from four months and persists throughout one's lifetime unless neurological damage occurs. It is also called the protective extension downward reflex. The onset of the standing tilting reflex is from 12 to 21 months, so an evaluation of this reflex is premature.

**Type of Reasoning: Evaluative**

One must weigh the possible options and then make a value judgment about the most accurate statement to make. This requires evaluative reasoning skill, which often utilizes guiding principles of action in order to arrive at a correct conclusion. For this case, because the child is displaying normal reflex development, the OTA should document this finding as normal. Review downward parachute reflex and age of integration if answered incorrectly.


## A44  C8

An OTA provides caregiver education to the family of an individual who is dependent in all self-care. During instruction on proper wheelchair positioning, where should the OTA advise the family to place the wheelchair seatbelt?

**Correct Answer: D. At hip level.**

**Incorrect Answers:**

A. At waist level.

B. Midway between waist and trunk.

C. At the widest point of the individual's midsection.

**Rationale:**

Wheelchair seat belts are to extend across the hips and into the lap at a 45 degree angle.

**Type of Reasoning: Deductive**

One must recall the proper positioning of a wheelchair seatbelt in order to arrive at a correct conclusion. This requires deductive reasoning skill, where factual knowledge is essential to choosing the correct solution. Standard practice is for the seatbelt to be placed at the hip level at a 45 degree angle. Review use of seatbelts in wheelchairs and proper positioning if answered incorrectly.

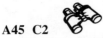

**A45 C2**

An occupational therapist and an OTA co-lead a work adjustment group. One member has become progressively more dependent on the OTA for directions, praise, and input throughout the group activities. Which action should the group leaders initially take in response to these behaviors?

**Correct Answer: C. Have the OTA work with the person during group sessions to develop independence in task completion.**

**Incorrect Answers:**

A. Schedule several individual sessions with the OTA and group member to examine the issues of dependency and transference.

B. Inform the attending psychiatrist that the group member is exhibiting signs of dependency and transference.

D. Have another therapist co-lead the group with the occupational therapist and reassign the OTA to another group.

**Rationale:**

The development of dependency is not uncommon in therapeutic relationships. The best approach is to utilize the situation and have the OTA function as a change agent. It is not necessary to devote individual sessions to this issue and this individualized attention could foster increased dependency. It is best addressed in the group setting during the activities. One can notify the psychiatrist but this does not address the potential to modify behavior in the group setting. Removing the OTA is not a good choice because the member does not have a chance to work through these issues. This does not give an opportunity for the OTA to use him/her self therapeutically.

**Type of reasoning: Inductive**

This question requires the test taker to problem solve a best course of action for a group member who shows dependency on the assistant. This requires inductive reasoning skill. For this case, the OTA should work with the person during group sessions to develop independence in task completion. If answered incorrectly, review group facilitation guidelines and the therapeutic relationship for persons with dependent-type behaviors.

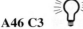

**A46 C3**

An OTA works with an individual with cubital tunnel syndrome who reports numbness and tingling. Which of the following is the most likely location for this person's sensory symptoms?

**Correct Answer: A. The ulnar aspect of the forearm and hand.**

**Incorrect Answers:**

B. Along the radial nerve distribution of the hand.

C. The medial aspect of the forearm and hand.

D. Along the ulnar nerve distribution of the hand.

**Rationale:**

Cubital tunnel syndrome is an ulnar nerve compression at the elbow. Its presenting symptoms are numbness and tingling along the ulnar aspect of the forearm and hand, pain at the elbow with extreme elbow flexion, weakness of power grip, and a positive Tinel's sign at the elbow.

**Type of Reasoning: Inferential**

One must have knowledge of cubital tunnel syndrome and presenting symptoms in order to arrive at a correct conclusion. This is an inferential reasoning skill where one must draw conclusions about a diagnosis. For this situation, the numbness and tingling would typically be reported along the ulnar aspect of the forearm and hand. If answered incorrectly, review symptoms of cubital tunnel syndrome.

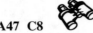

**A47  C8**

An adult diagnosed with multiple sclerosis over ten years ago experiences an exacerbation of symptoms. The individual's principle complaint is decreased strength and endurance. The person can ambulate short distances with a cane in the home and uses a wheelchair outside of the home. The client asks for suggestions to enable independent home maintenance. Which is the best positioning recommendation for the OTA to suggest the person use during meal preparation?

**Correct Answer: B. Sitting at the kitchen table.**

**Incorrect Answers:**

A.  Sitting in the wheelchair with a tray table.

C.  Leaning against the counter while standing.

D.  Leaning against a tall stool while standing.

**Rationale:**

Multiple sclerosis is characterized by fluctuations in abilities. The best choice for an activity that will be performed frequently is to perform the activity in an adequately supported position. The avoidance of fatigue is important in the management of MS. Doing meal preparation while sitting at the kitchen table achieves these aims and uses the person's natural context. There is no need indicated in this scenario for the use of a wheelchair and a tray. The client can do meal preparation activities with readily available supports. Standing might require using too much energy and does not provide good support or stability for performing the fine motor aspects of meal preparation. Leaning against the counter or a stool requires more energy, and does not provide good support or stability for performing the fine motor aspects of meal preparation, and may not be safe.

**Type of Reasoning: Inductive**

This question requires clinical judgment to determine which position would be optimal for a client with MS given the current status and symptoms presented. For this client, sitting at the kitchen table is best as it provides the appropriate stability and reinforces the natural context during meal preparation. If answered incorrectly, review meal preparation strategies for clients with MS.

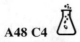

**A48  C4**

A middle school student with learning disabilities exhibits no behavioral problems in the classroom. However, whenever the class is in a line waiting to switch classrooms, the student becomes agitated and often pushes classmates. The OTA consultant advises the teacher that this behavior may be indicative of an underlying problem. Which of the following is most accurate for the OTA to identify as a potential disorder warranting further evaluation?

**Correct Answer: D. Tactile defensiveness.**

**Incorrect Answers:**

A.  Gravitational insecurity.

B.  A conduct disorder.

C.  Antisocial tendencies.

**Rationale:**

The tactile stimuli due to closeness of peers in a line can become overwhelming to an individual with tactile defensiveness. The behavior described in the scenario is not reflective of behavior indicative of the other disorders listed.

**Type of Reasoning: Analytical**

This question provides symptoms and the test taker must determine the likely cause for them. This is an analytical reasoning skill, as questions of this nature often ask one to analyze a group of symptoms in order to determine a diagnosis. In this situation the symptoms indicate tactile defensiveness, which should be reviewed if answered incorrectly.

## A49 C8

A nine year-old girl with the diagnosis of cystic fibrosis is hospitalized in a small rural hospital. Currently, there are no other children in the hospital and the hospital does not have a pediatric play area. The head nurse asks the OTA to suggest appropriate play activities that hospital volunteers can provide to the child. Which is the most age appropriate activity for the OTA to suggest?

**Correct Answer: C. Playing card games.**

**Incorrect Answers:**

A. Dressing paper dolls.

B. Coloring in coloring books.

D. Cutting and pasting pictures onto cards.

**Rationale:**

Children aged 7 – 12 are developmentally able to participate in games with rules, competition and social interaction. The other activities reflect creative play that is developed between ages the ages of 4 and 7. In addition, they are solitary activities and do not afford opportunities for competitive fun and socialization. Hospitalization can be lonely and frightening so having volunteers play with the child can be psychologically beneficial, as well as developmentally appropriate.

**Type of Reasoning: Inferential**

One must determine the most appropriate play activities for a child, given knowledge of the child's age and developmental ability. This requires inferential reasoning skill, where one must infer or draw conclusions about a best course of action. In this situation, the OTA should suggest playing card games. Review information on play activities for nine year-old children if answered incorrectly.

## A50  C9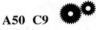

A three year-old with severe congenital anomalies and irreparable cleft palate has a do not resuscitate (DNR) order. While being fitted for a molded seat for a wheelchair, the child stops breathing and turns blue. The OTA determines that the child has a brachial pulse. Which of the following is the first action the OTA should take in response to this situation?

**Correct Answer: C. Implement the facility's emergency procedure.**

**Incorrect Answers:**

A. Inform the physician about the situation and the child's DNR order.

B. Call the supervising occupational therapist to discuss the best response.

D. Perform obstructed airway maneuver and monitor heart rate for five minutes.

**Rationale:**

The child is not breathing and the OTA should initiate the facility's plan for medical emergencies and cardiac codes. It is not the decision of the OTA to withhold actions because of the DNR order. The medical team that responds to emergency procedures must make the decision. It would be desirable to inform the physician, but the current situation requires emergency attention. The OTA can call the supervising occupational therapist to advise of the event and discuss the necessary follow-up after dealing with the event, but this is not the first action. Even a minute delay is too long to wait to notify the emergency team.

**Type of Reasoning: Evaluative**

This question requires one to make a value judgment about a best course of action, given the information presented. This necessitates evaluative reasoning where one must weigh the merits of the possible course of action in order to make a sound decision. For this situation, the OTA should implement the facility's emergency procedure. If answered incorrectly, review emergency management guidelines, especially for individuals with DNR orders.

## A51 C7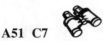

A ten year-old with congenital anomalies wears bilateral ankle-foot orthoses. The parents want the child to be able to don and doff shoes independently, but the child cannot tie shoes. Which is the best footwear recommendation for the OTA to make for the child to wear?

**Correct Answer: C. Running shoes with velcro shoe closures.**

**Incorrect Answers:**

A. Leather slip-on loafers.

B. Slip-on tennis shoes with no laces.

D. Hi-rise sneakers with sliding adapters on the laces.

**Rationale:**

Running shoes are the best option for use with ankle-foot-orthoses (AFOs) and velcro closures will help the child to be independent until tying is learned. Leather slip-on loafers are not feasible to correctly support the ankle-foot orthoses (AFOs). Slip-on tennis shoes that do not have laces do not have adequate support in the upper part of the foot to maintain the AFOs. The sliding adapters are a good option to replace the laces, but the hi-rise sneakers will not likely allow for placement of the AFOs on the feet.

**Type of Reasoning: Inductive**

Clinical knowledge and judgment are the most important skills needed for answering this question, which requires inductive reasoning skill. Knowledge of the diagnosis and most appropriate clinical outcomes is key to choosing the best solution. In this case, shoes with Velcro closures are best as it helps facilitate independence while providing the needed support when wearing AFOs. If answered incorrectly, review footwear adaptations to facilitate independence in fastening and tying.

## A52 C5

The population of an urban homeless shelter includes individuals with histories of chronic alcohol abuse who are at risk for developing peripheral neuropathy. The OTA consulting at this shelter monitors the residents' status to ensure early detection of this problem. Which is the most important observed status change for the OTA to report?

**Correct Answer: B. Progressive deterioration of sensorimotor functions of the lower extremities.**

**Incorrect Answers:**

A. Progressive deterioration in visual acuity.

C. Rapid onset of intention tremors.

D. Rapid loss of sensorimotor functions of the facial and neck muscles.

**Rationale:**

Peripheral neuropathy is a syndrome of sensory, motor, reflex, and vasomotor symptoms, with symptoms exhibited according to the distribution of the affected nerve. Its etiology includes diabetes, Lyme disease, multiple sclerosis, alcoholism, metabolic or infectious diseases. It has a slow and progressive onset and course. It does not result in a rapid loss of function, deterioration of visual acuity, or the onset of intention tremors. Treatment of the underlying systemic disorder (e.g., diabetes) can slow progression. In general, recovery takes extended time.

**Type of Reasoning: Inferential**

One must link knowledge of peripheral neuropathy to the symptoms presented in order to arrive at a correct conclusion. This requires inferential reasoning skill, where one must draw conclusions based on evidence presented. In this case the most important status change for the OTA to report is the progressive deterioration of sensorimotor functions in the lower extremities. Review symptoms of peripheral neuropathy if answered incorrectly.

## A53 C7

A person blinded in an accident begins an OT community re-entry program for persons with visual loss. The OTA collaborates with the individual to develop an intervention plan. Which should be included in the plan as an initial focus of intervention?

**Correct Answer:  D. Organizing the client's morning routine.**

**Incorrect Answers:**

A.  Developing computer skills.

B.  Adapting meal preparation techniques.

C.  Exploring vocational interests.

**Rationale:**

Organizing the morning routine is most appropriate as an initial goal to help the individual effectively and independently complete his/her personal activities of daily living. This can help the person feel confident, and serve as a basis for organizing the rest of the person's home and work routine. The development of meal preparation skills would initially focus on non-cooked foods and meals. Typically, one of the most frightening areas for the newly-blinded person is the use of the stove because of the risk of burns and danger of fire, so developing skills to cook hot meals would be a long term goal. The development of computer skills and the exploration of vocational interests would be better choices for long-term intervention, if the client identifies these as a personal goal.

**Type of Reasoning: Inferential**

One must infer or draw conclusions about the best initial focus for OT with a person who has experienced recent visual loss. The key to arriving at a correct conclusion is determining which approach fosters confidence and provides a starting point for future community re-entry activity. Organization of the morning routine is the best initial approach for achieving this goal. If answered incorrectly, review therapeutic approaches for patients with recent visual loss.

## A54 C8

An OTA working in a skilled nursing facility observes a resident with cognitive disabilities don slippers by putting them on the wrong feet. The resident plans to go visit a friend on another floor and does not seem aware that the slippers are on the wrong feet. Which is the best action for the OTA to take in response to this situation?

**Correct Answer: D. Approach the resident and advise the resident to reverse the slippers.**

**Incorrect Answers:**

A.  Say nothing for this error may embarrass the resident.

B.  Say nothing but follow the resident to the friend's room to ensure a safe arrival.

C.  Ask the resident to look at the slippers to see if the error is noticed.

**Rationale:**

The slippers must be immediately reversed to ensure safety and prevent a fall. Poor or inappropriate use of footwear is a primary cause of falls. Letting the resident walk with slippers on the wrong feet is an unacceptable risk. Since the resident has cognitive deficits, he/she may not be able to notice the error and self correct. A direct intervention done in a supportive manner is needed to ensure safety.

**Type of Reasoning: Evaluative**

This question requires professional judgment in a challenging situation, which is an evaluative reasoning skill. Because the resident is at risk for a fall wearing the slippers on the wrong feet, the OTA should advise the resident to reverse the slippers. In judgment situations such as these, where safety is a concern, test takers should often consider the safest, most prudent response as the best one. Review safe mobility guidelines if answered incorrectly.

**A55  C3**

A person fell and sustained bilateral Colles' fractures. The client wore bilateral short-arm casts for six weeks. After cast removal, the client began OT sessions to increase endurance and strength prior to returning to work. The client tends to work hard when performing resistive exercises with both wrists. The OTA monitors the client for overexertion. Which behavior indicates overexertion?

**Correct Answer: C. Complaints of pain in the wrist extensors.**

**Incorrect Answers:**

A.  Decreased respiration rate during resistive wrist flexion.
B.  Increased ability to achieve full ROM of the wrist.
D.  Consistent strength in wrist extension activities.

**Rationale:**

Complaints of pain can be a sign of overexertion. The others are signs of adequate performance, not overexertion.

**Type of Reasoning: Inferential**

The test taker must reason which observation would likely indicate overexertion. Inferential reasoning skill is used as one must draw conclusions about the statements provided based upon clinical knowledge of therapeutic exercise. For this situation complaints of pain often indicates overexertion. Review exercises approaches for Colles' fracture and signs of overexertion if answered incorrectly.

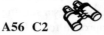

**A56  C2**

An OTA works in a school setting with adolescents with Asperger's syndrome. The need for a social skills training group is identified. One activity that the OTA plans to use in the group is role-playing. Which is the most effective way for the OTA to determine relevant scenarios for the role-play activities?

**Correct Answer: D. Ask the group members about their social concerns.**

**Incorrect Answers:**

A.  Survey the teachers on social difficulties displayed in class.
B.  Survey parents on social difficulties they have observed in the adolescents.
C.  Review literature on adolescent social skill development.

**Rationale:**

Directly asking members about their concerns will enable the OTA to identify areas of common concern that can serve as the basis of relevant role-play scenarios. This will foster Yalom's curative factor of universality. The ability to express one's concerns and needs is especially important to adolescents since their main developmental task is to separate from parents and develop their own self-identity. Surveying others provides information on their perceptions of the adolescents' needs. This may or may not be an accurate reflection of members' needs. Reviewing developmental literature can be helpful in understanding adolescent concerns but it cannot be used to plan role-play scenarios for a specific group of adolescents with unique needs.

**Type of Reasoning: Inductive**

This question requires one to determine the best approach for determining group members' needs. This requires inductive reasoning skill, where clinical judgment is paramount to arriving at a correct conclusion. For this situation, the OTA should ask the group members about their social concerns. If answered incorrectly, review group intervention techniques including role playing and the functional impact of Asperger's syndrome. The integration of this knowledge is required to answer the question correctly.

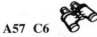

## A57 C6

An individual with developmental disabilities scores a Level 3 on the Allen Cognitive Level Test. The OTA collaborates with the occupational therapist to plan intervention. Which activities should the OTA and occupational therapist include in the intervention plan to help meet the client's functional needs?

**Correct Answer: C. Self-care activities such as brushing teeth.**

**Incorrect Answers:**

A. Community mobility activities such as taking a bus.

B. Home management activities such as preparing a food shopping list.

D. Leisure activities such as completing a 50 piece puzzle.

**Rationale:**

An individual who scores a Level 3 on the Allen's Cognitive Level Test can perform basic repetitive tasks. Level 3 is the beginning of using the hands to manipulate objects, but task completion requires proprioceptive cues (e.g. physical prompts to perform the hand to mouth movement needed to brush teeth). The other activities require cognitive skills that are not present at Level 3, according to Allen's model.

**Type of Reasoning: Inductive**

One must utilize clinical knowledge and judgment to determine the best activities for this individual. This requires inductive reasoning skill. In this case, because the individual is functioning at Level 3, the OTA and the occupational therapist should include self-care activities, such as brushing teeth in the intervention plan. If answered incorrectly, review Allen's cognitive disabilities model and intervention approaches for individuals functioning at Level 3.

## A58 C3

The occupational therapist and OTA collaborate to plan intervention for a client with a recent diagnosis of complex regional pain syndrome (CRPS) Type I. Which intervention approach is most effective to use to reduce pain and increase function?

**Correct Answer: B. Biofeedback.**

**Incorrect Answers:**

A. Hot packs.

C. Paraffin.

D. Passive range of motion

**Rationale:**

CRPS Type I is a vasomotor dysfunction which causes extreme hypersensitivity to touch, edema, intense burning pain, and dramatic temperature and color changes to the affected limb. Goals for treatment include reducing pain and edema, promoting normal positioning, and increasing function. Biofeedback is a technique where electrodes are used to measure muscle responses and stress levels. The goal is to train the individual to release tension, which can reduce pain and prepare the individual for increased tolerance to range of motion and functional movement. Hot packs and paraffin can be too painful to tolerate in the initial stages and are contraindicated if the affected limb demonstrates elevated temperature. Passive range of motion is usually not tolerated during the initial stages of the syndrome due to the severe pain and hypersensitivity to touch.

**Type of Reasoning: Inferential**

One must link the individual's diagnosis to the treatment approaches provided in order to determine which treatment approach would most effectively address the individual's deficits. This requires inferential reasoning, where one must draw conclusions about the potential treatment outcomes. In this case the occupational therapist and OTA should use biofeedback to reduce pain and promote tolerance to activity. Review treatment approaches for CRPS Type I if answered incorrectly.

## A59 C5

An individual recovering from hip replacement surgery prepares for discharge home. The client has a secondary diagnosis of gastric esophageal reflux disease (GERD). Which is the best bed position for the OTA to recommend to this client?

**Correct Answer: A. Supine with elevation of the shoulders and head.**

**Incorrect Answers:**

B. Sidelying with the neck in neutral.

C. Sidelying with elevation of the shoulders and head.

D. Supine with elevation of the hips.

**Rationale:**

In GERD, the stomach pyloric sphincter ineffectively closes and stomach contraction propels acid and acidic bolus back into the esophagus. Elevation of the head above the stomach when the person is reclined may decrease the upward retropulsion of the bolus from the stomach. The other positions are not effective for an individual with GERD and they are contraindicated for a person recovering from hip surgery.

**Type of Reasoning: Inferential**

One must infer or draw conclusions about a likely course of action, given the information presented. This is an inferential reasoning skill, where knowledge of a therapeutic approach, such as the appropriate bed positioning in this situation, is essential to choosing a correct solution. In this case, the OTA should recommend a supine position with elevation of the shoulders and head. Review bed positioning for individuals with GERD and post-hip replacement surgery if answered incorrectly.

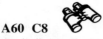

## A60 C8

An individual with left hemiplegia who is right hand dominant receives training to resume independent driving. Which adaptation is best for the OTA to recommend the client use?

**Correct Answer: C. A spinner knob on the steering wheel.**

**Incorrect Answers:**

A. "Palming" the steering wheel.

B. Hand controls for brake and gas pedals.

D. Left-sided accelerator pedal.

**Rationale:**

A person who is right hand dominant with left hemiplegia can drive one-handed using a spinner knob on the steering wheel. "Palming" the steering wheel is not recommended for one-handed drivers, for it is easier to lose control of the vehicle. It is difficult to maintain smooth handling and turns are made much more slowly, which can be dangerous in traffic situations. There is no functional need to change a car's existing pedal arrangement.

**Type of Reasoning: Inductive**

Clinical knowledge and judgment are the most important skills needed for answering this question, which requires inductive reasoning skill. Knowledge of the functional limitations and most appropriate equipment for driving is essential to choosing the best solution. In this case, a spinner knob on the steering wheel is the best recommendation. Review vehicle adaptations for one-handed drivers if answered incorrectly.

## A61  C1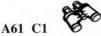

During a group session an older adult complains that everyone is mumbling. Which action should the OTA take after the group in response to these statements?

**Correct Answer: D. Notify the occupational therapist that the person may need an audiological evaluation.**

**Incorrect Answers:**

A.  Notify the client's physician that the person exhibited evidence of paranoia.

B.  Collaborate with the occupational therapist to remove groups from the client's intervention plan.

C.  Document objective data about the complaints in the person's charts.

**Rationale:**

It is common for older adults to experience hearing loss. The individual's report that people are mumbling is indicative of a potential hearing loss that warrants further evaluation. Interpreting the person's report as indicative of paranoia is subjective. Modifying the person's intervention plan to not include groups and documenting the individual's complaints does not deal directly with the issue at hand.

**Type of Reasoning: Inductive**

One must utilize clinical knowledge and judgment to determine the best action to take, given the individual's complaint. This requires inductive reasoning skill. In this case, the individual's complaint warrants notifying the occupational therapist that an audiological evaluation may be needed. If answered incorrectly, review symptoms of hearing loss in adults.

## A62  C4

An OTA implements intervention in a preschool program for children with tactile defensiveness. In the prior intervention session, the children had responded favorably when the OTA had rolled a large ball over their bodies as they lay supine on a mat. Which intervention method should the OTA use next?

**Correct Answer: A. Roll the large ball with increased pressure across the children's bodies.**

**Incorrect Answers:**

B.  Bounce the ball across the children's bodies.

C.  Have the children jump into a pool filled with small balls.

D.  Roll the large ball, as in the prior session, with the children prone.

**Rationale:**

Increasing pressure on the ball is the next gradation of the activity that has been reported to be successful. Children with tactile defensiveness respond well to firm pressure. Jumping into a pool with small balls is too large of a progression to make from comfort with a ball rolling over one's body for children who have tactile defensiveness. Bouncing a ball across their bodies can be frightening and it does not provide the desired deep pressure input. Changing the children's position from supine to prone does not provide an activity gradation related to intervention for tactile defensiveness.

**Type of Reasoning: Inferential**

One must have knowledge of tactile defensiveness in children and gradation of sensory activity in order to choose the next most appropriate gradation of activity. This is an inferential reasoning skill where knowledge of the diagnosis and progression of activity is pivotal to choosing the correct solution. If answered incorrectly, review sensory activities for children with tactile defensiveness, especially activities that provide deep pressure.

**A63 C1**

A school-based OTA receives a referral for a student who has illegible handwriting, poor attending behaviors, question-able visual skills, and problems with pencil management. After speaking with the teacher and occupational therapist, reviewing classroom work samples, and reading the student's history, which action should the OTA take next?

**Correct Answer: B. Directly observe the student during a naturally occurring writing time.**

**Incorrect Answers:**

A. Provide pencil grips and specialized paper as a trial to determine interventions.

C. Administer a standardized visual perceptual and visual motor assessment.

D. Administer a standardized handwriting assessment.

**Rationale:**

Skilled observation during a writing activity is an essential part of the evaluation process. Noting the student's performance in the classroom should precede standardized testing of performance components. These observations, review of the student's work and history, and the teacher interview can then be reviewed by occupational therapist and OTA to determine the need for further evaluation and the most appropriate standardized measures to use to evaluate the child, if needed.

**Type of Reasoning: Inductive**

This question requires one to determine a best course of action, given the information provided. This requires inductive reasoning skill, where one must use clinical judgment to determine the best approach for evaluating this child. In this situation, the OTA should directly observe the student during a naturally occurring writing time. If answered incorrectly, review observational guidelines for the evaluation of functional skills and the developmental skills required for effective classroom participation. The integration of this knowledge is required for the determination of a correct answer.

**A64 C6**

A child with attention deficit disorder with hyperactivity (ADHD) receives school-based occupational therapy services. During intervention sessions, which behaviors will the OTA most likely observe the child demonstrate?

**Correct Answer: D. Non-purposeful activity that interferes with function in age-appropriate skills.**

**Incorrect Answers:**

A. An excessively high energy level that can be lessened by eliminating consumption of caffeine or certain foods.

B. Symptoms of learning disabilities as evidenced by difficulties with reading and math.

C. Poor attention to school and play activities over the past three months.

**Rationale:**

One of the key behavioral characteristics for the diagnosis of ADHD is the presence of non-purposeful, hyperactive behavior that interferes with functioning in age-appropriate skills in school, play, and/or social settings. In the adolescent and adult, these behaviors must also interfere with work tasks. High energy levels that are relieved by elimination of foods are more likely food allergies or sensitivities rather than ADHD. Not all children with ADHD have learning disabilities. The two conditions are separate disorders. To be considered ADHD, the behaviors must last at least six months.

**Type of Reasoning: Inferential**

This question essentially asks one to infer the likely behavioral characteristics of a child with ADHD, which is an inferential reasoning skill. Of all the choices, non-purposeful activity that interferes with function in age-appropriate skills is consistent with ADHD and is most likely to be observed. If answered incorrectly, review behavioral characteristics and diagnostic criteria of ADHD.

**A65  C9**

The family of an individual being discharged from a spinal cord injury center offers the OTA a substantial cash gift. The OTA refuses the money but the family insists that the OTA take the cash gift. Which is the OTA's best response?

**Correct Answer: D. Decline the gift.**

**Incorrect Answers:**

A.  Donate the money to the hospital.

B.  Thank the family and donate the money to charity.

C.  Use the money to purchase an item on the OT department's "wish list."

**Rationale:**

Accepting a substantial cash gift would bring into question the ethical issue of financial gain; therefore, declining the gift is the best response. If the family continues to insist on concretizing their gratitude, it might be appropriate to suggest a donation to the department or facility. It is important to note that in some cultures, it is common practice to offer small tokens of appreciation to staff. It might be considered rude and offensive to some persons to refuse a small gift. Be aware that some facilities alter their policies about accepting small token gifts in these cases.

**Type of Reasoning: Evaluative**

This question requires one to weigh the merits of the four possible choices and determine the most ethical response to the situation. In keeping with hospital policy, the OTA should refuse the gift, citing hospital policy. Ethical questions often require evaluative reasoning skill, as there is not always a clear cut or simple answer to the situation. If answered incorrectly, review the AOTA Code of Ethics.

**A66  C8**

An older adult with a diagnosis of osteoarthritis in both knees is referred to inpatient occupational therapy. During screening, the patient expresses a desire to return home to live alone independently. Which should the OTA do first in response to the patient's stated goal?

**Correct Answer: B. Evaluate the patient's BADL and IADL using a standardized measure.**

**Incorrect Answers:**

A.  Recommend adaptations to the patient's home environment to increase safety.

C.  Teach the patient energy conservation techniques to use during IADL tasks.

D.  Train the patient in a home resistive exercise program to build strength and ROM.

**Rationale:**

The patient has just been screened for occupational therapy services so the next step in the OT process is to evaluate the person's functional abilities. OTAs can contribute to the evaluation process using standardized measures. Osteoarthritis is isolated to specific joints and is not systemic in nature. By evaluating the patient's BADL and IADL, the OTA can collaborate with the occupational therapist to determine the activity demands of the BADL and IADL the patient performs while keeping in mind the specific joints that are affected. Once this information is obtained, then the OTA and occupational therapist can make informed recommendations based upon their observations and clinical reasoning to decrease excessive loading and repetitive use of these joints. Simple adaptations, such as moving items higher (onto counters, etc.) can be recommended and energy conservation techniques can be taught based upon the evaluation results. Resistive exercise programs are contraindicated for persons with osteoarthritis.

**Type of Reasoning: Inferential**

One must determine the best approach for evaluation of this patient, given his/her stated desires and diagnosis. This requires inferential reasoning skill, where one must infer or draw conclusions about the approach that will result in the best functional outcome. In this case, evaluation of the patient's daily activities using a standardized measure is the best approach to learn about his/her ability to safely return home, managing the symptoms of osteoarthritis. Review evaluation guidelines and home management assessments if answered incorrectly. Integration of this knowledge with an understanding of the impact osteoarthritis has on BADL and IADL is required to determine a correct answer.

374

## A67 C1

A child with mild cerebral palsy receives OT intervention in a preschool setting. The OTA has collaborated with the occupational therapist to develop an intervention plan. Which intervention approach should the OTA employ to facilitate development of typical grasp patterns?

**Correct Answer: D. Grade the sizes and shapes of objects to be grasped.**

**Incorrect Answers:**

A. Place soft foam tubing around objects to be grasped.

B. Analyze the present components of the child's grasp.

C. Analyze the missing components of the child's grasp.

**Rationale:**

Gradation of the size and shape of items to be grasped enables the OTA to begin with items that are within the child's grasp capabilities and then add different items as the child's grasp abilities progress. There is no need to add soft foam tubing at this time. Soft tubing may be used as a compensation approach if the child does not develop typical grasp patterns. Analyzing the components of grasp is part of the evaluation and re-evaluation process, not intervention.

**Type of Reasoning: Inductive**

This question requires one to determine the most appropriate intervention for a child with mild CP. This requires inductive reasoning skill, where clinical judgment is paramount to arriving at a correct conclusion. For this situation, grading the size and shapes of objects to be grasped is most appropriate. If answered incorrectly, review development of grasp patterns for children.

## A68 C2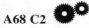

A single parent with rheumatoid arthritis and two school-aged children reports difficulty completing a home exercise program. The parent states that multiple familial, work, and home management responsibilities fill the day and additional activities cannot fit into the day. Which is the best action for the OTA to take in response to these realities?

**Correct Answer: C. Incorporate the parent's engagement in a diversity of role activities into the home program.**

**Incorrect Answers:**

A. Explain and reinforce the importance of active range of motion exercises for remediation of dysfunction.

B. Provide intervention for time management and temporal adaptation.

D. Increase the frequency of OT sessions to compensate for lack of follow-through on the home program.

**Rationale:**

The performance of role activities requires the individual to actively range joints which is the purpose of an exercise program. Incorporating AROM into one's daily routines can be more easily implemented than adding a specific exercise regimen. Some people find pure rote exercise uninteresting. In addition, since activity and the pursuit of occupational roles is the foundation of OT, this choice provides the most theoretically consistent action. Reminding the individual of the importance of AROM, providing time management intervention, and/or increasing the frequency of the OT sessions ignore the reality of a single parent's busy life. The person has reported nothing to indicate a lack of understanding of the importance of AROM, poor time management skills, or temporal dysfunction. Increasing the frequency of OT sessions would just add further demands to the parent's already busy schedule and is not indicated.

**Type of Reasoning: Evaluative**

This question requires a value judgment, which is an evaluative reasoning skill. In this situation, the patient has indicated that he/she has little time to complete a home exercise program. Therefore the test taker should look for a solution that addresses the client's concerns, but also still provides opportunities for functional activity. The only solution that addresses both concerns is to incorporate the client's engagement in a diversity of role activities into the home program. Review principles of client-centered practice and approaches to home program development if answered incorrectly.

**A69 C2**

An OTA works with adolescents who are survivors of child abuse. OT interventions can be provided in groups or on an individual basis. Which of the following would indicate to the OTA that intervention should be provided to an adolescent on an individual basis rather than in a group?

**Correct Answer: C. The adolescent desires greater control over the environment.**

**Incorrect Answers:**

A. The adolescent wants more socialization experiences.
B. The adolescent could benefit from feedback from peers.
D. The adolescent needs an opportunity to gain situational perspective.

**Rationale:**

The person who wants to have more control over the environment would benefit from working on an individual basis. Groups are unpredictable and effective group process requires trust and the sharing of control among all members. This may be difficult for an adolescent who has survived child abuse and is understandably seeking personal control. Someone who wants increased socialization would benefit from group interventions. A group is also the best intervention format to obtain peer feedback and to put one's own personal situation into perspective.

**Type of Reasoning: Inferential**

One must determine the benefits of individual therapy for adolescents who are survivors of abuse in order to arrive at a correct conclusion. This requires inferential reasoning, where one must draw conclusions based on the information provided. In this situation, if the client requires greater control over the environment, individual therapy is best, as a group situation can be unpredictable. If answered incorrectly, review the benefits of individual therapy versus group therapy and the characteristics of victims of abuse. Integration of this knowledge is required for a correct answer.

**A70 C3**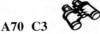

A school-aged child who is right-hand dominant complains of numbness and tingling after writing for more than 15 minutes. A neurological exam shows no reason for the numbness and tingling. Which action would be most beneficial for the OTA to recommend to the child?

**Correct Answer: C. Stretch the right upper extremity every 15-20 minutes during writing activities.**

**Incorrect Answers:**

A. Use a pencil held in a universal cuff.
B. Elevate the right upper extremity at night and whenever possible during the day.
D. Use a custom-molded pencil grip made of splinting material.

**Rationale:**

The neurological exam is negative. The best choice is to educate the child in active ROM and stretching of the upper extremity to increase circulation and to attempt to prevent numbness and tingling. The universal cuff and custom-molded grip are adaptations that do not address treatment of numbness and tingling. Elevation can reduce edema and edema is not a symptom here.

**Type of Reasoning: Inductive**

One must determine the reason for the child's symptoms in order to determine the best recommendation for the child to alleviate the symptoms. This requires inductive reasoning skill, where clinical judgment and diagnostic thinking are central to choosing a best solution. In this situation, stretching the right upper extremity every 15-20 minutes during writing is the best recommendation to increase circulation and prevent symptoms. Review intervention approaches for paresthesias if answered incorrectly.

376

**A71  C5**

A person recovering from a cerebral vascular accident has left-sided weakness and dysphagia. Which of the following is the most effective direct treatment approach to help the person successfully swallow ingested food?

**Correct Answer: D. Provide small, warm boluses.**

**Incorrect Answers:**

A.  Provide pureed, thick liquids.

B.  Provide thermal stimulation to the inferior faucial arches.

C.  Tilt the person's head back and towards the left side.

**Rationale:**

Direct treatment for oral motor control involves techniques that utilize a bolus. These techniques can involve modification of bolus amount, consistency, and temperature. Providing thermal stimulation to the inferior faucial arches using a chilled dental examination mirror can elicit a swallow response; however, this is considered an indirect treatment method. Tilting the head back is contraindicated because it increases choking risk.

**Type of Reasoning: Inferential**

One must infer or draw conclusions about a likely course of action, given the information presented. This is an inferential reasoning skill, where knowledge of a therapeutic approach, such as the direct treatment to swallow food in this situation, is essential to choosing a correct solution. In this case, the OTA should provide small, warm boluses. Review direct and indirect interventions for persons with oral motor disorders if answered incorrectly.

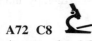

**A72  C8**

An entry-level OTA conducts an in-service at an outpatient wheelchair clinic for individuals with central nervous system dysfunction. According to the principles of wheelchair prescription, which of the following statements is accurate for the OTA to make during the presentation?

**Correct Answer: A. Firm seats are needed to provide stability.**

**Incorrect Answers:**

B.  Soft seats are needed to prevent decubiti.

C.  Back heights should be extended to facilitate weight shifting.

D.  Seat angles should be 45° to prevent falling forward.

**Rationale:**

Firm seats provide stability and a solid base for seating systems that can be used to prevent decubiti, contractures, and deformities, and to increase sitting tolerance, proper positioning, and functional abilities. Soft seats are contraindicated as they do not provide sufficient pressure relief. Soft seats can "collapse" under pressure and can increase the risk of decubiti. Extended back heights increase the difficulty of weight shifting because the person cannot hook his/her arm around the push handle. The recommended seat angle ranges from 80 to 110 degrees.

**Type of Reasoning: Deductive**

This question requires recall of guidelines and principles, which is factual knowledge. Deductive reasoning skills are utilized whenever one must recall facts to solve everyday problems. In this situation, the OTA is accurate in stating that firm seats are needed to provide stability. Review wheelchair prescription guidelines if answered incorrectly.

## A73 C5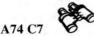

During an OT session, the OTA notes that a client who has a spinal cord injury at the C-5 level is flushed and sweating excessively. The client requests that the session end early. The client reports having a pounding headache that has become impossible to ignore. Which is the best initial action for the OTA to take in response to this situation?

**Correct Answer: A. Check the client's catheter line.**

**Incorrect Answers:**

B. Call the transporter to return the client to the client's room.

C. Report the client's symptoms to the client's unit head nurse.

D. Stop the session and recline the client in the wheelchair for a rest break.

**Rationale:**

The client's symptoms are indicative of autonomic dysreflexia. This is an extreme rise in blood pressure caused by a noxious stimulus. This complication is deemed a medical emergency that must be treated immediately by quickly removing the noxious stimulus that caused the problem. Common stimuli are a blocked catheter, sitting on sharp objects, a tight abdominal binder, pressure stockings that have rolled down or excess pressure on the buttocks. Symptoms of autonomic dysreflexia include profuse sweating and a pounding headache. The other choices do not deal with this medical emergency in an appropriate or timely manner. The client should remain in an upright position to help manage the rise in blood pressure.

**Type of Reasoning: Evaluative**

One must weigh the possible courses of action and then make a value judgment about the best course to take. This requires evaluative reasoning skill, where an understanding of what the symptoms indicate is pivotal to arriving at a correct conclusion. In this case, the symptoms indicate autonomic dysreflexia and the OTA's first action should be to check the catheter line to remove the noxious stimulus causing the dangerous rise in blood pressure. If answered incorrectly, review symptoms and management of autonomic dysreflexia.

## A74 C7

A teenage girl with juvenile rheumatoid arthritis (JRA) identifies a goal of applying her own makeup. Which adaptation is most beneficial for the OTA to recommend?

**Correct Answer: B. Enlarged soft foam handles on makeup applicators.**

**Incorrect Answers:**

A. Silver ring splints to hold makeup applicators.

C. Long thin handles on makeup applicators.

D. Taking a long hot shower to decrease stiffness prior to initiating the task.

**Rationale:**

Enlarged soft foam handles will facilitate independent grasp and increase independence in makeup application. Silver ring splints are not designed to hold objects. They are used on individual fingers to prevent boutonniere deformities which can contribute to improved functional grasp. However, there is no mention of the presence of boutonniere deformities in this item's scenario. Long thin handles would increase the difficulty of holding applicators. Taking a long shower prior to applying makeup may not be practical on a daily basis. In addition, the effort used to complete this activity can increase fatigue, which would be contraindicated in JRA.

**Type of Reasoning: Inductive**

Clinical knowledge and judgment are the most important skills needed for answering this question, which requires inductive reasoning skill. Knowledge of the diagnosis and most appropriate recommendations for the functional activity is essential to choosing the most beneficial solution. In this case, the OTA should recommend enlarged soft foam handles on the makeup applicators. Review self-care adaptations and adaptive devices for persons with rheumatoid arthritis if answered incorrectly.

378

## A75  C9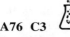

A patient has been discharged from a rehabilitation facility six months ago. An OTA who works at the facility sees the former patient and the occupational therapist that treated the patient in a dating situation. The occupational therapist confirms involvement in a personal relationship with the former patient. What is the OTA's best response to this situation?

**Correct Answer: C. Do nothing.**

**Incorrect Answers:**

A. Report the therapist to the NBCOT.

B. Advise the facility director.

D. Report the therapist to the OT supervisor.

**Rationale:**

A health care practitioner can date a former but not a current patient. This is no evidence that they dated while the person was a patient. The therapist is doing nothing wrong and there is no need to take any action.

**Type of Reasoning: Evaluation**

This question requires a value judgment in an ethical situation, which is an evaluative reasoning skill. In this situation, there is only evidence of a relationship between the therapist and patient after the patient was discharged, therefore no action needs to be taken. Ethical situations such as these often rely upon the AOTA Code of Ethics to provide guiding principles of action. Because there is no harm involved in dating a former patient, the therapist's actions do not constitute harm. Review the AOTA Code of Ethics if answered incorrectly.

## A76  C3

An adult participated in daily occupational therapy after incurring severe lacerations and median and ulnar nerve damage from shattered glass. The wounds have healed and the patient is being discharged. The final evaluation shows minimal limitations in palmar sensation, joint ROM lacking ten to 20 degrees of full ROM, and palmar scarring. The occupational therapist and OTA collaborate to prepare the home program for this patient. Instructions for which intervention are most important to include in this plan?

**Correct Answer: B. Tendon gliding exercises.**

**Incorrect Answers:**

A. Use of a resting splint.

C. Weight-bearing activities.

D. Home management tasks.

**Rationale:**

Tendon gliding exercises help to prevent adhesions of the tendons in the healing process. Initially after tendon repair or tendon transfer, a resting splint would be used and removed only for bathing and gentle active ROM. At the point of discharge from therapy, the client should be pursuing more active movement. A splint that allows the DIPs to be free for movement or a volar splint for day use that allows active finger and thumb use may be prescribed based on the client's needs. Weight-bearing activities help to strengthen the upper extremity, including the wrist extrinsic muscles. The focus after tendon trauma or surgery is prevention of adhesions with tendon gliding exercises and avoidance of heavy work to prevent tearing or re-injury. The answer choice of home management tasks is too vague. Some tasks may be appropriate, while others may be too stressful and require adaptations.

**Type of Reasoning: Analytical**

One must analyze the evaluation findings and match this to the most important intervention for the patient's home program, which requires analytical reasoning skill. For this case, the findings indicate that the patient would benefit most from a home program that incorporates tendon gliding exercise to prevent adhesions of the tendons. If answered incorrectly, review exercise guidelines for hand tendons post laceration.

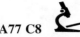

## A77 C8

A local pharmacy hires an OTA to consult on the redesign of the pharmacy's customer service area. Which height should the OTA recommend the pharmacy counter be no higher than?

**Correct Answer: D. 31 inches.**

**Incorrect Answers:**

A. 29 inches.

B. 33 inches.

C. 35 inches.

**Rationale:**

The recommended maximal height for countertops is 31 inches, according to the American National Standards Institute (ANSI) guidelines for buildings and facilities. The other choices do not meet these criteria.

**Type of Reasoning: Deductive**

This question requires recall of guidelines and principles, which is factual knowledge. Deductive reasoning skills are utilized whenever one must recall facts to solve novel problems. In this situation, following ANSI guidelines, the counter should be no higher than 31 inches. Review ANSI standards for buildings and facilities if answered incorrectly.

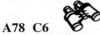

## A78 C6

Which is the most effective approach for an OTA to use when giving directions for a task to an individual with schizophrenia who is experiencing auditory hallucinations?

**Correct Answer: A. Written directions for making vanilla pudding.**

**Incorrect Answers:**

B. Verbal step-by-step directions for making a leather link belt.

C. General verbal directions for a group collage.

D. Demonstrate steps in a beginning level swing dance class.

**Rationale:**

Written directions with a structured, expected outcome are best to reinforce reality and to provide concrete feedback for the person experiencing hallucinations. Verbal directions are hardest to follow when someone is experiencing auditory hallucinations. Working near others with some interaction can help to decrease auditory hallucinations, but an unstructured open-ended group project like a collage may be too vague and ambiguous for this individual. Demonstration can be an excellent way to provide directions but the background music and the possibility of being touched by others during a dance activity may be conducive to increasing hallucinations. The quick movements of swing dancing may be contraindicated if the person is experiencing certain medication side effects, such as orthostatic hypotension.

**Type of Reasoning: Inductive**

This question requires one to assess the needs of the client based upon his/her diagnosis and knowledge of the symptoms of schizophrenia. This necessitates clinical judgment in determining a best course of action, which is an inductive reasoning skill. For this case, the therapist should choose structured activities with written directions to best ensure success and minimize the impact of auditory hallucinations. Review therapeutic approaches for patients with schizophrenia and auditory hallucinations.

380

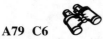

**A79  C6**

An individual receives treatment for major depression on an inpatient psychiatric unit. The patient has received an electroconvulsive treatment (ECT) treatment at 8 am. At 2 pm, the patient walks into the occupational therapy department stating a desire to participate in the leisure skills group. Which is the OTA's best response?

**Correct Answer: A. Encourage the client to select one of three structured leisure activities to complete.**

**Incorrect Answers:**

B.  Call nursing staff to escort the client back to the client's room.

C.  Commend the client's motivation but remind the client that rest is recommended for 24 hours after ECT.

D.  Provide the client with a leisure history questionnaire to complete.

**Rationale:**

Six hours after ECT, the individual is capable of engaging in a structured task. Giving the individual a choice of structured activities to complete can increase the likelihood that the person will be interested in the selected task. There is no need to return the client to his/her room and 24 hours of rest is not necessary after an ECT. However, there is some temporary memory loss after an ECT so it would not be appropriate to give the individual an activity that requires memory to complete.

**Type of Reasoning: Inductive**

This question requires one to determine the best response to a patient who had ECT treatment six hours ago. This requires inductive reasoning skill, where clinical judgment is paramount to arriving at a correct conclusion. For this situation, the test taker should recall the guidelines for activity after ECT treatment. Six hours after treatment the individual can engage in a structured task; therefore, the OTA should encourage the individual to engage in such a task. If answered incorrectly, review treatment guidelines for OT treatment post-ECT.

**A80  C3**

An OTA supervises a Level II Fieldwork student regarding the evaluation procedures of a work hardening program. The OTA explains that some individuals attending the program magnify their symptoms to retain benefits; therefore the validity of some evaluation measures may be compromised. Which assessment tool does the OTA identify as providing the most valid results?

**Correct Answer: A. A volumeter.**

**Incorrect Answers:**

B.  A dynamometer (all five positions).

C.  A standardized pegboard test.

D.  A total active motion (TAM) evaluation.

**Rationale:**

The volumeter is the only true objective assessment tool that occupational therapy practitioners utilize for it is based on the displacement law of physics. It is the only tool that a person cannot manipulate in any way to lead to an invalid conclusion.

**Type of Reasoning: Inferential**

One must have knowledge of all the assessment tools described and proper administration in order to arrive at a correct conclusion. This is an inferential reasoning skill where knowledge of clinical guidelines and judgment based on facts are utilized to reach conclusions. In this case, the only assessment that cannot be manipulated is volumeter measurements. If answered incorrectly, review volumeter assessment guidelines.

## A81  C9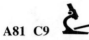

An OTA with 15 years of practice and administrative experience in a community mental health day program wants to work for a school system. Which position is the best match for the OTA's qualifications?

**Correct Answer: A. An entry level OTA.**

**Incorrect Answers:**

B.  A senior OTA.

C.  A director of the after-school activity programs.

D.  An OTA specialist in behavioral problems.

**Rationale:**

The OTA has 15 years practice and administrative experience, but no specific experience in the school system. As a result, the OTA is only qualified to apply for a position as an entry-level OTA. The OTA must be able to develop skills in school-based practice before applying for the other positions listed. The other positions require more school-based occupational therapy experience.

**Type of Reasoning: Deductive**

This question requires one to recall factual guidelines and knowledge, which is a deductive reasoning skill. The question essentially tests whether one understands what constitutes experienced versus entry-level practice. Because the OTA of 15 years has never practiced in a school system, his/her knowledge and skill is entry-level. If answered incorrectly, review standards of practice guidelines related to experienced versus entry-level practice.

## A82  C6

A graduate student with an anxiety disorder reports feeling confused about the future. During the OT evaluation, the client relates decreased feelings of competence for a chosen field of study and overall poor personal causation. Which is the best initial action for the OTA to take in response to the client's stated concerns?

**Correct Answer: D. Establish short-term goals with high potential for attainment.**

**Incorrect Answers:**

A.  Administer a vocational interest inventory.

B.  Provide activities related to the client's chosen field of study.

C.  Refer the client to the state office of vocational and educational services.

**Rationale:**

Decreased personal causation and feelings of incompetence are common symptoms of anxiety disorders. The establishment of short-term goals with high potential for attainment can provide the individual with the success experiences needed to develop a sense of competence and improve personal causation. Once these skills are developed, the need for further vocational exploration and/or services can be determined.

**Type of Reasoning: Inferential**

One must determine the best initial action for this student, given the symptoms described. This requires inferential reasoning, where one must draw conclusions based on the evidence presented. In this situation, the occupational therapist should establish short-term goals with high potential for achievement. If answered incorrectly, review intervention guidelines for individuals with anxiety disorders.

382

**A83  C7**

A client in the descending phase of Guillain-Barré syndrome has bilateral shoulder strength of 2/5. The client fatigues easily. Which equipment should the OTA recommend to enhance the person's performance of activities of daily living?

**Correct Answer: A. An overhead suspension sling.**

**Incorrect Answers:**

B.  Long-handled utensils and tools.

C.  Angled/curved-handled utensils and tools.

D.  An environmental control unit.

**Rationale:**

The overhead suspension sling is best suited for individuals presenting with proximal weakness with muscle grades in the 1/5 to 3/5 range. Long-handled and curved utensils and tools are useful for individuals with range of motion limitations. Environmental control units are used for individuals who have significant motor deficits, proximally and distally, and who cannot independently perform tasks such as controlling the switches on electronic equipment.

**Type of Reasoning: Inferential**

One must infer or draw conclusions about a likely course of action, given the information presented. This is an inferential reasoning skill, where knowledge of a therapeutic approach, such as providing equipment to enhance functioning in this situation, is essential to choosing a correct solution. In this case, the OTA should choose an overhead suspension sling. If answered incorrectly, review the diagnostic criteria and functional impact of Guillain-Barré syndrome and adaptive equipment for persons with proximal weakness. Integration of this knowledge is required to answer this item correctly.

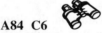

**A84  C6**

The parent of two elementary school-aged children receives home care hospice services due to metastasized bone cancer. The client is in pain and has poor endurance and decreased muscle strength. The client requires moderate assistance with self-care and dressing. Which is the best intervention for the OTA to incorporate into sessions with this parent?

**Correct Answer: D. Exploring play activities for the parent to do with the children.**

**Incorrect Answers:**

A.  Training in energy conservation techniques for self-care and dressing.

B.  Training in joint protection techniques for self-care and dressing.

C.  Using biofeedback to reduce the client's pain.

**Rationale:**

A major focus of hospice care is to maintain the individual's control over his/her life while enabling engagement in meaningful activities that are related to the person's valued roles. Although the person is dying, he/she is still a parent and will likely enjoy playing with his/her children when they are not in school. There are many play activities suitable for elementary school-aged children that can be completed by a person with decreased endurance and muscle strength. In addition, research has found that diversional activities can decrease the intensity of an individual's pain experience. There is no indication of a need to train the client in techniques for self-care or dressing. The client currently is in pain and requires moderate assistance due to functional deficits. It is likely that the client will continue to need this assistance due to the fact that his/her cancer is at the terminal stage. Even with training in energy conservation or joint protection, the individual would still need assistance with these tasks due to the effects of advanced cancer. Biofeedback is not effective in managing pain that results from metastasized bone cancer.

**Type of Reasoning: Inductive**

One must utilize clinical knowledge and judgment to determine the intervention approach that best incorporates control over the patient's life. In this case, because the patient is a parent of school-aged children, the OTA should incorporate play activities to do with the children after school. Review principles of hospice care and intervention approaches for patients with terminal illness if answered incorrectly.

**A85  C7**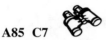

An elder resident of a skilled nursing facility becomes tearful during an OT session. The resident has a diagnosis of advanced osteoarthritis and relates that pain is causing discomfort during sexual activities. The resident expresses fear about "losing" a valued intimate relationship and asks the OTA for advice. Which is the most beneficial action for the OTA to take in response to the resident's expressed concerns?

**Correct Answer: B. Collaborate with the occupational therapist and resident to establish goals for sexual expression.**

**Incorrect Answers:**

A.  Refer the resident to social work for individual counseling.

C.  Refer the resident and the resident's significant other to social work for couples counseling.

D.  Advise nursing of the resident's statements to ensure that sexual behavior is monitored.

**Rationale:**

Sexuality and sexual expression are within the practice domain of occupational therapy. It is important for the OTA to create an atmosphere that enables the person to express his/her concerns. Once the individual's goals for sexual expression are established, strategies to attain these goals can be explored. These strategies can include the use of activity analysis, gradation, modification and simplification, non-medical methods to manage pain and stiffness (e.g. warm baths), positioning alternatives, adaptive equipment, energy conservation methods, and/or referral(s) to other professionals. It is inappropriate for staff to monitor consensual sexual expression of any individual, regardless of age or facility.

**Type of Reasoning: Inductive**

Clinical knowledge and judgment are the most important skills needed for answering this question, which requires inductive reasoning skill. Knowledge of the OTA's practice domain is essential for arriving at a correct conclusion. In this case, the OTA should collaborate with the occupational therapist to explore the resident's goals for sexual expression. Review guidelines for sexual expression if answered incorrectly.

**A86  C8**

An individual recovering from a total hip replacement is being discharged home. The individual is insured only by Medicare. For safety and independence in the bathroom, which adaptive equipment is best for the OTA to recommend?

**Correct Answer: C. A three-in-one commode.**

**Incorrect Answers:**

A.  A raised toilet seat.

B.  Grab bars.

D.  Non-skid mats.

**Rationale:**

A three-in-one commode will provide the additional height needed by the individual to maintain hip precautions. It is also the only item identified that is reimbursable by Medicare. Medicare does not cover any equipment that can be useful to individuals without a disability. Self-help items such as grab bars, raised toilet seats and non-skid mats are not considered medically necessary and are not reimbursable since other people can use them.

**Type of Reasoning: Inductive**

One must utilize clinical knowledge and judgment to determine the equipment that will be reimbursed by Medicare and provide safety and independence. In this case, a three-in-one commode is the only equipment reimbursed by Medicare and provides needed safety and independence. If answered incorrectly, review Medicare guidelines for reimbursement of durable medical equipment.

384

**A87 C6**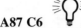

An OTA working in a skilled nursing facility conducts an inservice on validation therapy for the recently hired staff of a new psychogeriatric unit. Which fundamental principle of validation therapy is important for the OTA to include in this presentation?

**Correct Answer: A. Listen to the words an individual uses to ascertain the person's underlying message.**

**Incorrect Answers:**

B.  Provide highly structured activities to refocus the individual on reality.

C.  Provide unstructured activities to facilitate the expression of feelings.

D.  Listen to the words an individual uses and provide reality orientation for invalid statements.

**Rationale:**

Validation therapy is an approach to working with individuals with dementia founded on the principle that the unspoken messages an individual conveys in his/her speech are more important than the actual content of the speech. Individuals with dementia often make statements that are not based in reality. For example, an individual introduces a daughter as his/her mother. In validation therapy, the factual aspects of this familial relationship are irrelevant and do not need to be addressed at all. However, the underlying message that this relationship is valued and important is worthy of comment. The use of structured or unstructured activities is not a component of validation therapy. The focus of validation therapy is to facilitate communication with persons with dementia in a caring, respectful and empathetic manner.

**Type of Reasoning: Inferential**

This question requires one to determine the primary principle of validation therapy. This requires inferential reasoning skill, where one must infer or draw conclusions about a likely guideline or principle. For this case, the OTA should advise staff to listen to the words an individual uses to ascertain the person's underlying message. If answered incorrectly, review validation therapy principles and guidelines.


**A88 C3**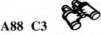

An individual with rheumatoid arthritis (RA) is currently in a stage of remission. During this inactive chronic phase of this disease, the OTA works with the client to maintain ROM and muscle strength. Which of the following is most effective for the OTA to recommend the client include in a daily home exercise program?

**Correct Answer: B. Active ROM.**

**Incorrect Answers:**

A.  Passive ROM.

C.  Isotonics.

D.  Progressive resistance.

**Rationale:**

Activities that use active ROM are indicated for the treatment of RA both in its acute and chronic phases. Passive ROM and progressive resistance are contraindicated in the treatment of RA. The use of isotonic exercises for individuals with RA is somewhat controversial. If isotonics are considered for an intervention, the occupational therapist must establish that the individual's joints are stable and would benefit from isotonic exercises without jeopardizing other joints. The individual's response to these exercises must be monitored; therefore, isotonics are not appropriate for an unmonitored home care program.

**Type of Reasoning: Inductive**

One must utilize clinical judgment in order to determine the best exercise approach for a patient with RA. Questions that require one to use knowledge of a diagnosis, coupled with therapeutic approaches often require inductive reasoning skill. For this situation, active ROM is indicated in both acute and chronic phases of RA. If answered incorrectly, review exercise guidelines for patients with RA.

**A89 C7**

A high school senior with Friedreich's ataxia is working on developing keyboarding skills in a school-to-work transition program. During the initial session, the OTA observes signs of dysmetria. Which is the most appropriate adaptation for the OTA to recommend to increase the effectiveness of the student's keyboarding skills?

**Correct Answer: B. A key guard overlay.**

**Incorrect Answers:**

A.  An eye-gaze input system.

C.  A voice-activated input system.

D.  A reduced size keyboard.

**Rationale:**

Dysmetria is the overshooting (hypermetria) or the undershooting (hypometria) of a target. It would be observed during a keyboarding activity as frequent misses of the desired key, either hitting keys above, below, or next to the targeted key. A key guard overlay provides raised separations between each key. This enables the individual to place his/her finger into the desired key space and prevents the person's finger from "jumping" to keys above, below, or next to the targeted key. An individual with Friedreich's ataxia has poor coordination of all muscles, including ocular muscles rendering an eye-gaze input system ineffective. Dysarthia is also characteristic of Friedreich's ataxia which limits the efficacy of a voice-activated system. A reduced size keyboard has smaller keys and controls. It is indicated for a person with decreased ROM and good fine motor skills.

**Type of Reasoning: Inferential**

One must have knowledge of Friedreich's ataxia and typical deficits in order to choose the best adaptation for keyboarding skills. This is an inferential reasoning skill where one must infer or draw conclusions based on information presented. For this case, a key guard overlay is the best recommendation to address the dysmetria during keyboarding skills. If answered incorrectly, review characteristics of Friedreich's ataxia and keyboarding adaptations for persons with mobility impairments. The integration of this knowledge is required to determine a correct answer.

**A90  C4**

A patient recovering from a CVA demonstrates hemiparesis of the right upper extremity and moderate flexion and extension synergies (i.e., flexion is stronger than extension). The intervention goal is to strengthen the shoulder muscles first. Which are the best movements for the OTA to promote during intervention?

**Correct Answer: A. Shoulder abduction with elbow extension.**

**Incorrect Answers:**

B.  Shoulder horizontal adduction with elbow extension.

C.  Shoulder horizontal adduction with elbow flexion.

D.  Shoulder abduction with elbow flexion.

**Rationale:**

Hemiplegic synergies are present and should not be reinforced. Shoulder abduction with elbow flexion is part of the flexion synergy, while adduction with elbow extension is part of the extension synergy. Adduction with elbow flexion is an out-of-synergy combination but this movement does not strengthen the deltoid. Shoulder abduction with elbow extension is the correct choice since it the only movement pattern that is out of synergy which also strengthens the shoulder muscles.

**Type of Reasoning:  Inductive**

One must evaluate the patient's symptoms and use knowledge of limb synergies to determine the best movements to promote during intervention. This necessitates clinical judgment, which is an inductive reasoning skill. Given the diagnosis and current status, shoulder abduction with elbow extension is best because hemiplegic synergies are discouraged using this approach. If answered incorrectly, review limb synergies with stroke and out-of-synergy movement patterns.

386

**A91  C7**

Several clients participate in an outpatient daily vocational rehabilitation group. Which is the main purpose of this group?

**Correct Answer: D. Affect changes in work skills.**

**Incorrect Answers:**

A.  Reduce costs by using an out-patient format instead of in-patient setting.

B.  Build each member's trust in a group for return to work.

C.  Enhance each member's self-esteem in the work setting.

**Rationale:**

The goal of a vocational rehabilitation group is to improve work skills. This increase in functional skills could improve clients' self-esteem in work and increase their trust of others. Reducing costs is likely achieved by the provision of services in an outpatient setting, but this is not the goal of the group treatment.

**Type of Reasoning: Inferential**

One must infer or draw conclusions about what is likely to be the primary purpose of a vocational rehabilitation group, which is an inferential reasoning skill. Improving work skills is the primary goal, though other secondary goals may exist, such as reducing costs or building trust. Questions of this nature may be challenging as all responses may seem correct. However, the question is ultimately asking for the main purpose of the group, rather than secondary benefits. Review the purposes of vocational rehabilitation if answered incorrectly.

**A92  C7**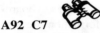

A child with spinal muscle atrophy can no longer reach beyond 90 degrees of shoulder abduction and 90 degrees of shoulder flexion. The parents state that the child can no longer don or doff a T-shirt. Which is the best approach for the OTA to recommend the child use to don a T-shirt?

**Correct Answer: C. Have the child support the elbows on a table at chest height to don the T-shirt over arms, then don over head.**

**Incorrect Answers:**

A.  Place the T-shirt directly on the child's lap, have the child don the arms first, then don the head of the T-shirt.

B.  Have the child wear front-opening shirts instead of T-shirts.

D.  Have the child sit with the trunk well-supported, lean to the right and don the right arm, repeat to the left, and then don the head of the T-shirt.

**Rationale:**

Spinal muscle atrophy is a progressive disorder and the OTA needs to prepare the child and family for progressive loss of skills. The best technique, as shoulder ROM decreases, is to use a table for support to don arms then over head.

**Type of Reasoning: Inductive**

This question requires one to consider the best approach for completing the ADL task, given an understanding of the diagnosis and limitations. This requires inductive reasoning skill, where the test taker must utilize clinical judgment based on knowledge of the diagnosis to arrive at a correct conclusion. For this case, the OTA should have the child support the elbows on a table at chest height to don the T-shirt over the arms, then don over head. If answered incorrectly, review information on spinal muscle atrophy and dressing skills.

**A93  C4**

An OTA constructs a splint for an individual with Erb's palsy. Which orthosis would be most effective for this condition?

**Correct Answer: B. An elbow lock splint.**

**Incorrect Answers:**

A.  A flail arm splint.

C.  A figure-of-eight splint.

D.  A deltoid sling.

**Rationale:**

Erb's palsy results from injury to the fifth and sixth cervical roots of the brachial plexus. The resulting clinical picture is that the arm hangs limp with the shoulder rotated inward due to atrophy and paralysis in the biceps, deltoid, brachialis, and brachioradialis muscles. This significantly limits functional movement. The elbow lock splint stabilizes the elbow to enable the individual to position the hand closer to or away from his/her body for functional use. A flail arm splint is recommended for a brachial plexus injury of C5-T1 resulting in whole upper extremity involvement. It provides the needed stability at both the shoulder and elbow for functional positioning of the hand. A figure-of-eight splint is used for a combined median ulnar nerve injury and to prevent MP hyperextension. A deltoid sling is used for upper extremity muscle weakness.

**Type of Reasoning: Inferential**

One must first determine the benefits and indications of each of the orthoses above in order to determine the orthosis that best addresses the patient's condition. This requires inferential reasoning, where one must draw conclusions based on the information provided. In this situation, an elbow lock splint is the ideal orthosis for Erb's palsy. If answered incorrectly, review Erb's palsy and appropriate orthoses.

**A94 C9**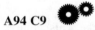

A non-English speaking family attends a discharge planning session. The assigned OTA does not share the language of the family. Which action should the OTA take first?

**Correct Answer: B. Obtain a translator to communicate with the family during the session.**

**Incorrect Answers:**

A.  Make a referral for a home-care therapist to visit the family to provide in-home education.

C.  Attempt to communicate with the family through non-verbal communication.

D.  Consult with the occupational therapist to develop a discharge plan.

**Rationale:**

The best choice to ensure the family involvement in the discharge planning process is to seek out a way to communicate directly and verbally with the family via a translator. The family is not included in these processes without a translator. Non-verbal communication does not transcend a language barrier for abstract concepts such as incorporating the individual's needs, values, and goals of treatment. There is no need for the OTA to consult with an occupational therapist if he/she has already been assigned this case. The OTA can independently get a translator to help communicate with the family. In addition, the OTA and occupational therapist should not develop a discharge plan without the family's input.

**Type of Reasoning: Evaluative**

This question requires one to determine the best course of action that considers the needs of the person and most effectively facilitates delivery of services. Questions that ask the test-taker to use judgment to determine a best course of action often utilize evaluative reasoning skills. In this situation, and in keeping with the AOTA Code of Ethics, the OTA should seek out a translator. Review cultural competency guidelines, including providing translation services.

388

## A95  C6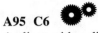

A client with a diagnosis of paranoid schizophrenia is participating in an initial evaluation session at a psychiatric day treatment program. Halfway through the completion of an activities configuration, the client states the referral to this day program is inappropriate and unnecessary because it was made by an incompetent psychiatrist. The client becomes visibly upset and loud when talking about the unfounded referral and the psychiatrist's incompetence. Which is the best initial action for the OTA to take in response to the client's statements?

**Correct Answer: C. Acknowledge that the client appears upset and ask if the client is able to focus on the remaining evaluation.**

**Incorrect Answers:**

A.  End the evaluation session and tell the client to call to re-schedule when feeling better.
B.  Assure the client of the referring psychiatrist's competence and advise the client to discuss concerns with the doctor.
D.  Contact the day program's chief psychiatrist to report the client's stated concerns about the referring psychiatrist's competence.

**Rationale:**

A simple acknowledgement of the client's concerns can validate his/her feelings in a non-threatening manner without validating potentially delusional thought content. Asking the person in a calm business-like manner if he/she can return to the task at hand can diffuse the situation. If the client states he/she is not able to regain focus, the OTA can then provide the needed support. Immediately ending the evaluation does not deal with the issue of potentially escalating behavior and does not provide the individual with the opportunity to engage in a therapeutic relationship. Continuing the evaluation can allow concrete opportunities for support and reality testing. Assuring the client of the doctor's competence could contribute to further escalation if the client's concerns are based on a delusional thought process, which is unshaken by external explanations. There is no need to report the client's concerns for there is no concrete evidence of physician incompetence at this time. The OTA should relay the client's expressed concerns at the next team meeting.

**Type of Reasoning: Evaluative**

One must weigh the possible courses of action and then make a value judgment about the best course to take. This requires evaluative reasoning skill, which often utilizes guiding principles of action in order to arrive at a correct conclusion. In this case, the client is upset and his/her feelings appear to be escalating. To address potential agitation and prevent escalation, the therapist should acknowledge the client's feelings and try to redirect him/her to the task at hand. Review redirection strategies for clients with escalating behavior if answered incorrectly.

## A96  C2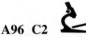

An OTA working for a home care agency provides an inservice to new employees on Medicare reimbursement guidelines for durable medical equipment (DME). Which item would the OTA describe as reimbursable by Medicare?

**Correct Answer: C. A walker for a person who cannot ambulate in the home without one.**

**Incorrect Answers:**

A.  A raised toilet seat for a patient after a hip replacement.
B.  A reacher for a person with arthritis in both hips.
D.  Grab bars in the bathroom for a person who cannot bathe or toilet without them.

**Rationale:**

The walker is covered by Medicare. The others are not. The criteria for durable medical equipment to be reimbursable by Medicare are that the item must be necessary and reasonable to treat an illness or incidence of decreased functioning. The item must have a medical purpose, be used repeatedly, and not useful in the absence of an illness.

**Type of Reasoning: Deductive**

This question requires one to recall Medicare reimbursement guidelines, which is factual knowledge. Deductive reasoning skills are utilized whenever one must recall concrete principles and guidelines to draw conclusions. The only item listed that is considered a medical necessity by Medicare is a walker when issued for a person who cannot ambulate in the home without one. Review Medicare guidelines for reimbursement of DME if answered incorrectly.

**A97  C9**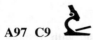

An OTA working in a school system must incorporate the Individuals with Disabilities Education Act (IDEA) into the program. In which of the following locations should the OTA provide intervention?

**Correct Answer: C. Regular classroom while general education classes are in session.**

**Incorrect Answers:**

A.  Regular classroom while general education classes are not in session.
B.  Special education classroom while other children with disabilities are present.
D.  Private occupational therapy room designed for children with disabilities.

**Rationale:**

The guidelines from IDEA emphasize that a child's needs be served in an inclusive manner that enables the child to have full access to the general education curriculum, focusing on participation in a general education classroom. The other options are too restrictive and do not facilitate inclusion in general education.

**Type of Reasoning: Deductive**

One must recall IDEA guidelines in order to arrive at a correct conclusion. This requires deductive reasoning skill, where knowledge of protocols and guidelines are paramount to choosing the correct answer. For this situation, therapy intervention in a regular classroom while general education classes are in session is the only location that provides inclusive treatment. If answered incorrectly, review IDEA guidelines and inclusive services in the classroom.

**A98  C5**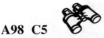

An individual with a spinal cord injury at C-7 reports noticeable redness on the ischial tuberosity during self-examination with a mirror. Which action is most effective for the OTA to recommend in response to client's observations?

**Correct Answer: A. Integrate weight shifting into daily activities.**

**Incorrect Answers:**

B.  Use a tilt-in-space wheelchair.
C.  Use an angled foam cushion.
D.  Self-direct caregivers to assist with weight shifting at least once every 30 minutes.

**Rationale:**

During rehabilitation, a person with a spinal cord injury must be instructed on the need to relieve pressure on a consistent basis. A person with a spinal cord injury at the level of C-7 can perform depression transfers so the ability to perform weight shifting for pressure relief is intact. The person is reporting the early signs of skin breakdown so it is vital that the person integrates weight shifting into daily activities. This is a very effective way to prevent decubitus ulcers. Since the person is able to weight shift independently, a tilt-in-space wheelchair and self-directing caregivers to assist with weight shifting are two modifications that are at too low a level for this scenario. An angled foam cushion would position the person in a manner that would increase weight on the ischial tuberosity. This would be contraindicated.

**Type of Reasoning: Inductive**

One must utilize clinical knowledge and judgment to determine the recommendation that best addresses the individual's issue. This requires inductive reasoning skill. In this case, the OTA should recommend the integration of weight shifting into daily activities to prevent pressure sores. If answered incorrectly, review pressure relief activities for individuals with cervical spinal cord injury and the functional abilities of the different levels of SCI. Integration of this knowledge is required for a correct answer.

390

**A99  C2**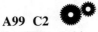

An OTA working in a skilled nursing facility conducts an initial therapeutic feeding session with an elder with dysphagia. During the session the resident consistently expresses a desire to return home. Which is the OTA's best response?

**Correct Answer: B. Acknowledge the resident's desire to return home.**

**Incorrect Answers:**

A.  Immediately redirect the conversation to the texture and taste of the food.

C.  End the session and report the resident's desire.

D.  Offer to contact the resident's family to convey this desire.

**Rationale:**

It is natural and normal for a new resident in a skilled nursing facility to express a desire to return home. This wish must be acknowledged and validated in order to establish therapeutic rapport. Ending the session or immediately redirecting the resident to the feeding activity ignores the validity of the resident's genuine feelings. This is counter-therapeutic. Once a person feels that he/she has been heard, he/she is often able to refocus on the activity. It is inappropriate for the OTA to offer to contact the family, for he/she cannot know the resident's relationship with his/her family.

**Type of Reasoning: Evaluative**

One must weigh the possible courses of action and then make a value judgment about the best course to take. This requires evaluative reasoning skill, which often utilizes guiding principles of action in order to arrive at a correct conclusion. For this case, the OTA should acknowledge the resident's desire to return home. Review validation techniques for individuals if answered incorrectly.

**A100  C6**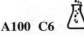

An individual recently lost significant functional abilities due to post-polio syndrome. The OTA works with the individual to develop compensation skills for performing daily tasks. During a meal preparation session, the person angrily throws all of the adaptive equipment onto the floor. At the next team meeting, which defense mechanism should the OTA report the individual appears to be demonstrating?

**Correct Answer: D. Displacement.**

**Incorrect Answers:**

A.  Acting out.

B.  Passive-aggressive behavior.

C.  Reaction formation.

**Rationale:**

Displacement occurs when an individual redirects an emotion from one "object" (in this case, the anger over the progression of the disease) to another "object" (i.e., the adaptive equipment). Acting out is a term used to describe behaviors that violate societal norms (e.g., sexually provocative behavior, physically assaultive behavior). Passive-aggressive behavior is characterized by indirect or unassertive aggression (e.g., being chronically late when meeting someone you had an argument with years ago). Reaction formation is the switching of an unacceptable impulse into its opposite (e.g., hugging someone you would like to hit).

**Type of Reasoning: Analytical**

This question provides a description of a behavior and the test taker must draw conclusions about what the behavior indicates. This is an analytical reasoning skill, as questions of this nature often ask one to analyze descriptors and symptoms in order to determine a diagnosis or draw a conclusion. In this situation the behavior indicates displacement. Review defense mechanisms if answered incorrectly.

**A101  C6**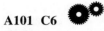

During a therapeutic feeding session, a 97 year-old resident with dementia, non-Alzheimer's type becomes upset and cries for his/her mother. What should the OTA say in response to the resident's statements?

**Correct Answer: B. "You must miss your mother, tell me about her."**

**Incorrect Answers:**

A. "Remember that you are now in a nursing home and your mother is not here."

C. "Remember your mother passed away years ago."

D. "I will tell the nurse that you want your mother contacted."

**Rationale:**

This response validates the person's feelings and provides him/her with the opportunity to reminisce about a pleasant memory. Even a few minutes of reminiscing can provide solace to the individual, which can help calm him/her. This can then enable the resident to reengage in the feeding activity. Individuals with dementia generally respond well to validation therapy and reminiscence activities. Asking the individual to recall that his/her mother is deceased and/or not available is inappropriate for they are asking the resident to remember something that is no longer part of his/her reality. Telling the person that that there is a potential for his/her mother to be contacted is offering an action that cannot be completed in reality. In addition, it does not address the individual's valid feelings which need to be addressed at the moment.

**Type of Reasoning: Evaluative**

This question requires professional judgment based on guiding principles, which is an evaluative reasoning skill. Most important in this situation is to validate the person's feelings. This way the OTA can provide an opportunity to reminisce without asking the person to recall something that is not part of reality. Review validation strategies for persons with dementia if answered incorrectly.

**A102  C1**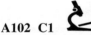

A five year-old is referred to OT. Upon the completion of a standardized test evaluation, the OTA determines that the child demonstrates age-appropriate cognitive and fine motor skills. Which activity would the child be able to complete at this developmental level?

**Correct Answer: C. Cutting simple figure shapes with scissors.**

**Incorrect Answers:**

A. Cutting long thin strips with scissors.

B. Holding and snipping with scissors.

D. Opening and closing scissors in a controlled fashion.

**Rationale:**

Cutting simple figure shapes is a four to six year-old cognitive and fine motor skill. Cutting strips is a three to four year-old skill. Holding and snipping with scissors and opening and closing scissors in a controlled fashion are 2-3 year old skills.

**Type of Reasoning: Deductive**

This question requires one to recall factual knowledge, which is a deductive reasoning skill. The question necessitates one to recall the developmental skills of a four year-old. In this situation, cutting simple figure shapes is a four year-old skill. If answered incorrectly, review the developmental sequence of scissor skills.

## A103 C8

An OTA provides caregiver training to the spouse of an individual with cerebellar cortical degeneration. The focus of the session is on community mobility using a wheelchair. The individual is dependent upon the spouse's assistance for mobility. Which of the following is most effective for the OTA to recommend the spouse do when descending a steep grade?

**Correct Answer: B. Go down backwards with all wheelchair wheels maintaining contact with ground surface.**

**Incorrect Answers:**

A. Tilt the wheelchair backward to its gravitational balance point and then go down forward.

C. Tilt the wheelchair backward to its gravitational balance point and then go down backward.

D. Push forward as on flat surfaces but lean body back for extra drag.

**Rationale:**

Proceeding down a steep grade backwards with all wheelchair wheels maintaining contact with the ground enables the spouse to use body weight to slow the chair's momentum. If the spouse tires, he/she can readily stop and use his/her body weight to hold the chair in place while putting the wheelchair brakes on. Pushing the chair in a forward position can be dangerous on a steep grade, for if the spouse loses his/her grip and/or tires, it could be very difficult to regain control of the situation. Maintaining the chair in a backward tilt position while going backwards is an unnecessary use of energy and can greatly contribute to caregiver's physical fatigue.

**Type of Reasoning: Inductive**

Clinical knowledge and judgment are the most important skills needed for answering this question, which requires inductive reasoning skill. Knowledge of safety guidelines in mobility utilizing a wheelchair is essential to arriving at a correct conclusion. In this case, the OTA should recommend descending a steep grade backwards with all wheelchair wheels in contact with the ground. Review community wheelchair mobility guidelines if answered incorrectly.

## A104 C4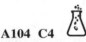

During an intervention session using a transfer of training approach, the OTA gives the client a list of items commonly found in a closet and asks the client to separate the items into grooming and dressing items. What skill is the OTA working on?

**Correct Answer: A. Categorization.**

**Incorrect Answers:**

B. Sequencing.

C. Problem solving.

D. Memory.

**Rationale:**

Separating items into two groups requires placing them into a category. Sequencing involves the planning, organization and implementation of the steps of a task in an appropriate order. Problem solving requires the recognition and definition of a problem and the selection and implementation of a plan. Memory is the registration, integration, recall and retrieval of information.

**Type of Reasoning: Analytical**

A descriptor of an activity is provided and the test taker must determine what these guidelines indicate, which is an analytical reasoning skill. One should determine that the description of this sorting activity most closely represents categorization. If answered incorrectly, review cognitive retraining guidelines, especially categorization activities.

## A105  C9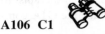

An OTA working in an outpatient clinic observes the clinic's administrative assistant leaving patient records open on the clinic's reception counter. The assistant has left the clinic to go for lunch. Which action is best for the OTA to take in response to this observation?

**Correct Answer: C. Pick up the records and place them in a location out of public view.**

**Incorrect Answers:**

A.  Remind the administrative assistant of the need to keep patient records private when the assistant returns from lunch.

B.  Contact the administrative assistant's direct supervisor to report this observation.

D.  Discuss the issue with the occupational therapist during their next scheduled supervision session.

**Rationale:**

The OTA must act to protect patient privacy. The HIPAA Privacy Rule requires that all providers protect patient confidentiality in all forms (i.e., oral, written, and electronic). Charts and any documentation with patients' names or other identifiers must be stored out of public view and in secure locations. Reminding the administrative assistant of documentation privacy requirements when the assistant returns, contacting the administrative assistant's direct supervisor, and discussing the issue with the supervising occupational therapist do not address the immediate need for the OTA to take action that makes sure no patient record is visible to anyone in the reception area.

**Type of reasoning: Evaluative**

This question requires the test taker to weigh the merits of the courses of action presented and determine the approach that will most effectively resolve the issue. This requires evaluative reasoning skill. For this situation, the OTA should pick up the records and place them in a location out of public view to protect patient privacy. If answered incorrectly, review HIPAA guidelines and the protection of patient privacy.

## A106  C1

A 21 month-old child with severe spastic quadriplegia has major sensorimotor deficits. The child is cognitively intact and exhibits age-appropriate cognitive skills. The OTA recommends a play activity to enhance these cognitive abilities and provide the child with a fun and pleasurable experience. Which is the best object for the OTA to recommend?

**Correct Answer: B. A mechanical toy with a chin controlled on/off switch.**

**Incorrect Answers:**

A.  A multi-colored mobile of objects of interest placed over the child's stroller.

C.  A shape sorter with foam squares, triangles, and circles.

D.  A battery controlled hammock swing.

**Rationale:**

At 21 months, a child is cognitively able to operate and control mechanical toys. The chin controlled switch will enable this child to self-direct his/her play despite the spastic quadriplegia. A mobile is cognitively too low for this child's abilities. It is a passive activity that would not provide active engagement of the child. The ability to identify and sort shapes does occur at 21 months, but the use of a shape sorter requires motor abilities beyond this child's capacities.

**Type of Reasoning: Inductive**

This question requires one to determine the best object for enhancing cognitive abilities of this child. This requires inductive reasoning skill, where clinical judgment is paramount to arriving at a correct conclusion. For this situation, a mechanical toy with a chin controlled on/off switch is most appropriate. If answered incorrectly, review developmental levels of cognition and play and treatment guidelines for children with spastic quadriplegia. The integration of this knowledge is required to answer this question correctly.

**A107 C7**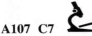

An OTA screens potential members for a vocational rehabilitation group according to established inclusionary and exclusionary criteria for membership. Functional deficits in which area would exclude persons from membership in this group?

**Correct Answer: D. Personal self-care.**

**Incorrect Answers:**

A. Problem-solving.

B. Self-awareness of strengths.

C. Social skills.

**Rationale:**

Personal self-care skills should be developed prior to attending a vocational rehabilitation group. A pre-vocational group would be appropriate for persons who exhibit self-care deficits. The other options can be addressed in a vocational rehabilitation group, as they are essential to success in the work setting.

**Type of reasoning: Deductive**

One must recall the guidelines for membership in a vocational group in order to arrive at a correct conclusion. This is factual information, which is a deductive reasoning skill. For this situation, personal self-care skills must be developed prior to attending a vocational rehabilitation group, therefore an individual would be excluded for this reason. If answered incorrectly, review vocational rehabilitation group guidelines.

**A108 C1**

An OTA completes a standardized early intervention screening of an 8 month-old child. The results indicate that the child is able to sit independently by propping forward on both arms. The OTA collaborates with the occupational therapist to determine the next step to take in working with this child. Which is the best action for them to determine the OTA complete next?

**Correct Answer: A. Evaluate the child's sensorimotor skills using a standardized evaluation.**

**Incorrect Answers:**

B. Inform the parents that the child exhibits typical behavior.

C. Develop goals to improve sitting balance.

D. Provide play activities to develop sitting balance.

**Rationale:**

The screening indicated a sensorimotor delay, which requires further evaluation. Sitting with arms propped forward is typical of a 5-6 month-old. At 8 months, a child typically sits without support; therefore, further evaluation of the child's sensorimotor status is indicated. The occupational therapist and OTA cannot collaborate to set goals or prescribe activities prior to the completion of a full evaluation. OTAs are able to perform standardized evaluations under the supervision of an occupational therapist.

**Type of Reasoning: Inferential**

One must determine the most likely next course of action for a child, given the diagnosis and functional ability described. This requires inferential reasoning skill, where one must draw conclusions based on the information presented. In this situation, the next step after screening is to complete a sensorimotor evaluation since the child is demonstrating a sensorimotor delay. Review motor development of infants, especially 6-8 month range, if answered incorrectly.

## A109  C6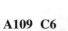

An individual hospitalized for the first time due to a brief psychotic episode attends an occupational therapy group. During task performance, the OTA notices that the person is restless with hand tremors and shaking legs. Which of the following should the OTA document that the person seems to be exhibiting?

**Correct Answer: C. Akathisia.**

**Incorrect Answers:**

A.  Akinesia.

B.  Pseudo-parkinsonism.

D.  Tardive dyskinesia.

**Rationale:**

Akathisia is a side-effect of anti-psychotic medications that is exhibited by restlessness, hand tremors, and shaky legs. Akinesia is also a potential side effect, but this is evident by a lack of movement. Akinesia is also a negative symptom of schizophrenia. Pseudo-parkinsonism is also a side-effect that appears as behaviors similar to the symptoms of advanced Parkinson's disease; that is, rigidity, pill-rolling tremors, masked face, and a shuffling gait. Tardive dyskinesia is an irreversible neurological condition caused by many years of taking neuroleptic medications. It would not be evident in someone being treated for a first break with neuroleptic medications.

**Type of Reasoning: Analytical**

This question provides symptoms and the test taker must determine the cause for such symptoms. This is an analytical reasoning skill, as questions of this nature often ask one to analyze a group of symptoms in order to determine a diagnosis. In this situation the symptoms indicate akathisia, which should be reviewed if answered incorrectly, along with other side-effects of psychotropic medications.

## A110  C4

An OTA is working with a child presenting with sensory seeking behaviors and under reactivity to touch and movement. The child has an unusually high activity level, inability to self calm, motor impulsivity, and frequent touching and handling of items in the environment.  Using Ayres classic sensory integrative (SI) approach which would be most effective for the OTA to use with this child to facilitate an adaptive response?

**Correct Answer: D. Individualized therapy based on the inner drive and interest of the child.**

**Incorrect Answers**

A.  A pre-determined schedule of sensory activities designed by the occupational therapist.

B. The child's passive participation in a variety of vestibular and proprioceptive experiences.

C.  Use of a sensory void environment to promote self regulation.

**Rationale:**

Classic Ayres SI treatment is based on the principles of inner drive and active involvement of the child.  Sensory systems are impacted by a sensory rich environment and the balance between structure and freedom in regards to activity and participation.  The OT practitioner is constantly vigilant and the interaction between the child and the practitioner is key to promoting the 'just right' challenge.

**Type of reasoning: Inductive**

One must utilize clinical judgment and knowledge of therapeutic guidelines in order to determine the most effective approach for a child with sensory seeking behaviors. This requires inductive reasoning skill. For this case, the OTA should provide individualized therapy based on the inner drive and interests of the child. If answered incorrectly, review the sensory integration frame of reference and therapeutic approaches for sensory seeking behaviors.

## A111 C7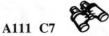

An OTA provides recommendations for play activities that a parent with a complete spinal cord injury at the C-7 level can do with children, aged eight and ten. Which is the best adapted activity for the OTA to recommend?

**Correct Answer: C. A board game using a tenodesis grasp.**

**Incorrect Answers:**

A.  An arts and crafts project using a mouthstick paint brush.

B.  A woodworking project using a universal cuff to hold tools.

D.  A computer game using a typing stick.

**Rationale:**

An individual with a C-7 SCI has a tenodesis grasp that can be effective for picking up and releasing game pieces. The other activity adaptations are appropriate for individuals with higher spinal cord injuries.

**Type of Reasoning: Inductive**

One must utilize clinical knowledge and judgment to determine the best activity for a patient with C7 injury. In this case, a board game using a tenodesis grasp is most appropriate given the person's level of injury. If answered incorrectly, review functional abilities and intact musculature for persons with C7 injury.

## A112 C5

An OTA receives a referral to provide home-based services to an elder adult who lives alone in a fourth floor walk-up apartment. Upon entering the apartment, the OTA notes the sweltering heat. The apartment has no fans or air conditioners. The client's skin is hot, dry, and red, and breathing is labored. The OTA offers the client a glass of water and places ice compresses on the arterial pressure points to help with cooling. Which is the most important action for the OTA to take next?

**Correct Answer: A. Cancel the intervention session and call for an ambulance to provide emergency medical services.**

**Incorrect Answers:**

B.  Proceed with the planned intervention session and include documentation about client's environmental conditions in the intervention report.

C.  Contact the home health agency's occupational therapist to report the client's environmental conditions and then proceed with the planned intervention session.

D.  Cancel the intervention session and advise the client to contact a doctor how to best address the impact of hot weather on personal health.

**Rationale:**

The client is exhibiting signs of heat stroke. The elderly are particularly at risk for heat-induced illnesses. Extended periods of intense heat can be life threatening to the elderly and must be treated as a medical emergency. While lowering the client's body temperature with ice on the arterial pressure points is an appropriate first-aid intervention, it is not sufficient to deal with this serious situation. Immediate medical care is required.

**Type of reasoning: Evaluative**

This question requires one to weigh the courses of action presented and determine the approach that will most effectively address the client's needs. This requires evaluative reasoning skill. For this case, based on the client's symptoms, the OTA should cancel the intervention session and call for an ambulance to provide emergency medical services. If answered incorrectly, review first aid approaches for heat stroke.

## A113  C4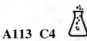

During the initial ADL evaluation, the OTA notes that the patient consistently spills food due to an inability to adjust movements while cutting food and moving the food from the plate to the mouth. Which deficit does this behavior most likely indicate?

**Correct Answer: D. Motor apraxia.**

**Incorrect Answers:**

A.  Ideational apraxia.

B.  Somatoagnosia.

C.  Tactile agnosia.

**Rationale:**

Motor apraxia (also known as ideomotor apraxia) is the loss of access to kinesthetic memory so that purposeful movement cannot be achieved due to ineffective motor planning; although sensation, movement and coordination are intact. Ideational apraxia is a breakdown in the knowledge of what is to be done or how to perform an action or use an object. Somatoagnosia is a body scheme disorder that results in diminished awareness of body structure and a failure to recognize body parts as one's own. Tactile agnosia, also known as astereognosis is the inability to recognize objects, forms, shapes and sizes by touch alone.

**Type of Reasoning: Analytical**

This question requires the test taker to determine the functional deficit of the patient, which is an analytical reasoning skill. Questions of this nature often call upon the test taker to determine a diagnosis based on a functional description of deficits. Based on this information, the symptoms of the patient indicate the deficit of motor apraxia, which should be reviewed if answered incorrectly.

## A114  C9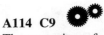

The supervisor of an acute inpatient unit requests that a recently hired entry-level OTA write summaries for several evaluation sessions that were completed by another OTA. The evaluating OTA had to leave work unexpectedly due to a medical emergency and is not expected to return to work. Which is the best response for the OTA to make in response to this request?

**Correct Answer: D. Suggest that the OTA's evaluation results be documented by the supervisor.**

**Incorrect Answers:**

A.  Comply with the supervisor's request but ask for the supervisor to co-sign the notes.

B.  Request time to complete an independent evaluation of each individual previously evaluated.

C.  Report the supervisor's request to the facility's administration.

**Rationale:**

It is not appropriate for a peer to document results of an evaluation session in which he/she did not participate. It is acceptable for a supervisor to provide documentation based upon staff's input, as long as the documentation reports that it is based upon the work of a given staff member. The supervisor must provide an accurate record of the situation (i.e., evaluation completed by OTA X found that...). In an acute inpatient setting, there is insufficient time to complete another evaluation. The entry-level OTA should communicate directly with his/her supervisor. There is nothing to report to the administration at this time.

**Type of Reasoning: Evaluative**

This question requires professional judgment based on guiding principles, which is an evaluative reasoning skill. In this situation, the OTA's most appropriate response is to suggest that the OTA's evaluation results be documented by the supervisor. Accuracy in record keeping is important in this situation and should be used as the guiding principle in finding the best solution to this situation. Review documentation guidelines if answered incorrectly.

398

## A115 C4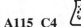

During an intervention session focused on the development of grasp and shoulder mobility, an OTA asks a client to move numerous identical one pound cans of vegetables from the counter top to the cabinet shelf above the counter. According to contemporary motor learning approaches, what type of practice has the OTA implemented for this client?

**Correct Answer: B. Blocked practice.**

**Incorrect Answers:**

A. Random practice.

C. Planned practice.

D. Contextual practice.

**Rationale:**

Blocked practice involves repeated performance of the same motor skill. Since the cans are identical and weigh the same, lifting each can requires the same motor skill. If the cans were of different sizes, shapes, and/or weights then different motor skills would be required for task performance. This would be an example of random practice which involves the performance of several tasks in random order to encourage the re-formulation of the solution to the presented motor problem. Planned practice and contextual practice are contrived terms.

**Type of Reasoning: Analytical**

This question requires one to analyze the information provided and determine the best descriptor for this functional activity. This requires analytical reasoning skill, where one must weigh all of the information provided in order to arrive at a correct conclusion. For this situation, the activity presented is that of blocked practice. Review principles of motor learning, especially blocked practice if answered incorrectly.

## A116 C4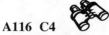

A child with a tactile defensive sensory modulation disorder attends a private early intervention clinic. The OTA collaborates with the child's parents to develop strategies and guidelines to help the child handle the symptoms of this disorder at home. Which is the best recommendation for the OTA to make to the parents?

**Correct Answer: C. Soften the child's clothing by repeated laundering and remove clothing tags.**

**Incorrect Answers:**

A. Avoid the use of swings and other moving equipment during play activities.

B. Encourage the use of swings and other moving equipment during play activities.

D. Provide a variety of textures in the clothing the child wears.

**Rationale:**

Children with tactile defensive sensory modulation disorder find stiff clothing, textured clothing, and clothing tags aversive. The use or avoidance of, swings and other moving play equipment is indicated for vestibular processing disorders.

**Type of Reasoning: Inductive**

This question requires one to determine the best recommendation for a child with tactile defensiveness. This requires inductive reasoning skill, where clinical judgment is paramount to arriving at a correct conclusion. For this situation, given knowledge of tactile defensive behaviors, the OTA should recommend softening clothing and removing clothing tags. If answered incorrectly, review treatment guidelines for children with tactile defensive behaviors.

## A117  C3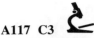

An individual has relocated to a new area and begins treatment at an outpatient OT clinic for follow-up after rotator cuff surgery. It is six weeks post-operation. Which is the most effective intervention for the OTA to implement at this time?

**Correct Answer: A. An isometric strengthening program.**

**Incorrect Answers:**

B.  Passive range of motion.

C.  Active assistive ROM.

D.  An isotonic strengthening program.

**Rationale:**

Strengthening should begin with isometrics at 6 weeks and then progress to isotonics. PROM progressing to AA/AROM is the intervention for 0-6 weeks post-operation.

**Type of Reasoning: Deductive**

This question requires recall of guidelines, which is factual knowledge. Deductive reasoning skills are utilized whenever one must recall facts to solve novel problems. In this situation, a patient who is six weeks post-operation for rotator cuff repair can begin an isometric strengthening program. Review treatment guidelines for post-surgical rotator cuff repair if answered incorrectly.

## A118  C6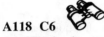

An OTA leads a social skills group for children aged 10-12 with conduct disorders. One of the children complains that the group activity is stupid and boring. Which is the most effective response for the OTA to provide in response to this complaint?

**Correct Answer: A. Encourage the child to complete the activity with the group.**

**Incorrect Answers:**

B.  Allow the child to leave the group since uninterested.

C.  Allow the child to suggest a different group activity.

D.  Tell the child the complaint will be discussed at the next family meeting.

**Rationale:**

Children between the ages of 10 and 12 are typically at the developmental age of cooperative play which emerges at 7 years of age. During this stage of development, children participate in games and learn to play according to rules in a cooperative manner. Encouraging the child to complete the activity with the group provides the child with the opportunity to develop age-appropriate social skills. Children with conduct disorders often show disregard for others and tend to violate rules; therefore, completing a planned activity with others is particularly relevant. Allowing the child to alter the group's in-progress activity or leave the group does not address these issues. There is no need for the behavior to be discussed at a family meeting.

**Type of Reasoning: Inductive**

This question requires one to determine the most appropriate response to a child with conduct disorder. This requires inductive reasoning skill, where clinical judgment is paramount to arriving at a correct conclusion. For this situation, the OTA should encourage the child to complete the activity with the group. If answered incorrectly, review the diagnostic criteria of conduct disorders and the typical developmental sequence of play. Integration of this knowledge is required for a correct answer.

## A119  C1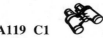

An OTA provides home-based early intervention services. The occupational therapist informs the OTA that an 18 month-old child is able to finger feed effectively but is not able to use a spoon or suck from a straw. The OTA puts together supplies to bring to the child's home and plans activities to use during the first intervention session. When selecting objects and activities to use during this initial session which developmental age is most important for the OTA to include?

**Correct Answer: D. 9-12 months.**

**Incorrect Answers:**

A.  6-9 months.

B.  12-18 months.

C.  18-20 months.

**Rationale:**

The information that the occupational therapist provided to the OTA indicates abilities that are typical at the age of 9-12 months. Therefore, the OTA should begin intervention by using activities that are at the child's developmental age. If the child's performance in certain parameters is more or less advanced than this developmental age, the OTA can adjust interventions accordingly. Since the child cannot use a spoon or a straw, activities that are typical of the developmental ages of 12-18 months and 18-20 months may be too difficult for the child. Spoon use typically develops at 12-18 months. Straw use typically develops at about 18 months. Since the child's finger feeding is noted to be effective, activities that are typical at 6-9 months would be too low developmentally for the child.

**Type of Reasoning: Inductive**

Clinical knowledge and judgment are the most important skills needed for answering this question, which requires inductive reasoning skill. Knowledge of the child's developmental age and most important activities to bring for the evaluation is essential to choosing the best solution. In this case, the OTA should bring objects and activities for the developmental age of 9-12 months. If answered incorrectly, review developmental milestones for feeding in infants.

## A120  C6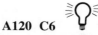

An individual with chronic undifferentiated schizophrenia is referred to a day hospital. The referring psychiatrist notes that the individual's positive symptoms have responded well to a new medication, but negative symptoms remain. During the evaluation, what will the OTA most likely observe?

**Correct Answer: B. Limited engagement in tasks due to anergia.**

**Incorrect Answers:**

A.  Inappropriate verbalizations due to delusions.

C.  Poor concentration and distractibility due to hallucinations.

D.  Immobility due to akathisia.

**Rationale:**

Limited engagement in tasks due to anergia is the only negative symptom listed. Delusions and hallucinations are positive symptoms. Akathisia results in restlessness, not immobility.

**Type of Reasoning: Inferential**

This question requires one to determine the likely symptoms of a patient displaying negative symptoms with schizophrenia. This requires one to infer or draw conclusions based upon the evidence provided, which is an inferential reasoning skill. In this situation, only limited engagement in tasks due to anergia is a negative symptom. If answered incorrectly, review information on negative symptoms associated with chronic schizophrenia.

**A121 C1**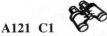

A school-based OTA is working with a child who has poor sitting posture, inefficient grasp, and excessive writing pressure into the paper. The OTA collaborates with the occupational therapist and determines that the best intervention approach requires integration of more than one intervention model. Which approaches will most effectively address all the child's deficits?

**Correct Answer: B. A combination of biomechanical and sensorimotor approaches.**

**Incorrect Answers**

A.  A combination of biomechanical and psychosocial approaches
C.  A combination of acquisitional and motor learning approaches
D.  A combination of psychosocial and neurodevelopmental approaches.

**Rationale:**

The task of writing is a complex process that requires graphomotor, cognitive, language, and visual processing abilities. OT intervention for handwriting problems often requires overlap and collaboration between multiple models and frames of reference. The biomechanical frame of reference is best suited to address the areas of posture, pencil grasp and possible compensatory strategies including environmental and tool adaptations.

**Type of reasoning: Inductive**

One must determine the best intervention approaches for a child with handwriting problems and poor sitting posture in order to arrive at a correct conclusion. This requires inductive reasoning skill. For this case, the approaches that will most effectively address the child's deficits are a combination of biomechanical and sensorimotor approaches. If answered incorrectly, review therapeutic approaches for addressing poor sitting posture and handwriting difficulties in children.

**A122 C4**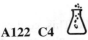

Following medical treatment for a brain tumor, a client is referred to OT home care services. During the initial interview with the OTA, the client reports difficulty locating desired items. For example, at lunchtime the client could not find a can of soup in the pantry. When discussing this self-report with the occupational therapist, which functional ability should the OTA identify as needing further evaluation?

**Correct Answer: A. Visual scanning.**

**Incorrect Answers:**

B.  Visual acuity.
C.  Spatial relations.
D.  Topographical orientation.

**Rationale:**

Visual scanning is the ability to systematically observe and locate items in the environment. Visual acuity is the clarity of both near and far. Spatial relations is the ability to relate objects to each other (i.e., above/below). Topographical orientation is the ability to find one's way in space.

**Type of Reasoning: Analytical**

This question provides symptoms and the test taker must determine the likely cause for them. This is an analytical reasoning skill, as questions of this nature often ask one to analyze a group of symptoms in order to determine a diagnosis. In this situation the symptoms indicate visual scanning deficits, which should be reviewed if answered incorrectly.

402

## A123 C7

An OTA leads a work group at a vocational rehabilitation program for persons with traumatic brain injuries. One member begins to make sexually suggestive comments to other group members. The OTA redirects the client to the work in progress but the member continues to make sexually suggestive statements. Which is the OTA's best initial response to this situation?

**Correct Answer: B. Explain to the client that such statements are not tolerated at work and the client must stop or leave the group.**

**Incorrect Answers:**

A. Explain to the client that such statements are not tolerated at work and call security to have the client removed from the group.

C. End the group before the situation escalates and reschedule the group to meet without the disruptive client.

D. Set the client up at a different work station so the client is not in contact with other group members and cannot disrupt the group's work.

**Rationale:**

This response reinforces the norms of a work environment and gives the individual the opportunity to practice making a decision about the most appropriate course of action. An important aspect of vocational rehabilitation for persons with traumatic brain injuries is the development of appropriate social interaction skills. Ending the group, removing the client from the group, or decreasing contact with others does not address the client's need to develop appropriate interaction skills for work. In addition, the role of the OTA in a vocational rehabilitation program is to act as a work supervisor, enforcing the realities of a work situation. Inappropriate sexual remarks are not tolerated in a work setting. If the client cannot comply with work norms in a vocational program, he/she may need to be referred to a pre-vocational program for basic social skills and work habit training. These basic skills are not the focus of vocational rehabilitation.

**Type of Reasoning: Evaluative**

One must weigh the possible courses of action and then make a value judgment about the best course to take. This requires evaluative reasoning skill, which often utilizes guiding principles of action in order to arrive at a correct conclusion. For this case, the OTA should explain that the client's statements are not tolerated and the client must either stop or leave the group. Refer to group leadership guidelines and reinforcement of group norms if answered incorrectly.

## A124 C8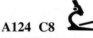

An OTA conducts a home evaluation for an individual with a complete T10 level spinal cord injury. The only entrance to the home has five steps, a total of 35 inches in height. Which ramp length is best for the OTA to recommend the family have constructed?

**Correct Answer: B. 35 feet.**

**Incorrect Answers:**

A. 17½ feet.

C. 48 feet.

D. 70 feet.

**Rationale:**

Accessibility guidelines state that the ramp should be constructed with one foot of ramp length for each inch of rise. The others do not meet these guidelines.

**Type of Reasoning: Deductive**

This question requires recall of guidelines, which is factual knowledge. Deductive reasoning skills are utilized whenever one must recall facts to find ideal solutions. In this situation, accessibility guidelines indicate that for every one inch of rise, there should be one foot of ramp. Review accessibility guidelines if answered incorrectly.

**A125 C8**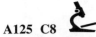

An OTA measures a person for a wheelchair. The widest point across the person's hips and thighs is 16 inches and the greatest length from the person's posterior portion of the buttocks to the popliteal fossa is 18 inches. Which wheelchair seat dimensions should the OTA recommend?

**Correct Answer: D. 18 inches wide by 16 inches deep.**

**Incorrect Answers:**

A. 18 inches wide by 20 inches deep.

B. 18 inches wide by 18 inches deep.

C. 16 inches wide by 18 inches deep.

**Rationale:**

To determine the width of a wheelchair seat, two inches are added to the measurement of the widest point across hips and thighs. This allows for clearance on the sides to prevent rubbing and to allow the individual to wear heavier material clothing without it being cumbersome. To determine the depth of a wheelchair seat, two inches are subtracted from the measurement of the length from the posterior portion of the buttocks to the popliteal fossa. This prevents rubbing and potential decubiti formation in the posterior knee region, while also allowing maximum swing length. In the case, the person's measurements were 16"W x 18"L; therefore, the resulting seat measurement is 18"W x 16"D.

**Type of Reasoning: Deductive**

One must recall the guidelines for wheelchair prescription. This is factual knowledge, which is a deductive reasoning skill. In this situation, because the individual's measurements were 16"W x 18"L, the seat dimensions should be 18"W x 16"L. If answered incorrectly, review wheelchair prescription guidelines.


**A126 C9**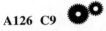

An OTA implements intervention with five patients using a group format. The OTA charges each patient's insurance provider for individual treatments. Which of the following does this action represent?

**Correct Answer: B. A violation of justice.**

**Incorrect Answers:**

A. An example of impairment.

C. An established, accepted practice.

D. A correct action, if group interventions are individualized.

**Rationale:**

Justice is the principle in the AOTA code of ethics which requires all occupational therapy personnel to comply with the laws and regulations guiding the profession and practice of occupational therapy. This includes being truthful in charging for services and meeting legal requirements for documentation. Impairment refers to being under the influence of alcohol, drugs or any substance that compromises judgment and abilities. It also includes personal issues, such as severe emotional distress, which impede the practitioner's abilities to fully engage in the OT process with clients. It is inappropriate and illegal to submit charges for individual treatments if treatment was actually performed in a group.

**Type of Reasoning: Evaluative**

This question requires a value judgment in an ethical situation, which is an evaluative reasoning skill. Following the AOTA Code of Ethics, all therapists should observe justice, which is to comply with all laws and rules, including being truthful in billing for services. Therefore, the billing is a potential violation of justice. Review the AOTA Code of Ethics if answered incorrectly, especially justice guidelines.

## A127 C2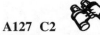

A caregiver support group meets weekly at a senior center. A new member attends the group for the third time and listens intently. The person nods in agreement when others speak, but does not participate verbally. Which action is most effective for the OTA to take to facilitate the individual's engagement in the group?

**Correct Answer: C. Invite the individual to join in the discussion, if the person would like.**

**Incorrect Answers:**

A. Reiterate the group's norm that active participation is expected from all group members.

B. Ask the individual several questions to encourage verbal participation.

D. Refer the individual to the center's social worker for individual, non-group counseling.

**Rationale:**

Inviting the individual to join the discussion acknowledges his/her membership and supports attention and active listening but it does not pressure the person to speak before ready. It can take time for an individual to feel comfortable sharing personal thoughts with a group of people who may have been just acquaintances (or even strangers) prior to this group membership. It is inappropriate to pressure for verbal participation before a person is ready. Individual counseling can be helpful, but it is no substitute for the therapeutic benefits of a group. In addition, group members can benefit from a group discussion without verbally participating. These benefits can include many of Yalom's curative factors including universality, instillation of hope, and the gaining of specific information.

**Type of Reasoning: Inductive**

One must utilize clinical knowledge and judgment to determine the best approach for this group situation. This requires inductive reasoning skill. In this case, because the new member has not initiated conversation, it is best to invite the member to join in the discussion if desired. If answered incorrectly, review group dynamics and methods of facilitating discussion.

## A128 C4

An OTA works with an individual with chest and upper extremity burns. During the intervention session, the client expresses vague fears about personal safety at home and asks the OTA to advocate for an extension in the discharge date. According to the medical record, the client had incurred the burns during a cooking accident. Which is the OTA's best initial response to the client's stated concerns?

**Correct Answer: D. Invite the client to expand upon the nature of these concerns.**

**Incorrect Answers:**

A. Encourage the client to speak to the occupational therapist about discharge plans.

B. Assure the client that pre-discharge fears are normal and expected.

C. Document the client's concerns and recommend an extension of the length of stay.

**Rationale:**

The OTA needs more information to determine the basis for the client's fears and evaluate for appropriate interventions. Referring the client to the occupational therapist can be helpful, but it will not address his/her concerns at this moment. A delay may result in the client deciding that his/her concerns are not worth mentioning. Many clients find it difficult to express fears so it is important to respond immediately when they do. This is of particular importance in cases of domestic violence, which this case (and any case) can have as a contributing and complicating factor. In addition, the client's fears may be functionally based and the OTA can address these immediately in the current intervention session. Assurance that fears are normal and expected does not address the issue at hand. A request to extend a client's length of stay requires a documented need for inpatient services. Client's stated concerns about home safety are not sufficient justification for a length of stay extension.

**Type of Reasoning: Evaluative**

This question requires professional judgment based on guiding principles, which is an evaluative reasoning skill. Because the OTA cannot determine the source of the patient's fears, the OTA should ask for the patient to elaborate on the nature of the concerns. This way the OTA can determine the best initial course of action based on further information. Without further information, clinical decision making is subject to being inaccurate or incomplete.

## A129  C4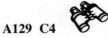

An individual presents with intention tremor, dysmetria, decreased equilibrium and nystagmus caused by a cerebellar lesion. The person expresses difficulty with routine tasks. Which intervention should the OTA provide?

**Correct Answer: D. Upper extremity weight bearing during self care routine at a sink.**

**Incorrect Answers:**

A. A cone and pegboard activity with wrist weights in a seated position to control tremors.

B. Quick stretch to lateral trunk muscles during a functional activity.

C. A power wheelchair to prevent falls during routine activities.

**Rationale:**

The treatment goals for persons with cerebellar dysfunction are focused on strengthening proximal muscles, improving postural responses, and increasing stability. Weight bearing of the upper extremities can increase shoulder girdle stability. A cone and pegboard activity does not describe a functional activity and would not generalize to activities of daily living. This activity is also very difficult to complete with dysmetria and intention tremor. Quick stretch to lateral trunk muscles describes a proprioceptive neuromuscular facilitation (PNF) technique that would be impractical to perform during a functional activity. A power wheelchair is not indicated nor will it help the person perform routine tasks with intention tremors and dysmetria.

**Type of Reasoning: Inductive**

Clinical knowledge and judgment are the most important skills needed for answering this question, which requires inductive reasoning skill. Knowledge of the diagnosis, its presenting symptoms, and the most appropriate clinical outcomes is essential to choosing the best solution. In this case, the OTA should provide upper extremity weight bearing during self care routine at the sink. Review the functional impact of cerebellar lesions and intervention approaches for persons with motor disturbances if answered incorrectly. The integration of this knowledge is required to determine a correct answer.

## A130  C6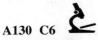

An OTA employed at a day treatment center for clients with psychiatric disorders is conducting a leisure planning group. The members of the group decide to take a day trip to the local sculpture garden. Which side effect of psychotropic medications is most important for the OTA to discuss preventative precautions for with the group?

**Correct Answer: C. Photosensitivity.**

**Incorrect Answers:**

A. Orthostatic hypotension.

B. Akathisia.

D. Tremors.

**Rationale:**

Photosensitivity results in severe sunburn which can occur during an outdoor trip. The other options are potential side effects of medications but they are not exacerbated by being outside.

**Type of reasoning: Deductive**

This question requires the test taker to recall the common precautions for clients using psychotropic medications in order to arrive at a correct conclusion. This requires deductive reasoning skill, where the recall of facts is utilized to draw a correct conclusion. For this situation, the most important precaution to discuss is photosensitivity. Review psychotropic medication side effects and preventative precautions for clients taking psychotropic medications if answered incorrectly.

406

**A131 C8**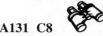

A rehabilitation hospital is interested in starting a driver rehabilitation program. Which must the occupational therapist and OTA hired to develop this program do first?

**Correct Answer: B. Learn the state's driving laws and requirements.**

**Incorrect Answers:**

A. Determine the cost of commercially available driving rehabilitation programs.

C. Develop admission criteria for program participants.

D. Develop a marketing plan to obtain referrals.

**Rationale:**

State laws and regulations regarding the mandatory reporting of driving ability post illness or injury are essential for an occupational therapist and an OTA developing a driver rehabilitation program. The occupational therapist and OTA would need to know state laws and regulations prior to setting admission criteria or a marketing plan. While cost is an important aspect of program development it is not the greatest priority. Knowledge and adherence to state laws are essential to avoid potential program liability.

**Type of Reasoning: Inductive**

Clinical knowledge and judgment are the most important skills needed for answering this question, which requires inductive reasoning skill. In this case, the OTA must first learn the state's driving laws and requirements in order to proceed with development of a driver rehabilitation program. Review program development guidelines, especially driver rehabilitation guidelines if answered incorrectly.

**A132 C3**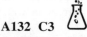

An OTA constructs a splint for a client with a low radial nerve injury to facilitate healing and promote function. What is the most effective splint for the OTA to fabricate for this individual?

**Correct Answer: A. A dynamic extension splint.**

**Incorrect Answers:**

B. A figure-of-eight splint.

C. A dynamic flexion splint.

D. A splint to support the functional position.

**Rationale:**

The presenting signs of a low level radial nerve injury includes incomplete extension of the fingers' and thumb's MP joints. The IP joints are extended by the interossei, but the MP joints rest in about 30 degrees flexion. A dynamic splint that provides wrist, MP, and thumb extension is indicated for radial nerve palsy to prevent over stretching of the extensor tendons during the healing phase. This splint also positions the hand for functional use. A figure-of-eight splint or a dynamic flexion splint is indicated for a combined median ulnar nerve injury. The functional position of wrist extension, MCP's flexion, IP's flexion and thumb abducted is not effective in radial nerve palsy intervention.

**Type of Reasoning: Analytical**

This question provides a description of an injury and the test taker must determine the most appropriate splint to address the injury. This is an analytical reasoning skill, as questions of this nature often ask one to analyze information in order to determine a proper course of action. In this situation the ideal splint to fabricate is a dynamic extensor splint. Review the diagnostic characteristics of nerve injuries and splinting guidelines nerve injuries if answered incorrectly.

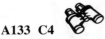

**A133  C4**

An OTA collaborates with the occupational therapist to complete the discharge plan for an individual with a right cerebral vascular accident (CVA) who has completed a three-week inpatient rehabilitation program. The patient is right hand dominant. The patient exhibits residual cognitive perceptual deficits but seems unaware of these problems. Which discharge recommendation is best for the OTA to discuss with the occupational therapist?

**Correct Answer: D. Supervision for cooking.**

**Incorrect Answers:**

A.  An extension of length of stay.
B.  A full-time home health aide.
C.  Assistance with personal care.

**Rationale:**

A right CVA results in left-sided deficits, decreased judgment, and diminished insight. The latter two deficits can pose a safety risk during cooking activities. Therefore, supervision is recommended. Since the person is right hand dominant, the ability to perform many personal tasks will likely remain intact. In addition, it is highly likely that the individual has received intervention to increase the functional abilities of his/her left UE and/or to develop unilateral functional skills during his/her three week rehabilitation program. Therefore, a full-time home health aide, personal care assistance, and an extension of length of stay are not warranted.

**Type of Reasoning: Inductive**

One must utilize clinical knowledge and judgment to determine the recommendation that best considers the person's limitations. This requires inductive reasoning skill. In this case, recommending supervision for cooking is best out of the choices provided as it poses the greatest risk to safety. If answered incorrectly, review intervention planning guidelines and IADL activity adaptations for persons with cognitive deficits and discharge options for persons with disabilities.

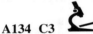

**A134  C3**

An OTA designs a dynamic splint for an individual recovering from a tendon repair. At which angle should the OTA position the outrigger?

**Correct Answer: B. 90 degrees to the joint.**

**Incorrect Answers:**

A.  45 degrees to the joint.
C.  60 degrees to the joint.
D.  110 degrees to the joint.

**Rationale:**

90 degrees is the appropriate angle of pull for it provides the most effective application of force. The application of a perpendicular force prevents unwanted traction on the joint and shearing stress. As the person's condition improves and mobility increases, the OTA must adjust the outrigger to maintain the 90 degree angle of pull.

**Type of Reasoning: Deductive**

One must recall the guidelines for dynamic splinting and angle of pull. This is factual knowledge, which is a deductive reasoning skill. 90 degrees is the appropriate angle of pull for this situation. If answered incorrectly, review guidelines for dynamic splinting, especially angle of pull after tendon repair.

408

## A135 C7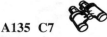

A client successfully completes a work hardening program to return to work as a cable installer and repair person. The client has residual moderate impairment in temperature perception. During the discharge planning session, the OTA discusses how this impairment may impact areas of occupation and suggests activity modifications to facilitate the client's occupational performance. What is the most appropriate recommendation for the OTA to make to the client?

**Correct Answer: C. Wear work gloves for activities involving extremes or variations in temperature.**

**Incorrect Answers:**

A.  Request reassignment to work activities that do not involve exposure to extreme temperatures.

B.  Mark all potentially hot objects at home and at work with bright stickers.

D.  Wear a protective splint during the work day and at home during home maintenance tasks.

**Rationale:**

The client should wear work gloves because of the danger of incurring a burn because of diminished temperature sensation. The work gloves can also protect the client's hands during extreme cold situations. As a cable installer and repair person, the essential functions of the client's job will frequently require him/her to work outdoors in all types of weather conditions. Reassigning the client is not needed since he/she developed the skills needed to adequately perform all essential work tasks in the work hardening program. During the performance of work tasks, the client can easily compensate for sensory deficits by wearing work gloves. Since there is no co-morbidity of a cognitive deficit, the client can be expected to be able to remember to don gloves to protect the hands when he/she judges a situation may involve extremes or variations in temperature. A splint would provide inadequate protection because it would not fully cover all surfaces of the hand.

**Type of Reasoning: Inductive**

The test taker must determine which recommendation most effectively addresses the client's current status and limitations. Because temperature perception is impaired, wearing work gloves when involved in activities that may involve extremes or variations in temperature is best to protect the client from injury. If answered incorrectly review recommendations for temperature impairments and guidelines for adaptations of work tasks.

## A136 C6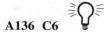

An OTA develops a task group for the patients of a psychiatric inpatient unit. The OTA considers several activities to use for the group's first session. Which activity is best for the OTA to present to the group members?

**Correct Answer: B. Decorating styrofoam cups and planting cuttings in them.**

**Incorrect Answers:**

A.  Planning a pizza party for the weekend.

C.  Publishing a weekly newsletter about city attractions for patients on the unit.

D.  Painting a large mural to cover one wall of the day room.

**Rationale:**

Decorating cups and planting cuttings is a simple concrete task, which can be structured to ensure successful completion by individuals with acute psychiatric disorders. In addition, individuals on an acute unit have a short length of stay and require activities that can be completed in one session. The other choices require multiple sessions, which are not realistic on an inpatient unit.

**Type of Reasoning: Inferential**

One must determine the most appropriate activity for an initial group session, given knowledge of the treatment setting. This requires inferential reasoning skill, where one must infer or draw conclusions about a best course of action. In this situation, the OTA should choose decorating Styrofoam cups and planting cuttings in them as a first activity. If answered incorrectly, review group activities for inpatient psychiatric settings.

## A137  C2

An OTA reviews the positioning protocol for a premature infant with severe spastic cerebral palsy with the infant's parents. The protocol is in a written format. During the review, the OTA notices that the parents do not seem able to follow along with the protocol's text. Which action is best for the OTA to take initially in response to this observation?

**Correct Answer: A. Ask the parents if they have any concerns about positioning their infant.**

**Incorrect Answers:**

B.  Ask the parents if they can read English.

C.  Include pictures of proper positioning in the protocol.

D.  Demonstrate proper positioning techniques.

**Rationale:**

This is an open-ended question that enables the parents to express any concerns that they may have about positioning their infant. These concerns may be comprehension related and/or task related. Caring for a child with severe physical disabilities can be overwhelming and the parents perceived difficulties in following the written protocol may be due to emotional stress, not limitations in literacy. The parents may welcome the opportunity to express their concerns. The other choices are close-ended and do not facilitate an open dialogue. If the parents have difficulty understanding English or if they could benefit from pictures and/or demonstrated positions, they can express this in response to the OTA's open invitation to express concerns.

**Type of Reasoning: Evaluative**

This question requires professional judgment based on guiding principles, which is an evaluative reasoning skill. Because the OTA cannot completely determine the source of the parents' difficulty, the OTA should ask if there are any concerns about positioning the infant. This way the OTA can invite the parents to share any concerns in an open-ended fashion without delineating the specific challenge.

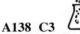

## A138  C3

An OTA evaluates a client's pain by asking the client which movements or activities elicit pain. Which of the following is the OTA assessing?

**Correct Answer: D. The triggers of pain.**

**Incorrect Answers:**

A.  The quality of pain.

B.  The location of pain.

C.  The intensity of pain.

**Rationale:**

Pain triggers are those activities and/or movements that result in pain. The quality of pain is determined by asking the person to describe the pain; common descriptors are sharp, throbbing, burning, tender, and shooting. The intensity of pain is measured by pain scales; a 0 to 10 scale is most commonly used. The location of pain is determined by having the person describe or point to the location.

**Type of Reasoning: Analytical**

This question provides a description of a functional activity and the test taker must determine the likely definition of such an activity. This is an analytical reasoning skill, as questions of this nature often ask one to analyze descriptors of functional skills to determine the overall skill involved. In this situation the activity is assessing pain triggers, which should be reviewed if answered incorrectly.

410

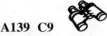

## A139 C9

An OTA recently attended a two-day splinting workshop. The OTA asks the OT supervisor for a caseload that includes more clients that require splinting interventions. Which action is best for the OTA's supervisor to take in response to this request?

**Correct Answer: C. Establish the OTA's service competency in splinting.**

**Incorrect Answers:**

A. Decline the request because splinting is an advanced practice skill.

B. Ask the OTA to give an in-service about splinting to demonstrate acquired knowledge.

D. Collaborate with the OTA and other members of the OT department to distribute the department's caseload to meet the OTA's request.

**Rationale:**

The establishment of service competency is required before the OTA takes on a new task. This ensures that the OTA will achieve the same intervention outcome as the occupational therapist. If service competency is established, splinting is not considered an advanced skill. Providing an in-service can demonstrate knowledge but it does not provide adequate information about the OTA's intervention abilities. Service competency must be established prior to revising the OTA's caseload.

**Type of Reasoning: Inductive**

This question requires one to determine the best approach for responding to the OTA's request. This requires inductive reasoning skill, where clinical judgment is paramount to arriving at a correct conclusion. For this situation, the OTA's supervisor should first establish that the OTA is competent to perform the delivery of splinting services. Review service competency and supervisory guidelines if answered incorrectly.

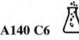

## A140 C6

An individual diagnosed with schizophrenia, undifferentiated type is referred to a partial hospitalization program. During the initial orientation session, the OTA observes that the client responds to each topic by consistently returning to the focus of the first topic. Each time the OTA introduces a new topic the client ignores this topic and returns to the original topical focus. When documenting the client's behavior, which of the following is most accurate for the OTA to report the client is demonstrating?

**Correct Answer: B. Perseveration.**

**Incorrect Answers:**

A. Thought blocking.

C. Obsessive thinking.

D. Poverty of speech.

**Rationale:**

Perseveration is a persistent focus on a previous topic or behavior after a new topic or behavior is introduced. Thought blocking is the interruption of a thought process before it's carried to completion. Obsessive thinking involves the persistence of an illogical thought. Poverty of speech is speech that is limited in amount and content.

**Type of Reasoning: Analytical**

This question provides symptoms and the test taker must determine the likely cause for them. This is an analytical reasoning skill, as questions of this nature often ask one to analyze a group of symptoms in order to determine a diagnosis. In this situation the symptoms indicate perseveration, which should be reviewed if answered incorrectly.

**A141  C5**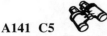

A person is diagnosed with chronic obstructive pulmonary disease (COPD). The OTA instructs the individual on breathing exercises to use to control respiration rate during activities. The OTA tells the person to inhale as if smelling roses. How should the OTA tell the person to exhale?

**Correct Answer: C. As if flickering a lit candle.**

**Incorrect Answers:**

A.  As if blowing out 20 lit candles on a birthday cake.

B.  As if blowing forcibly to relight a dying campfire.

D.  In quick short, multiple breaths.

**Rationale:**

When one exhales to flicker a lit candle, one uses pursed lip breathing. Pursed lip breathing is a method of controlled breathing which requires the individual to purse his/her lips while exhaling. This slows the exhalation process and improves the carbon dioxide exchange. This decreases one's rate of breathing and prevents airway collapse. The other descriptions do not result in pursed lip breathing.

**Type of Reasoning: Inductive**

This question requires one to determine the best approach for performing exercises for COPD. This requires inductive reasoning skill, where clinical judgment is paramount to arriving at a correct conclusion. For this situation, the person should exhale as if flickering a lit candle. If answered incorrectly, review breathing exercises, including pursed lip breathing, for persons with cardiopulmonary disorders.

**A142  C8**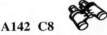

After six months of rehabilitation for a T-2 spinal cord injury, a patient is being discharged. The OTA conducts a home visit to evaluate accessibility. The individual lives with two roommates in an apartment in a private home. The doorway measurements currently range from 30 to 32 inches throughout the apartment. The patient's landlord is amenable to make changes in the apartment but has no financial resources. Which recommendation is best for the OTA to make for independent accessibility in the apartment?

**Correct Answer: A. Install offset hinges on all doors.**

**Incorrect Answers:**

B.  Remove doorframes of doorways less than 32 inches and install wider frames.

C.  Remove all doors except for the apartment's entrance door.

D.  Remove all doorframes and install 36 inch wide doorframes.

**Rationale:**

Offset hinges can increase a doorway's width by 2 inches, which would result in all doorways meeting or exceeding minimum accessibility standards. It is not necessary to widen the doorways any further. In addition, physically removing doorframes and then installing wider ones is costly. This extra expense is not warranted. While the removal of all doors can increase accessibility it also eliminates privacy, which may not be desirable when living with two other individuals.

**Type of Reasoning: Inductive**

Clinical knowledge and judgment are the most important skills needed for answering this question, which requires inductive reasoning skill. Reasoning the most realistic and cost effective solution to the problem at hand is important in choosing the best solution. In this case, the best solution is to install offset hinges on all doors. Review home adaptations for persons who use wheelchairs if answered incorrectly.

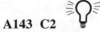

**A143 C2**

An OTA documents an individual's performance during a stress management group. According to established documentation standards, which statement should the OTA include in the daily progress note?

**Correct Answer: B. The client was able to identify three current life stressors.**

Incorrect Answers:

A. The client completed the checklist of stressors in an appropriate amount of time.

C. The client appeared upset and tense throughout the session.

D. The client stated walking is a relaxing and enjoyable activity.

**Rationale:**

Documentation must be specific, measurable and behavioral. In this scenario, it must provide information that is objective and related to the individual's performance in the group. Timely completion of an assessment does not include sufficient information about the client's performance. More specific information would need to be provided to meet documentation standards (e.g. client became upset when discussing the stress of single parenthood while having an exacerbation of multiple sclerosis). The identification of an enjoyable and relaxing activity can be relevant information to include in documentation but this statement does not directly address the person's performance in the group. In addition, more specific information would need to be provided to meet documentation standards (e.g., client states he/she goes for long walks when stressed). The report of a client appearing 'upset' is subjective and does not meet documentation standards.

**Type of Reasoning: Inferential**

One must determine the most appropriate statement to include in a progress note regarding a client in a stress management group. Established standards for documentation require notes to be specific, measurable, and behavioral. Therefore, the OTA would most appropriately document the client's ability to identify three current life stressors. If answered incorrectly, documentation guidelines should be reviewed.

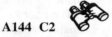

**A144 C2**

An OTA is asked, at the last minute, to assist another OTA with a problem-solving skills group. Which is the most helpful action for the OTA to take?

**Correct Answer: C. Support the leader with comments and questions that keep the group on focus.**

**Incorrect Answers:**

A. Split the group in two and have each OTA work with his/her own group.

B. Participate as a member of the group and supply the desired responses.

D. Act as an observer and take notes for documentation.

**Rationale:**

The role of assisting a group leader is to facilitate participation of the members and the achievement of the goals of the group. Splitting members into two groups would result in the assisting OTA having no knowledge of the group's history, process or goals. In addition, the existing leader would receive no input from a co-leader. The benefit of receiving feedback from a co-leader is likely the precipitant for the group leader asking the OTA to participate. Participating as a member, an observer, and/or a recorder also do not provide any co-leadership benefits.

**Type of Reasoning: Inductive**

Clinical knowledge and judgment are the most important skills needed for answering this question, which requires inductive reasoning skill. Knowledge of the group processes and effective co-leadership are essential to choosing the best solution. In this case, the OTA should support the leader with comments and questions that keep the group on focus. If answered incorrectly, review effective group co-leadership strategies.

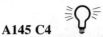

**A145 C4**

An occupational therapist and OTA plan intervention for an individual with cognitive perceptual deficits. In deciding whether to use a dynamic interactional approach or a deficit-specific approach which is most important for the occupational therapist and OTA to consider?

**Correct Answer: A. The client's auditory processing skills.**

**Incorrect Answers:**

B. The availability of familial support.

C. The client's social interaction skills.

D. The client's problem solving skills.

**Rationale:**

The dynamic interactional approach utilizes awareness questioning to help the individual detect errors, estimate task difficulty, and predict outcomes. Therefore, the occupational therapist and OTA must consider the client's level of auditory processing skills to determine if adaptations or modifications are needed when implementing this approach. If an individual has severe auditory processing deficits, it may indicate a need to use a deficit-specific approach, for cognitive perceptual remediation. Family support, social interaction skills and problem solving skills can all influence intervention, but they are not determining factors in selecting which theoretical approach to use in this case.

**Type of Reasoning: Inferential**

One must link the dynamic interactional approach to the functional skill in order to determine which skill is most important to consider. This requires inferential reasoning, where one must consider the primary features of the dynamic interactional approach and then determine the skill that is primarily utilized. In this case auditory processing is the most utilized skill. Review the dynamic interactional approach if answered incorrectly.

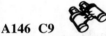

**A146 C9**

At a home care intervention planning meeting, the team discusses a client with a right CVA. The physical therapist states the individual's ambulatory status is now within functional limits. Physical therapy services will be discontinued because the person is no longer homebound. The OTA reports that the individual is frequently confused during home management task performance and becomes extremely anxious when community activities are discussed. Which recommendation should the OTA make?

**Correct Answer: B. Continue OT services as the person should continue to be considered homebound.**

**Incorrect Answers:**

A. Refer the individual to a psychiatrist for a mental status evaluation.

C. Discontinue OT services as they are nonreimbursable since the person is no longer considered homebound.

D. Contact the physician to discuss the need for OT services on an outpatient basis and for psychosocial counseling.

**Rationale:**

The individual can be considered homebound for cognitive and psychosocial deficits. Discontinuing services can place the individual at risk because the person will not receive evaluation or intervention for his/her demonstrated cognitive and psychosocial deficits. There is no need for a consultation with a physician at this point. OT practitioners can continue to provide services in this scenario without physician input.

**Type of Reasoning: Inductive**

Clinical knowledge and judgment are the most important skills needed for answering this question, which requires inductive reasoning skill. Knowledge of the diagnosis and best courses of action is essential to choosing the best solution. In this case, because the person is considered homebound for cognitive and psychosocial deficits, the team's best approach is to continue OT services. Review home health care treatment guidelines and criteria for homebound status if answered incorrectly.

414

## A147 C3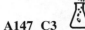

An OTA works with a survivor of a house fire. The client has burns on both hands that limit thumb mobility. The client identifies a personal goal of being able to pick up and hold cans to enable independent shopping and meal preparation activities. The OTA collaborates with the occupational therapist to establish a long-term goal for the client. Which movement of the thumb should the goal statement include as the desired functional outcome?

**Correct Answer: A. CMC palmar abduction.**

**Incorrect Answers:**

B.  CMC extension.

C.  MCP flexion.

D.  IP flexion.

**Rationale:**

CMC palmar abduction is the major movement required of the thumb to pick up cans. CMC extension places the thumb in a hitchhiking position which makes picking up a can very difficult. MCP and IP flexion alone will not expand the web space to pick up a can.

**Type of Reasoning: Analytical**

This question provides a description of a functional activity and the test taker must determine the major movement that is required in performing this functional activity. This is an analytical reasoning skill, as questions of this nature often ask one to analyze functional skills to determine the overall skill involved. In this situation the functional activity is performed using CMC palmar abduction and should be the focus of the long-term goal. Review movement patterns of the thumb if answered incorrectly.

## A148 C6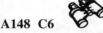

A recent high school graduate diagnosed with depression and anorexia nervosa attends an evening work adjustment group for 90 minutes each week. The client states that this group is the only activity engaged in outside of work. The OTA collaborates with the client to develop a plan to increase involvement in personally meaningful non-work activities. The client expresses interests in exercise and volunteerism and reports past roles to have included captain of the high school swim team, competitive tennis player, and volunteer in an after-school activities program for young children. Which of the following is the best resource for the OTA to recommend the client explore?

**Correct Answer: C. A local community center for volunteer opportunities.**

**Incorrect Answers:**

A.  A local fitness center for exercise classes.

B.  The town swimming pool for open swimming sessions.

D.  An area soup kitchen for volunteer opportunities.

**Rationale:**

This suggestion can facilitate the client's stated altruistic interests while providing a diversity of potential activity pursuits. Exercise and swimming can be contraindicated for persons with anorexia nervosa because they often engage in these activities in an excessive (sometimes self-abusive) manner that is counterproductive to healthy leisure. Volunteering in a soup kitchen is altruistic but persons recovering from eating disorders often find food-related activities difficult.

**Type of Reasoning: Inductive**

One must utilize clinical knowledge and judgment to determine the most best avocational resource for this patient. In this case, given an understanding of the nature of anorexia, the OTA should explore the local community center for volunteer opportunities. If answered incorrectly, review the diagnostic criteria and behavioral manifestations of eating disorders and depression and intervention guidelines for avocational/leisure activities. The integration of this knowledge is required to correctly answer this question.

**A149  C6**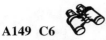

A young adult admitted to a locked inpatient psychiatric unit is referred to occupational therapy. The referral states that the client is exhibiting symptoms of bipolar disorder, manic episode, with anxiety. Which approach is best for the OTA to use to engage the client in the occupational therapy program?

**Correct Answer: D. In a cooking group, have the client cut shapes to construct a gingerbread house using templates and written directions.**

**Incorrect Answers:**

A. In a scrapbooking group, encourage the client to make a page using shared decorative paper, stickers, and pens to create a unique design.

B. Ask the client to help decorate the unit for an upcoming holiday using supplies from a storage box of last year's decorations.

C. Monitor how the client engages in the unit chores of tidying magazines in the day room, replacing furniture, and cleaning the dining table.

**Rationale:**

Choosing a structured activity with clearly defined task steps is a good choice. Because bipolar disorder interferes with executive functions of the brain, structuring the activity with directions and patterns would lessen information processing demands and lend itself to greater potential for success. Additionally, this activity can be individualized so the client works on the task alone in a parallel group or in an assembly line fashion in a project group. This action would allow for the activity to be meaningful, graded for task demands and social interaction, and organized to minimize stress. The client in a manic phase of bipolar disorder would approach the tasks of scrapbooking and decorating the unit in a disorganized manner. During scrapbooking, the client would have difficulty negotiating for shared materials and supplies, making the task difficult for other group members. The resulting psychosocial reactions would present a challenging group dynamic for the OTA to manage using therapeutic use of self. This action would not be helpful to the client or group members. The task of decorating the unit has not been structured to facilitate goal attainment for this client. Instead, it can contribute to the client's mania by its lack of structure, unclear definition of roles for client participation, and laissez-faire leadership approach. The aim of inpatient hospitalization is to facilitate symptom management, so this is not a good action. Unit chores simulate home management activities, but in this action, they are not structured as a therapeutic intervention. Instead, there is little structure other than the outcome needed to keep the unit in order. Monitoring is not a therapeutic role, so this would not be a good example of occupational therapy.

**Type of reasoning: Inductive**

This question requires one to determine the best therapeutic approach for a client to promote engagement in OT programming. This is an inductive reasoning skill; as clinical judgment is utilized in determine a therapeutic course of action. For this case, the OTA should have the client cut shapes to construct a gingerbread house using templates and written directions in a cooking group. If answered incorrectly, review structured activities for clients with bipolar disorder.

**A150  C3**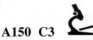

An OTA constructs a dorsal forearm splint. Which is the most appropriate length for this splint?

**Correct Answer: C. Two thirds of the forearm.**

**Incorrect Answers:**

A. One fourth of the forearm.

B. One third of the forearm.

D. One half of the forearm.

**Rationale:**

A major splinting principle is to decrease pressure and distribute weight by having a long wide splint base. The two-thirds length accomplishes this goal. The other measurements are too short.

**Type of Reasoning: Deductive**

One must recall the guidelines for construction of dorsal forearm splints, which is factual knowledge. This requires deductive reasoning skill. In this situation, a forearm based splint should be two thirds the length of the forearm. Review splinting principles for constructing forearm based splints if answered incorrectly.

416

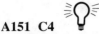

## A151 C4

An adult with multiple sclerosis receives home-based OT intervention to address IADL deficits and functional mobility impairments. During intervention, which of the following should the OTA do?

**Correct Answer: A. Observe the individual for signs of visual difficulties.**

**Incorrect Answers:**

B. Treat the individual in the afternoon.
C. Increase activity tolerance just beyond the point of fatigue.
D. Encourage consistent performance from day to day.

**Rationale:**

Individuals with MS often experience visual difficulties, including partial blindness, nystagmus, eye pain, and/or diplopia. Since these visual difficulties can significantly impact on the safe performance of IADL and functional mobility, the OTA should consistently observe the client for any indications of a visual impairment. There is nothing in the scenario to indicate what time of day is best for this person's intervention sessions. Patients with MS tend to have periods of fatigue during the day. For many persons, this fatigue will occur in the afternoon. OT services are best provided when the patient has more energy. In MS, fatigue inhibits recovery and can contribute to exacerbations; therefore, it should be avoided. The OTA should stop activities prior to reaching the point of fatigue to allow recovery and prevent exacerbations. MS is characterized by fluctuations in performance so consistency is not a realistic goal. The OTA should accommodate intervention sessions to allow for daily changes in the person's functional level and fluctuating abilities.

**Type of Reasoning: Inferential**

One must have knowledge of multiple sclerosis and the visual limitations that often occur with the diagnosis in order to choose the approach that will have the most beneficial outcome. This is an inferential reasoning skill where one must infer or draw conclusions about a potential course of action. For this situation, the OTA should monitor the client for signs of visual difficulties. If answered incorrectly, review treatment approaches for patients with MS.

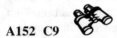

## A152 C9

An OTA accepts a position at an adult day care and respite program for elders with a variety of physical and cognitive disabilities. The OTA only has clinical experience in school-based practice. Which is the most effective way for the OTA to prepare for the professional responsibilities this new position will entail?

**Correct Answer: B. Review current literature on evidence-based elder care.**

**Incorrect Answers:**

A. Attend caregiver support group meetings.
C. Review area demographic information on elders with disabilities.
D. Confer with the program's administrative director.

**Rationale:**

The OTA must update his/her knowledge base about current evidence-based practices in the care of the elderly with an emphasis on physical and cognitive disabilities. A review of the professional literature can provide relevant information about effective evaluation and intervention approaches for the setting's population. Attending a caregiver group will provide information about caregiver needs but this is not the most important area for the OTA to acquire knowledge about for this new position. Information about demographics is too broad. The program's administrative director can provide relevant information about the setting's policies, but he/she would not be able to provide information on the practice of occupational therapy.

**Type of Reasoning: Inductive**

This question requires one to determine the most effective approach for preparing for an entry-level job role. This requires inductive reasoning skill, where clinical judgment is paramount to arriving at a correct conclusion. For this situation, the OTA should prepare by reviewing current OT literature on evidence-based elder care. Review importance of evidence-based practice if answered incorrectly.

**A153 C2**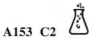

A cooking group meets for 1½ hours each week at a partial hospitalization program. During the group, members do not smoke, they wait for everyone to be served before eating, and they clean up after the meal. When reporting these observations, which of the following is the most accurate statement for the OTA to make?

**Correct Answer: B. Group norms are being followed.**

**Incorrect Answers:**

A. The group protocol is clear.

C. Group sanctions are effective.

D. A diversity of group roles is evident.

**Rationale:**

Group norms are the expected and accepted behaviors in a group. These norms establish an atmosphere of mutual respect, safety, and support. Sanctions are implemented only in a group if members' behaviors fall outside of the group's norms and are considered deviant. The scenario does not provide sufficient information to determine members' group roles. A group protocol outlines the group's membership criteria, goals, and activities.

**Type of Reasoning: Analytical**

This question provides a description of a functional activity and the test taker must determine the likely definition of such an activity. This is an analytical reasoning skill, as questions of this nature often ask one to analyze descriptors of functional skills to determine the overall skill involved. In this situation the activity demonstrates that group norms are being followed. Review guidelines for establishing group norms if answered incorrectly.

**A154 C9**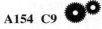

An adult with hereditary ataxia receives home care occupational therapy services. Recently, the client has become more withdrawn and the client's spouse has become more verbal about caregiver strain. During an intervention session, the OTA works with the client on attaining the goal of dressing independently. The OTA notices and comments on several large bruises on the middle section of the client's back. The client tearfully states that a bad fall that morning had caused these and that the progression of the ataxia is becoming too difficult to handle. Which action is best for the OTA to take in response to the observed bruises and the client's statements?

**Correct Answer: D. Supportively question the client about the incident.**

**Incorrect Answers:**

A. Provide reassurance and support of the client's legitimate feelings of loss.

B. Conduct an evaluation of the home to remove items that can contribute to falls.

C. Report the incident to the local domestic violence hotline.

**Rationale:**

While persons with ataxia often do fall resulting in bruises, it would require a very unusual fall to incur bruises in the middle of the back. The possibility that the injuries were the result of an incident of domestic violence must be seriously considered given the location of the injury and the increasing evidence of caregiver strain. The client may respond to the OT's supportive questioning and share concerns. Due to the serious nature of domestic violence, the OT must provide the client with this opportunity to disclose. Providing reassurance and conducting a home evaluation may be relevant to the case, but they do not assess the immediate need to determine if the individual is a victim of domestic violence. Contacting the domestic violence hotline when a client has not disclosed this as a problem is premature since a shelter can only work with persons who self-disclose. This action could increase the client's fear of disclosure and escalate the situation.

**Type of Reasoning: Evaluative**

This question requires a value judgment in an ethical situation, which is an evaluative reasoning skill. In this situation, there is evidence of injury, which could be caused by abuse rather than a fall. Ethical situations such as these often rely upon guiding principles of action to choose best courses of action. Because the potential for abuse exists, the OTA's best course of action is to supportively question the client about the incident. Review guidelines for addressing and following up on suspected abuse if answered incorrectly.

**A155 C1**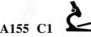

During an occupational therapy session, the OTA observes that a child bangs objects on a tabletop but has difficulty physically letting go of a toy upon request. The OTA documents these behaviors. Which developmental level would be most accurate for the OTA to report the child's observed behaviors indicates?

**Correct Answer: D. 3-4 months.**

**Incorrect Answers:**

A. 7-8 months.

B. 9-10 months.

C. 11-12 months.

**Rationale:**

At 3-4 months, children are able to bang toys on a tabletop but they do not have a voluntary release. At 7-8 months children begin to be able to give up objects with an assisted release, and at 9-10 months there is more efficient release. One-year children have a voluntary release.

**Type of Reasoning: Deductive**

One must recall the developmental guidelines for children in banging toys and lack of a voluntary release. This is factual knowledge, which is a deductive reasoning skill. The functional activity described is a skill at 3-4 months developmentally. If answered incorrectly, review developmental milestones of infants in gross motor and fine motor skills.

**A156 C8**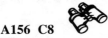

An OTA provides caregiver education to the spouse of a client with Alzheimer's disease and a secondary diagnosis of left CVA. The client is dependent upon a wheelchair for mobility and has been deemed cognitively incompetent. The spouse reports that the client becomes restless at meal times, consistently undoes the lap belt, and tries to get up from the wheelchair. The spouse reports that the need to constantly say "sit down" is personally exhausting and often increases the client's agitation. Frequently, neither one eats dinner. Which is the most effective recommendation for the OTA to make to the spouse?

**Correct Answer: B. Use a wheelchair lap tray to serve several smaller meals to the client at intervals throughout the day.**

**Incorrect Answers:**

A. Allow the spouse to get up when restless and provide dinner to the client at a later time.

C. Hire a home care attendant to assist the client at meal times and provide some respite to the spouse.

D. Use a wheelchair lap tray to serve the client large meals at breakfast, lunch, and dinner.

**Rationale:**

The client must be considered at risk for falling if he/she is allowed to get up because a person deemed dependent upon a wheelchair for mobility has significant motor deficits. A lap tray is a permissible and reasonable restraint if it is necessary to maintain a person's safety, if it allows for increased function, and if less restrictive restraints have been attempted. A family member can approve the use of this device if a person is not cognitively intact. These criteria apply to this case. A lap belt has been applied but it has not been successful. A lap tray with food on it can provide physical and sensory cues necessary to keep the client seated for a time that is sufficient for eating a small meal. It is advisable to provide small meals at frequent intervals rather than three large meals when a person has significant cognitive impairments. Hiring a home care attendant can relieve the spouse's caregiver stress, but it does not address the client's risk of falling when attempting to get up from the wheelchair. It is unlikely that this behavior would cease for a home care attendant.

**Type of Reasoning: Inductive**

Clinical knowledge and judgment are the most important skills needed for answering this question, which requires inductive reasoning skill. Knowledge of the diagnosis and most effective recommendations is essential to choosing the best solution. In this case, recommending use of a lap tray to serve several smaller meals throughout the day is most appropriate. If answered incorrectly, review treatment guidelines for persons with Alzheimer's disease and principles of fall prevention and restraint reduction.

## A157 C3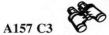

A person incurred a traumatic above elbow amputation to the non-dominant upper extremity. The client establishes a goal to be independent in all ADL using the residual limb without a prosthesis; however, the limb is painful and very sensitive. What should the OTA include in the OT intervention program?

**Correct Answer: A. Train the client in the use of adaptive strategies and/or equipment to perform ADL.**

**Incorrect Answers:**

B. Refer the client to an amputee support group to facilitate acceptance of the need for a prosthesis to attain ADL independence.

C. Implement an exercise program to focus on strengthening muscles that will enable the effective use of a prosthesis.

D. Teach the client to protectively wrap the residual limb with an elastic bandage in a circular manner to decrease pain and manage hypersensitivity.

**Rationale:**

There are many techniques that the client can learn to independently perform ADL. The client can learn to use the dominant intact UE to perform unilateral tasks using adaptive equipment such as a rocker knife to cut meat. Instruction on the use of the residual non-dominant UE as a stabilizer and/or assist during task performance can also be very effective (e.g., stabilizing clothing to enable the fastening of closures) in attaining independence in ADL. Many unilateral amputees function independently without a prosthesis and this is the client's stated goal. Ignoring this preference by referring the person to a support group or implementing an exercise program is a violation of the OT ethical principle of autonomy. Wrapping a residual limb with an elastic bandage in a circular manner is a major contraindication in amputee care. This action would cause a tourniquet effect and dangerously restrict the limb's circulation. The wrapping of a residual limb should be done in a figure-of-eight diagonal pattern going from a distal to proximal direction with greater pressure applied at the distal end of the limb. The OTA should treat the client's pain and hypersensitivity with established intervention methods. Pain management techniques can include relaxation techniques, alternative exercise programs (e.g., aquatics, Tai Chi), and physical agent modalities. Methods of desensitization can include the application of diverse textures to the limb, massage, and tapping.

**Type of reasoning: Inductive**

This question requires one to determine a best course of action, based on knowledge of upper extremity amputations and adaptive strategies without use of a prosthesis. This necessitates clinical judgment, which is an inductive reasoning skill. For this case, the OTA should train the client in the use of adaptive strategies and/or equipment to perform ADL. If answered incorrectly, review principles of pre-prosthetic and prosthetic training for patients with upper extremity amputations.

## A158 C9

An OTA provides early intervention services to a three year-old child with left spastic hemiplegia due to cerebral palsy. During a session, the OTA observes behaviors that seem to indicate the presence of visual deficits. In discussing these observations with the occupational therapist, which recommendation should the OTA make?

**Correct Answer: D. A referral of the child to an optometrist.**

**Incorrect Answers:**

A. The completion of a motor-free visual perceptual assessment.

B. The completion of a developmental vision assessment.

C. A referral of the child to an optician.

**Rationale:**

Prior to conducting a visual perceptual evaluation, an anatomical visual assessment to determine visual acuity is required. Optometrists are the professionals who are qualified to perform eye examinations to determine visual acuity, level of visual impairments, and damage to or disease in the visual system.

**Type of Reasoning: Evaluative**

One must weigh the possible courses of action and then make a value judgment about the best course to take. This requires evaluative reasoning skill, which often utilizes guiding principles of action in order to arrive at a correct conclusion. For this case, because the child demonstrates visual deficits, the OTA should discuss with the occupational therapist the need to refer the child to an optometrist.

## A159 C4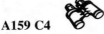

A person who incurred a traumatic brain injury and multiple fractures in a motor vehicle accident has been receiving hospital-based OT services for four weeks. Currently, the patient is highly distractible, forgetful, and confused and often repeats the same questions throughout the day. The patient's family and friends visit consistently and have asked the OTA for an activity recommendation that they can do with the patient during visiting hours. Which activity is best for the OTA to recommend?

**Correct Answer: C. Reviewing the patient's memory picture book of familiar people and activities.**

**Incorrect Answers:**

A. Playing a simple board game that is familiar from the patient's childhood.

B. Watching a TV show that the patient had enjoyed prior to the accident with the patient.

D. Playing a matching card game that includes pictures of the patient's past interests.

**Rationale:**

The individual's behavior is indicative of Stage V, Confused-Inappropriate on the Rancho Level of Cognitive Functioning Scale. Due to the presence of confusion and the patient's high level of distractibility playing a board or card game or watching TV are activities that are too high level at this point. Reviewing the patient's memory book enables family and friends to reinforce the patient's identification of pictures that are meaningful to him/her and can serve as a precipitant to relevant focused conversation about familiar people and favorite activities. This review can help with the patient's cognitive rehabilitation as it can answer many of his/her repeated questions. Introducing activities that are stimulating (watching TV) or multi-step (games) may increase confusion which can contribute to agitation.

**Type of Reasoning: Inductive**

One must utilize clinical knowledge and judgment to determine the best activity for this client. This is an inductive reasoning skill. In this case, reviewing the patient's memory picture book of familiar people and activities is best. If answered incorrectly, review characteristics of Stage V Rancho Level of Cognitive Functioning and effective activities for persons with cognitive impairments.

## A160 C5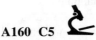

An OTA provides services to a homeless shelter which includes residents who are HIV positive. The OTA conducts several activity groups. Which should the OTA do while working with this population?

**Correct Answer: A. Wash hands before and after each group session.**

**Incorrect Answers:**

B. Always wear latex gloves during groups.

C. Wear latex gloves when handling food.

D. Implement transmission-based precautions.

**Rationale:**

Health professionals should use standard precautions at all times, regardless of clients' diagnoses. Washing hands is a basic precautionary step all individuals should take to prevent the spread of infections and diseases (even in their own homes). The diagnosis of HIV is irrelevant to the question's correct answer for HIV is transmitted only through the exchange of body fluids. See Chapter 9. Wearing gloves while handling food is a health department regulation but it only addresses sessions involving food. One must still wash one's hands before and after glove use. In addition, due to potential latex allergies, health care environments must be latex-free. Transmission-based precautions are used when the route(s) of transmission is (are) not completely interrupted using standard precautions alone. For some diseases that have multiple routes of transmission (e.g., SARS), more than one transmission-based precaution category may be used. Transmission-based precautions have three categories: contact precautions, droplet precautions, and airborne precautions. None of these are indicated for HIV. See Chapter 3 for comprehensive information about standard and transmission-based precautions

**Type of Reasoning: Deductive**

This question requires recall of guidelines and principles, which is factual knowledge. Deductive reasoning skills are utilized whenever one must recall facts to solve everyday problems. In this situation, the OTA should follow standard precautions, which includes washing hands before and after each group session. Review standard precautions if answered incorrectly.

## A161 C9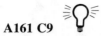

An OTA wants to develop an after-school program for obese adolescents who have diabetes or who are at risk for developing diabetes. Which program development action should the OTA take first?

**Correct Answer: B. Collaborate with the occupational therapist to survey the adolescents about their occupational performance.**

**Incorrect Answers:**

A.  Obtain statistical data about adolescent obesity to support the need for the program to the school administrators.
C.  Collaborate with the occupational therapist to survey occupational therapy practitioners about services they provide to obese adolescents.
D.  Review the professional literature to obtain ideas for the program's activities.

**Rationale:**

The development of new services would require a needs assessment to determine the necessity and focus of services. The information obtained from surveying potential participants is an excellent way to ensure that the program developed will meet a real unmet need. While statistics can support the rationale for a program, specific information about the target population is more relevant. In addition, prior to marketing a program, one should first determine its focus. Practitioner viewpoints and professional literature do not substantiate an unmet need that would require a program to be developed.

**Type of reasoning: Inferential**

This question requires one to utilize knowledge of program development guidelines in order to determine the first approach for development of a program. This requires one to reason which action will have the most effective outcome, which is an inferential reasoning skill. For this situation, the OTA should collaborate with the occupational therapist to survey the adolescents about their occupational performance in order to determine the adolescents' needs. If answered incorrectly, review program development guidelines.

## A162 C7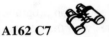

An OTA meets with a patient scheduled for a right hip total arthroplasty (THA) to review post-surgery hip precautions. The client has expressive aphasia resulting from a cerebral vascular accident incurred four years ago. How can the OTA most reliably determine that hip precautions will be effectively implemented post-discharge?

**Correct Answer: A. Have the patient demonstrate the techniques that have been taught.**

**Incorrect Answers:**

B.  Ask the family to observe the patient once home.
C   Ask the patient to point to pictures of the hip precautions being used during activities.
D.  Have the patient demonstrate positions that should be avoided.

**Rationale:**

Expressive aphasia interferes with the person's ability to verbally express him/herself. Therefore, the most effective method for assessing the individual's understanding of teaching is via demonstration. The OTA must observe the person performing the precautions during activities to ensure that the person has generalized the precautions to actually implement them during functional activities. Asking the family to observe the client may be helpful to assess carry-over, however, this source can be unreliable. Family members are not trained in assessment or activity analysis and they may not accurately report details of activity performance. Pointing to pictures provides limited information. The person may recognize precautions but not use them during the performance of an activity. Therefore, the OTA still does not know for sure that the individual can perform the activity appropriately. Having the individual demonstrate positions that should be avoided is contraindicated and could cause harm.

**Type of Reasoning: Inductive**

One must utilize clinical knowledge and judgment to determine the educational approach that best determines effectiveness and competence. This requires inductive reasoning skill. In this case, having the client demonstrate the skills that have been taught is most reliable. If answered incorrectly, review educational training guidelines for persons with CVA and aphasia.

422

## A163 C5

An OTA provides bed mobility training for an individual recovering from a left CVA. The OTA notes that the person's right calf is swollen and warm. The person complains that it is painful. Which action should the OTA take initially?

**Correct Answer: D. Contact the charge nurse immediately to report symptoms.**

**Incorrect Answers:**

A.  Elevate the leg and provide retrograde massage.

B.  Advise the person to tell the physician about the symptoms during the physician's next bedside visit.

C.  Continue with the training and document the symptoms in the medical record.

**Rationale:**

The signs and symptoms in this scenario are indicative of deep vein thrombosis (DVT). DVT, an inflammation of a vein in association with the formation of a thrombus and, is often a complication of CVAs or the result of prolonged bed rest. DVT is a medical emergency that must be handled immediately by medical staff. While it would be appropriate to elevate the legs, massage is contraindicated. The other answers are inappropriate because they delay the acquisition of needed medical care.

**Type of Reasoning: Evaluative**

This question requires a value judgment in an urgent situation, which is an evaluative reasoning skill. In this situation, the symptoms indicate a DVT, which is a medical emergency. Essential to arriving at a correct conclusion in situations such as these, is determining when symptoms indicate an emergency and recognizing appropriate measures to remedy the situation. For this situation, the OTA should contact the charge nurse immediately to report the symptoms. Review symptoms of DVT, especially appropriate courses of action if answered incorrectly.

## A164 C7

A 19 year-old with spastic diplegia and an IQ in the range of 55 to 69 is graduating from a special education program. The student has been involved in transitional programming since the age of 14. The OTA collaborates with the occupational therapist and the student to complete a discharge plan to meet the student's post-secondary goals. Which of the following should the OTA recommend be included as a post-discharge referral?

**Correct Answer: B. State vocational rehabilitation services.**

**Incorrect Answers:**

A.  A vocational rehabilitation workshop.

C.  A community college.

D.  A transitional employment program.

**Rationale:**

The purpose of state vocational rehabilitation services is to provide "one-stop" access to a multitude of vocational and educational evaluation and training programs. Since this student has been involved with transitional programming at school, a full assessment of vocational potentials and interests is warranted. Based upon this evaluation, the state vocational rehabilitation counselor can work with the individual to determine the best course of action to attain desired vocational goals. The student's IQ of 55-69 is reflective of mild intellectual disability (formerly termed mental retardation); therefore, the student's functional level is higher than the functional level appropriate for a vocational rehabilitation workshop (formerly called sheltered workshop). A transitional employment program and/or community college classes may be appropriate for the student but a complete evaluation is needed to determine the desired intervention program. In addition, since the student has been involved in transitional services since 14, he/she may have the skills necessary for competitive employment with or without reasonable accommodations, or additional training.

**Type of Reasoning: Inferential**

One must determine the benefits of the possible referral choices, given the student's age, current status, and needs. This requires inferential reasoning, where one must draw conclusions based on the evidence provided. In this situation, the best recommendation is to refer the student to the state vocational rehabilitation service. If answered incorrectly, review guidelines for transition planning for students with disabilities and programming options across the continuum of care. The integration of this knowledge is required to determine a correct answer.

**A165  C8**

An individual with amyotrophic lateral sclerosis requires the use of an environmental control unit (ECU) to access electrical devices and a personal emergency response system. The individual lives alone and self-directs personal care attendants to perform personal activities of daily living. During instruction to the individual on the capabilities and use of the ECU, which is most important for the OTA to discuss with the client?

**Correct Answer: A. The ECU's back-up power source and charging instructions.**

**Incorrect Answers:**

B.  Additional assistive technology available.

C.  Augmentative alternative communication options.

D.  Funding for assistive technology.

**Rationale:**

Back-up systems for electronic devices must be specified, especially if the device is used to access emergency assistance. Batteries used as back-up systems often have very strict schedules for charging (e.g. water cell batteries must be regularly checked for adequate water levels). Information about additional assistive technology, augmentative alternative communication, and funding can be helpful but they are not the most important area for consumer education in this case.

**Type of Reasoning: Inferential**

One must determine the most important information to provide for an individual about an ECU, given an understanding of the individual's diagnosis. This requires inferential reasoning skill, where one must infer or draw conclusions about a best course of action. In this situation, the OTA should provide information about a back-up power source and charging instructions as the device may be used to access emergency assistance. If answered incorrectly, review information on ECUs and patient training.

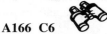

**A166  C6**

In an acute in-patient psychiatric facility, the OTA conducts an activity group for individuals with poor orientation to reality. Which is the best activity choice for the OTA to provide in this group?

**Correct Answer: B. The assembly of wooden toys for a children's unit.**

**Incorrect Answers:**

A.  A discussion of the effects of hospitalization on occupational roles.

C.  Guided imagery for stress management.

D.  Structured verbalizations of personal assets and limitations.

**Rationale:**

On an acute inpatient psychiatric unit, activities should be structured, easily completed in one session, and provide a concrete result to reinforce reality. Wooden toy kits meet these criteria and donating them to the children's unit facilitates Yalom's curative factor of altruism. Discussions and verbal activities are abstract and even if presented in a structured format, they would be difficult for persons with poor orientation to reality to follow. They also involve personal issues that require time to process feelings, adequate verbal skills, and adequate level of insight. This time allotment is not available in a setting with a short length of stay Guided imagery can be difficult for a disoriented person to focus on and can be frightening to an acutely ill person. Unstructured types of activities can actually increase hallucinations and reinforce poor reality orientation.

**Type of Reasoning: Inductive**

One must determine which activity best meets the needs of persons who are acutely ill and disoriented. This requires inductive reasoning skill, where the test taker must utilize clinical judgment to determine a best course of action. In this situation, assembly of wooden toys for a children's unit is the best choice for individuals with poor orientation to reality as it provides structured activity that is easily completed in one session. If answered incorrectly, review Mosey's taxonomy of groups and recommended therapeutic activities for acutely ill individuals in inpatient psychiatric settings.

**A167  C3**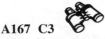

A carpenter complains of tingling of the left thumb, index, and middle finger, weakened grasp, and night pain secondary to carpal tunnel syndrome. The left thenar eminence appears smaller and more flattened compared to the right thenar eminence. The OTA collaborates with the client and the occupational therapist to develop an intervention plan. Which recommendation is best to include in this plan?

**Correct Answer: B. Modification of techniques used to hold a hammer.**

**Incorrect Answers:**

A.  Wrapping wrists with elastic bandages to provide support.

C.  Application of hot packs upon waking to decrease pain.

D.  Performance of wrist flexion and extension exercises with progressively increasing repetitions.

**Rationale:**

The symptoms provided are indicative of carpal tunnel syndrome (CTS). CTS includes sensory and motor deficits associated with median nerve compression, which can lead to permanent loss of motor and sensory functions. An important aspect in the treatment of CTS is modification of repetitive motions, especially those involved in everyday activities such as work. Elastic wraps are not supportive enough. Soft or semi-rigid splints are helpful to allow minimal wrist movement while providing sufficient stability for day use. Sometimes positional night splints may be helpful. The administration of physical agent modalities (PAMS) such as hot packs should be done under the supervision of an OT or PT practitioner. In occupational therapy, PAMS are used to prepare the person for functional performance of meaningful occupations. Repetitive motions should be limited as they can exacerbate symptoms.

**Type of reasoning: Inductive**

One must determine the best recommendation for a carpenter with carpal tunnel syndrome, based on an understanding of the client's occupation and diagnosis. This requires inductive reasoning skill. For this situation, the best recommendation for the intervention plan is to provide modification of techniques used to hold a hammer. Review activity adaptations for carpal tunnel syndrome if answered incorrectly.

**A168  C9**

A young adolescent with right hemiplegic cerebral palsy demonstrates a strong flexor synergy of the hand. The child does not use the hand for grasp, pinch, or release and often maintains the thumb flexed in the palm. The orthopedic hand surgeon recommends a flexor tendon release followed by several weeks of hand therapy and splinting. The family is very anxious about surgery and they ask the OTA what to do. Which is the OTA's best response?

**Correct Answer: A. Advise the family to review all the information to make an educated decision.**

**Incorrect Answers:**

B.  Recommend that the child follow the surgery presented by the doctor.

C.  Suggest a pre-operative course of intensive therapy and static and dynamic splinting.

D.  Encourage the family to get a second opinion.

**Rationale:**

The OTA should offer unbiased, objective support and not give medical or other advice. The OTA does not make the decision for the family. The surgery is an option that the family can choose. This is an elective procedure. The suggestion about pre-operative treatment should be first presented to the physician to be sure that it is an appropriate choice. It is not in the realm of occupational therapy to encourage the family to get a second opinion.

**Type of Reasoning: Evaluative**

One must weigh the potential course of action and determine the best response to the parent's concerns. Following guidelines for the AOTA Code of Ethics, the OTA should observe nonmaleficence, which includes doing no harm, and duties, practicing within the parameters of the profession. The only response in this situation that follows guidelines of practice is to advise them to review all the information in order to make an educated decision. Review the AOTA Code of Ethics and principles of team communication if answered incorrectly.

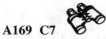

## A169  C7

A person diagnosed with dementia, Alzheimer type is evaluated by an occupational therapist and an OTA. Although the client demonstrates diminished memory skills, the occupational therapist and OTA determine that the patient is still able to live at home with supportive structure. They collaborate with the client to identify activities to include in a structured routine that enables the client's continued occupational performance. Which activity is best for the occupational therapist and OTA to recommend to the client?

**Correct Answer: C. Walking with a neighbor.**

**Incorrect Answers:**

A. Cooking dinner.

B. Doing laundry.

D. Watching television.

**Rationale:**

Walking with a neighbor can meet the person's needs for social participation and physical exercise. This is an activity that can be safely pursued even with memory deficits. Cooking is unsafe for a person with memory deficits. Leaving the stove on due to memory loss can be a fire hazard. Doing laundry requires memory of multiple steps that would make this task difficult. While watching television is safe for a person with a cognitive deficit, it is passive activity that does not support the use of intact abilities.

**Type of reasoning: Inductive**

One must utilize clinical judgment in order to determine the best activity to recommend for a client with Alzheimer's disease. This requires knowledge of the diagnosis and best activities to promote social participation and physical exercise, which necessitates inductive reasoning skill. For this situation, the occupational therapist and OTA should recommend walking with a neighbor. If answered incorrectly, review therapeutic activity guidelines for persons with Alzheimer's disease, especially activities that promote socialization and physical exercise.

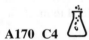

## A170  C4

A client recovering from a left CVA demonstrates increased flexor tone in the dominant right upper extremity while trying to re-learn to write with the left hand. Which of the following is most accurate for the OTA to state the client is exhibiting when documenting this observation?

**Correct Answer: A. An associated reaction.**

**Incorrect Answers:**

B. A crossed flexion reaction.

C. A tonic labyrinthine reflex with unilateral upper extremity flexion.

D. An asymmetrical tonic neck reflex.

**Rationale:**

Providing resisted voluntary movements to the unaffected limb facilitates an associated reaction in the affected limb. A tonic labyrinthine response results from changes in the orientation of the head, leading to bilateral flexor or extensor posturing of the arms/legs. The asymmetrical tonic neck reflex response is facilitated by rotation of the head, and results in limb extension on the face side, and limb flexion on the skull side. Crossed flexion reaction is a made up term.

**Type of Reasoning: Analytical**

This question requires the test taker to determine the functional deficit of the patient, which is an analytical reasoning skill. Questions of this nature often call upon the test taker to determine a deficit based on a functional description. Based on this information, the symptoms of the person indicate the deficit of associated reaction, which should be reviewed if answered incorrectly.

426

## A171 C9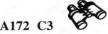

A 19 year-old with diagnoses of dysthymic disorder and narcissistic personality disorder attends a vocational rehabilitation program. When the client arrives for the work adjustment group, the OTA notes that the client has an unsteady gait, slurred speech, and alcohol-smelling breath. Which is the best action for the OTA to take in response to these observations?

**Correct Answer: D. Arrange for transportation to bring the client home.**

**Incorrect Answers:**

A.  Include the topic of alcohol's effect on work performance in the scheduled group's session.
B.  Refer the client to the social worker to discuss treatment options for potential alcohol abuse.
C.  Contact the client's parents to transport the client home.

**Rationale:**

The person is showing signs of being under the influence of alcohol. It is not appropriate to use the group or an individual session to discuss the client's behavior and/or potential treatment needs. In the client's current state, he/she is impaired and cannot be a full participant in this discussion. The client is a young adult so there is no need to contact the client's parents.

**Type of Reasoning: Evaluative**

This question requires professional judgment based on guiding principles, which is an evaluative reasoning skill. Because the person is showing signs of being under the influence of alcohol, the OTA should arrange for transportation back to his/her home. Questions such as these are challenging to answer as clear cut answers may not be readily available. Essential to choosing the correct conclusion is to do what is in the best interest of the individual.

## A172 C3

An older teenager with a congenital right below-elbow amputation had never wanted a prosthesis before. Now the teen wants a prosthesis "to look good at the prom and for going on dates." Which action would be most beneficial to meet the client's expressed need?

**Correct Answer: C. Recommend a prosthesis with a myoelectrically controlled hand.**

**Incorrect Answers:**

A.  Recommend a prosthesis with a cosmetic passive hand.
B.  Recommend a prosthesis with a voluntary opening hook.
D.  Recommend counseling to explore the client's sudden preoccupation with body image.

**Rationale:**

The best choice is a prosthesis that meets the teen's expressed need for a cosmetically appealing device which can also be used to perform functional age-appropriate bilateral fine motor activities, such as text messaging, or playing video games. Although a prosthesis can be used for purely cosmetic reasons, it would be best to provide the teen with a device that he/she could use to increase functional performance. A passive cosmetic hand can be used for grasping large objects like a beach ball or to hold an object on a table but has no moving parts for grasp and release, so it would not be the most functional choice. Although a voluntary opening hook would enable the teen to perform functional activities, recommending this would not respect the teen's expressed desire for a cosmetically appealing device. Recommending counseling based on an interpretation of the teen's request as a preoccupation with body image is judgmental. This action also violates the person's rights of autonomy.

**Type of Reasoning: Inductive**

This question requires the test taker to determine through clinical judgment which course of action will best address the client's request and provide optimal functioning. This requires inductive reasoning skill, where clinical judgment plus prediction of how a course of action will result in future benefit is accentuated. For this case, a prosthesis with a myoelectrically controlled hand is the best choice to facilitate function and fulfill the client's wishes. Review upper extremity prosthetic options if answered incorrectly.

## A173  C9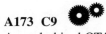

A newly hired OTA is instructed by the director of rehabilitation to supervise two hospital volunteers as they learn how to assist patients in safely completing bed to wheelchair transfers. Which is the first action the OTA should take in response to this request?

**Correct Answer: D. Explain to the director of rehabilitation why the request is inappropriate.**

**Incorrect Answers:**

A.  Recommend the hospital develop a transfer training program for volunteers.

B.  Inform the OT supervisor of the director's request.

C.  Supervise the volunteers during the transfers to ensure patient safety

**Rationale:**

Volunteers are not trained health care professionals and they cannot perform transfers with patients. Therefore, the OTA cannot comply with the director's request to supervise volunteers in performing transfers nor should the hospital provide transfer training to volunteers. The OTA must immediately inform the director of rehabilitation of the inappropriateness of this request. An explanation of the OTA's rationale for refusing to comply with the director's request is needed to prevent future inappropriate requests of the OTA and/or other hospital staff. After declining the director's request, the OTA should next inform the OT supervisor of this request so that the OT supervisor can follow-up with the director of rehabilitation to ensure that the director clearly understands the appropriate use of volunteers and OT staff.

**Type of Reasoning: Evaluative**

One must weigh the possible courses of action and then make a value judgment about the best course to take. This requires evaluative reasoning skill, which often utilizes guiding principles of action in order to arrive at a correct conclusion. For this case, because the request to supervise volunteers in transfer training is an inappropriate request, the OTA should first speak to the director to explain why the request is inappropriate. Review guidelines for supervision of personnel if answered incorrectly.

## A174  C3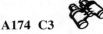

A carpenter recovering from injuries incurred during a fall from a ladder has decreased strength in the triceps, bilaterally. The most recent manual muscle test indicated that the triceps' muscle strength is 3. The OTA provides the client with a tabletop wood project to complete. To develop triceps' muscle strength, how should the OTA position the tabletop when the person sands the project?

**Correct Answer: A. At a 45 degree incline angled so that the individual's hands are above the elbows when the elbows are flexed.**

**Incorrect Answers:**

B.  At the individual's waist height so that the individual's hands and elbows are on the same plane when the elbows flex.

C.  At the individual's chest height so that the individual's hands and elbows are on the same plane when the elbows flex.

D.  At a 45 degree incline angled so that the individual's hands are below the elbows when the elbows are flexed.

**Rationale:**

This position requires the triceps to perform movement against gravity, which is possible at a muscle strength of 3 (fair). The sanding activity will provide slight resistance, which is the next level of muscle strength (3+, fair plus). Sanding wood placed on a table at waist or chest height, or inclined so that the hand is below the elbow when it is flexed, uses gravity-eliminated or gravity-assisted positions. These positions are too low of an activity for a person with fair muscle strength who can perform complete range of motion against gravity and they will not increase strength.

**Type of Reasoning: Inductive**

One must utilize clinical knowledge and judgment to determine the exercise approach that provides gravity-resisted movement. This requires inductive reasoning skill. In this case, the tabletop should be at a 45 degree inclined angle so the hands are above the elbows when the elbows are flexed. If answered incorrectly, review activity analysis principles and strengthening guidelines. The integration of this knowledge is needed to determine the correct answer.

428

**A175 C9**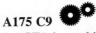

An OTA is working in a skilled nursing facility. The OTA is documenting current patient progress for the past fourteen days and realizes that a required seven day progress report to the client's insurance carrier had not been documented. What should the OTA do in response to this omission?

**Correct Answer: B. Write a note describing the patient's progress after seven days of treatment and sign with the current date.**

**Incorrect Answers:**

A.  Document the patient's status as of fourteen days and back date the note one week.

C.  Call the insurance company to explain the documentation was lost due to a computer failure.

D.  Describe the patient's progress after seven days of treatment and back date the note one week.

**Rationale:**

It is important to accurately document therapy progress in a timely manner. It is possible for an OTA to inadvertently miss a documentation deadline. If this occurs, the OTA should follow the AOTA Code of Ethics for veracity and document the patient's progress for the first seven days and date it with the current date. Notes should never be back dated.

**Type of Reasoning: Evaluative**

This question requires one to determine a best course of action in an ethical situation. This requires evaluative reasoning skill, where one must evaluate the merits of the potential courses of action and choose the one course of action that best provides resolution, while still adhering to the Code of Ethics. For this situation, the OTA should write a note that describes the patient's progress after seven days of treatment, dating the note with the current date. If answered incorrectly, review the AOTA Code of Ethics, especially veracity.

**A176 C4**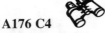

A client has right-sided weakness and decreased motor control. The OTA uses the proprioceptive neuromuscular facilitation (PNF) approach to help the client increase use of the right upper extremity and hand. Which of the following actions should the OTA have the client do during an intervention session to apply PNF principles?

**Correct Answer: D. Take items out of a dishwasher on the right side and reach across the body to place them in the upper cabinet on the opposite side.**

**Incorrect Answers:**

A.  Reach overhead with the right hand to retrieve a dish out of a higher cabinet and set it down on the countertop in front.

B.  Reach to the right side to retrieve an item out of refrigerator at hip height and place it into the left hand to set it on the countertop to the left.

C.  Use both hands together to pour juice out of a heavy pitcher into a glass on a countertop.

**Rationale:**

Pproprioceptive neuromuscular facilitation (PNF) is a technique which involves use of diagonal patterns of movement and involves rotational trunk movement. Using the right upper extremity to reach down to one side to take items out of a dish-washer and reaching across one's body (trunk rotation) to place these items into a higher cabinet on opposite side of body creates this diagonal pattern and encourages use of the affected side to increase motor control and volitional movement.

**Type of Reasoning: Inductive**

This case requires the test taker to first recall PNF guidelines and then determine the approach that will best facilitate improved functioning given the deficits. This necessitates inductive reasoning skill, where clinical judgment is paramount to arriving at a correct conclusion. For this situation, the OTA should have the patient take items out of a dishwasher on the right side and then place the items above and to the left side. If answered incorrectly, review PNF patterns and treatment guidelines, especially D1 pattern.

## A177  C2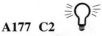

A home-care OTA seeks to enhance an elder's compliance with the occupational therapy intervention program. After discussing the goals of the program with the person, which intervention is most effective for the OTA to use?

**Correct Answer: C. Integrate previously learned strategies into new activities to facilitate generalization.**

**Incorrect Answers:**

A.  Provide the individual with limited opportunities for practice of skills to decrease boredom.

B.  Use multiple, variable instructions to ensure retention of new learning.

D.  Teach the family positive techniques to reinforce activity performance in the home.

**Rationale:**

The integration of previously learned strategies will increase compliance with intervention. Investment in treatment is an important factor in motivation and compliance. Providing the individual with limited practice of new skills can decrease compliance because he/she will have a smaller number of successful experiences. This can increase feelings of hopelessness. The use of multiple and variable instructions will increase the complexity of intervention. This can be difficult for the client to follow which will be frustrating and decrease the likelihood of success during the intervention session. Discussing the person's goals with his/her family and providing them with methods of positive reinforcement can be helpful but this can only be done with the individual's permission. Additionally, this does not directly address the individual who is the person that the OTA needs to engage.

**Type of Reasoning: Inferential**

One must determine the most effective method for enhancing compliance with a treatment program, given the information provided. This requires inferential reasoning skill, where one must infer or draw conclusions about a best course of action. In this situation, the OTA should discuss the goals of the program with the person and integrate previously learned strategies into new activities to facilitate generalization. If answered incorrectly, review approaches to increase compliance with therapy programs.

## A178  C9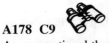

An occupational therapy administrator implements a continuous quality improvement program at a large private hand therapy clinic. The administrator determines that the OTA staff is not completing their assigned initial standardized screenings in a timely manner which has resulted in scheduling delays for complete functional evaluations. Which initial action is most effective for the administrator to take in response to this situation?

**Correct Answer: B. Examine the organizational structure of the screening process.**

**Incorrect Answers:**

A.  Counsel the OTAs on the need to adhere to screening schedules.

C.  Assign the occupational therapists to complete all screenings.

D.  Redesign the screening process.

**Rationale:**

A fundamental principle of continuous quality improvement (CQI) is to view problems and limitations as opportunities to explore organizational improvement needs. Blame for identified problems is not attributed to any person within the organization. Counseling the OTAs, reassigning screening to the occupational therapists, and/or redesigning the screening process may not effectively address the underlying reason for the delays in screening. The administrator must first examine the organizational structure of the screening process to be able to identify the needed organizational change.

**Type of Reasoning: Inductive**

This question requires one to determine the most effective initial action for addressing delays in completing initial screenings. This requires inductive reasoning skill, where clinical judgment is paramount to arriving at a correct conclusion. For this situation, the administrator should examine the organizational structure of the screening process. If answered incorrectly, review CQI guidelines.

430

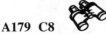

## A179 C8

An OTA working in a school has been asked to recommend technological devices for a student with severe spastic quadriplegia and dysarthria. Which action should the OTA take prior to recommending specific equipment?

**Correct Answer: D. Determine intervention goals in collaboration with the occupational therapist.**

**Incorrect Answers:**

A. Determine access capabilities in collaboration with the speech language pathologist.

B. Identify funding source(s) in collaboration with the social worker.

C. Obtain family support in collaboration with the psychologist.

**Rationale:**

Establishing the goals of technological interventions is essential to ensure that all equipment recommendations are meaningful and relevant to the student's needs. For example, technology can facilitate communication, functional mobility, and/or the completion of schoolwork. Determining access capabilities is an important step to take after the goal of the device is established. Funding for a device would be provided by the school in accordance with IDEA. While obtaining family support is always important and is required by IDEA, the OTA and occupational therapist must be able to explain the need and rationale for the recommended equipment to effectively obtain this support.

**Type of Reasoning: Inductive**

This question requires one to determine the best approach for recommending assistive technology. This requires inductive reasoning skill, where clinical judgment is paramount to arriving at a correct conclusion. For this situation, the OTA should collaborate with the occupational therapist to determine the intervention goals in order to ensure that the equipment recommendations are relevant to what the student needs. If answered incorrectly, review assessment guidelines for assistive technology.

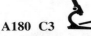

## A180 C3

An individual with post-polio syndrome receives an occupational therapy re-evaluation. How should the OTA initiate sensory testing with this client?

**Correct Answer: C. Demonstrate the test with the client's vision not occluded.**

**Incorrect Answers:**

A. Demonstrate the test with the individual's vision occluded.

B. Proceed proximal to distal.

D. Proceed distal to proximal.

**Rationale:**

Sensory testing must begin with a demonstration of the test with the client being able to visually observe the demonstration. If the client's vision is impaired, the OTA must verbally explain each step of the demonstration to ensure that the individual understands the testing process. After this demonstration is complete, the testing proceeds with vision occluded. Sensory testing for individuals with spinal cord injuries proceeds from proximal to distal. Sensory testing for individuals with peripheral nerve injuries proceed from distal to proximal.

**Type of Reasoning: Deductive**

One must recall the testing guidelines for sensory testing in order to arrive at a correct conclusion. This requires deductive reasoning skill, where factual knowledge is essential to choosing the correct solution. In this case, all sensory testing must begin with demonstration of the test that the patient can visualize. Review guidelines for administration of sensory testing if answered incorrectly.

**A181 C7**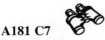

A young adult with a diagnosis of schizophrenia, paranoid type is scheduled to be discharged from an inpatient setting to a halfway house and psychosocial clubhouse. The OTA is assisting the team with the discharge plan. What is the most important information for the OTA to provide to the team about this person?

**Correct Answer: A. The person's instrumental ADL skills.**

**Incorrect Answers:**

B.  The possible effects of medication on the person's functional performance.

C.  The person's vocational potential.

D.  The person's social interaction skills.

**Rationale:**

Knowledge of the person's level of skills for the performance of IADL is essential for the OTA to share with the team. This can provide the halfway house staff with information that can be used to determine the level of structure and support this person may need to make a successful transition. In a halfway house, residents are typically responsible for the maintenance of their rooms and personal items (e.g., laundry). They are also expected to contribute to the maintenance of the entire household (e.g., cleaning and cooking). Successful adjustment to the halfway house will require the performance of instrumental ADL, whether independently or with assistance. In addition, the IADL of community mobility will be needed to travel from the halfway house to the clubhouse. OT practitioners are the only members of the team who are able to assess the specifics of the individual's functioning in these areas. While the OTA's input on the other areas identified in the answer choices can be helpful, it is not as essential as the individual's IADL status. Nursing can provide information on the functional effects of medications. All team members can provide information on social skills. The individual's vocational potential can be assessed at the clubhouse because an inherent component of the clubhouse model is vocational services.

**Type of Reasoning: Inductive**

This question requires one to determine the most important information to provide to the discharge planning team. This requires inductive reasoning skill, where clinical judgment is paramount to arriving at a correct conclusion. For this situation the OTA should provide information about the person's instrumental ADL skills, since the person will be transitioning to a halfway house. If answered incorrectly, review discharge planning guidelines for persons in inpatient settings and the expectations of community-based settings. Answering this question correctly requires the integration of this knowledge.

**A182 C3**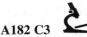

An OTA provides a wellness and prevention education series to the members of a community senior center. The topic of the week is joint protection. Which joint protection principle should the OTA include in the presentation?

**Correct Answer: D. Start an activity only if it can be immediately stopped when it requires capacities beyond existing capabilities.**

**Incorrect Answers:**

A.  Stand diagonally to the side of containers to be opened or closed to maximize torque.

B.  Work through the pain experienced during activities by performing stretching exercises.

C.  Preserve joint ROM and muscle strength by using the minimal effort required to perform an activity.

**Rationale:**

A key principle of joint protection is that a person should only start an activity if it can be immediately stopped when it requires capacities beyond existing capabilities. The other choices are counter to joint protection principles. These principles include that one should stand directly in front of items to be opened or closed; pain should be a warning sign indicating that an activity should be modified or stopped; ROM and muscle strength can be maintained by using maximal ROM and maximal strength during activities.

**Type of Reasoning: Deductive**

One must recall joint protection principles in order to arrive at a correct conclusion. This requires deductive reasoning skill, where factual knowledge is paramount to choosing the correct solution. For this scenario, the only principle that is in keeping with proper joint protection is to start an activity only if it can be immediately stopped when it requires capacities beyond existing capabilities. Review joint protection principles if answered incorrectly.

### A183  C2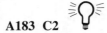

A person recently diagnosed with multiple sclerosis begins an outpatient program. During the initial intervention session, the client expresses difficulty concentrating on daily tasks due to chronic fatigue. What should the OTA do in response to the client's stated concerns?

**Correct Answer: C. Inquire about the client's fatigue level during different tasks.**

**Incorrect Answers:**

A.  Reassure the client that these are typical symptoms of this diagnosis.

B.  Reassure the client that medications will ease these symptoms.

D.  Inform the occupational therapist of the need to evaluate the client's endurance and cognition.

**Rationale:**

The OTA must obtain further information about the individual's fatigue levels and activity patterns. This information is essential to plan intervention for energy conservation and fatigue management. In addition, this action supports the validity of the client's concern and can be helpful in providing the foundation for a therapeutic relationship. Reassurance does not acknowledge the reality of the client's concern and does not deal with the stated problem. In addition, medications may not ease the client's symptoms. The client has just begun the program so the client's abilities would have been evaluated during the admission process. There is no information provided in this exam item to indicate a need to re-evaluate the client's status at this time.

**Type of Reasoning: Inferential**

One must have knowledge of multiple sclerosis and typical symptoms of the disease in order to choose the best response in this situation. This is an inferential reasoning skill where one must infer or draw conclusions about the information provided. For this situation, the OTA should inquire about the patient's fatigue level during various tasks. If answered incorrectly, review symptoms of multiple sclerosis.

### A184  C8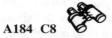

An OTA works with a child who has developmental delay and unintelligible speech to develop the child's functional communication skills using a communication board. The child has attained 100% accuracy in pointing to "yes" and "no" on the communication board in response to questions. The OTA and occupational therapist collaborate and determine that the child should be provided with the opportunity to expand communication skills. Which action should the OTA take to help attain this goal?

**Correct Answer: A. Add two more choices such as "play" and "snack" to the communication board.**

**Incorrect Answers:**

B.  Reverse the positions of "yes" and "no" on the communication board to assure competence.

C.  Add the options of "play," "thirsty," hungry and "TV" to the communication board.

D.  Recommend the occupational therapist evaluate the child's ability to use a joystick to access a computer.

**Rationale:**

The best choice for a child with developmental delay is to maintain the consistency of the original selections and add one or two new options at a time. The best choices are to pick concrete items that the child prefers and enjoys and would therefore be interested in communication. Reversing the position of the items will test the child's memory and ability to generalize, but would not improve his/her communication skills. With a developmental delay, it is important to be consistent in intervention to retain desired behaviors. Four new options would be too many to add at this time. Evaluating the child's ability to use a joystick does not address his/her communication skills. Using a joystick requires the ability to understand directionality, access four directions, and understand cause and effect.

**Type of Reasoning: Inductive**

One must determine the next step in communication after determining competency in pointing to yes and no. This requires inductive reasoning, where the test taker must utilize clinical judgment to determine the next course of action. For this scenario, adding two more choices to the board is the best next step. If answered incorrectly, review the characteristics of children with developmental delays and the use of augmentative communication devices for persons with communication difficulties. The integration of this knowledge is required for the determination of a correct answer.

**A185  C4**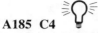

The parents of a school-aged child with Rett syndrome ask the OTA for activities that can help their child regain lost skills. The OTA collaborates with the occupational therapist to design a home program. Which of the following should the OTA recommend be included in the home program for the parents to do with their child?

**Correct Answer: D. Perform passive ROM to prevent contractures.**

**Incorrect Answers:**

A.  Encourage the child to use pressure distribution techniques.

B.  Use four-step sequencing cards to increase attention.

C.  Give positive feedback for active ROM performance.

**Rationale:**

Rett syndrome is a genetic progressive disorder in which motor, cognitive, social, and language skills deteriorate. If the child is school-aged, it is highly likely that the child has experienced significant functional decline. Regardless of the child's current functional level, children with this progressive condition cannot regain lost skills. Therefore, the home program must focus on maintaining function and preventing complications. Passive ROM is an activity that the parents can do to prevent contractures, which are a complication of this progressive condition. The child will not be able to respond to encouragement to use pressure distribution techniques. Since pressure relief is important to prevent the complication of skin breakdown, a more appropriate approach is to make sure that the parents are aware of correct positioning and the need to change positions frequently. The child in this scenario will not be able to attend to sequencing cards to increase attention or independently perform ROM.

**Type of Reasoning: Inferential**

One must link the child's diagnosis to the activities presented in order to determine which activity would be the most likely recommendation for a home program. This requires inferential reasoning, where one uses knowledge of a diagnosis to choose a best course of action. In this case passive ROM to prevent contractures is the best recommendation. Review symptoms of Rett syndrome if answered incorrectly.

**A186  C7**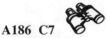

A woman with a complete spinal cord injury at the C-5 level has given birth to a daughter. The client seeks suggestions on methods to facilitate independent and safe parenting. Which of the following is most beneficial for the OTA to recommend the mother use to help her independently feed her child?

**Correct Answer: A. A pillow to support the mother's arms during breast feeding.**

**Incorrect Answers:**

B.  Pre-measured formula.

C.  Bottles that have molded easy to grip shapes.

D.  A sling to support the infant's head during breast feeding.

**Rationale:**

Providing support of the mother's upper extremities will enable her to independently breast feed her child. Breast feeding is physically the easiest method for feeding an infant and it is the healthiest for the infant. The individual with a C-5 spinal cord injury has sufficient upper extremity function to be able to support the infant's head without the use of a sling, especially since the mother's arms will be supported by a pillow to decrease fatigue. Pre-measured formula is not indicated in this case. The individual would need a splint or other piece of adaptive equipment to hold a baby's bottle.

**Type of Reasoning: Inductive**

Clinical knowledge and judgment are the most important skills needed for answering this question, which requires inductive reasoning skill. Knowledge of the diagnosis and most effective courses of action are essential to choosing the best solution. In this case, a pillow to support the mother's arms is the best recommendation to enable independent breast feeding. Review child care adaptations for individuals with disabilities if answered incorrectly.

434

## A187 C9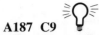

An adult who incurred a severe traumatic brain injury (TBI) is entering the second week of care at a long-term TBI rehabilitation center. The patient's family visit regularly and frequently asks multiple questions of the treatment team. A team and family conference is planned to address family concerns. Which is the most important information for the team to share with the family?

**Correct Answer: A. Realistic and clear information about the individual's current status and care plan.**

**Incorrect Answers:**

B. Each team member's expert opinion about the expected prognosis and discharge recommendations.

C. Reimbursement information about each professional service to assist in determining treatment choices.

D. Community resources for family support and respite care.

**Rationale:**

The family needs to understand the individual's current status and what is being done in treatment to facilitate recovery. This information can help the family support the team's care plan. Since the individual has only been in rehabilitation for two weeks, it is not possible for the team to know the prognosis or discharge plan. Reimbursement is always pertinent to the provision of care, but it is not the primary basis for determining interventions. Providing the family with community resources is important; but it is premature at this time. Community-based support programs are focused on individuals with TBI who have completed the acute rehabilitation phase. Most (if not all) TBI rehabilitation centers offer on-site support programs for families, which would be more relevant to this family's current needs. Respite services may or may not be needed by the family, depending upon the individual's level of recovery, which cannot be determined at this point.

**Type of Reasoning: Inferential**

One must determine the benefits of providing the information described in order to determine which information would be most important. This requires inferential reasoning, where one must draw conclusions of the benefits to the family based on the information provided. In this situation, providing realistic and clear information about the individual's current status and care plan is most important. Review the purposes of family conference meetings and the guidelines for client-centered care if answered incorrectly.

## A188 C2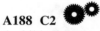

A child with attention deficit with hyperactivity disorder (ADHD) and conduct disorder attends an after-school program that utilizes sensory-integrative and behavioral management approaches to achieve intervention goals. Snacks are provided and occasionally used as rewards. A parent insists that a child not be given any foods containing sugar. Which is the OTA's best response to this request?

**Correct Answer: C. Comply with the parent's request.**

**Incorrect Answers:**

A. Discontinue providing sugary snacks but continue their use as rewards in the behavioral management program.

B. Provide the parent with recent research that refutes the link between sugar and problem behaviors.

D. Inform the parent that the OTA will discuss the issue with the occupational therapist to determine the best course of action.

**Rationale:**

The parent's request must be respected and honored. While an OTA may provide a parent with research information related to a child's condition, it is not the OTA's role to attempt to prove the parent wrong in his/her beliefs. The OTA can directly address the issue with the parent and does not need to discuss the issue with the occupational therapist prior to responding. Behavioral rewards and appropriate snacks that do not contain sugar can be used in the program. The use of non-sugar items can also be beneficial for children at risk with a secondary diagnosis of diabetes or other medical conditions.

**Type of Reasoning: Evaluative**

One must weigh the possible courses of action and then make a value judgment about the best course to take. This requires evaluative reasoning skill, which often utilizes guiding principles of action in order to arrive at a correct conclusion. For this case, because the mother has requested no foods containing sugar, the OTA should comply with the mother's request.

**A189 C2**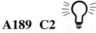

An individual with myasthenia gravis is being discharged home after a hospitalization for the treatment of pneumonia. The person's spouse has expressed concern about caregiving responsibilities and the client's ability to function in the home. The OTA collaborates with the occupational therapist to address the spouse's concerns and the client's needs. Which is the most beneficial recommendation for the OTA and occupational therapist to make?

**Correct Answer: D. A referral to a home care agency for a functional evaluation and home assessment.**

**Incorrect Answers:**

A. The extension of client's length of stay to allow for caregiver training.

B. The extension of client's length of stay to provide intervention to develop ADL skills.

C. A referral for the client to an adult day care program to relieve caregiver stress and to develop functional skills.

**Rationale:**

A functional evaluation in the client's home and an assessment of the home environment is the most beneficial choice listed to provide accurate information about the client's functional status and caregiver needs. This information will enable the home care team to collaborate with the family to develop an appropriate intervention plan to address their identified needs. An extension of length of stay is very difficult to justify because the individual was hospitalized for the medical treatment of pneumonia. Once this illness is effectively treated, discharge must occur. In addition, it is more effective to provide caregiver and ADL training in the person's home environment. A referral to adult day care may be determined based on the home care evaluation.

**Type of Reasoning: Inferential**

One must determine the most beneficial recommendation for this patient, given the caregiver's stated concerns. This requires inferential reasoning skill, where one must draw conclusions based upon presented evidence. In this situation, referral to a home care agency for a functional evaluation and home assessment is the most appropriate recommendation. Review home care services for individuals with disabilities and the functional impact of myasthenia gravis if answered incorrectly. The integration of this knowledge is needed to determine the best answer.

**A190 C9**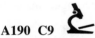

An OTA applies for the position of activities program director in a skilled nursing facility (SNF). During the job interview, the OTA discusses supervisory requirements for this position with the SNF administrator. Which amount of supervision from an occupational therapist should the OTA expect to be needed for this position?

**Correct Answer: C. None.**

**Incorrect Answers:**

A. Daily.

B. Weekly.

D. Monthly.

**Rationale:**

According to AOTA standards of practice and Medicare guidelines, an OTA who works strictly as an activities program director is not providing occupational therapy. While OTAs who work as activities program directors likely use their OT knowledge (e.g., the impact of client factors on activity performance) and skills (e.g., activity analysis, adaptation, and gradation) in this position; they are not providing OT services. Rather they are providing directorship to the SNF's activity program. Therefore, they do not require the supervision of an occupational therapist.

**Type of Reasoning: Deductive**

One must recall the supervisory guidelines for OTAs in the role of activities program director. This is factual knowledge, which is a deductive reasoning skill. Because OTAs can perform duties as an activities director without supervision, no supervision from an occupational therapist is required. If answered incorrectly, review supervisory guidelines for OTAs and Medicare guidelines for activity program director positions in SNFs.

**A191 C8**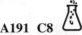

An individual with hemiplegia has inadequate ankle dorsiflexion on the affected side. Which of the following equipment is best for the OTA to recommend the person use to compensate for this deficit and facilitate safe and effective ambulation?

**Correct Answer: A. An ankle-foot orthosis (AFO).**

**Incorrect Answers:**

B. A wide-based quad cane (WBQC).

C. A narrow-based quad cane (NBQC).

D. A knee-ankle-foot orthosis (KAFO).

**Rationale:**

An AFO will provide the needed stability to the ankle joint to enable safe and effective ambulation. In this case, the knee is not involved so a KAFO is not indicated. A WBQC and a NBQC would be indicated for an individual with poor balance. Although canes can be very helpful ambulation aids, the concern in this case was to provide equipment to compensate for the lack of ankle dorsiflexion.

**Type of Reasoning: Analytical**

This question provides a description of a functional devices and the test taker must determine the best device to address the patient's deficits. This is an analytical reasoning skill, as questions of this nature often ask one to analyze descriptors or equipment to determine the best match for an individual's deficits. In this situation an AFO is the best recommendation. Review guidelines for use of AFOs if answered incorrectly.

**A192 C8**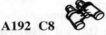

An OTA providing home-based occupational therapy services implements a bed positioning plan for a person recovering from a cerebral vascular accident. The person is receiving care from family members and personal care assistants employed by a home-care agency. Which action should the OTA take to ensure the accurate implementation of this plan by the client's caregivers?

**Correct Answer: C. Post pictures of the desired positions next to the bed's headboard.**

**Incorrect Answers:**

A. Provide verbal step-by-step directions of the desired positions to the client's caregivers.

B. Post written step-by-step directions of the desired positions on the wall by the client's bed.

D. Require each caregiver to demonstrate the replication of the desired positions.

**Rationale:**

A visual representation of the exact positions desired can decrease any misinterpretations of a written description. Placing this picture by the bed's headboard will ensure that it is visible to all caregivers. It is the most effective method provided to ensure compliance. Providing verbal step-by-step directions for positioning is reliant on the caregiver's memory which can be incomplete or faulty. Posting written step-by-step directions is reliant on the initiation of all caregivers to read the documented procedures and on the caregivers' accurate interpretation of the written word. These methods may also assume a knowledge base (e.g. 30 degrees of shoulder abduction) that is beyond the level of some of the client's caregivers. Requiring caregivers to demonstrate replication of the positions can be helpful but it is highly unlikely that the OTA would be able to access every personal care assistant who will be providing direct care to this client. In addition, home care agencies often use on-call per diem staff that would not be available to participate in a demonstration session.

**Type of Reasoning: Inductive**

This question requires one to determine the best approach for implementing a bed positioning plan. This requires inductive reasoning skill, where clinical judgment is paramount to arriving at a correct conclusion. For this situation, posting a picture of the person in the desired bed position next to the person's bed's headboard is best to ensure effective carryover. Review caregiver training guidelines if answered incorrectly.

**A193  C9**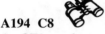

The residents of a halfway house plan a community leisure activity for a Saturday. Two residents state that they cannot participate in Saturday activities due to religious observances. The other residents express strong interest in the activity. Which is the OTA's best response to this situation?

**Correct Answer: B. Explore with the group an alternative schedule for a community leisure activity.**

**Incorrect Answers:**

A.  Schedule an in-house Saturday leisure activity for the two residents.

C.  Schedule an in-house Saturday leisure activity for all residents.

D.  Recommend the two members seek approval from their religious leadership to attend the Saturday activity.

**Rationale:**

All residents should be provided with the opportunity to engage in the community leisure activity. Facilitating the group's exploration of alternative scheduling can result in all residents' needs being met. Engaging in an on-site activity is not congruent the residents' statement that they could not participate in activities on Saturday. It is inappropriate to advise group members to seek the approval of their religious leadership to engage in an activity that is inconsistent with their religious beliefs. Finding an alternative schedule for a community activity that all residents can participate in does not prevent the other residents from engaging in community activities of interest on a Saturday.

**Type of Reasoning: Evaluative**

One must weigh the possible courses of action and then make a value judgment about the best course to take. This requires evaluative reasoning skill, which often utilizes guiding principles of action in order to arrive at a correct conclusion. For this case, because not all residents can attend the leisure activity due to religious observances, the best recommendation is for the group to explore an alternative schedule for the activity.

**A194  C8**

An OTA conducts a group in a forensic facility. Which of the following would be best for the OTA to focus on during the group?

**Correct Answer: C. Leisure management techniques.**

**Incorrect Answers:**

A.  Vocational planning strategies.

B.  Remedial educational activities.

D.  Money management skills.

**Rationale:**

Persons in a forensic setting have a significant amount of time that is not filled by productive or meaningful activity. A group focused on the development of leisure management skills would be an appropriate focus for a group of individuals living in an environment with limited leisure opportunities. Moreover, since most residents in a forensic setting are there for extended time periods or indefinitely, the development of skills to effectively manage leisure time would benefit them on an ongoing basis. Vocational planning and money management skills would be appropriate group foci for persons who are nearing their release. They would be not the most relevant group focus for persons with time remaining on their sentences. Remedial educational activities would be the focus of services provided by an educational professional, not by an OTA.

**Type of Reasoning: Inductive**

One must consider the information provided determine the best focus for the group in this facility, which is an inductive reasoning skill. For this situation, leisure management techniques are best to address in a group within a forensic facility. If answered incorrectly, review information on the characteristics of forensic settings and the focus of OT interventions in these settings.

438

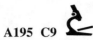

## A195 C9

The OTA collaborates with the occupational therapist to review the use of the occupational therapy department's resources to determine medical necessity and cost efficiency. Which service management task is the OTA working on with the occupational therapist?

**Correct Answer: A. Utilization review.**

**Incorrect Answers:**

B. Retrospective peer review.

C. Total quality management.

D. Risk management.

**Rationale:**

Utilization review is a plan to review the use of resources within a facility to determine medical necessity and cost efficiency. It is often a component of a continuous quality improvement (CQI) or a performance assessment and improvement (PAI) system. Total quality management is the creation of an organizational culture that enables all employees to contribute to an environment of continuous improvement. Risk management is a process that identifies, evaluates and takes corrective action against risk; and plans, organizes and controls the activities and resources of OT services to decrease actual or potential losses. Retrospective review involves the auditing of medical records by third-party payers to ensure appropriate care was rendered. Peer review is a system in which the quality of work of a group of health professionals is reviewed by their peers.

**Type of Reasoning: Deductive**

One must recall the definition of a utilization review for this question. This requires deductive reasoning skill, where factual knowledge is vital in choosing the correct solution. Utilization review is defined as a plan to review the use of resources in a facility, which should be reviewed if answered incorrectly.

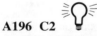

## A196 C2

An OTA collaborates with an occupational therapist to design a new day treatment program for individuals with dementia. Which groups are best for the OTA to recommend the program include?

**Correct Answer: D. Instrumental groups.**

**Incorrect Answers:**

A. Reality orientation groups.

B. Cognitive-behavioral groups.

C. Parallel groups.

**Rationale:**

According to Mosey's taxonomy of groups, instrumental groups help individuals function at their highest possible level for as long as possible. They provide supportive structured environments and appropriate activities that prevent regression, maintain function, and meet mental health needs. Activities can include reminiscence, arts and crafts, music, exercise, dance, and any other activity that is interesting and enjoyable to the members. Reality orientation groups are contraindicated for persons with dementia who cannot remember basic facts like dates, people, or places. Groups that focus on the use of memory can be very frustrating and counter-therapeutic for persons with dementia. Cognitive-behavioral groups require intact cognition and are at too high a level for persons with dementia. Parallel groups can be indicated for individuals with dementia but a schedule should not be comprised primarily of parallel groups for they are limiting in their potential for social interactions.

**Type of Reasoning: Inferential**

One must link the symptoms of the provided diagnosis to the type of groups presented in order to determine which group is best for individuals with dementia. This requires inferential reasoning, where one must draw conclusions about the features and benefits of each of the groups. In this case an instrumental group is best. Review Mosey's taxonomy of groups, especially instrumental groups if answered incorrectly.

**A197  C6**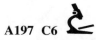

A homemaker and parent is hospitalized for depression and prescribed Parnate to treat depressive symptoms. The patient's hobbies are gardening and jogging. Upon discussing the functional effects of medications with the patient, which is the most important precaution for the OTA to review?

**Correct Answer: B. Dietary restrictions.**

**Incorrect Answers:**

A.  Photosensitivity.

C.  Orthostatic hypotension.

D.  Amenorrhea.

**Rationale:**

Parnate is a monoamine oxidase inhibitor (MAOI). It has serious side effects when a person eats foods that contain the amino acid tyramine. Tyramine increases blood pressure and may lead to stroke or other cardiovascular reactions. Photosensitivity, orthostatic hypotension, and amenorrhea can be side effects of psychiatric medications but they are not typically a major concern of MAOIs. These side effects are more of a concern with anti-psychotic medications.

**Type of Reasoning: Deductive**

One must recall the precautions for psychotropic medications in order to arrive at a correct conclusion. This requires deductive reasoning skill, where factual knowledge is essential to choosing the correct solution. Dietary restrictions are common when taking an MAO inhibitor, such as Parnate. Review precautions for MAO inhibitors if answered incorrectly.

**A198  C5**

A person is five days post coronary artery bypass graft (CABG). The patient expresses anxiety about performing any type of activity and reports chest pain during ambulation. The cardiologist has approved activities at a MET level of 2-3. Which activity is best for the OTA to use when initiating intervention with this person?

**Correct Answer: A. Grooming while standing at the sink.**

**Incorrect Answers:**

B.  Grooming in sitting.

C.  Showering in standing.

D.  Performing light housework.

**Rationale:**

Grooming while standing at the sink is at a MET level of 2-3. Grooming in sitting is at a 1-2 MET level. Showering in standing and light housework are at the 3-4 MET level.

**Type of Reasoning: Deductive**

One must recall MET level guidelines for cardiac rehabilitation. This is factual knowledge, which is a deductive reasoning skill. In this situation, the only activity that falls within the range of the 2-3 MET level is grooming while standing at the sink. If answered incorrectly, review MET level guidelines, especially 2-3 level.

440

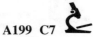

**A199 C7**

A patient is recovering from a right total hip replacement (posterolateral incision, cementless fixation). Which is the best type of bed-to-wheelchair transfer for the OTA to teach the patient to use?

**Correct Answer: B. Stand-pivot transfer to the non-surgical side.**

**Incorrect Answers:**

A. Stand-pivot transfer to the surgical side.

C. Lateral slide transfer using a transfer board.

D. Squat-pivot transfer to the surgical side.

**Rationale:**

During initial healing, it is important to protect the hip from dislocation or subluxation of the prosthesis. With a posterolateral incision, excessive hip flexion, internal rotation and adduction past neutral are contraindicated. This is minimized by transferring to the non-surgical side. Full ROM of the operated hip is also contraindicated.

**Type of Reasoning: Deductive**

This question requires one to recall posterolateral hip precautions and the guidelines for bed to wheelchair transfers of patients with total hip replacements in order to arrive at a correct conclusion. The recall of factual guidelines and information necessitates deductive reasoning skill. For this case, the OTA should perform a stand-pivot transfer to the non-surgical side. Review guidelines for transferring patients with hip replacements if answered incorrectly.

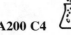

**A200 C4**

An OTA works with a patient who incurred a right CVA and has homonymous hemianopsia. Which is the most effective compensatory strategy for the OTA to use initially with this patient?

**Correct Answer: A. Teach the patient to turn the head to the affected left side.**

**Incorrect Answers:**

B. Provide printed notes on the left side telling the patient to look to the left.

C. Place the patient's plate and eating utensils on the left side of the bed tray.

D. Rearrange the patient's room so while the patient is in bed the left side is facing the doorway.

**Rationale:**

Homonymous hemianopsia results in the loss of ½ of the visual field in each eye (nasal half of one eye and temporal half of other eye) which corresponds to the side of the sensorimotor deficit incurred by the CVA. A patient with a right CVA will have left homonymous hemianopsia. Left homonymous hemianopsia results in an inability to receive information from left side. Initially, the patient needs to be made aware of his/her deficit and instructed to compensate by turning the head to the affected left side. Providing printed notes on the left side and placing the patient's eating utensils on the left side will not be effective as these items will not be within the person's intact visual field. Initially, items should be placed on the person's right (unaffected side) so that the patient can successfully complete tasks and interact with the environment. As the person develops awareness of the deficit, additional compensatory strategies including moving items to the midline and then to the affected left side and teaching the person to scan from the right to midline to the left.

**Type of Reasoning: Analytical**

For this question, the test taker must consider the best initial strategy for a patient with homonymous hemianopsia in order to arrive at a correct conclusion. This requires analytical reasoning skill, where deficits are analyzed in order to determine a most effective approach to addressing the deficits. For this case, teaching the patient to turn his/her head is what needs to occur first when compensating for the functional effects of homonymous hemianopsia. Review intervention approaches for homonymous hemianopsia if answered incorrectly.

## *Examination B*

**B1 C1**

An OTA provides intervention for a four-year old with developmental delays characterized by the persistence of primitive postural reflexes. The child demonstrates age-appropriate cognitive skills. Which is the best play activity for the OTA to incorporate into the child's intervention?

**Correct Answer: D. Pretending to be an explorer crawling through caves.**

**Incorrect Answers:**

A. Spinning on a swing.

B. Putting a puzzle together.

C. Lying on the floor and playing a game of marbles.

**Rationale:**

Pretending to crawl through caves can help facilitate the integration of primitive postural reflexes. It is also imaginative, which is appropriate play for a 4 year-old. Spinning on a swing is a fast vestibular activity indicated for treatment of sensory integration dysfunction. This activity could increase abnormal reflex activity in this child. Putting a puzzle together and playing marbles require fine motor skills and dexterity and would be too advanced for a child with the persistence of primitive postural reflexes.

**Type of Reasoning: Inductive**

One must utilize clinical knowledge and judgment to determine the therapeutic approach that would be best for the child. In this case, pretending to be an explorer crawling through caves is best given the child's age and limitations. If answered incorrectly, review the developmental levels of play and the impact of primitive postural reflexes on motor function. The integration of this knowledge is required to determine the correct answer.

**B2 C8**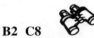

During a wheelchair evaluation, an individual with limited functional mobility expresses concern about the ability to continue volunteer work at a local church. The church's doorways are 31 inches wide. The client knows (from a recent home remodeling project) that 32 inches is the minimum width recommended for wheelchair access. After the evaluation, the OTA reviews the client's concerns with the occupational therapist and they determine the most effective way to address the client's concerns and functional mobility needs. Based on this review, what is the best recommendation for the OTA to make to the client?

**Correct Answer: B. Order a wheelchair with wrap-around armrests.**

**Incorrect Answers:**

A. Have the church widen its doorways to comply with ADA requirements.

C. Have the client explore alternative volunteer activities in accessible locations.

D. Order a customized narrow adult wheelchair.

**Rationale:**

Wraparound armrests (also called space saver armrests) reduce the overall width of a wheelchair by one inch. A customized chair can be very expensive. The case does not indicate the individual's measurements, so it is not possible to ascertain if a narrow wheelchair would actually fit the person. Religious organizations are exempt from ADA accessibility requirements. The individual does not need to explore alternative volunteer experiences since valued established activities can continue with an appropriate wheelchair.

**Type of Reasoning: Inductive**

Clinical knowledge and judgment are the most important skills needed for answering this question, which requires inductive reasoning skill. Knowledge of available mobility equipment to remedy the issue of a narrow doorway is paramount to arriving at a correct conclusion. In this case, the most appropriate recommendation is to order a wheelchair with wraparound armrests, which should be reviewed if answered incorrectly.

**B3  C7**

An adolescent with Duchenne muscular dystrophy can no longer close snaps or zip zippers on jeans. Which recommendation is best for the OTA to make to this client?

**Correct Answer: A. Replace snaps and zippers with Velcro.**

**Incorrect Answers:**

B.  Replace snaps and zippers with large buttons.

C.  Use a zipper pull to zip jeans and leave the snaps unsnapped.

D.  Purchase elastic waist pants.

**Rationale:**

Muscular dystrophy is a progressive condition. The OTA must be able to assist the person in adjusting to its progressive nature and provide options that maintain independence as long as possible. Velcro can be more easily managed than snaps or zippers. It can also be easily sewn into the jeans and pants that the adolescent already owns. Buttoning large buttons and using a zipper pull are not the best solutions due to the progressive loss of dexterity, coordination, and strength that occurs with Duchenne muscular dystrophy. Elastic waist pants facilitate the process of donning pants but they do not address the identified difficulty of fastening jeans. This recommendation would not allow the adolescent to continue wearing jeans and pants in his current wardrobe. In addition, the style of elastic waist pants may not be acceptable to a teenaged boy. Recall that Duchenne muscular dystrophy is sex-linked and only affects males.

**Type of reasoning: Inductive**

This question requires one to determine a best adaptation for an adolescent with Duchenne muscular dystrophy in order to arrive at a correct conclusion. This requires clinical judgment, which is an inductive reasoning skill. For this scenario, the OTA should recommend replacing snaps and zippers with Velcro. Review self-care adaptations for persons with Duchenne muscular dystrophy if answered incorrectly.

**B4  C5**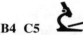

A child with spastic quadriplegic cerebral palsy demonstrates a consistent gag reflex. Which technique should the OTA use to help inhibit this reflex?

**Correct Answer: C. Press a spoon down firmly on the center of the tongue.**

**Incorrect Answers:**

A.  Move a spoon from side to side on the tongue.

B.  Walk a spoon down the tongue, going from proximal to distal with even pressure.

D.  Stroke the tongue in a circular motion with a firm object.

**Rationale:**

The best approach to decrease a gag reflex is to press down firmly on the center of the tongue and to apply pressure from distal to proximal. Lateral and circular movements can facilitate the gag reflex.

**Type of Reasoning: Deductive**

This question requires recall of guidelines for feeding children with spastic cerebral palsy, which is factual knowledge. Deductive reasoning skills are utilized whenever one must recall facts to solve clinical problems. In this situation, the OTA can inhibit the gag reflex by pressing down firmly on the center of the tongue. Review feeding guidelines for children with a persistent gag reflex if answered incorrectly.

**B5 C7**

A middle school aged child with right upper extremity amelia attends occupational therapy to learn how to dress independently. Which of the following is most beneficial for the OTA to focus on during intervention?

**Correct Answer: A. Donning and doffing a variety of shirt types of personal preference.**

**Incorrect Answers:**

B.  Donning and doffing only shirts that can be donned overhead.

C.  Donning and doffing shirts that button in the front.

D.  Donning and doffing shirts with velcro tabs sewn on to replace buttons.

**Rationale:**

A child with amelia, or absence of one arm, can easily learn to use a diversity of techniques to independently don and doff a variety of shirt types. This is the best way to engage a pre-adolescent and to allow the pre-adolescent to make decision about clothing. This choice reflects incorporation of the child's developmental levels, motivation level, and therapeutic use of self to work with the child's interests. There is no need to limit the child's shirt choices. Velcro tabs are appropriate for someone with decreased fine motor skills and/or strength but are not needed in this case.

**Type of Reasoning: Inductive**

This requires one to understand the nature of amelia, and based on this knowledge; choose the most appropriate dressing activity. This requires inductive reasoning skill, where clinical judgment is paramount to arriving at a correct conclusion. In this case, working on a variety of shirt types of personal preference is the best recommendation for this patient. If answered incorrectly review information on amelia in children and dressing activities.

**B6 C6**

During an intervention session, a client complains of dry mouth due to prescribed medications. What is the most effective strategy for an OTA to suggest to the client to manage this side effect?

**Correct Answer: D. Sip water.**

**Incorrect Answers:**

A.  Suck on ice.

B.  Suck on hard candies.

C.  Drink iced tea.

**Rationale:**

Sipping water is the best choice to relieve dry mouth. Sucking ice and/or hard candies presents a possible choking risk. Hard candies might present a dietary risk for some clients. Iced tea contains caffeine, which can increase dehydration. Tea can cause serious, even fatal reactions, when taken with certain medications such as MAO inhibitors.

**Type of Reasoning: Evaluative**

This question requires one to evaluate the merits of the four possible choices and determine which will most effectively remedy the clients' symptoms. This requires evaluative reasoning skill. For this situation, sips of water is the best and the safest remedy for dry mouth. If answered incorrectly, review information on side effects of psychotropic medications and compensatory techniques.

## B7 C8

An individual who had a CVA one year ago continues to demonstrate unilateral neglect. The individual drives daily to therapy despite several suggestions from the OTA to discontinue this activity. The OTA is concerned that the client is an unsafe driver. What is the best approach for the OTA to take in response to this situation?

**Correct Answer: C. Report the information to the occupational therapist.**

**Incorrect Answers:**

A. Report the individual to the department of motor vehicles.

B. Suggest that the individual attend a driver training program.

D. Tell the individual's family that the client is at risk for injuring self and others while driving.

**Rationale:**

The OTA must report the information to the occupational therapist, who can then determine the need for further evaluation to assess the individual's ability to drive. The department of motor vehicles addresses issues related to the administration of licenses but it does not provide cognitive evaluation or address remedial issues concerning driving. A driver training program is a good suggestion to help the person improve skills but it does not address the need to evaluate if the person is an unsafe driver. The option to inform the family can be presented in the context of the skills that occupational therapy addresses, such as unilateral neglect. However, it does not directly address the safety issue.

**Type of Reasoning: Evaluative**

One must weigh the merits of each of the four possible courses of action in order to determine the best response to the situation. This necessitates evaluative reasoning skill, where guiding principles of action are paramount to arriving at a correct conclusion. In this situation it is best to report the information to the occupational therapist, who can then determine a need for further evaluation. If answered incorrectly, review driver re-education guidelines and reporting potential unsafe driving.

## B8 C8

An elder adult lives in a second floor apartment in a private home. The individual is experiencing sensory losses that are consistent with the aging process. All other abilities are within normal limits. Which action is best for the OTA to recommend to the client?

**Correct Answer: D. Install light switches at the top and bottom of the stairway.**

**Incorrect Answers:**

A. Acquire a first floor apartment.

B. Initiate an application to an assistive living facility.

C. Install a stair glide system.

**Rationale:**

With normal aging there is decreased visual acuity (presbyopia), reduced night vision, and impaired depth perception. These deficits can make ascending and descending stairs dangerous. To decrease the risk of falls, it is advisable to install light switches at both ends of a stairway so that the person can independently illuminate the stairs. There is no information provided in this case to indicate a need for a stair glide or for movement to another apartment.

**Type of Reasoning: Inferential**

One must link the individual's diagnosis to the recommendations presented in order to determine which recommendation is best for this individual. This requires inferential reasoning, where one must draw conclusions about the deficits in order to make a sound recommendation. In this case the best recommendation would be the installation of light switches at the top and bottom of the stairway. Review home adaptations for sensory loss if answered incorrectly.

**B9 C6**

An adult with obsessive-compulsive disorder is hospitalized due to the exacerbation of symptoms. During the patient's first occupational therapy group, which is the most beneficial activity for the OTA to employ with this person?

**Correct Answer: B. Repotting plants.**

**Incorrect Answers:**

A. Sanding a cutting board.

C. Stringing small beads into a necklace.

D. Lacing a wallet with the double cordovan stitch.

**Rationale:**

Persons with obsessive-compulsive disorders exhibit behaviors that are characterized by orderliness, perseverance, and driven by a pursuit for perfection. Repotting plants is the activity choice that offers an opportunity to break away from the repetitive behavioral patterns of obsessive-compulsive disorder. The other activities all have elements that could reinforce the repetitive behavioral components of the disorder; i.e., sanding back and forth, stringing bead after bead, and lacing the stitch over and over. In addition, these activities could be held to a standard of perfection; i.e., a perfectly smooth surface, the perfect bead pattern, a complex stitch with no twists.

**Type of Reasoning: Inferential**

One must determine which activity is most beneficial, given an understanding of the client's diagnosis. This requires inferential reasoning skill. In order to arrive at a correct conclusion, the test taker should infer that activities that encourage repetitive patterns of behavior and perfectionism should be avoided. Repotting plants is the only activity that does not encourage such behavior. If answered incorrectly, review the behavioral characteristics of OCD and principles of activity analysis.

**B10 C1**

An eight month-old child with myelomeningocele at the L1 level shows cognitive function within normal limits. Which of the following activities would the OTA most likely focus on with this child during intervention?

**Correct Answer: B. Increasing trunk balance when placed in sitting.**

**Incorrect Answers:**

A. Doffing sleeves of overhead shirts with assistance.

C. Transferring objects from one hand to the other.

D. Transitioning from sitting to supine and from supine to sitting.

**Rationale:**

Working on trunk balance is within normal limits for the eight month-old. The development of gross motor skills in the child with myelomeningocele parallels those of the typical child. The difference is that upright mobility at the 12-18 month level concentrates on the use of assistance devices. Doffing sleeves overhead is a skill consistent at the ten to 12 month level. Transferring objects from one hand to another is found at the six to eight month level. Transitioning from sitting to supine comes after working on trunk balance after being placed in sitting, from nine to 11 months.

**Type of Reasoning: Inferential**

One must infer or draw conclusions about the likely activities a child will be working on with myelomeningocele at eight months of age. The key to arriving at a correct conclusion is matching the child's age with the spinal level of myelomeningocele. For this scenario, increasing trunk balance when placed in sitting is the most likely skill to be addressed for this child. If answered incorrectly, review information on myelomeningocele in infants and gross development.

**B11  C1**

An OTA works in a school system with a child with developmental delays. One of the goals of treatment is to develop pre-writing skills. The child exhibits the ability to grasp a pencil proximally with crude approximation of the thumb, index, and middle fingers and the ring and little fingers slightly flexed. The OTA collaborates with the occupational therapist to develop an intervention plan. Which grasp should be the focus for the implementation of intervention?

**Correct Answer: C. Dynamic tripod grasp.**

**Incorrect Answers:**

A.  Digital pronate grasp.

B.  Static tripod posture grasp.

D.  Palmar supinate grasp.

**Rationale:**

The grasp pattern described in the case is static tripod posture grasp. The next grasp pattern to be mastered after this grasp is the dynamic tripod grasp. The other grasp patterns are precursors to the static tripod grasp.

**Type of Reasoning: Inferential**

This question requires one to infer the intervention goal that will develop appropriate grasp for this child. This requires inferential reasoning skill, where one must draw conclusions about the described grasp pattern. For this situation, dynamic tripod grasp is the next pattern to be mastered after static tripod grasp. If answered incorrectly, review grasp patterns of the hand in children, especially dynamic tripod.

**B12  C6**

A patient in an acute psychiatric inpatient unit with a diagnosis of major depressive disorder is placed on suicide precautions. The OTA has scheduled 30 minute individual sessions in the patient's room to begin intervention. Which is the most beneficial activity for the first intervention session?

**Correct Answer: D. Decorating cookies to contribute to the patients' lounge.**

**Incorrect Answers:**

A.  Tooling a leather wallet.

B.  Writing in a personal journal.

C.  Building a sand terrarium in a plastic globe.

**Rationale:**

Decorating cookies is a safe, "non-fail" project. The end product fosters the curative factor of altruism which can be therapeutic. Also the end product is not dangerous or potentially harmful to the patient. Tooling uses tools that can be used to harm oneself. The OTA should be careful during the work process to count all tools, but it is potentially high risk. While writing in a journal can be therapeutic, it may reinforce negative feelings and poor self-esteem. The globe of the sand terrarium can be broken and sharpened into an object that one can use to harm self.

**Type of Reasoning: Inductive**

One must utilize clinical judgment for a best course of action in order to arrive at a best conclusion. This requires considerations of the client's diagnosis and current status in order to choose the best activity. In this situation, decorating cookies is best as it creates the least potential for harm and is a no fail activity. If answered incorrectly, review therapeutic activities for patients with major depressive disorders and principles of activity analysis. The integration of this knowledge is required to determine the correct answer.

**B13  C9**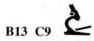

A mental health facility provides inpatient and outpatient services for a catchment area that encompasses five counties. The occupational therapy department meets to design a continuous quality improvement (CQI) project. Which is the best focus for this CQI project?

**Correct Answer: D. The follow-up process after discharge from the hospital.**

**Incorrect Answers:**

A.  Keeping services that are rated positively on a satisfaction survey.
B.  Cost reduction in specific service areas.
C.  Methods to educate staff on new wellness services.

**Rationale:**

Continuous quality improvement (CQI) involves a prospective analysis of specific services to improve service quality and meet the needs of a population. Since this program serves a broad geographic area, evaluating post-discharge follow-up services would be an appropriate focus for a CQI project. The determination that services be maintained should be made according to the efficacy of service outcomes in meeting the needs of a population, not based on client perspectives. Making changes in service delivery to reduce costs is a fiscal management task, not the focus of CQI. Wellness services are offered to employees as a benefit. CQI focuses on improving service quality and patient care, not on promoting employee benefits.

**Type of Reasoning: Deductive**

This question requires one to recall the guidelines for CQI, which is a factual (deductive) skill. Understanding the nature of CQI is key to arriving at a correct conclusion. Focusing on the follow-up process after discharge is most likely to be the focus out of all the choices provided. If answered incorrectly, review guidelines for CQI, especially in hospital settings.

**B14  C7**

A middle school aged child with osteogenesis imperfecta reports feelings of low self-esteem, social isolation, boredom and lethargy. The OTA collaborates with the child to identify resources for after-school leisure activities to promote social-ization and community participation. Which of the following activities is most beneficial for the OTA to explore with the child?

**Correct Answer: D. Computer clubs.**

**Incorrect Answers:**

A.  Team sports.
B.  Public park programs.
C.  Scouting programs.

**Rationale:**

Osteogenesis imperfecta results in brittle bones that fracture easily. Fracture prevention through activity restrictions is a primary focus. This can result in social isolation, decreased self-efficacy, and depression. Exploring different computer clubs can provide the child with a number of viable options for leisure activities that he/she can successfully pursue after school without risking fractures. The other options involve more physically-based activities that would be difficult for the child to safely pursue. These activities would highlight what the child is unable to do, rather than his/her abilities. This would be contraindicated in the treatment of depression. In computer clubs, physical abilities are not needed because physical deficits can be readily compensated for with adaptations and modifications.

**Type of Reasoning: Inferential**

One must determine the most appropriate activity recommendation, given knowledge of the presenting diagnosis. This requires inferential reasoning skill, where one must infer or draw conclusions about a best course of action. In this situation, the OTA should recommend that the child join a computer club. If answered incorrectly, review symptoms of osteogene-sis imperfecta and developmentally appropriate leisure activities. The integration of this knowledge is required to answer this question correctly.

448

**B15  C3**

An individual is recovering from deep partial thickness burns on both upper extremities, chest, and lower neck. The OTA provides equipment to prevent positions that can result in contractures. Which are the most important positions for the OTA to prevent?

**Correct Answer: A. Positions of comfort.**

**Incorrect Answers:**

B.  Anti-deformity positions.

C.  Positions resulting in edema.

D.  Positions of discomfort and pain.

**Rationale:**

The position of comfort is often assumed by individuals recovering from burns. This position occurs when the person assumes the protective postures of adduction and flexion of the upper extremities, flexion of the hips and knees, and plantar flexion of the ankles. This position does decrease discomfort but it is nonfunctional and can result in contractures. The anti-deformity position is the desired position. It is the opposite of the position of comfort. While preventing edema is important in burn rehabilitation, the question is about the prevention of contractures. Positions of pain and discomfort are unavoidable for persons recovering from deep partial thickness burns. These burns involve the epidermis and deep portion of the dermis, hair follicles, and sweat glands, and are often very painful.

**Type of Reasoning: Inductive**

Clinical knowledge and judgment are the most important skills needed for answering this question, which requires inductive reasoning skill. Knowledge of the diagnosis and most appropriate positioning given the severity of the burns is essential to choosing the ideal solution. In this case, the patient should avoid positions of comfort. If answered incorrectly, review positioning guidelines for patients with full thickness burns.

**B16  C4**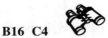

An individual recovering from a traumatic brain injury is assessed to be at Level VI of the Rancho Level of Cognitive Functioning Scale. What should the OTA use to implement treatment?

**Correct Answer: D. Simple meal preparation tasks such as making a sandwich.**

**Incorrect Answers:**

A.  Sensory stimulation activities such as moving to music.

B.  Repetitive self-care tasks such as brushing hair.

C.  Community re-entry activities such as taking a bus.

**Rationale:**

At Level VI the individual is appropriate and goal-directed but can become confused. Cues are required. Community re-entry activities are too high-level for an individual at Level VI. They are more appropriate for Level VII and VIII. Sensory stimulation activities such as moving to music would be appropriate for Level III. Repetitive self-care tasks would be appropriate for Level V.

**Type of Reasoning: Inductive**

One must utilize clinical knowledge and judgment to determine the approach that provides appropriate therapeutic challenge for a patient at Level VI. In this case, the therapist should implement treatment by having the individual prepare a simple meal, such as a sandwich. If answered incorrectly, review treatment guidelines for patients at Level VI on the Rancho Level of Cognitive Functioning Scale.

**B17  C8**

An adolescent incurred a C-4 spinal cord injury. During the initial session, the patient refuses to speak to the OTA. The OTA supportively acknowledges the client's response. Which action should the OTA take next?

**Correct Answer: A. Set up a chin-operated bed-side ECU.**

**Incorrect Answers:**

B.  Provide passive range of motion.

C.  Explain what OT can offer the adolescent to adjust to decreased abilities.

D.  Ask the adolescent to tell nursing staff when personally ready for OT.

**Rationale:**

The individual immediately needs a method to access the environment. Being able to call staff, operate a TV and/or radio, answer the phone, turn on/off lights, and other basic ECU functions are important tasks for the adolescent to self-control. It is not necessary to explain what OT can offer. Some of the benefits of OT will likely become self-evident as the adolescent learns to use the ECU. This explanation can be expanded on as the adolescent begins to engage in intervention. Providing PROM ignores the patient's feelings. PROM can be provided by direct care staff. The individual may not be ready for quite a while to collaborate with the OTA due to the need to adjust to disability. While this is occurring, the OTA can still provide meaningful supportive interventions and work on developing a therapeutic relationship.

**Type of Reasoning: Inductive**

One must utilize clinical knowledge and judgment to determine the best action that addresses the adolescent's needs in the absence of his/her input. In this case, a chin-operated bedside ECU is the best course of action out of the choices provided as it provides access to the environment. If answered incorrectly, review treatment guidelines, especially equipment needs for persons with a C4 injury.

**B18  C6**

An employed individual is completing an inpatient program for substance abuse. What would be most beneficial for the OTA to recommend as part of the individual's discharge plan?

**Correct Answer: B. Regular attendance at one or more Narcotics Anonymous meetings weekly.**

**Incorrect Answers:**

A.  Assignment to a member of a local Narcotics Anonymous group.

C.  Attendance at the psychosocial clubhouse for leisure skills groups.

D.  Referral to the state vocational rehabilitation services.

**Rationale:**

Narcotics Anonymous (NA) is based on the same 12-step principles as AA (Alcoholics Anonymous) and has been found to be an effective resource for those in recovery. NA and AA provide critical support to maintain abstinence. NA and AA stress that the individual seek out meetings and enlist a sponsor independently. Psychosocial clubhouses provide a diversity of supportive services for persons with serious and persistent mental illnesses. Since the person is employed and has no secondary diagnosis of mental illness, this setting would not be an appropriate referral recommendation. Psychosocial clubhouses do not specifically address the abstinence needs of substance abusers. Based on the information provided, one cannot assume that vocational rehabilitation is a potential goal or need for this person.

**Type of Reasoning: Inferential**

One must consider the information provided and make certain assumptions about that information, including what is most beneficial for the client. Judgment based on facts and assumptions utilizes inferential reasoning skill. In this case, the OTA should recommend regular attendance at NA meetings. Questions such as these can be challenging, as one may be tempted to assume information not found in the question. Therefore, be careful that conclusions drawn from questions such as these only consider the facts given. Review intervention guidelines for persons with substance abuse if answered incorrectly.

450

## B19 C4

During an occupational therapy intervention session, a client with a left CVA demonstrates extinction to the right and a tendency to ignore items on the right side. When documenting this behavior what should the OTA report?

**Correct Answer: B. Unilateral inattention.**

**Incorrect Answers:**

A. Agnosia.

C. Poor right/left discrimination.

D. Poor visual scanning.

**Rationale:**

Unilateral inattention is a situation in which the individual neglects the side of the body contralateral to the CVA site and the environment on that side. The other options describe cognitive-perceptual deficits with different manifestations. Agnosia can be the inability to identify body parts. Right/left discrimination is the differentiation of one side of the body from the other. Visual scanning is the engagement and disengagement of visual attention as the eye moves its focus from one object to another.

**Type of Reasoning: Analytical**

This question provides symptoms and the test taker must determine the likely cause for them. This is an analytical reasoning skill, as questions of this nature often ask one to analyze a group of symptoms in order to determine a diagnosis. In this situation the symptoms indicate unilateral inattention, which should be reviewed if answered incorrectly.

## B20 C5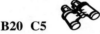

An OTA is discussing the recommended activity regimen with an individual who is at Stage II of cardiac rehabilitation. Which activity should the OTA recommend?

**Correct Answer: C. Doing a tabletop craft of interest.**

**Incorrect Answers:**

A  Completing isometric exercises.

B. Light gardening.

D. Checking emails on a lap top computer.

**Rationale:**

Tabletop craft activities are at the appropriate MET level for a person in Stage II of a cardiac rehabilitation program. Checking emails on a lap top computer is a Stage I activity and light gardening is a Stage IV activity. Isometric exercises are contraindicated for all stages of cardiac rehabilitation.

**Type of Reasoning: Inductive**

One must utilize clinical judgment combined with knowledge of cardiac rehabilitation guidelines to determine the best activity to recommend for a client in Stage II of recovery. This necessitates inductive reasoning skill, where knowledge of cardiac clinical guidelines is paramount to arriving at a correct conclusion. For this case, the OTA should recommend a tabletop craft of interest. If answered incorrectly, review cardiac rehabilitation guidelines, especially MET level activity.

**B21  C4**

A seven year-old with complete spina bifida at the T10 level attends out-patient OT weekly. The child's parent reports that the child is losing bladder control. The OTA notes that the child shows a minimal decrease in strength of bilateral lower and upper extremities and an increase in the equinovarus position of the feet. The OTA suspects that the child may have which of the following?

**Correct Answer: D. Tethered cord.**

**Incorrect Answers:**

A.  Shunt malformation.
B.  A recent growth spurt.
C.  Arnold-Chiari formation.

**Rationale:**

Tethered cord is noted by all of the symptoms listed. The spinal cord of the child with spina bifida is sometimes attached to the spinal column and becomes taut as the child grows. The child requires a surgical release of the tethered cord. Shunt malformation is marked by intermittent headaches, shortened attention span, increased paralysis, decreased upper extremity strength, noticeable decrease in school performance, and increased irritability. Young children often demonstrate increased head size, nausea, and vomiting. The tethered cord presents whether the child has an even rate of growth or goes through a recent growth spurt. Arnold-Chiari formation occurs in the process of development and involves the part of the lower portion of the brain slipping or being pushed through the foramen ovale.

**Type of Reasoning: Analytical**

One must recall the signs and symptoms of tethered cord in order to arrive at a correct conclusion. Questions that provide a group of symptoms and the test taker must determine the cause requires analytical reasoning skill. In this case the symptoms indicate tethered cord with spina bifida, which should be reviewed if answered incorrectly.

**B22  C7**

An individual with mild cognitive deficits takes medications for multiple medical conditions. The OTA works with the individual to develop the ability to safely self-administer medications. Which equipment and/or strategy should the OTA train the client to use?

**Correct Answer: C. A daily pill holder with time-labeled slots for each dosage.**

**Incorrect Answers:**

A.  Easy open caps on the medication bottles.
B.  A chart listing medication dosages and administration times on the refrigerator.
D.  Family caregiver supervision of medication administration

**Rationale:**

The use of a pill holder with slots for each dose of medication labeled with its administration time can provide the needed structure for safe self-administration of medications. A chart on a refrigerator is not as useful because the individual cannot take the chart with him/her during daily activities. Easy open caps do not provide any organizational structure for the identified cognitive deficits. Family caregiver supervision could be needed if the person was not able to benefit from organizational strategies. The individual needs to be provided with the opportunity to develop abilities to self-administer medications to maintain autonomy. In addition, one cannot assume that there is a family caregiver available who would be able to provide the appropriate support.

**Type of Reasoning: Inferential**

One must determine the best recommendation for an individual with cognitive deficits. This requires inferential reasoning skill, where one must infer or draw conclusions about a best course of action. In this situation, the OTA should recommend a daily pill holder with time-labeled slots to aid in appropriate administration of medication. Review adaptive strategies for medication management if answered incorrectly.

452

## B23  C5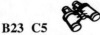

An OTA advises a parent of an 18 month-old with developmental delays on techniques to facilitate feeding. The child has a reflexive bite. Which utensil is most beneficial for the OTA to recommend the parent use when feeding the child?

**Correct Answer: B. A narrow shallow coated spoon.**

**Incorrect Answers:**

A.  A deep bowled soupspoon.

C.  A traditional teaspoon.

D.  A plastic spork.

**Rationale:**

The use of a narrow shallow coated spoon will help the food slide off. Deeper spoons or a spork will make it more difficult for the food to slide off, which would not be indicated for a child with a reflexive bite. In addition, the prong edges of the spork may hurt the child as he/she bites.

**Type of Reasoning: Inductive**

One must have knowledge of reflexive bite in children in order to choose the best feeding utensil. This is an inductive reasoning skill where knowledge of the diagnosis coupled with an understanding of the benefits of each of the utensils is essential to arriving at a correct conclusion. In this situation the OTA should suggest a narrow shallow coated spoon. If answered incorrectly, review guidelines for issuing utensils for children with reflexive bite.

## B24  C4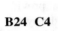

An adult who incurred a traumatic brain injury three months ago receives home care OT services. During meal preparation tasks the client ignores items on the left side of the counter. Which is the best remediation approach for the OTA to use with this client to enhance performance?

**Correct Answer: A. Place a brightly colored placemat on the left side of the counter.**

**Incorrect Answers:**

B.  Encourage bilateral activities.

C.  Place all items on the right side of the counter.

D.  Practice scanning activities.

**Rationale:**

The placemat provides an external cue, which the client can be taught to look for during meal preparation. This anchoring technique is a basic remediation approach. The other interventions would not remediate the performance deficit caused by the client's unilateral neglect. Practicing scanning activities can develop visual scanning skills but these would not directly address the functional deficit resulting from the unilateral neglect.

**Type of Reasoning: Inferential**

This question requires one to draw conclusions and make certain assumptions about clinical situations based on evidence, which is an inferential reasoning skill. For this scenario, placing a brightly colored placemat on the left side of the counter utilizes a remediation approach to the patient's deficit. If answered incorrectly, review information on remediation of deficits after traumatic brain injury.

**B25  C3**

A carpenter incurred a short below-elbow amputation. The client plans to return to work. Which components would be most important for the OTA to recommend for the client's prosthesis?

**Correct Answer: C. A fixed elbow socket and a heavy duty serrated grip terminal device.**

**Incorrect Answers:**

A.  A fixed elbow socket and a lightweight Teflon coated terminal device.

B.  A cable driven elbow socket and a heavy duty serrated grid terminal device.

D.  A cable driven elbow socket and lightweight Teflon coated terminal device.

**Rationale:**

An individual with a short below-elbow amputation will require a fixed elbow socket to provide stability because natural forearm rotation is not possible. A carpenter will need a heavy duty serrated grid terminal device to hold tools and nails.

**Type of Reasoning: Inferential**

One must link the individual's diagnosis to the prostheses presented in order to determine which prosthesis would best meet the individual's needs. This requires inferential reasoning, where one must draw conclusions about the likely needs of an individual based on an understanding of the carpenter's occupation. In this case a fixed elbow socket and heavy duty serrated grip terminal device would best meet the carpenter's needs. Review prosthetic options and features for below-elbow amputations if answered incorrectly.

**B26  C7**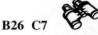

An individual with bilateral proximal weakness identifies a goal of independence in self-feeding. Which equipment is most beneficial for the OTA to recommend for goal attainment?

**Correct Answer: D. Mobile arm supports.**

**Incorrect Answers:**

A.  Extended long-handled utensils.

B.  Built-up handled utensils.

C.  An electric feeder.

**Rationale:**

Mobile arm supports can effectively compensate for upper extremity weakness. Extended long-handled utensils are indicated for individuals with decreased ROM. Built up handled utensils are indicated for individuals with decreased grasp. An electric feeder is indicated for individuals with no functional use of the upper extremities.

**Type of Reasoning: Inductive**

This question requires one to determine the most appropriate equipment for an individual based on the person's limitations. This requires inductive reasoning skill, where clinical judgment is paramount to arriving at a correct conclusion. For this situation, mobile arm supports are most effective in order to enhance self-feeding. If answered incorrectly, review indications for use of mobile arm supports.

454

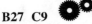

**B27  C9**

A person recovering from hip replacement surgery wants to begin meal preparation. The client refuses to use the walker that was ordered by the physician. The physician is unavailable for consultation. Which is the best initial action for the OTA to take in response to this situation?

**Correct Answer: A. Work on meal preparation activities with the client sitting at a table.**

**Incorrect Answers:**

B.  Work on meal preparation activities with the client standing without the walker.

C.  Delay working on meal preparation activities until the physician can be contacted.

D.  Tell the client the walker must be used until the physician changes the order.

**Rationale:**

There are many meal preparation activities that can be done while seated so there is no need to delay meal preparation activities. The OTA should not conduct the session without the prescribed walker or ambulatory aid until a written or verbal order is received. This is not negotiable as the client's safety is the paramount concern. Telling the client that the walker must be used violates the client's rights to self-determination.

**Type of Reasoning: Evaluative**

One must make a judgment call based on values and ethical principles, which is an evaluative reasoning skill. Situations such as these are challenging as one must weigh the interests of all the parties involved. The only solution that considers the safety and needs of the client is to work on meal preparation activities with the client sitting at the table. Review safety guidelines for clients with total hip arthroplasty if answered incorrectly.

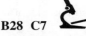

**B28  C7**

An intervention plan for a person with a complete lesion of the spinal cord at the C6 level has been developed by the client, occupational therapist, and OTA. Which activity should be included in this plan as a goal for the client to develop the ability to independently perform?

**Correct Answer: C. Donning pants while in bed.**

**Incorrect Answers:**

A.  Typing with a mouth stick.

B.  Transferring from bed to wheelchair using a sliding board.

D.  Feeding using a suspension sling or mobile arm support.

**Rationale:**

A person with a C6 spinal cord injury can independently don underwear and pants while lying in bed. Minimal assistance is needed to don socks and shoes. Therefore, intervention would focus on developing the ability to don pants while lying in bed. The client with a complete spinal cord injury at the C6 level does not need a mouth stick to type, a sliding board for transfers, or a suspension sling/mobile arm support to feed. Therefore, intervention is not needed to develop these abilities.

**Type of Reasoning: Deductive**

This question requires factual recall of functional abilities according to spinal level lesions. Specifically, one must recall the expected outcomes of a patient with C6 complete injury. This is factual information, which is a deductive reasoning skill. Donning pants while in bed is most aligned with C6 functioning. Review functional outcomes of cervical level injuries if answered incorrectly.

**B29  C6**

A young adult recently diagnosed with undifferentiated schizophrenia is referred to an OT day treatment program. What should the OTA do first with the client?

**Correct Answer: C. Have the person complete an occupational interest inventory**

**Incorrect Answers:**

A.  Determine short-term and long-term goals for program participation.

B.  Model desired behaviors during OT and therapeutic recreation groups.

D.  Encourage the client to maintain a daily log of medication intake.

**Rationale:**

Upon referral, the first step in the OT process is screening. The OTA can contribute to this process by having the person complete a screening tool. Determining the person's occupational interest can help identify areas requiring further evaluation. One cannot establish short-term and long-term goals with the client until an evaluation is completed. It is unknown if the client has deficits in medication management. Modeling behavior is a component of the intervention process.

**Type of Reasoning: Inductive**

One must draw conclusions about a best approach based on the diagnosis of the client in order to arrive at a correct conclusion. This requires inferential reasoning skill. For this case, the OTA should have the person complete an occupational interest inventory. If answered incorrectly, review client-centered approaches in psychosocial practice, especially during the screening process.

**B30  C7**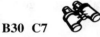

An individual is recovering from lumbar surgery. The patient must remain flat in bed during the initial recovery stages. The patient expresses an interest in reading from a personal collection of classic comics. Which adaptation is best for the OTA to recommend the client use for reading?

**Correct Answer: A. Prism glasses.**

**Incorrect Answers:**

B.  A page magnifier.

C.  Audiotapes of books of interest.

D.  Large print books of interest.

**Rationale:**

Prism glasses are eyeglasses that bend light by 90 degrees. This angle enables a person who is lying on his/her back to read anything that is resting on his/her lap. This recommendation enables the individual to read his/her collection of classic comics independently, as the client wanted. The use of audiotaped books does not meet the client's expressed interest in reading comics. Large print books and a page magnifier do not address the issue that the client must remain flat on his/her back.

**Type of Reasoning: Inductive**

Clinical knowledge and judgment are the most important skills needed for answering this question, which requires inductive reasoning skill. Knowledge of the diagnosis and most appropriate equipment to address the patient's limitations are essential to arriving at a correct conclusion. In this case, prism glasses is the most appropriate recommendation as it is the only device that addresses the individual's needs while maintaining the lumbar restrictions. If answered incorrectly, review information on the use of prism glasses.

## B31  C9

An older client with a diagnosis of late onset dementia of the Alzheimer type lives with family members. On the last three occasions, the client attended OT sessions with bruises and cuts on both legs. When asked about these, the client replies that a family member caused these injuries. What is the first action the OTA should take?

**Correct Answer: B. Immediately report potential abuse according to the facility policy.**

**Incorrect Answers:**

A.  Confirm the client's statements with the family.

C.  Call the police to report elder abuse.

D.  Discuss the situation with the OT supervisor at their next scheduled supervisory session.

**Rationale:**

This might be elder abuse. The OTA must report the findings according to the facility policy immediately. It is not the realm of the OT practitioner to confirm, investigate, or judge child, adult, and/or elder abuse. The role of the OT practitioner is to report suspected abuse to professionals who investigate the incident. Even though the person claims the injuries were caused by a family member, the OTA should not call the police. A professional skilled in abuse investigation must investigate the situation and decide the most appropriate action. Waiting for the next supervisory session to discuss this situation with the occupational therapist can be dangerous to the elder if this is indeed an abuse situation.

**Type of Reasoning: Evaluative**

This question requires one to determine a best course of action, given the information provided by the person. The test taker must understand that the elder's disclosure of potential abuse needs to be reported for investigation by appropriate agencies. The person's diagnosis of dementia, Alzheimer's type does not mitigate this requirement. Questions that require one to weigh the merits of each choice often require evaluative reasoning skills. If answered incorrectly, review guidelines on reporting suspected elder abuse.

## B32  C2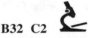

An OTA conducts a communication group in a wellness program for a large corporation. In this mature level group, what should the OTA do?

**Correct Answer: B. Participate as a member.**

**Incorrect Answers:**

A.  Help to develop the group norms of conduct.

C.  Actively resolve group conflicts.

D.  Maintain a leader role.

**Rationale:**

In a mature group, the group leader participates at the level of a member and does not act as a designated leader except in special circumstances such as a member becoming destructive to the group process. The members decide formally and informally the norms for behavior. The group leader does not usually participate in conflict resolution except to facilitate the member's participation in extreme situations, such as deadlocked conflicts. The group leader functions in a variety of task, maintenance, or egocentric roles as needed to show members how these roles function in the group.

**Type of reasoning: Deductive**

This question requires one to recall the guidelines for conducting a mature level group and the role of the group leader in order to arrive at a correct conclusion. This necessitates the recall of factual guidelines, which is a deductive reasoning skill. For this case, the OTA participates as a member in a mature level group. Review group levels and the role of the group leader in facilitating groups if answered incorrectly.

**B33  C8**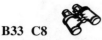

An individual cannot independently get from a supine position to a sitting position. The client has good scapular, shoulder, and elbow muscle strength. Which of the following should the OTA recommend as the most effective for the client to use to improve bed mobility?

**Correct Answer: D. A rope ladder.**

**Incorrect Answers:**

A. A leg lifter.
B. A bed rail assist.
C. A log roll technique.

**Rationale:**

A rope ladder or bed loops enable the individual to loop the arm(s) into the first 'rung'/loop, and then into the next 'rung'/loop, and so on until he/she has achieved a sitting position. The other options do not assist with independently moving from supine to sitting. A leg lifter is used to lift a leg that cannot move independently. A bed rail assist is used to help with rising from sitting to standing. A log roll technique can be used to help a person go from supine to sitting but this technique requires the assistance of another person. It is indicated for an individual who cannot use the rope ladder technique.

**Type of Reasoning: Inductive**

This question requires one to determine the most effective device to improve bed mobility in supine to sit. This requires inductive reasoning skill, where clinical judgment is paramount to arriving at a correct conclusion. For this situation, the OTA should recommend a rope ladder to assist with moving to a sitting position. If answered incorrectly, review adaptive devices for bed mobility, especially rope ladders.

**B34  C1**

A child with congenital anomalies has severe developmental delay. The child demonstrates motor and cognitive skills at the nine-month level. Which is the best adaptation for the OTA to use during intervention to develop the child's visual and auditory awareness?

**Correct Answer: C. A button switch that activates a CD player when the switch is pressed.**

**Incorrect Answers:**

A. A hand-held rattle of the child's favorite cartoon character.
B. A wrist bracelet with blinking lights that makes noise when moved.
D. A communication device that offers selections of "yes" and "no."

**Rationale:**

The button switch encourages the child to begin to develop cause and effect and provides auditory stimulation as well as a visual component in focusing on the device to access it. The rattle is a tool for the child at the three to six month level. The wrist bracelet is for the child at the three to six month level. The communication device is at the level of 12 to 18 months.

**Type of Reasoning: Inferential**

One must infer or draw conclusions about each of the four possible choices. The key to answering this question correctly is matching an activity to the child's developmental age and current needs. For this situation, a button switch that activates a CD player helps to develop cause and effect for this child who functions at a nine month level. If answered incorrectly, review developmental milestones and appropriate activities for the nine month level.

458

**B35 C8**

An individual with scleroderma has limited upper extremity ROM. Coordination is within functional limits. The person wants to improve efficacy in computer inputting capabilities. Which adaptation would be most effective for this person?

**Correct Answer: D. A contracted keyboard.**

**Incorrect Answers:**

A.  An expanded keyboard.
B.  A concept keyboard.
C.  A key guard.

**Rationale:**

A contracted keyboard decreases the ROM required to strike the keys. It is indicated for someone with limited ROM; however, due to smaller key size coordination must be functional. An expanded keyboard requires increased ROM to strike the keys. A key guard is an overlay on the keyboard used for individuals with poor coordination who frequently miss or overshoot keys. A concept keyboard is used for individuals with cognitive impairments. It replaces the keyboard's letters and numbers with pictures, symbols, or words to represent the concepts that are needed by a software program.

**Type of Reasoning: Inductive**

One must utilize clinical knowledge and judgment to determine the keyboard adaptation that is most effective for the individual, given the diagnosis and limitations. In this case, a contracted keyboard is most appropriate. If answered incorrectly, review modifications for increasing computer accessibility and indications for issuing a contracted keyboard.

**B36 C9**

Which task can OTAs perform when working in a subacute rehabilitation department?

**Correct Answer: A. Document the results of an ADL evaluation.**

**Incorrect Answers:**

B.  Decide which information to include in the client's medical record.
C.  Design a research project to measure the efficacy of interventions.
D.  Evaluate clients with the Allen Cognitive Level Test and interpret results.

**Rationale:**

An OTA can document the results of an ADL evaluation. Such documentation must be co-signed by the supervising occupational therapist. An occupational therapist makes the decision about what to include in the medical record. An OTA can contribute to the implementation of a research project but the occupational therapist is in charge of the design of a research protocol. An OTA can administer the Allen Cognitive Level Test but an OTA cannot interpret the evaluation results. Occupational therapists are responsible for the interpretation of evaluations.

**Type of Reasoning: Inferential**

This question requires one to recall the standards of practice for the OTA. Inferential reasoning skills are utilized as the test taker must determine, based on knowledge of practice guidelines, what is likely to be true. For this situation an OTA can document the results of an ADL evaluation. If answered incorrectly, review information on standards of practice for the OTA.

**B37  C7**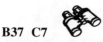

Several homeless veterans with a post-traumatic stress disorder attend an OT community re-entry group in a shelter. Which should be the primary focus of the initial group session?

**Correct Answer: C. Identification of local resources such as soup kitchens and thrift stores.**

**Incorrect Answers:**

A. Development of home management skills such as clothing care and meal preparation.

B. Determination of financial assets and money management skills.

D. Exploration of vocational interests and employment possibilities.

**Rationale:**

Locating basic resources is the most essential survival skill listed. Initial sessions at a homeless shelter would likely focus on basic survival and personal self-care skills prior to focusing on vocational interests, employment opportunities, or instrumental activities of daily living (IADL) such as laundry, cooking and money management skills. Subsequent sessions may focus on the development of IADL and vocational skills.

**Type of Reasoning: Inductive**

One must consider the needs of the group and benefits of each of the four possible courses of action. This necessitates inductive reasoning skill, where the test taker must use clinical judgment to determine the merits of each of the four choices, based on client needs. In this case, location of resources is the most beneficial topic, as it is the most essential survival skill for this group. If answered incorrectly, review guidelines for working with homeless individuals and appropriate community resources.

**B38  C7**

Several individuals participate in a work hardening program with a goal to resume working on a production line that utilizes electrical equipment and conveyers. Which functional deficit would the individuals participating in this program most likely demonstrate?

**Correct Answer: C. Decreased task speed.**

**Incorrect Answers:**

A. Poor judgment skills.

B. Incoordination.

D. Visual disturbances.

**Rationale:**

Decreased task speed is the only characteristic listed that is not a contraindication for working with electrical equipment, conveyers, or other potentially dangerous equipment. Poor judgment skills can cause serious problems in this work setting. Incoordination and/or visual disturbances can impair the clients' ability to perform the job safely or effectively.

**Type of Reasoning: Inferential**

One must infer or draw conclusions about what is likely to be true about the group members given the setting they are in and the characteristics of the task at hand. For this case, decreased task speed should be inferred as most likely to be present, as the other deficits would not be indicative for placement in a group of this nature due to safety issues. If answered incorrectly, review guidelines and goals for work conditioning and rehabilitation.

**B39 C9**

A co-worker in the occupational therapy department complains excessively during working hours of personal problems. Which action is best for the OTA to take in response to this situation?

**Correct Answer: D. Inform the supervising occupational therapist of the situation.**

**Incorrect Answers:**

A. Call the employee assistance program for the co-worker.

B. Talk with the co-worker using a client-centered approach.

C. Tactfully and firmly redirect the co-worker to work issues.

**Rationale:**

The OT supervisor should be informed in the best interests of the co-worker, all other staff, and the facility. This falls in the area of the supervisor's responsibility. One should not call the employee assistance program or counseling service for the co-worker. This decision for action falls to the co-worker. Co-workers are not responsible to and should not treat fellow workers. Tactfully redirecting the co-worker is a common technique to avoid being drawn into the problems of others. This is the second best answer, but will not address the problem in the department.

**Type of Reasoning: Evaluative**

One must make a decision based on ethical guidelines and value judgment, which is an evaluative reasoning skill. In this situation, the OTA should inform the supervising occupational therapist of the issue, as it is in the best interests of everyone involved. Questions of this nature can be challenging to answer as a simple solution is not often found and clear cut guidelines are not always at hand to refer to in situations such as these. Review standards of practice and team collaboration guidelines if answered incorrectly.

**B40 C4**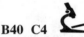

A patient who is status-post left frontal lobe ischemia has difficulty bearing weight through the right lower extremity during reaching activities (e.g., standing at a sink during morning self-care routine). The OTA implements a Motor Re-Learning Program (MRP). Which is the best intervention for the OTA to provide according to this approach?

**Correct Answer: D. Verbal and visual feedback while practicing reaching.**

**Incorrect Answers:**

A. Therapeutic handling to affect the central nervous system.

B. A stool to sit on during reaching activities.

C. Light joint compression throughout the trunk and right lower extremity during reaching activities.

**Rationale:**

A MRP approach provides verbal and visual feedback to give a person the input needed to make postural and limb adjustments. Therapeutic handling to affect the central nervous system is consistent with a neurodevelopmental therapy approach. Providing a stool to sit on during reaching activities can be used for safety purposes. This is consistent with a compensatory approach. Light joint compression throughout the trunk and right lower extremity during reaching is consistent with the Rood approach.

**Type of Reasoning: Deductive**

One must recall the guidelines of a Motor Re-Learning Program in order to arrive at a correct conclusion. This is factual knowledge, which is a deductive reasoning skill. For this situation, the most appropriate intervention is verbal and visual feedback while practicing reaching. If answered incorrectly, review Motor Re-Learning Program guidelines.

**B41  C3**

An OTA works with a person who incurred full thickness burns to both arms. Which intervention to approach would be most effective for the OTA to provide to control hypertrophic scar formation?

**Correct Answer: B. Compression garments.**

**Incorrect Answers:**

A. Axillary splints applied in the airplane position.

C. Wound grafting.

D. Elevation of the areas just above heart level.

**Rationale:**

Custom made compression garments provide equal pressure over the entire area to prevent scarring. They must be worn 23 hours a day for approximately 12 months, or until the scar and wound maturation is complete. Airplane splints are used to prevent tightening of the axilla area which would result in the inability to horizontally abduct the arm. Wound grafting is used as biological dressing to provide wound covering and pain relief. Elevation of the areas just above heart level is a technique to reduce upper extremity edema.

**Type of reasoning: Inferential**

One must determine the most effective approach to control hypertrophic scar formation in order to arrive at a correct conclusion. This requires one to determine what course of action will result in the best therapeutic outcome, which is an inferential reasoning skill. For this case, compression garments are most effective. Review intervention approaches for burns if answered incorrectly.

**B42  C9**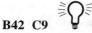

An occupational therapist and an OTA establish a program for a new acute psychiatric unit at a community hospital. The OTA assists with the design of the physical layout of the occupational therapy department. Which of the following should the OTA recommend to store arts and crafts materials?

**Correct Answer: A. A ventilated locked metal cabinet accessible only to staff.**

**Incorrect Answers:**

B.  Open shelving accessible to patients.

C.  Shelving next to a sink for easy clean up.

D.  A locked closet outside of the intervention area to ensure safety.

**Rationale:**

Arts and crafts materials include flammable, hazardous materials such as paint, stain, and thinners. These must be kept in ventilated metal cabinets in accordance with fire safety guidelines. Since these supplies are also toxic and potentially dangerous, access to them must be controlled by staff; therefore, a locked storage unit is required. The other options do not meet fire safety needs.

**Type of Reasoning: Inferential**

One must have knowledge of safety guidelines given the clinical setting in order to arrive at a correct conclusion. This is an inferential reasoning skill where knowledge of clinical guidelines and judgment based on facts are utilized to reach conclusions. In this case, the OTA should recommend a ventilated locked metal cabinet accessible only to staff. If answered incorrectly, review safety guidelines for storage of equipment in acute psychiatric settings.

462

## B43  C7

During a topical work preparation group for individuals recovering from mental illness, a member expresses concern about answering questions related to personal psychiatric history during a job interview. Which action is best for the OTA to take in response to these expressed concerns?

**Correct Answer: C. Lead a group discussion on the legal rights afforded in the interview process.**

**Incorrect Answers:**

A.  Refer the client to a vocational rehabilitation counselor.

B.  Encourage the other members of the group to share their interview experiences.

D.  Support the client in not disclosing past psychiatric history.

**Rationale:**

A primary purpose of a topical group is to develop knowledge about a particular area of occupational performance. Since members of the group may not be aware of all of their legal rights in an interview, it is most important for the OTA to lead a discussion about this issue. ADA protection concerning the disclosure of medical histories is invaluable knowledge for all members to acquire. This information can help the individual make an informed decision about disclosure. For example, if the person can perform the essential functions of a job, there is no compelling reason to disclose a past medical history. There is no need to refer the individual to a vocational rehabilitation counselor as this area is within OT's domain of practice. While encouraging members to share experiences and supporting a client's decision are both relevant, it is more important for the OTA to share information about ADA.

**Type of Reasoning: Evaluative**

This question requires a value judgment, which is an evaluative reasoning skill. Having an understanding of the Americans with Disabilities Act (ADA), the test taker should conclude that the best response in this situation is to discuss the legal rights afforded in the interview process with the group members. Review ADA regulations related to job interviewing if answered incorrectly.

## B44  C6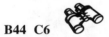

The most complex behavior an individual is able to perform on the Allen Cognitive Level Test is the running stitch while imitating an example. According to the Cognitive Disabilities model, this behavior is indicative of level 3 of Allen's Cognitive Levels. Which activity is best for the OTA to use when implementing intervention with this patient?

**Correct Answer: C. Sanding wooden bookends.**

**Incorrect Answers:**

A.  Exercises that require the imitation of another's posture.

B.  Sorting laundry by matching the colors of clothing items.

D.  Planning a three course meal.

**Rationale:**

According to Allen's Cognitive Disability model, people at level 3 of Allen's Cognitive Levels can use their hands to manipulate objects and they are able to perform a limited number of simple tasks that are repetitive. Sanding wood is a skill consistent with level 3 of Allen's Cognitive Levels. Sanding bookends will result in the completion of a tangible object that has functional use which can facilitate the person's feelings of self-efficacy. The imitation of posture is reflective of a level 2 skill according to the Cognitive Disabilities model, so exercises that require postural imitation would be too low for this individual. Sorting laundry by matching clothing colors is a level 4 skill. Planning a three course meal would require the level 5 skills of problem solving. This is too high of a level for this person.

**Type of reasoning: Inductive**

One must determine a functional activity that is best to implement for an individual functioning at Level 3 of Allen's Cognitive Levels. This requires knowledge of the Cognitive Disability model as well as functional abilities within each level. For this case, sanding wooden blocks is an ideal approach, as it provides a repetitive task within the capabilities of this individual. If answered incorrectly, review the Allen Cognitive Levels and characteristics of Level 3 functioning.

**B45 C1**

An OTA provides intervention to develop independent feeding skills in an 18 month-old child with significant developmental delays. The child can hold and suck on a cracker. The child has also mastered the ability to hold a spoon and bang it on the tray of the high chair. Which activity is best for the OTA to provide next during intervention?

**Correct Answer: A. Finger-feeding soft foods.**

**Incorrect Answers:**

B. Scooping food and bringing it to the mouth.
C. Taking cereal from a spoon held by the OTA.
D. Bringing a filled spoon to the mouth.

**Rationale:**

The next developmental milestone after holding and banging a spoon is finger-feeding soft foods. Due to the child's developmental delay, an OTA would work on the acquisition of feeding skills according to normal developmental milestones. The typical developmental sequence of feeding is: taking cereal from a spoon (5-7 months), self-feeding by sucking a cracker (6 - 9 months), holding and banging a spoon (6 - 9 months), finger-feeding soft foods (9 -13 months), bringing a filled spoon to mouth (12-14 months), scooping food and bringing it to the mouth (15- 18 months). See Table 5-4 in Chapter 5 for more details on the developmental sequence of self-feeding. In working with a child with developmental disabilities, it is the child's developmental age, not his/her chronological age which guides intervention.

**Type of Reasoning: Deductive**

One must recall the developmental guidelines for feeding infants with developmental delays. This is factual knowledge, which is a deductive reasoning skill. First, the test taker must determine what developmental age the child is performing feeding and then determine the next developmental milestone for that skill. In this case, the child is developmentally at 9 months and finger-feeding soft foods is the next milestone for feeding. If answered incorrectly, review developmental milestones of infant feeding.

**B46 C9**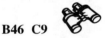

An OTA observes an aide having difficulty transferring a client with athetoid movements from a mat to a wheelchair. Before the OTA can cross the room to help with the transfer, the aide slides with the client to the floor. The OTA assists the aide in safely returning the client to the wheelchair. They assess that the client appears to be unharmed and return the client to the unit for a medical evaluation. Which action should the OTA take next?

**Correct Answer: D. Complete an occurrence report according to facility standards.**

**Incorrect Answers:**

A. Counsel the aide on the need to ask for assistance with difficult transfers.
B. Require the aide to attend a transfer training inservice.
C. Document the aide's unsafe actions in the personnel record.

**Rationale:**

Immediately after an incident occurs, the OTA must complete documentation according to setting's standards. Counseling an aide to ask for assistance and requiring attendance at a workshop can be appropriate aspects of risk management but they are not the first steps. In addition, there is no information provided to clearly identify that the aide was acting unsafely. There are transfer situations that unexpectedly become beyond a person's ability to successfully complete. During those situations, the person should guide the patient to the floor in a controlled manner. This is often done by using one's own body to support the patient and can give the appearance of "sliding". More information is needed to determine if the aide's actions were actually unsafe.

**Type of Reasoning: Inductive**

This question requires one to determine the best course of action. This requires inductive reasoning skill, where clinical judgment is paramount to arriving at a correct conclusion. For this situation, after returning the client to the unit for a medical evaluation, the OTA should complete an occurrence report according to the facility standards. If answered incorrectly, review guidelines for completing facility incidence reports.

464

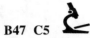

## B47  C5

An OTA implements intervention for individuals on an inpatient cardiopulmonary rehabilitation unit. The OTA assesses a patient's heart rate during intervention sessions by palpating a peripheral pulse. Which of the following most accurately describes the timing the OTA should use to complete this assessment?

**Correct Answer: B. 1-2 minutes prior to, during, and at cessation of the activity and 5 minutes post activity.**

**Incorrect Answers:**

A.  30 seconds prior to, during, and at cessation of the activity.
C.  1-2 minutes prior to, during, and at cessation of the activity.
D.  30 seconds prior to, during, and at cessation of the activity and 5 minutes post activity.

**Rationale:**

On an inpatient cardiopulmonary rehabilitation unit, the OTA must monitor a patient's heart rate before, during, and immediately after an activity and a few minutes (e.g., 5 minutes) post activity. Heart rate should be assessed using palpation of peripheral pulses. The most common monitoring site is the radial artery. Individuals with normal heart rhythms require only 30 seconds of palpation. Individuals receiving treatment in an inpatient cardiopulmonary rehabilitation unit may likely have irregular heart rhythms which require 1-2 minutes of palpation.

**Type of Reasoning: Deductive**

This question requires recall of guidelines and principles, which is factual knowledge. In this situation, the guideline for inpatient cardiac monitoring is to monitor a patient's heart rate before, during and immediately after an activity, plus a few minutes post activity. Review cardiac monitoring guidelines for inpatient rehabilitation if answered incorrectly.

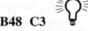

## B48  C3

An individual is being treated in an outpatient clinic for complex regional pain syndrome, type I. Which activity is best for the OTA to recommend the person complete at home?

**Correct Answer: D. Washing a car.**

**Incorrect Answers:**

A.  Doing light handwork in a craft of choice.
B.  Playing cards or a table-top game.
C.  Performing visualization relaxation exercises.

**Rationale:**

Washing a car involves scrubbing and the carrying of buckets of water, which are stress loading activities. Stress loading is a recommended intervention for complex regional pain syndrome, type I (formerly known as reflex sympathetic dystrophy or RSD). Light crafts, cards, a table-top game, and/ or visualization relaxation exercises can be meaningful and relevant to the person, but they do not provide any weight bearing. Therefore, these activities are not indicated as the primary intervention approach for this disorder.

**Type of Reasoning: Inferential**

This question requires the test taker to recall characteristics of CRPS Type I and then match this to a home program that most effectively addresses the patient's symptoms. In this situation, washing a car would provide the best approach to address the symptoms, which allows for stress loading activity. If answered incorrectly, review treatment guidelines for CRPS, especially Type I.

## B49 C6

An OTA implements a group for adolescents newly admitted to an eating disorders unit. Which activity is most beneficial for the OTA to use to develop the clients' task and social skills?

**Correct Answer: D. Completion of a group collage about personal interests.**

**Incorrect Answers:**

A.  Discussion of reasons for admission to the unit.
B.  Cooking a three course dinner to be eaten family-style.
C.  Watching a teen reality show and discussing problem scenarios.

**Rationale:**

A group collage is an activity that requires both task and social skills for completion. The OTA can provide interventions during this group to develop needed skills and reinforce observed skills. Discussion groups do not require task skills. A cooking and dining group does require task and social skills; however, it is not an appropriate activity for persons with eating disorders who are just beginning treatment.

**Type of Reasoning: Inferential**

One must have knowledge of eating disorders and of task and social skills groups in order to arrive at a correct conclusion. This is an inferential reasoning skill where knowledge of clinical guidelines and judgment based on facts are utilized to reach conclusions. In this situation, completion of a group collage reflecting personal interests is the best choice. If answered incorrectly, review the diagnostic criteria of eating disorders and the foci of different therapeutic groups. The integration of this knowledge is required to answer this question correctly.

## B50 C8

An individual prepares for discharge home following rehabilitation for a left CVA. Residual difficulties include fair dynamic balance, decreased upper extremity (UE) strength, and poor dexterity. The individual's stated priority is to be able to ambulate safely to the senior center located in the client's apartment building. Which ambulatory aid would be most effective for the OTA to recommend to this client?

**Correct Answer: B. A rolling walker.**

**Incorrect Answers:**

A.  A hemi-walker.
C.  A side-stepper walker.
D.  A standard walker.

**Rationale:**

A rolling walker is indicated for a person who cannot lift a standard walker due to impaired balance or upper extremity weakness. A hemi-walker and side-stepper are indicated for individuals who do not have use of both hands. This individual has poor dexterity in the affected UE, but only gross grasp is needed to hold a walker.

**Type of Reasoning: Inferential**

One must determine the most appropriate ambulatory aid, given knowledge of the presenting symptoms and limitations. This requires inferential reasoning skill, where one must infer or draw conclusions about a best course of action. In this situation, the OTA should recommend a rolling walker. Review guidelines for use of a rolling walker and other ambulatory aides if answered incorrectly.

**B51  C9**

An OTA provides home care services to a person recovering from a recent CVA. The client lives alone and receives home care Medicare benefits. The OTA arrives at the client's house at the scheduled session time, but there is no response to the knocking on the door. A neighbor reports seeing the client leave with a friend. Which is the best action for the OTA to take in response to this situation?

**Correct Answer: A. Document that no one answered the door and that the appointment will be rescheduled.**

**Incorrect Answers:**

B.  Call the supervising occupational therapist to discuss the missed appointment.

C.  Document that no one was home and that the appointment will be rescheduled.

D.  Document that the client is engaged in community mobility activities and should be evaluated for discharge.

**Rationale:**

Documentation must state that no one answered the door. This is factually correct and allows the individual to continue to receive home care service reimbursement from Medicare. To receive Medicare home care reimbursement, an individual must be homebound which means he/she can only leave home according to specific criteria. See Chapter 4 for these criteria. The client may have left for a reason that would meet these criteria. It is best not to document any behaviors that may jeopardize a person's homebound status. The OTA is capable of providing this documentation and does not need to discuss the missed appointment with the occupational therapist prior to completing the documentation.  The OTA follow up directly with the individual. One missed appointment is not a basis for discharge.

**Type of reasoning: Evaluative**

This question requires one to use guiding principles in order to determine a best course of action. This necessitates evaluative reasoning skill, as one must weigh the merits of the courses of action in order to arrive at a correct conclusion. For this scenario, the OTA should document that no one answered the door and that the appointment will be rescheduled. Review Medicare guidelines for homebound status if answered incorrectly.


**B52  C8**

Upon evaluating a client for a wheelchair, the OTA determines that a standard narrow adult wheelchair would be suitable for the individual. Which dimensions most accurately identify this chair?

**Correct Answer: C. 16 inches wide x 16 inches deep x 20 inches high.**

**Incorrect Answers:**

A.  18 inches wide x 18 inches deep x 20 inches high.

B.  16 inches wide x 16 inches deep x 18.5 inches high.

D.  14 inches wide x 16 inches deep x 18.5 inches high.

**Rationale:**

These are the standard dimensions for a narrow adult chair. The other choices do not identify measurements consistent with standard adult wheelchairs. These measurements would reflect a customized chair. A regular adult chair has dimensions of 18 inches wide x 16 inches deep x 20 inches high. A slim adult standard chair has dimensions of 14 inches wide x 16 inches deep x 20 inches high and a junior standard chair has dimensions of 16 inches wide by 16 inches deep by 18.5 inches high.

**Type of reasoning: Deductive**

One must recall the standard measurements for a narrow adult wheelchair in order to arrive at a correct conclusion. This is factual recall of guidelines, which is a deductive reasoning skill. For this case, the standard measurements are 16 inches wide x 16 inches deep and 20 inches high. Review standard narrow adult wheelchair guidelines if answered incorrectly.

**B53 C1**

An OTA is scheduled to give a one-hour presentation to a support group of parents of infants with a diversity of developmental disabilities. Which of the following is the most important focus for the OTA's presentation?

**Correct Answer: B. Discussion of typical areas of concern addressed by OT practitioners.**

**Incorrect Answers:**

A. Demonstration of infant positioning techniques.

C. Demonstration of different types of developmental assessments.

D. Discussion of the Individual Family Service Plan (IFSP).

**Rationale:**

An overview of the domain of concern addressed by OT for infants with developmental disabilities is the most appropriate topic for a one-hour presentation to an audience with diverse needs. Demonstration of infant positioning techniques and developmental assessments can be informative, but these techniques and assessments must be tailored to the individual child. A discussion about the IFSP can also be informative, but this information should be provided by the family's early intervention service provider.

**Type of Reasoning: Evaluative**

One must weigh the possible courses of action and then make a value judgment about the best course to take. This requires evaluative reasoning skill, which often utilizes guiding principles of action in order to arrive at a correct conclusion. For this case, given the audience the OTA is speaking to and the range of diagnoses of the infants, the OTA should discuss typical areas of concern addressed by OT practitioners.

**B54 C5**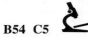

An adult with chronic schizophrenia attends a transitional employment program. The individual has a secondary diagnosis of Class I heart disease. The OTA meets with the client and the client's work supervisor to discuss the work activities the client can safely complete. Which of the following most accurately describes the client's capacity for work?

**Correct Answer: B. Work with no limitations.**

**Incorrect Answers:**

A. Work with minimum limitations.

C. Work with reasonable accommodation of frequent rest breaks.

D. Work with reasonable accommodation of no heavy lifting.

**Rationale:**

Class I heart disease requires no limitations on activities; therefore, no reasonable accommodations are needed.

**Type of Reasoning: Deductive**

One must recall the guidelines for activity and potential restrictions with Class I heart disease. This is factual knowledge, which is a deductive reasoning skill. For this case, the patient with Class I heart disease has no limitations. If answered incorrectly, review Class I heart disease activity guidelines.

**B55  C9**

A young adolescent with right hemiplegic cerebral palsy demonstrates a strong flexor synergy of the hand. The child does not use the hand for grasp, pinch, or release and often maintains the thumb flexed in the palm. The orthopedic hand surgeon recommends a flexor tendon release followed by several weeks of hand therapy and splinting. The family is very anxious about surgery and they ask the OTA what to do. Which is the OTA's best response?

**Correct Answer: C. Advise the family to review all the information to make an educated decision.**

**Incorrect Answers:**

A. Recommend that the child follow the surgery presented by the doctor.

B. Suggest a pre-operative course of intensive therapy and static and dynamic splinting.

D. Encourage the family to get a second opinion.

**Rationale:**

The OTA should offer unbiased, objective support and not give medical or other advice. The OTA does not make the decision for the family. The surgery is an option that the family can choose. This is an elective procedure. The suggestion about pre-operative treatment should be first presented to the physician to be sure that it is an appropriate choice. It is not in the realm of occupational therapy to encourage the family to get a second opinion.

**Type of Reasoning: Evaluative**

One must weigh the potential course of action and determine the best response to the parent's concerns. Following guidelines for the AOTA Code of Ethics, the OTA should observe nonmaleficence, which includes doing no harm, and duties, practicing within the parameters of the profession. The only response in this situation that does not create potential harm (physical or psychological) and follows guidelines of practice is to advise them to review all the information in order to make an educated decision. Review the AOTA Code of Ethics and principles of team communication if answered incorrectly.

**B56  C4**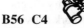

A five year-old attends an after-school program for children with sensory processing disorders. Intervention activities are designed to provide deep proprioceptive input. Which activity is most effective for the OTA to use during intervention?

**Correct Answer: A. Playing tug of war.**

**Incorrect Answers:**

B. Drawing with crazy foam on a mirror.

C. Finding objects in a paper bag.

D. Finger painting.

**Rationale:**

Playing tug of war is the only activity listed that has a proprioceptive component. Drawing with crazy foam on a mirror, finding objects in a paper bag, and finger painting are primarily tactile activities. Finding objects in a paper bag also has a strong stereognosis component.

**Type of Reasoning: Inductive**

One must determine the most effective intervention approach for the child, given the diagnosis provided. This requires inductive reasoning skill, where one must utilize clinical judgment to draw conclusions based on the information presented. In this situation, because deep proprioceptive input is best, the OTA should choose the game of tug of war. If answered incorrectly, review deep proprioceptive activities for children with sensory processing disorders.

**B57 C2**

During an individual session with an OTA, a client states, "I don't know what I want to work on. I don't really know what my goals are." What is the best action for the OTA to take in response to the client's concerns?

**Correct Answer: D. Initiate a discussion with the individual about what is personally important.**

**Incorrect Answers:**

A. Defer the development of an intervention plan until the individual has self-determined goals.

B. Establish a short-term goal related to improving goal-setting skills.

C. Contact the client's psychiatrist to request a medication evaluation.

**Rationale:**

It is best for the OTA to employ therapeutic use of self to establish rapport with the individual and engage him/her in the goal-setting process by exploring personal priorities. This answer choice is client-centered and incorporates patient's rights. Deferring the development of an intervention plan does not provide the client with the opportunity to participate in this planning process nor does it provide the opportunity to facilitate the ability to articulate his/her preferences. Setting up a short-term goal to improve goal setting skills without the input of the individual is vague and would not contribute to a client-directed intervention plan. This is a violation of the ethical principle of autonomy. There is nothing in the scenario to indicate the need for a medication evaluation.

**Type of Reasoning: Evaluative**

One must determine which of the four possible courses of action will best establish a therapeutic rapport and incorporate the patient's rights. This requires evaluative reasoning, where the test taker must determine which course of action is most valuable and effective. In this situation, the OTA should initiate discussion about what the client finds important. If answered incorrectly, review information on client-centered treatment planning.

**B58 C9**

A school-based OTA is providing per diem coverage for an OTA on a disability leave. Upon reviewing the caseload, the OTA notes that ten students have had evaluations completed during the past month. Five of these students' individualized education plans (IEPs) have also been completed by the team and approved by their families. Which is the best initial action the OTA to take as a contract practitioner?

**Correct Answer: A. Consult with the team and family to complete the IEPs for the remaining children.**

**Incorrect Answers:**

B. Conduct independent evaluations of each child under the supervision of the school's occupational therapist.

C. Implement the IEPs that have been established and approved under the supervision of the school's occupational therapist.

D. Report to the supervisor of the contract agency that the school has failed to comply with IEP guidelines.

**Rationale:**

The Individuals with Disabilities Act (IDEA) mandates that an IEP be written within 30 days of evaluation. This must be done as a team effort with the professionals providing their recommendations to the team and the child's family. Family consent is an essential part of the IEP process and is required by IDEA. There is nothing in the scenario to indicate a need for an additional evaluation or the reporting of the school. While it is important to implement IEPs, the first priority is to ensure that all students have an IEP within 30 days of evaluation. In addition, many aspects of the IEP can be implemented by teachers and other school personnel (e.g., resource room aides, behavioral specialists, speech-language pathologists).

**Type of Reasoning: Inferential**

One must infer or draw conclusions about a likely course of action, given the information presented. This is an inferential reasoning skill, where knowledge of IDEA guidelines is essential to choosing a correct solution. In this case, the OTA should consult with the team and family to complete the remaining IEPs. Review IDEA guidelines for completion of IEPs if answered incorrectly.

470

## B59 C3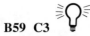

A client is being discharged after recovery from hip replacement surgery to live at home alone. Which is the most important equipment for the OTA to review with the client prior to discharge?

**Correct Answer: B. A long handled reacher.**

**Incorrect Answers:**

A. A rolling walker.

C. A bedside commode.

D. An emergency call system.

**Rationale:**

The client will need to observe hip precautions for several weeks. These precautions include not flexing the hip beyond 90°, which can make retrieving items very difficult. A long handled reacher can facilitate safety and independence in numerous tasks throughout the home. A rolling walker, bedside commode, and emergency call system can be helpful to many individuals with a variety of diagnoses. However, they are not necessary for an individual recovering from hip replacement surgery with no secondary diagnosis; therefore, they are not indicated in this case.

**Type of Reasoning: Inferential**

One must have knowledge of hip replacement and functional activities in the home setting in order to choose the most important equipment to recommend. This is an inferential reasoning skill where knowledge of the diagnosis coupled with the benefits of each of the described equipment is pivotal to choosing the correct solution. If answered incorrectly, review the benefits of a long-handled reacher and other adaptive aides for clients with post-hip replacement precautions.

## B60 C8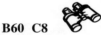

The transition plan for an 18 year-old with developmental delay includes a referral to a vocational rehabilitation (sheltered) workshop job setting. The student has set a goal to live independent of family. Which is the best living environment for the OTA to recommend for this student?

**Correct Answer: D. A group home with daily on-site supervision.**

**Incorrect Answers:**

A. An apartment in a subsidized housing project.

B. A group home with case managers available on-call.

C. A supported apartment with a roommate.

**Rationale:**

A person with developmental disabilities who meets the referral criteria for a vocational rehabilitation (formerly called sheltered) workshop will typically have cognitive deficits that require structure and supervision to successfully and safely complete tasks. A group home with on-site staff would provide this type of support. In addition, since this student has lived with family for all of his/her life, it is likely that he/she will need training to develop instrumental activities of daily living skills (IADL). Upon the attainment of IADL skills in the group home and vocational skills in the vocational rehabilitation (sheltered) workshop, the person may be able to progress to a higher level of independence in work and home management. The person would have to first develop IADL skills to live more independently in a housing project apartment, unsupervised group home, or supported apartment.

**Type of reasoning: Inductive**

This question requires clinical judgment in order to determine the best living environment for an individual with developmental delay. This requires inductive reasoning skill, where knowledge of the diagnosis and ability to live independently are paramount to arriving at a correct conclusion. For this situation, the OTA should recommend a group home with daily on-site supervision. If answered incorrectly, review community living options for individuals with developmental disabilities.

**B61 C8**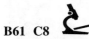

Occupational therapy services are provided to the clients of a psychogeriatric unit in a skilled nursing facility. An OTA presents an inservice on restraint reduction to the unit's direct care staff. Which of the following would the OTA identify as a permissible use of a restraint?

**Correct Answer: C. A lapboard to enhance a resident's self-directed functional behavior.**

**Incorrect Answers:**

A.  A bed guardrail to prevent a confused resident from wandering in the evening.

B.  Prescribed medication to control a resident's agitated behavior.

D.  A wheelchair with a lap belt to prevent a person with ataxic gait from falling.

**Rationale:**

A restraint is defined as anything that prevents access to the environment or to one's self. A restraint such as a lapboard can enhance functional performance and is permissible with a resident's informed consent. The correct answer choice states that the individual can self-direct; indicating that the person has the ability to give the required informed consent and that he/she can direct the staff on its removal and its desired use. The other purposes of restraints are not permissible and alternatives such as the provision of meaningful activities, adaptive aids and/or environmental modifications must be actively pursued as preventative measures.

**Type of Reasoning: Deductive**

This question requires recall of guidelines and principles, which is factual knowledge. Deductive reasoning skills are utilized whenever one must recall facts to solve novel problems. In this situation, the use of a lapboard is the only choice that does not constitute a restraint as it does not prevent access to the environment or one's self. Review guidelines for use of restraints if answered incorrectly.

**B62 C4**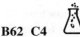

During an intervention session focused on developing home management skills, a client made a grocery list. The client grouped needed items together to make shopping easier and listed eggs separately from all of the other items. When explaining how the list was composed, the client stated, "Eggs break, they should be on top". Which of the following is the most accurate for the OTA to report that the client's approach to this task represents?

**Correct Answer: B. Concreteness.**

**Incorrect Answers:**

A.  Diminished insight.

C.  Anosognosia.

D.  Poor sequencing.

**Rationale:**

The statement reflects concrete thinking which is concerned with the actual properties of things and the realities of situations, rather than abstract properties or situational potentialities. In this situation, it is a functional strength. Insight is an awareness and understanding of oneself and behavior. Anosognosia is unawareness or denial of deficits. Sequencing is the ability to determine the proper ordering of steps in a task.

**Type of Reasoning: Analytical**

This question provides a description of a behavior and the test taker must determine the definition of the behavior displayed. This requires analytical reasoning skill where one must analyze the behavior in order to correctly determine the appropriate behavioral characteristic. In this situation, the behavior indicates concrete thinking. Review concrete thinking behaviors if answered incorrectly.

472

## A63 C1

A six year-old begins prosthetic training with a right below-elbow myoelectric prosthesis. To learn to operate the terminal device, the OTA implements intervention using age-appropriate play activities. Which activity is best for the OTA to first include during intervention?

**Correct Answer: A. Assembling building blocks.**

**Incorrect Answers:**

B. Squeezing a squeeze toy.
C. Playing board games.
D. Stacking one inch blocks.

**Rationale:**

In prosthetic training, the person first learns to open and close the terminal device. Assembling building blocks provides the opportunity to develop this skill and it is the most appropriate activity for the child of this age. A squeeze toy is appropriate for a child up to two years of age. The pieces of board games are small and will require an advanced level of skill in operating the terminal device. Stacking blocks is appropriate for a pre-school child.

**Type of Reasoning: Inferential**

One must determine the best activity for a child with a below-elbow myoelectric prosthesis. The key is to choose the activity that is age appropriate and focuses on opening and closing the terminal device. In this situation, assembling building blocks provides opportunities to practice opening and closing the device and is age appropriate for a six year-old. If answered incorrectly, review functional prosthetic training activities for children.

## B64 C7

A tool and die designer develops bilateral carpal tunnel syndrome. The local work hardening program does not have the exact equipment that the designer uses in the job setting. Which action is best for the OTA to take in response to this situation?

**Correct Answer: D. Duplicate the job task components as closely as possible.**

**Incorrect Answers:**

A. Refer the client to another work hardening program that has the equipment.
B. Advocate to the occupational therapist about the need to order and install the equipment necessary to duplicate the work setting.
C. Perform some necessary aspects of rehabilitation in the client's work setting.

**Rationale:**

Work hardening programs can use real or simulated tasks that duplicate, as closely as possible, the components of each client's job tasks. It is not realistic for all programs to have every possible piece of equipment related to clients' job tasks. Consequently, OT practitioners become skilled at activity analysis and adept at simulating job tasks with the equipment that they have available. An OTA who is experienced in work hardening can provide effective intervention without equipment that exactly matches the client's work. Therefore, there is no reason to refer the client to another facility A reason to refer a client to another facility is the therapy staff's lack of experience and inability to provide effective intervention. It may be helpful to perform some aspects of rehabilitation during a site visit, but the logistics of this can be difficult and the OTA's ability to provide intensive therapy on in a work environment would likely be limited. Therefore, the best answer is to duplicate the job tasks in the clinic.

**Type of Reasoning: Evaluative**

This question requires the test taker to weigh the merits of each of the possible courses of action. This necessitates evaluative reasoning skill, where value judgments are paramount to arriving at a correct conclusion. In this situation, the most appropriate action is for the OTA to duplicate the job task components as closely as possible. Questions of this nature can be challenging, as value judgments often do not have clear cut answers. Review therapeutic approaches to job simulation in work hardening settings if answered incorrectly.

**B65  C3**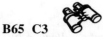

A restaurant employee incurred a fracture to the left humerus. After cast removal, the patient received OT and now demonstrates 3/5 strength of the left triceps and full ROM of the left elbow. To increase elbow function in order to perform work-related tasks, which activity is most effective for the OTA to next include during intervention?

**Correct Answer: A. Storing plates and glasses on shelves at chest height.**

**Incorrect Answers:**

B.  Wiping off a table while standing.

C.  Carrying a tray of dishes from the table to the sink.

D.  Wiping off a counter at chest height.

**Rationale:**

Storing plates at chest height is a resistive activity against gravity, one of the best ways to increase strength in a muscle to attain full elbow ROM. Wiping the table at stomach level is an isotonic activity, gravity assisted. Carrying a tray of dishes is an isometric activity. Wiping a counter at chest height is isotonic with the effects of gravity decreased.

**Type of Reasoning: Inductive**

One must utilize clinical knowledge and judgment to determine the functional activity that would provide resistive activity of the triceps. In this case, storing plates and glasses on shelves at chest height is the ideal way to implement a resistive activity for the triceps. If answered incorrectly, review resistive and strengthening exercises.


**B66  C4**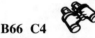

Following a left CVA, an individual receives OT services at a sub-acute rehabilitation facility. The patient's personal goal is to be independent in dressing. The patient demonstrates decreased memory, poor sequencing skills, and ideational apraxia. Which of the following is most effective for the OTA to provide when teaching one-handed dressing techniques to this patient?

**Correct Answer: C. Physical prompts to initiate the steps in dressing.**

**Incorrect Answers:**

A.  Step-by-step verbal instructions.

B.  Sequenced photographs of the steps in dressing.

D.  A full length mirror for the client to observe self-dressing performance.

**Rationale:**

Ideational apraxia is the breakdown in the knowledge of what is to be done and how to perform specific activities. This means that one cannot perform a task either spontaneously or upon request. However, the sensorimotor aspects needed to perform the activity can be intact. Providing physical prompts to initiate dressing may be a sufficient cue for the individual to begin and then complete the task. Providing verbal instructions or sequenced photographs will not address the fundamental deficit of ideational apraxia and therefore will not enhance performance. Observing one's self dressing in front of a mirror results in a view opposite of actual performance. This can increase confusion, especially with apraxia.

**Type of Reasoning: Inductive**

One must utilize clinical knowledge and judgment to determine the best approach for teaching one-handed dressing techniques, given the patient's symptoms. In this case, because the patient has ideational apraxia, it is best to provide physical prompts to initiate dressing tasks. If answered incorrectly, review ideational apraxia symptoms and ADL intervention guidelines.

**B67  C9**

During an accreditation self-study, the OT department personnel review all charts. An OTA notices that a colleague fills out the review forms without reading the charts. Which action is best for the OTA to take in response to this observation?

**Correct Answer: D. Report the observation to the OT supervisor.**

**Incorrect Answers:**

A. Talk to the colleague directly.
B. Report the incident to the director of medical records.
C. Report the colleague to the accrediting agency.

**Rationale:**

Reporting the observation to the supervisor is the best choice since the OTA directly observed a colleague committing an act that directly violates the AOTA Code of Ethics. Any overt violation of the Code of Ethics should be reported to the direct supervisor of the practitioner. The supervisor is the person who is responsible for dealing with the situation. The OTA does not need to personally talk directly to the colleague and find out what is happening. It is not necessary to report the incident to the accrediting agency.

**Type of Reasoning: Evaluative**

This question requires a value judgment in an ethical situation, which is an evaluative reasoning skill. In this situation, the colleague has violated the Code of Ethics of veracity, which is to be truthful in duties. Therefore, the OTA should report the colleague's actions to the supervisor. If answered incorrectly, review the AOTA Code of Ethics, especially veracity.

**B68  C4**

An individual recovering from a head trauma exhibits a motor pattern indicative of being influenced by the symmetrical tonic neck reflex. Which is most likely for the OTA to observe the client having difficulty with during functional mobility?

**Correct Answer: B. Moving from lying supine to sitting.**

**Incorrect Answers:**

A. Moving both arms to midline when supine.
C. Flexing the head from the supine position.
D. Extending the head from the prone position.

**Rationale:**

Moving from lying to sitting is initiated by flexion of the neck. The presence of a symmetrical tonic neck reflex will cause this flexion to result in increased hip extension, making it difficult to assume a sitting position. The presence of the asymmetrical tonic neck reflex can decrease the ability to bring both arms to midline when supine. Flexing the head from a supine position would be more difficult in the presence of the tonic labyrinthine supine reflex because this reflex increases extensor tone. Extending the head from a prone position would be more difficult in the presence of the tonic labyrinthine prone reflex because this reflex increases flexor tone.

**Type of Reasoning: Inferential**

One must have knowledge of symmetrical tonic neck reflex (STNR) and influence of the reflex on functional activity. This is an inferential reasoning skill where knowledge of clinical guidelines and judgment based on facts are utilized to reach conclusions. In this case the presence of a STNR can affect moving from supine to sitting. If answered incorrectly, review STNR reflex and its influence on functional activities.

**B69 C5**

A child with developmental delay has poor oral motor control. What should the OTA do to facilitate lip closure?

**Correct Answer: D. Give a slight upward sweep of the index finger from the lower jaw to the lower lip.**

**Incorrect Answers:**

A. Give pressure with the index finger under the jaw.

B. Place food on a spoon and firmly place the spoon on the back part of the tongue.

C. Place the thumbs on the lateral ends of the mandibles.

**Rationale:**

Providing a slight upward sweep of the index finger from the lower jaw to the lower lip can facilitate lip closure. Pressing down on the space between the nose and upper lip is also facilitative for lip closure. Placing pressure with the index finger under the jaw and placing each thumb on the lateral end of the mandibles facilitates jaw closure. Placing food on a spoon and firmly placing the spoon on the back part of the tongue can facilitate the gag reflex.

**Type of Reasoning: Inferential**

One must determine the most likely intervention approach for a child, given the diagnosis provided and skill described. This requires inferential reasoning skill, where one must draw conclusions based on the information presented. In this situation, the OTA would give a slight upward sweep of the index finger from the lower jaw to the lower lip to facilitate lip closure. If answered incorrectly, review oral motor control techniques for children.

**B70 C2**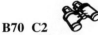

To develop social interaction skills, an OTA implements a group program for students with Asperger's syndrome. Which group is best for the OTA to include in this program?

**Correct Answer: C. A developmental group.**

**Incorrect Answers:**

A. A directive group.

B. A topical group.

D. A task-oriented group.

**Rationale:**

A developmental group's focus is to teach the social interaction skills needed for group participation in a sequential manner. It provides relevant group structure and activities along a continuum that is consistent with how interaction skills develop normally. Asperger's syndrome is a pervasive developmental disorder. Individuals with Asperger's often have normal intelligence but significant deficits in social interaction skills. A directive group uses a highly structured 5 step approach to help low functioning patients (e.g., persons with dementia or serious and persistent mental disorders) develop basic skills. This group is too low functioning for students with Asperger's. A topical group is a discussion group that focuses on activities performed outside of the group (e.g., vocational planning). A task-oriented group's focus is to increase members' awareness of their values, ideas, and feelings as revealed through group activity. This emphasis on intra-psychic functioning would be inappropriate for individuals with Asperger's syndrome.

**Type of reasoning: Inductive**

This question requires the test taker to determine the best group focus for students with Asperger's syndrome and the need to focus on social interaction skills. This requires clinical judgment and knowledge of Asperger's syndrome symptoms in order to arrive at a correct conclusion, which is an inductive reasoning skill. For this case, the OTA should use a developmental group focus. Review appropriate group focuses for individuals with Asperger's syndrome, especially developmental groups, if answered incorrectly.

476

## B71 C5

An individual recovering from hepatitis, type C has decreased upper and lower extremity muscle strength and hypertension. Six months ago the client had an angioplasty and is very fearful of having a heart attack. Which should the OTA advise the client to perform to increase muscle strength?

**Correct Answer: A. Isotonic exercises.**

**Incorrect Answers:**

B. Isometric exercises.

C. Contract-relax exercise.

D. Muscle contractions and holds.

**Rationale:**

Isotonics are the only exercises listed that are not contraindicated for a person with hypertension or heart disease. The other choices describe isometric exercises or activities which include isometric elements and are contraindicated in this case.

**Type of Reasoning: Inferential**

One must determine the most appropriate exercise for an individual, given knowledge of the presenting diagnoses. This requires inferential reasoning skill, where one must infer or draw conclusions about a best course of action. In this situation, the OTA should recommend isotonic exercises, as this is the only exercise listed that is not contraindicated for individuals with hypertension or heart disease. Review exercise guidelines for individuals with hypertension and heart disease if answered incorrectly.

## B72 C4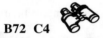

A child who incurred a head trauma exhibits moderate to severe spasticity throughout the trunk. Both upper extremities exhibit increased flexor tone. Which is the most effective generalized technique of controlled sensory input for the OTA to use to decrease tone?

**Correct Answer: B. Slow rolling supine to prone position.**

**Incorrect Answers:**

A. Facilitation of the triceps through tapping.

C. Inhibition of the biceps through pressure to the tendon insertion.

D. Fast rocking over a therapy ball to elicit protective extension.

**Rationale:**

Slow rolling is a generalized inhibitory technique. Facilitation of the triceps and inhibition of the biceps are not generalized techniques for they act on specific muscles. Fast rocking is contraindicated for it is facilitation technique that would increase spasticity.

**Type of Reasoning: Inductive**

Clinical knowledge and judgment are the most important skills needed for answering this question, which requires inductive reasoning skill. Knowledge of generalized inhibitory techniques is essential to choosing the best solution. In this case, slow rolling in supine to prone position is the only generalized inhibitory technique. Review generalized techniques for inhibiting flexor tone if answered incorrectly.

**B73 C3**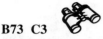

An OTA meets with a client to ensure compliance with a prescribed splinting protocol. Which is the most important outcome of this session?

**Correct Answer: C. The client's understanding of the purpose(s) and procedure(s) of the splint protocol.**

**Incorrect Answers:**

A. The client's adherence to a written splint wearing schedule.

B. The client's ability to independently don and doff the splint.

D. The completion of functional training in the use of the splint.

**Rationale:**

If a client understands the purposes and procedures of the splint protocol he/she will become a collaborative partner in the intervention programs. The other choices are important components of a splinting intervention program and may be required by accrediting bodies (e.g., JCAHO requires documentation of functional training and the individual's ability to don/doff a splint). However, the success of these interventions and the attainment of client compliance rely on the client's understanding of the splint protocol's purposes(s) and procedure(s).

**Type of reasoning: Inductive**

This question requires one to determine the most important approach for ensuring clients' compliance with a splinting program in order to arrive at a correct conclusion. This necessitates clinical judgment, which is an inductive reasoning skill. For this situation, the OTA should ensure the clients understand the purpose(s) and procedure(s) of the splint. If answered incorrectly, review guidelines for improving compliance with splinting programs.

**B74 C4**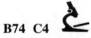

An adolescent incurred a spinal cord injury at the C-5 level. During a family caregiver education session, the OTA instructs family members in the provision of passive range of motion (PROM) to the patient's wrist and fingers. Which method of PROM should the OTA teach the family members to perform?

**Correct Answer: D. Flex the fingers with the wrist fully extended and extend the fingers with the wrist fully flexed.**

**Incorrect Answers:**

A. Extend the fingers with the wrist extended.

B. Flex the fingers with the wrist flexed.

C. Flex and extend the fingers with the wrist in a neutral position.

**Rationale:**

A major goal of OT for a person with a SCI at C-5 or C-6 is to enhance the development of a tenodesis grasp. Family caregivers can perform PROM to enhance achievement of this goal. Ranging the finger flexors with the wrist extended and the finger extensors with the wrist flexed will result in shortening of the flexor tendons without compromising joint ROM. This shortening will enhance the tenodesis grasp. The other ROM patterns do not do this.

**Type of Reasoning: Deductive**

One must recall the guidelines for ranging in a tenodesis pattern. This is factual knowledge, which is a deductive reasoning skill. The proper ranging in this pattern is to flex the finger with the wrist fully extended and extend the fingers with the wrist fully flexed. Review tenodesis pattern and PROM if answered incorrectly.

478

**B75  C4**

A young adult with Down syndrome exhibits poor motor planning and gross motor incoordination. Which activity should the OTA use during intervention to increase functional skills?

**Correct Answer: B. Line dancing.**

**Incorrect Answers:**

A.  Riding a stationary bicycle.

C.  Walking on a treadmill.

D.  Playing a board game.

**Rationale:**

Line dancing requires motor planning to follow the dance steps. The steps repeat themselves in an established pattern, which can help develop gross motor coordination. Bicycling on a stationary bicycle and walking on a treadmill do not require significant motor planning. Playing a board game does not require gross motor coordination.

**Type of Reasoning: Inferential**

One must determine the most appropriate intervention approach for a person, given the diagnosis provided. This requires inferential reasoning skill, where one must draw conclusions based on the information presented. In this situation, given the diagnosis of Down syndrome and deficits presented, the most appropriate activity would be line dancing. If answered incorrectly, review motor planning and gross motor coordination activities and principles of activity analysis. The correct answer requires the integration of this knowledge.

**B76  C5**

An occupational therapist and an OTA design a dining rehabilitation program in a long-term care facility. The OTA instructs paraprofessional staff in proper feeding techniques. Which point is most important for the OTA to include in this staff training?

**Correct Answer: A. Meals should occur in a home-like environment with staff conversing with the elders being fed.**

**Incorrect Answers:**

B.  Individuals with swallowing difficulties should be fed in a group so that staff can remind them to swallow at the beginning of each meal.

C.  Placing three fingertips on the throat and pressing firmly will stimulate a swallow response.

D.  The head should be tilted slightly backward during feeding to facilitate an assisted swallow.

**Rationale:**

Proper feeding techniques include a facilitative environment. Dining in a homelike setting with staff who are attentive to the elders' needs and interests during feeding/mealtimes will facilitate eating and socialization during the activity. Grouping individuals with swallowing difficulties diminishes the individualized approach that is essential to quality long-term care. In addition, reminding people to swallow does not effectively deal with the reasons for their swallowing difficulties. If an individual does forget to swallow food, he/she must be reminded/cued throughout the meal to prevent aspiration/choking. Reminding/cueing only at the beginning of a meal is not sufficient. Placing three fingertips on the throat and pressing firmly does not stimulate a swallow response. Tilting the head back may facilitate aspiration and is contraindicated.

**Type of Reasoning: Inferential**

One must determine the most important feeding instruction to provide to staff, given knowledge of the clinical setting and feeding guidelines. This requires inferential reasoning skill, where one must infer or draw conclusions about a best course of action. In this situation, the OTA should inform staff of the importance of meals occurring in a home-like environment with staff conversing with the elders being fed. Review feeding guidelines in long-term care settings if answered incorrectly.

**B77 C3**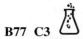

An individual is status post carpal tunnel release. When the OTA conducts a sensory test for sharp/dull (pain), the person reports dull as sharp on the palmar surface of the thumb and index finger. All other responses were correct. Which is accurate for the OTA to document about the individual's sensation?

**Correct Answer: C. Hypersensitive along the median nerve distribution of the thumb and index fingers.**

**Incorrect Answers:**

A. Impaired for pain along C5 and C6 dermatomes.

B. Hypersensitive along the ulnar nerve distribution of the palmar surface of the hand.

D. Absent for pain along the median nerve distribution.

**Rationale:**

The individual is so sensitive that when touched with a dull stimulus he/she reports it as "sharp". Therefore, the sensation is not absent, but rather impaired at the median nerve distribution. Impairment at C5 and C6 would also involve the loss of sensation in the upper arm and forearm. Ulnar nerve distribution involves the ring and little fingers.

**Type of Reasoning: Analytical**

This question provides symptoms and the test taker must determine the likely cause for them. This is an analytical reasoning skill, as questions of this nature often ask one to analyze a group of symptoms in order to determine a diagnosis. In this situation the symptoms indicate hypersensitivity in the median nerve distribution of the thumb and index finger. Review symptoms of median nerve disorders if answered incorrectly.

**B78 C8**

A resident of a skilled nursing facility (SNF) is severely dehydrated after a viral illness. The resident is agitated and confused. The doctor has prescribed intravenous (IV) fluid infusions, but the nursing staff is concerned that the individual will pull out the infusion line. They request that the OTA provide a restraint for this resident. Which is the best action for the OTA to take in response to this request?

**Correct Answer: A. Provide soft fleeced mittens for the person's hands.**

**Incorrect Answers:**

B. Report the request to the occupational therapist as a violation of restraint-free standards.

C. Decline the referral and explain that restraints are no longer allowed to be used in SNFs.

D. Provide a lap board as this is the least restrictive restraint.

**Rationale:**

Wearing mittens will help prevent the individual from pulling out the IV lines. Providing ones that are soft and fleeced can provide tactile input that is not noxious. While recent federal guidelines (i.e., OBRA) emphasize restraint reduction and the provision of a restraint-free environment, they also recognize the potential need to provide restraints in certain circumstances. A restraint is permissible and acceptable if it is medically necessary and temporary for lifesaving treatment. These criteria apply in this case; therefore, the OTA should not decline the request. The wearing of mittens can sufficiently deter the person from pulling out the IV line. If the person begins to rub the IV line with his/her hands even while wearing the mittens, the OTA may need to recommend the use of bilateral soft elbow splints that fix the elbows at 20-30 degrees of flexion. The splints would prevent the person from accessing the IV line. However, this is a more restrictive solution so it would only be allowed after the failure of less restrictive methods. A lap tray would not limit the person's upper extremity mobility and thus would not be effective.

**Type of Reasoning: Inductive**

Clinical knowledge and judgment are the most important skills needed for answering this question, which requires inductive reasoning skill. Knowledge of the federal guidelines for use of restraints and most appropriate courses of action are essential to choosing the best solution. In this case, the OTA should provide soft fleeced mittens for the person's hands. Review restraint utilization guidelines in SNFs if answered incorrectly.

480

**B79  C3**

An individual with a traumatic above-elbow (transhumeral) amputation has received a body-powered prosthesis. To train the person in the operation of the terminal device (TD), which of the following should the OTA do initially during intervention?

**Correct Answer: D. Lock the elbow in 90° of flexion and teach only TD control.**

**Incorrect Answers:**

A. Teach the person how to control the elbow joint.
B. Combine training of TD use with training for elbow joint movement.
C. Lock the elbow in full extension and teach only TD control.

**Rationale:**

Locking the elbow joint into flexion places the TD in a functional position for the completion of activities with the TD. Locking the elbow in extension would not place the TD in a position suitable for the completion of most functional activities. The question specifically asks about training for TD operation, not control of the elbow joint. Control of the elbow joint would occur independent of TD control training, because the elbow joint must be locked for TD use in an above-elbow (transhumeral) prosthesis.

**Type of Reasoning: Inductive**

One must utilize clinical knowledge and judgment to determine the training approach for an individual with an above-elbow amputation (AEA). This requires inductive reasoning skill. In this case, the OTA should lock the elbow in 90° of flexion and teach only TD control. If answered incorrectly, review training guidelines for individuals with AEA and body-powered prostheses.

**B80  C7**

An individual with a complete C-5 spinal cord injury prepares for discharge. The client plans to return to work as an editor of children's books. Which adaptive equipment is best for the OTA to recommend the client use to access desktop publishing programs?

**Correct Answer: A. A wrist splint in the functional position with a slot to hold a typing stick.**

**Incorrect Answers:**

B. A balanced forearm orthosis with a slot to hold a typing stick.
C. A wrist-driven flexor hinge splint with a slot to hold a typing stick.
D. A universal cuff to hold a typing stick.

**Rationale:**

A wrist splint in the functional position will provide the support needed due to absence of wrist extensors and wrist flexors. A person with a C-5 spinal cord injury can perform keyboarding tasks with a typing stick inserted into a splint. A balanced forearm orthosis (BFO) is used to compensate for upper extremity muscle weakness. BFOs are also called deltoid aids or suspension slings. BFOs and similar equipment solely support the upper extremity and do not provide any options for holding items as a substitute for hand function. A person at C-5 does not have active wrist movements so a wrist-driven flexor hinge splint and a universal cuff would be ineffective.

**Type of Reasoning: Inferential**

One must have knowledge of C5 spinal injury and effective adaptive devices for this level of injury in order to choose the best device to enhance participation in computer skills. This is an inferential reasoning skill where knowledge of the diagnosis coupled with knowledge of the functional ability to use devices with residual upper extremity musculature is key to choosing the correct solution. If answered incorrectly, review C5 injury, intact musculature, and available adaptive devices for computer skills.

**B81  C4**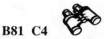

An OTA uses a motor learning intervention approach to develop prehension patterns with a child recovering from a brain tumor. The OTA places small toys on a table and asks the child to pick up the toys and put them into a storage box that is also on the table. The OTA uses random practice during this activity. Which types and arrangement of toys are most effective for the OTA to provide according to the motor learning approach?

**Correct Answer: D. Toys of different shapes, sizes, and weights in a mixed arrangement on the table.**

**Incorrect Answers:**

A.  Toys that are exactly the same shape, size, and weight in a mixed arrangement on the table.
B.  Toys that are exactly the same shape, size, and weight placed in a straight line on the table.
C.  Age-appropriate toys arranged in a developmental sequence according to the child's developmental age.

**Rationale:**

According to a motor learning approach, random practice involves the performance of several motor tasks in random order to encourage the re-formulation of the solution to the presented motor problem. Each time the child picks up a small toy of a different shape, size and/or weight his/her grasp pattern must be different. This activity is consistent with random practice. Having the child pick up toys that are of the same shape, size, and weight involves repeated performance of the same motor skill. This activity reflects blocked practice according to the motor learning approach. The motor learning approach does not utilize a developmental sequence.

**Type of Reasoning: Inductive**

This question requires one to determine the best approach for arrangement of toys for prehension according to motor learning approach and utilization of random practice. This requires inductive reasoning skill, where clinical judgment is paramount to arriving at a correct conclusion. For this situation, the toys of different shapes, sizes, and weights should be placed in a mixed arrangement on the table. If answered incorrectly, review motor learning approach, especially the principle of random practice.


**B82  C1**

An ambulatory elder adult with hemiparesis and presbycusis is moving in with a daughter. The daughter requests information from an OTA that can maintain the elder's functional ability in the home. Which should the OTA recommend?

**Correct Answer: B. Speak directly, clearly, and slowly to the elder.**

**Incorrect Answers:**

A.  Remove knobs from the stove when the elder is home alone.
C.  Add bright color strips to the edge of each stair tread.
D.  Provide lists of the sequence of routine tasks.

**Rationale:**

Presbycusis is an age-related sensorineural loss that results in decreased hearing. Speaking directly, clearly, and slowly can help ensure that the elder hears what the family is saying. This will enable the elder to participate fully in family interactions. There is nothing in the situation to indicate the need for any of the other suggestions, as no cognitive or visual deficits are noted.

**Type of Reasoning: Inferential**

One must have knowledge of presbycusis and presenting symptoms in order to determine the best recommendation for this situation. This is an inferential reasoning skill where knowledge of clinical guidelines and judgment based on facts are utilized to reach conclusions. In this situation, the OTA should recommend speaking directly, clearly, and slowly to the elder. If answered incorrectly, review presbycusis and compensation approaches.

482

**B83  C2**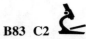

An OTA administers a standardized cognitive-perceptual assessment to a client. The client demonstrates difficulty performing the first two tasks of the evaluation. Which is the most appropriate action for the OTA to take?

**Correct Answer: C. Continue the evaluation according to the established administration protocol.**

**Incorrect Answers:**

A.  Continue the evaluation and provide additional verbal cues during task performance.

B.  Continue the evaluation and model each task.

D.  Discontinue the evaluation to avoid frustrating the client.

**Rationale:**

A standardized assessment must be administered according to its established protocol to be reliable. Providing additional cues or modeling would compromise the reliability of the assessment tool. Discontinuing the evaluation would not enable the OTA to obtain needed information about the person's cognitive-perceptual status. Since most cognitive-perceptual assessments measure several skills, one cannot assume that poor performance on the first two tasks will mean poor performance on the other tasks. OTAs are able to administer standardized assessments under the supervision of the occupational therapist. For specialized evaluations, the OTA must establish service competence. The occupational therapist is responsible for the interpretation of the evaluation.

**Type of Reasoning: Deductive**

This question requires recall of guidelines, which is factual knowledge. Deductive reasoning skills are utilized whenever one must rely on facts to solve problems. In this situation, because the OTA is administering a standardized assessment, the established protocol must be followed. Review guidelines for administering standardized assessments if answered incorrectly.

**B84  C4**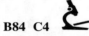

A patient had a brain tumor removed one month ago and exhibits residual cognitive-perceptual deficits. The OTA uses a neurofunctional approach to remediate the client's cognitive dysfunction. Which of the following is best for the OTA to include in the intervention program?

**Correct Answer: A. Functional activities in their real contexts.**

**Incorrect Answers:**

B.  Client education on strategies to remediate deficits.

C.  Tabletop activities to practice remediation strategies.

D.  Computer games to develop performance component skills.

**Rationale:**

A neurofunctional approach emphasizes functional activity performance in the actual environment. The other options reflect a transfer of training approach.

**Type of Reasoning: Deductive**

One must recall factual knowledge of the neurofunctional approach to rehabilitation in order to choose the correct solution. This is a deductive reasoning skill. A typical neurofunctional approach emphasizes functional activity performance in a real-life context. If answered incorrectly, review guidelines for providing treatment under a neurofunctional approach.

**B85 C7**

A parent recovering from brain cancer is preparing to be discharged home from a rehabilitation center. The client has residual cognitive deficits in problem solving. Sensori-motor abilities are within functional limits. To develop requisite problem solving skills for independent functioning at home, which task should the OTA work on with the client during OT intervention?

**Correct Answer: C. Washing the family's laundry.**

**Incorrect Answers:**

A. Performing routine morning self-care.

B. Making a shopping list of grocery staples.

D. Reading a bedtime story to the client's children.

**Rationale:**

Problem solving is the ability to recognize and define a problem, identify alternative plans for solving the problem, select a plan, organize steps in the plan, implement the plan, and evaluate the plan's outcome. Doing laundry can present a number of potential problems that must be solved (i.e., stain removal, appropriate care for different textured and/or colored fabrics). The other task choices are more structured and have less of a problem-solving component.

**Type of Reasoning: Inferential**

One must infer or draw conclusions about the likely intervention approach needed at home, given the information presented. This is an inferential reasoning skill, where knowledge of a therapeutic skill, such as problem solving in this situation, is essential in choosing a correct solution. In this case, the person will mostly likely require intervention for developing independence in laundry skills. If answered incorrectly, review problem solving skills after brain injury and instrumental ADL. The integration of this knowledge is required to answer to this question correctly.

**B86 C4**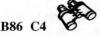

After a right cerebral vascular accident (CVA), an individual has a subluxed left shoulder. Which is the most effective approach for the OTA to use to treat this subluxation?

**Correct Answer: D. Position the person's arm to avoid shoulder traction while in bed and in the wheelchair.**

**Incorrect Answers:**

A. Rest the person's arm on the wheelchair's lapboard throughout the day.

B. Rest the person's arm in an inclined arm trough attached to the wheelchair throughout the day.

C. Have the person wear a shoulder sling 24 hours per day to reduce stress at the shoulder joint.

**Rationale:**

Proper positioning during the day and evening is most effective in treating subluxations. Positioning must avoid shoulder traction and weight on the shoulder. Wearing a shoulder sling 24 hours per day is contraindicated as long-term use can result in soft-tissue contractures, edema and the development of pain syndromes. Shoulder slings can be used to support a flaccid shoulder for short and controlled periods of time. Lap boards and arm troughs can be used for proper daytime positioning when a person is in a wheelchair but positioning in bed must also be considered.

**Type of Reasoning: Inductive**

This question requires one to determine the best approach for treating subluxation of the shoulder. This requires inductive reasoning skill, where clinical judgment is paramount to arriving at a correct conclusion. For this situation, positioning the arm to avoid should traction while in bed and the wheelchair is best. If answered incorrectly, review treatment guidelines and positioning recommendations for patients with shoulder subluxation.

484

## B87  C3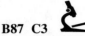

An individual recovering from myasthenia gravis has fair minus (F-) muscle strength in both upper extremities. The occupational therapist and OTA develop an intervention plan to include the goal of increasing muscle strength. According to the biomechanical approach, which should the OTA work on with the patient during intervention?

**Correct Answer: B. Complete active ROM against gravity.**

**Incorrect Answers:**

A. Complete active ROM with gravity decreased.
C. Incomplete active ROM against gravity.
D. Complete active ROM against gravity and slight resistance.

**Rationale:**

The next muscle grade after a minus Fair (F-) is fair (F) which indicates the ability of the body part to actively move through its complete ROM against gravity. An F- muscle grade indicates a body part can move through its incomplete ROM (more than 50%) against gravity. An F+ muscle grade indicates a body part can move through its complete ROM against gravity and slight resistance. The ability to move a body part through complete ROM with gravity decreased is indicative of a poor (P) muscle grade.

**Type of Reasoning: Deductive**

This question requires recall of guidelines and principles, which is factual knowledge. Deductive reasoning skills are utilized whenever one must recall facts to solve problems. In this situation, one should recall the definition of the next grade above F- in order to arrive at a correct conclusion. Review muscle grades obtained from manual muscle testing if answered incorrectly.

## B88  C6

An individual attends an outpatient parenting skills group. The person has a history of serious recurrent depression and is taking Nardil. The client complains of recurrent headaches and difficulty focusing during the day (e.g. when helping children with their homework). Which action is best for the OTA to make in response to the client's expressed concerns?

**Correct Answer: D. Tell the client you will be notifying the psychiatrist of these complaints.**

**Incorrect Answers:**

A. Instruct the client in stress reduction techniques.
B. Ask the group for suggestions on how to deal with the parenting stress of homework.
C. Suggest that the individual consult with a nurse practitioner for headache relief strategies.

**Rationale:**

Nardil is a monoamine oxidase inhibitor (MAOI). It has serious side effects when a person eats foods that contain the amino acid tyramine. Tyramine increases blood pressure and may lead to stroke or other cardiovascular reactions. Headache and heart palpitations are the first sign of a problem. This must be considered a serious medical situation and the physician must be contacted. To assume that the headaches are stress-related is dangerous. Suggesting that the person contact a nurse practitioner does not guarantee follow through. The individual needs to collaborate with the psychiatrist to determine if an MAOI is the best medication, given its restrictions. Chapter 10 in this text provides these restrictions.

**Type of Reasoning: Evaluative**

One must weigh the possible courses of action and then make a value judgment about the best course to take. This requires evaluative reasoning skill, which often utilizes guiding principles of action in order to arrive at a correct conclusion. For this case, because the patient is describing potentially serious side effects of the medication, the OTA must notify the person's psychiatrist. Questions of this nature can be challenging. Essential to arriving at a correct conclusion is concern for the person's well-being and safety.

**B89  C4**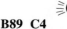

A seven year-old with spastic diplegia holds a pencil by using a tight static tripod grasp and hyperextension of the index DIP and the thumb IP. Which of the following is best for the school-based OTA to provide to improve the child's grasp on the pencil?

**Correct Answer: A. A soft built-up pencil grip.**

**Incorrect Answers:**

B.  Activities to relax and stretch the fingers prior to writing.

C.  A plastic triangular pencil grip.

D.  Application of heat packs prior to writing.

**Rationale:**

A soft pencil grip will help to inhibit the increased tone of the fingers. Relaxation and stretching activities can be helpful but the child still needs a soft grip on the pencil. Seven year old children are required to hold a pencil for great deal of time to complete school assignments, so the most effective intervention is an adaptation to the activity. A plastic grip is hard, which may increase tone. Heat packs are not helpful and would typically not be provided in a school setting for improving grasp.

**Type of Reasoning: Inferential**

One must have knowledge of spastic diplegia in children in order to choose the best recommendation. This is an inferential reasoning skill where one must draw a conclusion about a best course of action based on the information presented. In this situation a soft built-up pencil grip is the best recommendation as it will help to inhibit the increased tone. If answered incorrectly, review characteristics of spastic diplegia in children and adaptive techniques for writing.

**B90  C9**

An OTA leads a transitional planning group for high school students with conduct disorders. The school fire alarm goes off five minutes before the group's scheduled termination. There have been six false alarms during the past three days at the school. Several of the students laugh and say, "There it goes again". Which is the OTA's best response to this situation?

**Correct Answer: B. Escort the students to the nearest fire exit.**

**Incorrect Answers:**

A.  Call the school's main office to determine the validity of this alarm.

C.  Continue with the group's planned wrap-up, adding a discussion about the implications of false alarms.

D.  Escort the students back to their homeroom classrooms to await directions.

**Rationale:**

All alarms must be taken seriously to ensure safety. In the event of an actual fire, any delay can be deadly. All the other choices are incorrect for they place students at potential risk.

**Type of Reasoning: Evaluative**

This question requires a value judgment in an emergency situation, which is an evaluative reasoning skill. In this type of situation, the safest procedure should be followed, which is to escort the students to the nearest fire exit. Question such as these, that inquire about a course of action in a potential emergency often require the test taker to respond in the safest, most effective manner possible.

## B91 C3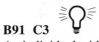

An individual with rheumatoid arthritis has developed several boutonniere deformities. Which of the following is the most accurate description for the OTA to include in documentation of the individual's presenting signs?

**Correct Answer: C. Flexion of the PIP joint and hyperextension of the DIP joint.**

**Incorrect Answers:**

A. Hyperextension of the PIP joint and flexion of the DIP joint.
B. Ulnar deviation and subluxation of the MCP joints.
D. Heberden's nodes at the DIP joints and Bouchard's nodes at the PIP joints.

**Rationale:**

A boutonniere deformity occurs when there is hyperextension of the DIP joint with flexion of the PIP joint. A swan neck deformity is evident when there is hyperextension of the PIP joint and flexion of the DIP joint. Ulnar deviation and subluxation of the MCP joints are additional deformities that can result from rheumatoid arthritis. Heberden's nodes and Bouchard's nodes are types of bone spurs that can result from osteoarthritis.

**Type of Reasoning: Inferential**

One must link the individual's diagnosis to the signs presented in order to determine which presenting signs are most representative of boutonniere deformities. This requires inferential reasoning, where one must draw conclusions about the likely presentation of a diagnosis. In this case the diagnosis would present with flexion of the PIP joint and hyperextension of the DIP joint. Review signs and symptoms of boutonniere deformity if answered incorrectly.

## B92 C6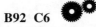

A 17 year-old student with a diagnosis of bipolar disorder and a history of self-abusive behaviors attends a transitional school-to-work program conducted by an OTA and an occupational therapist. During the vocational skills group, the student expresses feelings of hopelessness about the future and questions the point of participating in the program. The student asks to leave the group due to being too tired to concentrate as a result of sleepless nights. The occupational therapist asks the OTA to address the student's concerns while the therapist works with the other group members. Which action is best for the OTA to take in response to the student's statements?

**Correct Answer: A. Pull the student aside from the group and ask if the student is feeling self-destructive.**

**Incorrect Answers:**

B. Allow the student to leave the group after reminding the student to relay concerns to the guidance counselor.
C. Support the validity of the student's feelings and encourage the student to remain in group.
D. Remind the student that in a work setting the norm is to work even if fatigued.

**Rationale:**

All statements of hopelessness and a lack of future vision must be taken seriously, as they can indicate a suicide risk. This is especially important in this case since there is a history of self-destructive behavior. Pulling the student aside from the group allows for the maintenance of confidentiality. The student's reports of sleep disturbances, concentration difficulties, and feelings of hopelessness can reflect an increase in depression. If the student is allowed to leave the group, there is a risk that self-destructive behavior (or even suicide) may occur. Validating the student's feelings and reinforcing work place norms do not deal safely with a potential immediate crisis.

**Type of Reasoning: Evaluative**

This question requires professional judgment based on guiding principles, which is an evaluative reasoning skill. Because the student is stating feelings of hopelessness and lack of future vision, the OTA should ask the student if there are feelings of self-destructiveness. This way the OTA can determine the most appropriate course of action based on this information. Review symptoms of suicidal ideations if answered incorrectly.

**B93  C5**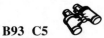

An OTA works with the new foster parent of a two year-old child diagnosed with major developmental delays and severe hypotonia. The OTA advises the foster parent to position the head in midline during feeding. Which additional positioning recommendations for feeding are best for this child?

**Correct Answer: C. Semi-reclined with neck in neutral.**

**Incorrect Answers:**

A.  Sitting with hips and knees at 90 degrees flexion, neck in neutral.

B.  Sitting with hips and knees at 90 degrees flexion, neck in extension.

D.  Semi-reclined with neck in extension.

**Rationale:**

This semi-reclined position can be easily maintained with the use of a commercially available child seat and it allows for correct postural alignment during the feeding activity. The support of positioning equipment is needed due to the child's severe hypotonia which prevents the child from independently maintaining a sitting position. Although it is possible to design equipment to support a seated position, the child's severe hypotonia would require equipment that is over-restrictive (e.g., a chest restraint). Feeding in a semi-reclined position is the least restrictive and most comfortable option for the child. It is not safe to feed anyone with neck in extension for this can result in choking.

**Type of Reasoning: Inductive**

One must utilize clinical knowledge and judgment to determine the best position for feeding the child, given knowledge of the diagnosis. In this case, positioning the child semi-reclined with the neck in neutral is the best position for feeding. If answered incorrectly, review positioning guidelines for children with hypotonia and for feeding. Integration of this knowledge is required to answer this question correctly.

**B94  C3**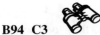

A child with moderate arthrogryposis complains of profuse sweating when wearing bilateral night resting splints. Which of the following should the OTA suggest to the child?

**Correct Answer: B. Wear a cotton stockinet liner under the splints.**

**Incorrect Answers:**

A.  Wear only one splint each night, rotating from left to right.

C.  Wear volar cock-up splints instead.

D.  Wear a splint with several one centimeter perforations in the splinting material.

**Rationale:**

A stockinet liner helps to absorb sweat. It is also helpful to wash and thoroughly dry the hands prior to donning splints. Wearing only one splint each night does not address sweating and cuts wearing time in half, making splints less effective. Volar cock-up splints do not address the position of the MPs and IPs and might result in increased MP and IP flexion contractures. Perforations might decrease the strength and integrity of the splinting material.

**Type of reasoning: Inductive**

One must utilize clinical judgment in order to determine the best recommendation for a child with sweating while wearing night splints. This requires inductive reasoning skill. For this case, the OTA should suggest wearing a cotton stockinet liner under the splints to absorb sweat. If answered incorrectly, review splinting adaptations and addressing sweating while wearing splints.

488

**B95  C4**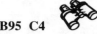

An OTA working in early intervention meets with the parents of an infant who cries a lot and has difficulty being soothed. The parents are concerned that they are unable to comfort their child. Which is the most effective strategy for the OTA to recommend to the parents?

**Correct Answer: D. Tightly wrap the infant in a blanket.**

**Incorrect Answers:**

A. Loosely wrap the infant in a blanket.

B. Provide frequent and rapid changes in movement.

C. Do nothing, as the infant's behavior is typical.

**Rationale:**

Tightly wrapping an infant in a blanket can provide controlled and consistent firm pressure that is non-aversive and soothing. The crying behavior whether typical, or indicative of a difficulty, will likely respond to this strategy. Loosely wrapping the infant provides inconsistent and variable input that can increase discomfort. Frequent and rapid changes in movement are contraindicated because they can increase tone and stimulate arousal. Whether the child's behavior is considered typical or not is irrelevant; the parents are concerned and can benefit from suggestions.

**Type of Reasoning: Inductive**

This question requires one to determine the best approach for an infant with difficulty being soothed. This requires inductive reasoning skill, where clinical judgment is essential to arriving at a correct conclusion. For this situation, the OTA should recommend tightly wrapping the infant in a blanket. If answered incorrectly, review treatment guidelines for infants with difficulties in being soothed.

**B96  C2**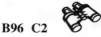

An adolescent with Duchenne muscular dystrophy refuses to use mobile arm supports (MAS) because "they look so big and stupid." Which action should the OTA take first in response to the client's statement?

**Correct Answer: B. Explore other options with the client to perform activities that do not use the MAS.**

**Incorrect Answers:**

A. Collaborate with a rehabilitation engineer to design a more compact device.

C. Provide several logical reasons for using the MAS to enhance functional performance.

D. Discharge the client and follow up with after one month to re-assess interest in the MAS.

**Rationale:**

The most appropriate first action is exploring ways the client can do activities without requiring the use of the mobile arm supports. This response is an example of therapeutic use of self and a client-centered approach. Developing a different design for a mobile arm support is a long-term option that may not be feasible. Providing logical reasons for using the mobile arm supports is not the best initial response as it ignores the client's feelings of frustration and is not a client-centered approach. There is no need to discharge the client from treatment. The issue needs to be addressed now, not in one month.

**Type of Reasoning: Inductive**

This question requires one to determine the best approach for addressing the client's concerns about using mobile arm supports. This requires inductive reasoning skill, where clinical judgment is paramount to arriving at a correct conclusion. For this situation, the OTA should explore other options for activity performance that do not use the arm supports. If answered incorrectly, review treatment guidelines for persons with Duchenne muscular dystrophy, especially the use of mobile arm supports.

**B97  C7**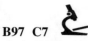

An individual admitted to a psychosocial day treatment program has a diagnosis of a major depressive disorder. The client reports having difficulty performing home management tasks and caring for two young children. The occupational therapist determines that the recently hired, entry-level OTA can contribute to the evaluation process. Which evaluation will the OTA complete with this client?

**Correct Answer: D. An activities of daily living evaluation.**

**Incorrect Answers:**

A.  A cognitive evaluation.

B.  A mental status examination.

C.  An occupational history interview.

**Rationale:**

OTAs are trained and qualified to perform ADL evaluations during their entry-level education. The ability to complete a cognitive evaluation, mental status examination, and an occupational history interview require the establishment of the OTA's service competence prior to the assignment of these evaluation tasks. The establishment of service competency requires the acquisition of experience and continuing training. The OTA in this scenario has been recently hired and is an entry-level practitioner; therefore, service competency for these additional evaluations would not have yet been established.

**Type of Reasoning: Deductive**

This question requires recall of guidelines and principles, which is factual knowledge. Deductive reasoning skills are utilized whenever one must recall facts to solve clinical problems. In this situation, the OTA can contribute to the evaluation process by performing an ADL evaluation. Review supervisory guidelines for OTAs, especially the evaluation process if answered incorrectly.

**B98  C4**

A client at the Rancho Los Amigos Level VII of automatic-appropriate is attending a vocational rehabilitation program three days a week. The client is frequently late due to difficulties with getting ready in the morning. The client asks the OTA for suggestions to address this problem. What is the most effective action for the OTA to take in response to the client's request?

**Correct Answer: A. Develop a visual chart with the client, depicting the necessary sequence of morning activities.**

**Incorrect Answers:**

B.  Advocate that the vocational program provide the client with a flexible start time.

C.  Advise the client to call the vocational program to tell staff when running late.

D.  Advise the client to wake up one hour earlier on vocational rehabilitation program days.

**Rationale:**

Individuals at Rancho Los Amigos Level VII have cognitive abilities that are automatic-appropriate. They are able to initiate and attend to highly familiar tasks (e.g., BADL) in a distraction-free environment, but have shallow recall of what has been completed. Creating a visual chart of the necessary sequence for routine morning activities will provide the person with a tool that the client can use each morning to check off his/her ADL task completion. This visual cueing device can also help the client refocus if he/she gets distracted. Increasing the time available in the morning to do the daily routine is not needed. In this scenario, the client does not have any reported sensorimotor deficits that require extended time for ADL performance. In addition, having extra time can increase the potential for distractions and can decrease focus. While it is polite to call when one is going to be late, this action is not addressing the client's need to develop an organized effective routine. Changing the vocational rehabilitation program schedule is also inappropriate for this reason.

**Type of Reasoning: Inductive**

One must utilize clinical knowledge and judgment to determine the most appropriate action to address an individual's unique challenge. This requires inductive reasoning skill. In this case, given the client's current level of recovery, the OTA should develop a visual chart with the individual, depicting the sequence of morning activities. If answered incorrectly, review scales and activities for the different cognitive levels, especially activity completion for individuals at Level VII.

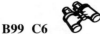

**B99  C6**

An individual with schizophrenia continues to experience hallucinations. Which action should the OTA take when the individual begins to actively hallucinate during an OT project group?

**Correct Answer: A. Redirect the individual's attention back to the project.**

**Incorrect Answers:**

B.  Provide tactile reassurance to the individual.

C.  Verbally reassure the individual that the hallucination is not real.

D.  Use humor to divert the individual's attention away from the hallucination.

**Rationale:**

The best action to take is to redirect attention back to the project. Additional effective strategies for responding to hallucinations are to reinforce all misinterpretations of environmental noises and events, use a calm tone, avoid sarcasm, avoid arguing about the reality of the hallucinations, and help the client to find a reassuring phrase, word, and/or action to focus on reality. The client may not respond favorably to the tactile reassurance since touch can be threatening during hallucinations. The other choices are ineffective ways to reinforce reality for the client who is hallucinating.

**Type of Reasoning: Inductive**

One must determine a best course of action through clinical judgment, based on the information provided, which is an inductive reasoning skill. For this situation, the question inquires about the best way to help a patient who is actively hallucinating. The best response would be to redirect the individual back to the activity at hand. If answered incorrectly, review information on schizophrenia and management of hallucinations.

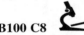

**B100  C8**

An OTA provides an accessibility consultation to a business that has hired a new employee who uses a wheelchair for mobility. The only entrance to the business has four steps, each seven inches high. Which ramp length is best for the OTA to recommend the business have constructed?

**Correct Answer: B. 28 feet.**

**Incorrect Answers:**

A.  14 feet.

C.  35 feet.

D.  46 feet

**Rationale:**

Accessibility guidelines state that the ramp should be constructed with one foot of ramp length for each inch of rise. The total rise for these steps is 28 inches; therefore the ramp should be 28 feet long. The other options do not meet these guidelines.

**Type of Reasoning: Deductive**

This question requires recall of guidelines, which is factual knowledge. Deductive reasoning skills are utilized whenever one must recall facts to find ideal solutions. In this situation, accessibility guidelines indicate that for every one inch of rise, there should be one foot of ramp; therefore the ramp should be 28 feet long. Review accessibility guidelines, especially ramp construction, if answered incorrectly.

## B101 C9

An OTA working in an outpatient pediatric clinic has been seeing a child for sensory processing deficits. After 12 treatment sessions a denial letter for services has been received. The letter states that the diagnosis and the treatment do not meet the requirements of the policy. The parents who are aware of the denial want the OTA to change the child's diagnosis code in order to receive reimbursement. What is the best way for the OTA to respond?

**Correct Answer: C. Explain to the parents that the current diagnosis cannot be changed in order to receive reimbursement.**

**Incorrect Answers**

A.  Collaborate with the occupational therapist to plan the child's discharge from OT and develop a home sensory program for follow up by the parents.
B.  Encourage the parents to seek an alternate insurance carrier to receive improved coverage for services.
D.  Encourage the parents to set up a payment plan with the clinic's accounting department.

**Rationale:**

It is against the AOTA Code of Ethics of veracity to change a diagnosis in order to receive payment from an insurance company. If there was an error in the diagnosis when the bill was submitted for payment to the insurance company or if the OTA actually assigned an incorrect diagnosis code by mistake, then the diagnosis could be corrected and resubmitted with a letter of explanation. However, in this scenario, there is nothing to indicate the code was incorrect. Therefore the code cannot be changed. Discharging the child deprives the child of needed skilled treatment. It is not the OTA's place to suggest changes in insurance carriers and it also does not solve the current situation. While setting up a payment plan may be needed, it does not address the parent's request to change the code.

**Type of reasoning: Evaluative**

This question requires one to weigh the merits of the course of actions presented and determine which action effectively addresses the issue at hand. This requires judgment based on guiding principles, which is an evaluative reasoning skill. For this situation, the OTA should explain to the parents that the current diagnosis cannot be changed in order to receive reimbursement as it violates ethical principles. If answered incorrectly, review the AOTA Code of Ethics, especially veracity.

## B102 C5

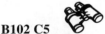

An adult recently diagnosed with scleroderma receives occupational therapy services to deal with the functional changes caused by this disease. Which recommendation is best for the OTA to make to this individual?

**Correct Answer: B. Dress in layers for neutral warmth.**

**Incorrect Answers:**

A.  Dress in lightweight clothing for thermal comfort.
C.  Use pull-on clothing to ease donning and doffing.
D.  Use Velcro/or a button hook to ease fastening.

**Rationale:**

Scleroderma is a systemic disease of unknown etiology. Symptoms are grouped into the CREST syndrome which includes calcinosis, Raynaud's phenomenon, esophageal dysfunction, sclerodactyly of fingers and toes, and telangiectasis or red spots covering the hands, feet, forearms, face and hips. The systemic sclerosis of internal organs can be life threatening. A common early (and ongoing) symptom of scleroderma is poor circulation. This phenomenon usually affects the hands, and at times the feet. It is often precipitated by exposure to cold. Dressing in layers can compensate for this problem. Lightweight clothing would not address the person's need for warmth. The use of pull on clothing, Velcro fasteners and/or a button hook may be indicated if the disease progresses to the point that the individual develops contractures. However, these are not indicated for a person recently diagnosed with the disorder.

**Type of Reasoning: Inductive**

One must utilize clinical knowledge and judgment to determine the best recommendation for the patient with scleroderma. Knowledge of scleroderma and guidelines to minimize effects of the condition are critical in order to arrive at a correct conclusion. In this case, the best recommendation is for the patient to dress in layers for neutral warmth. If answered incorrectly, review characteristics of scleroderma.

492

**B103 C2**

A three year-old with recurring headaches and decreased gross and fine motor skills is hospitalized for a diagnostic work-up. Just prior to the OT evaluation session, the parents have been told that the child has cancer. The parents are upset when they bring the child to OT. The OTA provides support. Which are the next best actions for the OTA to take in response to this situation?

**Correct Answer: A. Refer the parents to their spiritual advisor or the social worker and proceed with the OT session.**

**Incorrect Answers:**

B. Cancel the OT session and refer the parents to their spiritual advisor or the social worker.
C. Ask the supervising occupational therapist to participate in the session and spend it addressing the parents' acceptance of the diagnosis.
D. Reschedule the OT session for later in the day so that the family can speak with the supervising occupational therapist and their spiritual advisor or the social worker.

**Rationale:**

The best actions are to refer the family to a source of help and comfort and proceed with the session. The OTA can provide this referral in a supportive and empathetic manner and then complete the scheduled evaluation. The child needs an occupational therapy evaluation as part of the diagnostic work-up. The OTA can help the family adjust to and accept the diagnosis via therapeutic activities during the OT session without direct OT supervision. However, the provision of counseling is most appropriately provided by pastoral care and/or social work practitioners. Moreover, in a medical model setting, these services would not be reimbursable if administered by an OTA. Canceling or rescheduling the session is not necessary and in a hospital setting it is highly unlikely that immediate re-appointments would be available.

**Type of Reasoning: Evaluative**

One must weigh the possible courses of action and then make a value judgment about the best course to take. This requires evaluative reasoning skill, which often utilizes guiding principles of action in order to arrive at a correct conclusion. For this case, because the parents are obviously upset, the OTA should refer the family to their spiritual advisor or the social worker and proceed with the session. Refer to guidelines for helping families cope with grief if answered incorrectly.

**B104 C9**

An OTA employed in a pediatric clinic participates in a performance appraisal. The OT supervisor identifies the area for the OTA's improvement as handling skills in working with children with various types of cerebral palsy. Which is the most effective way for the OTA to improve handling skills?

**Correct Answer: C. Participate in a beginning level experiential course on handling skills with children with cerebral palsy.**

**Incorrect Answers:**

A. Observe an experienced occupational therapist using handling techniques with a diversity of children with cerebral palsy.
B. Complete an extensive literature review of evidence-based practice for children with cerebral palsy.
D. Attend a teleconference on handling skills for the child with cerebral palsy.

**Rationale:**

Participating in an experiential handling skills course provides opportunities to interact with other therapists and benefit from visual and kinesthetic learning. Observing a skill is helpful but does not offer opportunity to develop hands-on skills and obtain feedback on the application of learned techniques. A literature review and a teleconference can cover a variety of information about best practices and handling techniques for children with cerebral palsy but these offer little opportunity to learn handling skills, which is a hands-on competence rather than knowledge-based.

**Type of reasoning: Inferential**

This question requires one to determine what course of action will be most effective for an OTA that requires improvement in handling skills with children with cerebral palsy. This requires inferential reasoning skill, as one must determine what action will have the most beneficial outcome. For this situation, the OTA should participate in a beginning level experiential course on handling skills with children with cerebral palsy. If answered incorrectly, review approaches to improve therapeutic techniques and competency.

## B105  C5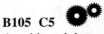

An older adult recovering from a myocardial infarction is referred to occupational therapy for a home care evaluation. The referral states that the client has high blood pressure and medication-related orthostatic hypotension. Which precaution is most important for the OTA to observe with this client?

**Correct Answer: D. Avoidance of activities that require sudden postural changes.**

**Incorrect Answers:**

A.  Adherence to dietary restrictions during meal preparation activities.

B.  Avoidance of activities that require movement against gravity.

C.  Delay of the OT evaluation until the client's medications are stabilized.

**Rationale:**

Orthostatic hypotension or postural hypotension is an excessive drop in blood pressure that occurs upon assuming an upright position. All functional activities have components that are against gravity so these cannot be avoided in treatment. Adherence to dietary restrictions during meal preparation activities is important, but the question is about an evaluation session not an intervention session. The side effect of orthostatic hypotension may not be remediated and the patient's need for OT evaluation cannot wait.

**Type of Reasoning: Evaluative**

This question requires one to weigh the merits of each of the possible courses of action, which is an evaluative reasoning skill. After weighing the patient's symptoms and current status, the test taker should determine that avoidance of activities that require sudden postural changes is most important. If answered incorrectly, review activity precautions and treatment guidelines for orthostatic hypotension.

## B106  C3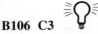

An individual recently had a left transfemoral amputation as a result of the complications of diabetes. The client is two years status-post a right transtibial amputation as a result of the same precipitant. The client is referred to OT for pre-prosthetic interventions. The referral notes that the complications of neuromas and phantom limb pain are present in left residual limb. Which intervention is best for the OTA to implement during the first OT session?

**Correct Answer: C. Upper extremity strengthening with emphasis on the triceps.**

**Incorrect Answers:**

A.  Upper extremity strengthening with emphasis on the biceps.

B.  Percussion to the left lower extremity's residual limb.

D.  Lower extremity dressing with emphasis on donning and doffing prostheses.

**Rationale:**

Strengthening the upper extremities, especially the triceps, will facilitate independence in transfers. Neuromas are nerve endings that are adhered to scar tissue. Since neuromas can be very painful, percussion to the left residual limb and donning/doffing of the left prosthesis is contraindicated at this time. Given that the right amputation is two years status-post, it is likely that the client has achieved independence in donning and doffing the right prosthesis.

**Type of Reasoning: Inferential**

One must link the patient's diagnosis and current symptoms to the interventions presented in order to determine which intervention would be best to address current deficits. This requires inferential reasoning, where one must infer or draw conclusions based on facts and evidence. In this case, upper extremity strengthening, especially the triceps is most important in order to facilitate independence in transfers. Review intervention approaches for clients with lower extremity amputations if answered incorrectly.

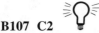

**B107  C2**

An OTA conducts an initial home visit to a family with a premature infant who, at four months and 5 lbs., has just been sent home. The child has multiple disabilities and has been evaluated by the occupational therapist. Which is the best primary goal for the OTA to work on with the family during this first session?

**Correct Answer: A. Communicate effectively to develop a therapeutic relationship with the family.**

**Incorrect Answers:**

B.  Teach the family proper body mechanics for lifting the child.

C.  Teach the family assertiveness training to develop advocacy skills.

D.  Determine whether adaptive aids or positioning equipment is needed.

**Rationale:**

During the first visit, it is essential that the OTA practice effective communication and work on developing a therapeutic relationship with the family. Since the child has multiple disabilities, the OTA will need to work closely and frequently with the family to address their child's needs over an extended period of time. The other choices can be addressed when, and if the need evolves. In addition, one cannot assume that the family will need assertiveness training.

**Type of Reasoning: Inferential**

One must determine the most likely intervention approach for a child on an initial home visit. This requires inferential reasoning skill, where one must draw conclusions based on the information presented. In this situation, practicing effective communication and developing a therapeutic relationship is the primary goal. If answered incorrectly, review guidelines for family centered practice and home health care of premature infants.

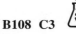

**B108  C3**

In measuring the ROM of a client's elbow, the OTA records a flexion measurement of 145 degrees. Which is most accurate for the OTA to document based on this measurement?

**Correct Answer: D. Normal elbow ROM.**

**Incorrect Answers:**

A.  Hypomobility.

B.  Dysfunctional elbow ROM.

C.  Hypermobility.

**Rationale:**

Normal elbow ROM is zero degrees to 135-150 degrees. Individual variation in the end range of elbow flexion is normal due to differences in muscle mass of the biceps and the forearm as they meet at the end range. Having 145 degrees of flexion is normal. ROM outside of these parameters would be atypical. Hypermobility would be evident if the person extended the elbow beyond zero and hypomobility would be indicated if the person could not flex within the normal range.

**Type of Reasoning: Analytical**

This question provides a functional description and the test taker must determine the likely indicator of the description. This is an analytical reasoning skill, as questions of this nature often ask one to analyze a group of symptoms or functional indicators in order to determine a diagnosis or outcome. In this situation the description indicates typical ROM of the elbow, which should be reviewed if answered incorrectly.

## B109  C8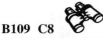

During a clubhouse vocational support group, a client reports difficulty keeping track of the job tasks that need to be completed each day. What is the most effective recommendation for the OTA to make to the client?

**Correct Answer: C. Develop and use a checklist of tasks to be completed each day.**

**Incorrect Answers:**

A. Write down directions for each task that needs to be completed.

B. Keep a daily log of completed tasks.

D. Ask the work supervisor to provide verbal cues through the workday.

**Rationale:**

Developing a daily "to do" checklist provides a clear visual cue of what needs to be accomplished. The client can check off each job task as he/she completes it and immediately see what job tasks must still be accomplished. This can provide the needed organizational structure to complete all job tasks each day. There is nothing in the scenario to indicate that the person does not know how to perform his/her job tasks; therefore, there is no need for the person to write down directions for each task. Keeping a log of each completed job task will help the person to know what has been accomplished, but it provides no organizational cue regarding what remains to be done. There is nothing in the scenario to indicate that the person cannot independently perform his/her daily work tasks; therefore, there is no need for the supervisor's cueing.

**Type of Reasoning: Inductive**

This question requires one to determine the approach for assisting a client in keeping track of job tasks. This requires inductive reasoning skill, where clinical judgment is paramount to arriving at a correct conclusion. For this case, the OTA's most effective recommendation is to develop and use a checklist of tasks to be completed each day. If answered incorrectly, one should review vocational training guidelines, especially organizational behaviors and compensatory strategies.

## B110  C4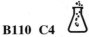

During a home visit, a client who had incurred a CVA reports difficulty finding objects during BADL and IADL. The client reports that the directions family members provide (e.g., look on the refrigerator's door, look in the medicine cabinet) are not helpful. When discussing this behavior with the occupational therapist, which cognitive perceptual ability should the OTA report as requiring further evaluation?

**Correct Answer: D. Visual closure.**

**Incorrect Answers:**

A. Stereognosis.

B. Organization.

C. Spatial relations.

**Rationale:**

This behavior may be evidence of difficulties with visual closure since the person may not be able to find an item if it is in its incomplete form (i.e., covered partially by other objects in the refrigerator or cabinet). The other options describe cognitive-perceptual deficits with different manifestations. Stereognosis is the ability to recognize objects by touch alone. Organization is the ability to structure thoughts and actions. Spatial relations are the ability to relate objects in relationship to each other or the self (e.g., up/down, front/back, under/over).

**Type of reasoning: Analytical**

This question provides a description of a functional deficit and the test taker must determine the likely cause for this deficit. This requires analysis of symptoms, which is an analytical reasoning skill. For this case, the client is reporting difficulties with visual closure. If answered incorrectly, review signs and symptoms of visual closure dysfunction.

## B111  C5

An individual with a C3 spinal cord injury is participating in a community mobility group at a shopping mall. The client expresses the desire to return to the rehabilitation center due to a pounding headache. The OTA notices the client is sweating profusely. What should the OTA do first in response to this observation and request?

**Correct Answer: A. Check the client's urinary catheter and collecting bag.**

**Incorrect Answers:**

B.  Call the rehabilitation center's transportation department to relay the client's request

C.  Escort the client to outside of the mall to cool off in the fresh air.

D.  Immediately activate the recline feature of the patient's tilt-in–space wheelchair.

**Rationale:**

Profuse sweating and headaches are signs of autonomic dysreflexia. This is an extreme rise in blood pressure caused by a noxious stimulus, which must be treated immediately by removing the stimulus. A blocked catheter and overfilled urine bag are common precipitants to this complication and could result in a medical emergency in persons with a spinal cord injury. Other common stimuli include sitting on sharp objects, a tight abdominal binder, pressure stockings that have rolled down or excess pressure on the buttocks. The patient should be placed in an upright position to help manage the rise in blood pressure.

**Type of Reasoning: Evaluative**

One must weigh the possible courses of action and then make a value judgment about the best course to take. This requires evaluative reasoning skill, where an understanding of what the symptoms indicate is pivotal to arriving at a correct conclusion. For this case, the symptoms indicate autonomic dysreflexia and the OTA's first action should be to check the urinary catheter and collecting bag. If answered incorrectly, review symptoms of autonomic dysreflexia and appropriate intervention approaches.

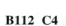

## B112  C4

A three year-old child with hypotonia presents with delayed motor milestones and immature grasping patterns. The OTA begins each session with preparatory activities and positioning. This includes quadruped weight bearing and shoulder girdle compression to promote muscle activity and postural alignment. Which frame of reference is the OTA primarily using during these intervention sessions?

**Correct Answer: D. Neurodevelopmental.**

**Incorrect Answers:**

A.  Sensory integration.

B.  Motor learning.

C.  Acquisitional.

**Rationale:**

The NDT frame of reference relies heavily on preparation and facilitation prior to active movement and task performance. Facilitation of alignment using NDT handling and facilitation techniques, key points of control, and positioning is meant to increase the potential for appropriate muscle activation.

**Type of reasoning: Analytical**

This question provides a description of a functional activity and the test taker must determine the most like frame of reference being utilized in the intervention approach. This requires analytical reasoning skill. For this scenario, the OTA is primarily using the neurodevelopmental frame of reference. Review NDT frame of reference and therapeutic approaches if answered incorrectly.

## B113 C3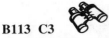

An individual with degenerative joint disease (DJD) incurred an injury to the right hand. The client complains of severe pain, stiffness, and extreme temperature changes in the hand. The OT referral states that the person has pitting edema and blotchy, shiny skin. At this time, which evaluation tool should the OTA use to assess this client?

**Correct answer: C. Volumeter.**

**Incorrect answers:**

A. Vigormeter.
B. Dynamometer.
D. Sphygmomanometer.

**Rationale:**

One of the client's major presenting problems is edema. The volumeter is an assessment tool that objectively measures edema based on the displacement law of physics. A dynamometer, vigormeter, and sphygmomanometer are tools used to measure grip strength. An evaluation using these measures would be contraindicated at this time due to the client's secondary diagnosis of degenerative joint disease (DJD) and the presenting complaints of severe pain and stiffness.

**Type of Reasoning: Inductive**

One must have knowledge of all the assessment tools described and reasons for administration in order to arrive at a correct conclusion. This is an inductive reasoning skill where knowledge of clinical guidelines and clinical reasoning are utilized to reach conclusions. If answered incorrectly, review volumeter assessment guidelines and evaluation approaches for individuals with DJD and edema.

## B114 C6

A patient with a diagnosis of borderline personality disorder attends a stress management group on an inpatient psychiatric unit. During the group, the patient's roommate states that there is a pocket knife in the patient's backpack. The patient says the roommate is exaggerating and that the item is only a keychain. What should the OTA do in response to these statements?

**Correct Answer: A. Immediately inform the charge nurse.**

**Incorrect Answers:**

B. Immediately check the patient's backpack.
C. Check the patient's backpack after the group session.
D. Inform the occupational therapist after the group session.

**Rationale:**

The possibility that there is any item on an inpatient psychiatric unit that could be used by a person to harm him/herself or others presents a danger to all; therefore, the charge nurse must be immediately notified of the situation. Searching the backpack may or may not produce the item and it is not the OTA's role to conduct a room or person search. Informing the occupational therapist after the group session keeps a potentially dangerous item in a place where others could access it. This is not acceptable on an inpatient unit.

**Type of Reasoning: Evaluative**

One must weigh the possible courses of action and then make a value judgment about the best course to take. This requires evaluative reasoning skill, which often utilizes guiding principles of action in order to arrive at a correct conclusion. For this case, because the object could harm the patient or others, the OTA should immediately contact the charge nurse. Review safety protocols for inpatient psychiatric facilities if answered incorrectly.

**B115  C5**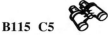

An individual with an incomplete C6 spinal cord injury has a secondary diagnosis of thromboangiitis obliterans. The OTA conducts a pre-discharge home evaluation of the patient's rented apartment. Which is the most important area for the OTA to assess?

**Correct Answer: B. The apartment's water temperature.**

**Incorrect Answers:**

A.  The apartment's electrical capacity for an environmental control unit.

C.  The apartment's electrical capacity for an emergency call system.

D.  The landlord's willingness to modify the bathroom.

**Rationale:**

Thromboangiitis obliterans, also known as Buerger's disease, results in diminished temperature sense, paresthesias, pain and cold extremities. It is most common in young men who smoke. Poor or absent temperature sense can place a person at serious risk for scalding burns. If the apartment's water temperature is higher than 102 degrees, an anti-scalding faucet and/or valve must be installed. An individual with a C6 SCI is independent in many tasks and does not require an environmental control unit to access the environment. A special emergency call system is also not needed because this person can independently access a telephone to call 911 with minimal modifications (i.e., large push buttons, speaker phone). Structural bathroom modifications are not needed. A person with a C6 SCI can bathe with minimal assistance using a tub bench, a sliding board transfer and a hand-held shower. None of these modifications would require a landlord's permission.

**Type of Reasoning: Inductive**

One must utilize clinical knowledge and judgment to determine the most important area for assessment based on the individual's diagnosis. In this case, the OTA should assess the apartment's water temperature to prevent scalding burns from hot water due to the individual's diminished temperature sense. If answered incorrectly, review safety skills for patients with impaired sensory function, especially impaired thermosensation.

**B116  C2**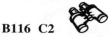

A client expresses interest in playing a computer game with another group member during a leisure skills group. The OTA and the occupational therapist review the client's cognitive evaluation and agree that the game is a good choice for the client's cognitive level. After 15 minutes of engaging in the computer game, the client rubs both eyes, looks around, and reports trouble focusing. What should the OTA do?

**Correct Answer: D. Suggest the client and the other member talk about the game's progress in between completing their turns.**

**Incorrect Answers:**

A.  Provide verbal encouragement for the client to complete the game before taking a break.

B.  Suggest the client and the other member play a different video game that is easier for the client.

C.  Discontinue the session and advise the client to select a different leisure activity to do with the other member.

**Rationale:**

The client appears to be experiencing visual strain which can be caused by staring at a computer screen without a break. Consequently, the best choice is to decrease the visual strain by providing periodic brief breaks from looking intently at the screen. Having the clients talk between taking turns will facilitate them looking at each other rather than the computer screen. Providing verbal encouragement and suggesting a new game that is easier does not address the visual fatigue/strain issue. There is no need to discontinue the session at this point. Ending the session would be inappropriate because it would not enable the OTA to use the client's experience to teach ways to effectively manage discomfort and successfully engage in activities of interest. This could leave the client with a feeling of failure and contribute to a low self-esteem, which would be counterproductive to leisure skill development.

**Type of Reasoning: Inductive**

This question requires clinical judgment to determine a best course of action for the OTA, which is an inductive reasoning skill. For this situation, the behavior exhibited by the client indicates that a decrease in visual stimuli is warranted; therefore the client should talk about the game's progress with the other member in between completing turns. If answered incorrectly, review information on visual fatigue in computer use.

**B117  C6**

An individual with peripheral neuropathies due to diabetes is scheduled for a bilateral lower extremity (transfemoral) amputation. During an OT session to develop upper extremity strength to assist with post-amputation transfers, the patient happily chats about plans to go shopping for new clothing to wear to a grandchild's wedding. After the session, which defense mechanism should the OTA document that the person seems to be exhibiting?

**Correct Answer:  A. Suppression.**

**Incorrect Answers:**

B.  Regression.

C.  Displacement.

D.  Projection.

**Rationale:**

Suppression is a defense mechanism that allows an individual to divert uncomfortable feelings (in this case, fear of an undesirable event) into socially acceptable feelings (in this case, anticipation of a desirable event) in order to avoid thinking about a disturbing issue.  Regression is the returning to an earlier stage of development to avoid tension or conflict (e.g., an individual becomes needy or childlike during a period of stress).  Displacement is the redirection of an emotion or reaction from one object to a similar but less threatening one (e.g., a child who is angry with his parents yells at his younger sister). Projection is the attribution of unacknowledged characteristics or thoughts to others (e.g., someone who feels guilty interprets the statements of others as blaming him/her).

**Type of Reasoning: Analytical**

This question provides symptoms and the test taker must determine the likely cause for them. This is an analytical reasoning skill, as questions of this nature often ask one to analyze a group of symptoms in order to determine a diagnosis. In this situation the symptoms indicate the defense mechanism of suppression, which should be reviewed if answered incorrectly.

**B118  C8**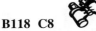

An individual with Charcot-Marie-Tooth disease receives services at a wheelchair clinic. The client reports difficulty keeping both feet on the wheelchair's footrests. What is the most effective action for the OTA to take to address the client's stated concerns?

**Correct Answer: D. Provide ankle straps on the foot rests.**

**Incorrect Answers:**

A.  Implement an exercise routine to strengthen lower extremities.

B.  Elevate the foot rests.

C.  Provide heel loops on the foot rests.

**Rationale:**

Ankle straps are used to prevent feet from slipping off the footrests. Charcot-Marie-Tooth disease is a neuropathic muscular atrophy characterized by progressive weakness of the distal muscles of the arms and feet. It does not respond to strengthening exercises. Elevating footrests are indicated for edema control, LE extension contractures and long leg casts. They do not prevent the lower extremity from slipping off the rest. In fact, the increased pull of gravity would likely exacerbate the problem. In addition, elevated footrests greatly extend the length of a wheelchair, making it very cumbersome to maneuver in the environment. Heel loops on foot rests prevent the feet only from slipping posteriorly which would not be an adequate solution in this case.

**Type of Reasoning: Inductive**

One must utilize clinical knowledge and judgment to determine the most effective recommendation for this individual. In this case, ankle straps on the foot rests is most effective to prevent the feet from slipping off the footrests. If answered incorrectly, review footrest equipment for wheelchairs, especially ankle straps.

**B119 C3**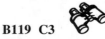

An adult is referred to an outpatient hand clinic for treatment of DeQuervain's syndrome. Which is the most beneficial splint for the OTA to construct for this client?

**Correct Answer: C. A forearm-based thumb spica splint.**

**Incorrect Answers:**

A. A dorsal wrist splint with the wrist in neutral.

B. A volar wrist splint with the wrist in 30 degrees of extension.

D. A resting hand splint.

**Rationale:**

De Quervain's syndrome is a stenosing tenosynovitis of the abductor pollicis longus and the extensor pollicis brevis. The forearm-based thumb spica splint would immobilize the wrist, thumb CMC and MCP joints which places the involved tendons at rest. A resting hand splint is not indicated as the entire hand does not have to be immobilized. A wrist splint, of any type or with the wrist in any position, would not immobilize the involved two tendons.

**Type of Reasoning: Inductive**

Clinical knowledge and judgment are the most important skills needed for answering this question, which requires inductive reasoning skill. Knowledge of the diagnosis and most beneficial splinting procedures is essential to choosing the best solution. In this case, the OTA should construct a forearm-based thumb spica splint. Review splinting procedures for DeQuervain's syndrome if answered incorrectly.

**B120 C5**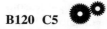

A client attends a work hardening program. The client arrives on time for the scheduled session but complains of significant substernal pain, extreme discomfort in the epigastric area, indigestion and nausea. What is the best action for the OTA to take in response to the client's expressed complaints?

**Correct Answer: B. Cancel the session and call emergency medical services.**

**Incorrect Answers:**

A. Initiate the session and provide support, breaks, and activity modifications as needed.

C. Cancel the session and tell the client to call to reschedule when feeling better.

D. Ask the client to wait while the OTA consults with the occupational therapist to determine the best course of action.

**Rationale:**

The client is complaining of symptoms that can be the presenting signs for a myocardial infarction. This is a medical emergency and must be handled as such. The OTA must call for emergency medical services to address the situation. The OTA should not delay this action by having the client wait until after the OTA speaks to the occupational therapist. The OTA can (and should) act independently in this medical emergency.

**Type of Reasoning: Evaluative**

One must weigh the possible courses of action and then make a value judgment about the best course to take. This requires evaluative reasoning skill, which often utilizes guiding principles of action in order to arrive at a correct conclusion. For this case, because the patient's symptoms are indicative of a myocardial infarction, the OTA should cancel the session and call emergency medical services. Review symptoms of myocardial infarction if answered incorrectly.

**B121 C5**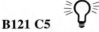

A client with myasthenia gravis shows increasing difficulty with speech and oral-motor control during swallowing. Which behavior is most accurate for the OTA to document as indicative of a swallowing disorder?

**Correct Answer: B. Coughing while swallowing thin liquids.**

**Incorrect Answers:**

A.  A tendency to spit out foods of mixed textures.

C.  A deep voice during oral speech.

D.  Loud noises in the throat during swallowing.

**Rationale:**

Coughing, and choking are signs of swallowing difficulties. It is important to determine the type and viscosity of foods that cause choking and coughing. Spitting out foods tends to reflect an oral problem such as hypersensitivity and is not a component of a swallowing dysfunction. The symptoms of a swallowing dysfunction include a gurgly quality of speech, not a deep voice. Loud noises are not specific signs of swallowing trouble.

**Type of Reasoning: Inferential**

One must infer or draw conclusions about the symptoms that indicate swallowing dysfunction. Questions that ask what to expect from a certain diagnosis often require inferential reasoning skill. In this situation coughing while swallowing thin liquids indicates the presence of swallowing dysfunction. Review symptoms of swallowing dysfunction if answered incorrectly.

**B122  C4**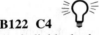

An individual who has Parkinson's disease presents with poor trunk rotation during ambulation and while performing activities of daily living. Which is the most effective therapeutic intervention for the OTA to use with this person?

**Correct Answer: C. Activities of daily living using D1 flexion patterns.**

**Incorrect Answers:**

A.  Facilitation of rotation using neurodevelopmental (NDT) handling techniques.

B.  Slow rolling with the person supine with knees and hips flexed.

D.  Provision of a rolling walker to compensate for limited rotation and to enhance mobility.

**Rationale:**

The person is presenting with poor trunk rotation during ADL and functional mobility. This is typical in individuals with Parkinson's disease. The most appropriate approach is to use a technique to facilitate rotation during activity performance. PNF diagonals are the best choice because many activities (e.g., loading/unloading the dishwasher, putting away groceries) can be performed using diagonal patterns. NDT handling techniques and the Rood technique of slow rolling can facilitate rotation; however, they do not incorporate functional activities. Therefore, they are not the best choice. A rolling walker does not address the effects of poor rotation on the person's performance of activities of daily living.

**Type of Reasoning: Inferential**

One must determine the most appropriate intervention approach, given knowledge of the presenting diagnosis and incorporation of functional activity. This requires inferential reasoning skill, where one must infer or draw conclusions about a best course of action. In this situation, the OTA should choose ADL approaches incorporating D1 flexion patterns. Review information on intervention approaches for Parkinson's disease and PNF intervention techniques. Answering this question correctly requires integration of this knowledge.

502

## B123  C8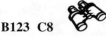

An OTA prepares to transfer an individual. The OTA cannot locate the transfer belt that the OTA had planned to use during the transfer. Which is the OTA's best course of action?

**Correct Answer: A. Locate a transfer belt and then complete the transfer.**

**Incorrect Answers:**

B.  Instruct the individual in a stand pivot transfer.

C.  Instruct the individual in a sliding board transfer.

D.  Complete the transfer slowly and carefully.

**Rationale:**

The OTA had determined that a transfer belt was needed to complete a transfer; therefore, a transfer belt should be used. Not following the original plan would be unsafe and a liability risk. A person requiring the assistance of an OTA using a transfer belt would be an inappropriate candidate for learning to transfer independently via a stand pivot or sliding board transfer.

**Type of Reasoning: Inductive**

This question requires one to determine the best course of action when considering a transfer without a transfer belt. This requires inductive reasoning skill, where clinical judgment is essential to arriving at a correct conclusion. For this situation, because safety is paramount, the OTA should locate a transfer belt and then complete the transfer. If answered incorrectly, review transfer safety procedures.

## B124  C4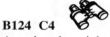

A patient has right homonymous hemianopsia. The OTA provides recommendations to modify the patient's room to enhance independence. What are the most effective recommendations for the OTA to make for the placement of the patient's telephone and radio?

**Correct Answer: D. Telephone on the left side and the radio on the right side.**

**Incorrect Answers:**

A.  Telephone on the left side and the radio on the left side.

B.  Telephone on the right side and the radio on the right side.

C.  Telephone on the right side and the radio on the left side.

**Rationale:**

The telephone must be placed within the person's intact visual field (which, in this case, is left) so that the person can readily access it in case of emergency. However, the radio can be placed outside of the person's visual field (right, in this case), to encourage the person to scan the environment. If the person initially has trouble locating the radio, it will not pose any danger to him/her. The OTA can use the radio as a tool to increase scanning skills during intervention sessions.

**Type of Reasoning: Inductive**

Clinical knowledge and judgment are the most important skills needed for answering this question, which requires inductive reasoning skill. Knowledge of the diagnosis and most effective clinical outcomes is essential to choosing the best solution. In this case, the OTA should recommend that the telephone is placed on the left and the radio on the right side. This best addresses the person's safety as well as improving function in scanning the environment.

**B125  C8**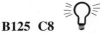

An adolescent with a complete spinal cord injury at C-8 is a client at an outpatient rehabilitation center. The client has met all goals for functional performance in activities of daily living. Which of the following actions should the OTA do next?

**Correct Answer: C. Establish community participation goals with the client.**

**Incorrect Answers:**

A.  Provide an obstacle course activity for the client to work on community mobility.

B.  Discharge the client from OT with a referral to the local school-based OT program.

D.  Discharge the client from OT and provide a home maintenance program for the family.

**Rationale:**

The focus of intervention after attainment of ADL goals is community re-integration. Establishing community participation goals can address both the physical and psychosocial adjustment to disability. The client likely has relevant needs that can be addressed in OT; therefore, discharge is premature. Functional mobility is a component of ADL and the case scenario states all ADL goals have been met. In addition, applying functional mobility skills into different community participation activities can strengthen these skills and facilitate generalization to real-life situations that the client will encounter upon discharge.

**Type of Reasoning: Inferential**

One must have knowledge of intervention goals for persons with cervical spinal cord injury in order to arrive at a correct conclusion. This is an inferential reasoning skill where knowledge of clinical guidelines and judgment based on facts are utilized to reach conclusions. For this client, after achieving goals in ADL, community participation would become the focus of intervention. Consequently, the OTA should initiate community participation activities. If answered incorrectly, review occupational performance interventions, especially leisure and community pursuits.

**B126  C6**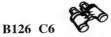

Children with autism participate in an after-school playgroup which uses a behavioral frame of reference. The playgroup is conducted by Level I occupational therapy assistant students who are each partnered with a child to facilitate the development of play and social interaction skills. What should the supervising OTA advise the students to do when working with their assigned child?

**Correct Answer: A. Be consistent and reinforce developmentally appropriate behaviors.**

**Incorrect Answers:**

B.  Speak loudly and repeat directions frequently.

C.  Give detailed descriptions about the goals of each activity.

D.  Provide a diversity of sensory stimulation activities.

**Rationale:**

According to a behavioral frame of reference, consistency and reinforcement are used to develop skills. This approach can be effective in developing play and social interaction skills for children with autism. Speaking loudly, repeating directions, and/or giving detailed descriptions rely on the children's ability to process and respond to auditory input. These skills are often limited in children with autism. Sensory stimulation activities are often used with children with autism, but this approach employs the sensory integration frame of reference, not a behavioral one. Consequently, this option is not the best choice for the scenario provided.

**Type of Reasoning: Inductive**

This question requires one to determine the best approach for conducting a group session with children who have autism using a behavioral frame of reference. This requires inductive reasoning skill, where clinical judgment and knowledge of the behavioral frame of reference is paramount to arriving at a correct conclusion. For this situation, the OTA should advise the students to be consistent and reinforce developmentally appropriate behaviors. If answered incorrectly, review behavioral guidelines for working with children with autism.

**B127  C3**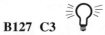

A client who incurred a nerve laceration exhibits maximum motor and sensory losses consistent with a radial nerve laceration below the supinator. Which deformity should the OTA note the client is exhibiting?

**Correct Answer: D. Wrist drop.**

**Incorrect Answers:**

A.  'Claw' hand.

B.  'Ape' hand.

C.  'Saturday night' palsy.

**Rationale:**

The presenting signs of a radial nerve laceration are weakness or paralysis of the extensors of the wrist, MCPs, and thumb with a characteristic wrist drop. 'Ape' hand, which presents as a flattening of the thenar eminence, is indicative of a median nerve palsy. A 'claw' hand is indicative of ulnar nerve palsy. Saturday night palsy is a term used to denote a radial nerve palsy that results from a position that compresses the radial nerve against the humerus.

**Type of Reasoning: Inferential**

One must link the diagnosis provided to the symptoms presented in order to determine which definition most accurately represents a radial nerve laceration. This requires inferential reasoning, where one must infer or draw conclusions about a diagnosis. In this case symptoms of radial nerve laceration include weakness of the wrist, MCP, and thumb extensors. Review symptoms of radial nerve injury if answered incorrectly.

**B128  C2**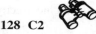

An OTA implements a transitional program for a 15 year-old high school student with a history of numerous school-related failures. Which is the most important principle of intervention for the OTA to use with this student? :

**Correct Answer: B. Grade an activity of interest into achievable steps to facilitate successful completion.**

**Incorrect Answers:**

A.  Utilize activities that are typically at the developmental level of a 12 year-old to ensure successful completion.

C.  Introduce several activities during each session and change them frequently to decrease boredom.

D.  Terminate the activity during a treatment session when there is difficulty with activity completion to eliminate frustration.

**Rationale:**

Grading an activity to be presented in achievable steps is the most appropriate intervention principle for a person with a history of diminished success experiences. Employing activities appropriate for a younger child and terminating the activity will not address the teen's need for transitional services. Introducing several activities during one session can be overwhelming and decrease the ability to work in a focused manner on the attainment of transition goals.

**Type of Reasoning: Inductive**

Clinical knowledge and judgment are the most important skills needed for answering this question, which requires inductive reasoning skill. Knowledge of the student's limitations and most appropriate interventions to foster success is essential to choosing the correct solution. In this case, the most important principle for intervention planning is to grade the activity of interest into achievable steps to ensure successful completion. Review treatment planning guidelines for students in transitional programs if answered incorrectly.

**B129  C1**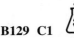

During an intervention session in a school, the OTA observes a young child turn the pages of a book. The OTA identifies this behavior as an example of an in-hand manipulation task. What task should the OTA report to the occupational therapist that the child is capable of performing?

**Correct Answer: A. Shift.**

**Incorrect Answers:**

B.  Simple rotation.

C.  Translation.

D.  Translation without stabilization.

**Rationale:**

Turning the pages of a book involves a linear movement of each page on the finger surface. This allows for repositioning of the page relative to the pads of the fingers while the thumb remains opposed. Simple rotation is not correct as this involves a turning/rolling of an object held at the finger pads with the fingers acting as a unit and the thumb in opposition (e.g., unscrewing a bottle cap). Translation is incorrect as this involves linear movement of an object from the palm to the fingers or fingers to the palm. The activity of turning pages does not use the palm with stabilization or without stabilization.

**Type of Reasoning: Analytical**

This question provides a description of a functional activity and the test taker must determine the likely definition of such an activity. This is an analytical reasoning skill, as questions of this nature often ask one to analyze descriptors of functional skills to determine the overall skill involved. In this situation the activity is that of the in-hand manipulation task of shift, which should be reviewed if answered incorrectly.

**B130  C4**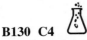

An OTA provides home-based services to a homemaker who incurred a right CVA eight months ago. The individual and the OTA have chosen to focus on kitchen activities during the intervention session. The OTA has the client stand in front of the counter with an open dishwasher to the left. The OTA asks the client to put the clean dishes into an open overhead cabinet to the right of the client. By setting up the activity in this manner, which proprioceptive neuromuscular facilitation (PNF) technique is the OTA using?

**Correct Answer: D. Diagonal patterns of D1 flexion/extension.**

**Incorrect Answers:**

A  Approximation during reaching.

B.  Rhythmic rotation to facilitate hand grasp/release.

C.  Diagonal patterns of D2 flexion/extension.

**Rationale:**

In this example, the D1 flexion pattern moves the person's left upper extremity "up and away" as the person grasps the dishes from the dishwasher on the left and puts them away in the cabinet above the counter to the right. Approximation and rhythmic rotation are treatment techniques used during PNF extension patterns. Approximation involves the manual compression of the joint and is used to stimulate joint receptors. Rhythmic rotation is utilized when the OTA feels restriction during range of motion. When the restriction is felt, the OTA repeats rotation of all of the components of the diagonal at the point of restriction, slowly and gently. As the relaxation occurs, the movement is continued throughout a larger range. D2 is the PNF extension diagonal which moves the UE "down and in".

**Type of Reasoning: Analytical**

For this question, a description of a functional activity is provided and the test taker must determine the functional activity that is being performed. This requires analytical reasoning skill, as questions of this nature often ask one to analyze descriptors of functional tasks to determine the overall skill involved. In this situation the activity being performed is that of D1 flexion/extension. Review PNF patterns, especially D1 if answered incorrectly.

506

### B131  C6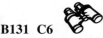

An OTA collaborates with the occupational therapist to plan individual and group activities for a child with oppositional defiant disorder. Which is most important for the OTA to address during group activities?

**Correct Answer:  B. The child's ability to attend to and complete a task.**

**Incorrect Answers:**

A.  The child's willingness to take on a variety of group roles.

C.  The child's distorted body image.

D.  The child's self-regulation of energy and activity levels.

**Rationale:**

Children with oppositional defiant disorder tend to have difficulties with impulse control, attention span, and short-term memory and exhibit argumentative and resentful behaviors. These deficits often affect the ability to complete tasks and can hinder adaptive role functioning. A child does not have to be willing to take on a variety of roles to benefit from group activities. Some find security and stability in the same type role. This stability can be healthy as long as the role contributes to productive behavior. Distorted body image is more indicative of anorexia nervosa, bulimia nervosa, or body dysmorphia. Difficulties with energy and activity levels relate more to hyperactivity disorder than to oppositional defiant disorder.

**Type of Reasoning: Inductive**

This question requires one to recall the typical features of a client with oppositional defiant disorder and then to determine what would be an important skill to address in therapy. This necessitates inductive reasoning skill, where the test taker must couple knowledge of the diagnosis with clinical judgment to arrive at a correct conclusion. For this case, it is most important for the OTA to address the child's ability to attend to and complete a task. If answered incorrectly, review symptoms of oppositional defiant disorder and therapeutic approaches.

### B132  C2

During a parallel task group, one of the members appears agitated and fidgety. The member gets up and looks out the window for a few minutes and then sits back down and quietly returns to the task. This behavior continues throughout the group. What is the OTA's best response when the group member stands again?

**Correct Answer: C. Say nothing to the group member.**

**Incorrect Answers:**

A.  Tell the group member to remain seated or leave the group.

B.  Ask the other members if the group member is bothering them.

D.  Inform the group member that the observed behaviors indicate a lack of readiness for this group.

**Rationale:**

Many individuals, due to the symptoms of their illness and/or medication, have difficulty remaining still. They can, however, benefit from attending a group. A parallel group does not require any interaction for task completion. Therefore, if the group member's behavior is not disturbing or disruptive to the group he/she should be allowed to benefit from this form of treatment.

**Type of Reasoning: Evaluative**

This question requires professional judgment based on guiding principles, which is an evaluative reasoning skill. Because the person is not disturbing the other group members with his/her behavior, the OTA should say nothing to the person. Questions such as these can be challenging. However, essential to arriving at a correct conclusion is determining if the behavior is expected or typical of the person, given their diagnosis. In this situation, it is typical behavior; therefore no action needs to be taken.

## B133  C8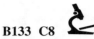

An OTA provides consultation services to members of a town chamber of commerce who are interested in improving their businesses' accessibility. What is the minimum door width that the OTA should recommend to the chamber members as accessible and not requiring modification?

**Correct Answer: B. 32 inches.**

**Incorrect Answers:**

A.  28 inches.

C.  30 inches.

D.  34 inches.

**Rationale:**

The minimum clearance width for doorways to allow for wheelchair access is 32 inches. Measurements less than 32 inches must be modified. Measurements equal to or greater than 32 inches are acceptable.

**Type of Reasoning: Deductive**

One must recall the minimum clearance width for doorways in order to arrive at a correct conclusion. This requires deductive reasoning skill, where factual knowledge is essential to choosing the correct solution. Thirty-two inches is the minimum clearance for door widths in this situation. Review accessibility guidelines, especially door width measurements if answered incorrectly.

## B134  C6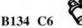

An OTA leads an outpatient wellness program. An individual with obsessive-compulsive disorder asks for suggestions to manage symptoms that are interfering with life satisfaction. Which is the most beneficial recommendation for the OTA to make to the individual?

**Correct Answer: C. Redirect thoughts and energies into meaningful activities.**

**Incorrect Answers:**

A.  Approach activities in a nonchalant manner without high expectations.

B.  Engage in concrete activities that can be broken down into simple steps.

D.  Set limits on the number of activities done in a day.

**Rationale:**

The focus of OT in a wellness program is to help individuals attain and maintain life satisfaction through the engagement in meaningful activities. Individuals with obsessive-compulsive disorder have recurring and persistent thoughts (obsessions) and the need to engage in repetitious or ritualistic behaviors (compulsions) that interfere with functional activities; therefore, redirecting thoughts and energy into meaningful activities can be an effective behavior management strategy. Approaching activities in a nonchalant manner without high expectations and limiting the number of activities performed during a day would not address the person's need to refocus thoughts and behaviors away from his/her obsessions and compulsions. Engaging in activities that can be broken down into simple steps is helpful for persons with cognitive deficits. Individuals with obsessive-compulsive disorders typically do not have cognitive deficits.

**Type of Reasoning: Inductive**

This question requires one to determine the most beneficial recommendation for a person with obsessive-compulsive disorder. This requires inductive reasoning skill, where clinical judgment is paramount to arriving at a correct conclusion. For this situation, the OTA should suggest redirecting thoughts and energies into meaningful occupations. If answered incorrectly, review treatment guidelines for persons with obsessive-compulsive disorder.

508

## B135 C1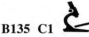

An occupational therapy assistant education program provides an after-school play program for typically developing children to help the OTA students understand development. The students observe a child who is beginning to use blunt scissors to snip paper. The child opens and closes the scissors and moves them in a controlled forward motion, but the child cannot cut circles or figure shapes. At which age are these behaviors typical?

**Correct Answer: D. 3 years-old.**

**Incorrect Answers:**

A. 2 years-old.

B. 4 years-old.

C. 5 years-old.

**Rationale:**

The described activities are typical of three year-old children. The behaviors described in this scenario are too advanced for 2 year-old children. While older children can perform the described activities, they typically are cutting circles at $3^1/2$-$4^1/2$ years and cutting simple figure shapes at 4-6 years.

**Type of reasoning: Deductive**

One must recall developmental motor milestones of children in order to arrive at a correct conclusion for this question. This necessitates the recall of factual guidelines, which is a deductive reasoning skill. For this scenario, the behaviors described are typical of three year-old children. Review motor skills and developmental milestones of children, especially skills of three year-olds, if answered incorrectly.

## B136 C6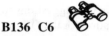

During an occupational therapy group, a person receiving electroconvulsive therapy (ECT) treatments complains about short-term memory loss. What should the OTA do in response to the client's stated concerns?

**Correct Answer: A. Provide cues during activities to compensate for memory loss.**

**Incorrect Answers:**

B. Immediately contact the psychiatrist to inform him/her of this symptom development.

C. Tell the person to inform the psychiatrist of this symptom development.

D. Reassure the person that short-term memory loss is a typical response to ECT.

**Rationale:**

Short-term memory loss is typical after ECT; therefore, there is no need to inform the psychiatrist. However, reassuring the person that this loss is typical does not address the problem at hand. Providing cues can effectively help the individual deal with this memory loss and allow effective engagement in meaningful activities.

**Type of Reasoning: Inductive**

This question requires one to determine the best approach for assisting a person who is dealing with short-term memory loss after ECT. This requires inductive reasoning skill, where clinical judgment is paramount to arriving at a correct conclusion. For this situation, the OTA should provide cues during activities to compensate for the loss. If answered incorrectly, review effects of ECT treatment on cognitive functioning.

## B137 C7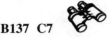

An elder with peripheral neuropathies resulting from the chronic effects of diabetes expresses concern over the ability to have a satisfying sexual relationship with a partner. What is the most beneficial recommendation for the OTA to make to the elder?

**Correct Answer: B. Focus on intact senses and areas of intact sensation.**

**Incorrect Answers:**

A. Experiment with different positions during sexual expression activities.

C. Schedule sexual expression activities after rest periods.

D. Advise the elder to accept decreased abilities in sexuality expression as a normal part of aging.

**Rationale:**

Peripheral neuropathies result in sensory loss; therefore, focusing on intact senses and intact areas of sensation can help the elder and his/her partner achieve satisfying methods for sexual expression. Experimenting with different positions during sexual expression activities is an effective recommendation for individuals with neuromuscular or musculoskeletal deficits. Scheduling sexual expression activities after rest periods is effective for persons who experience fatigue that limits activity (e.g., multiple sclerosis). While the effects of aging may decrease some abilities in sexuality expression, the desire to engage in sexual expression does not necessarily diminish with age. Sexual desire and interest in pursuing sexual expression activities is deeply personal and highly individualized. Advising the elder to accept decreased abilities in sexual expression as a normal part of aging reflects an ageist bias. Moreover, in this situation the elder has expressed concerns which should be directly addressed by the OTA.

**Type of Reasoning: Inductive**

This question requires one to determine the best recommendation for a person according to the current deficits and diagnosis. This requires inductive reasoning skill, where clinical judgment is paramount to arriving at a correct conclusion. For this situation the OTA should recommend focusing on intact senses and areas of intact sensation. If answered incorrectly, review sexual expression guidelines for individuals with disabilities or chronic impairments.

## B138 C4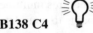

An adult with right hemisphere damage resulting from a CVA is referred to occupational therapy. The OTA contributes to the screening and evaluation process. Which deficits will the patient most likely demonstrate upon evaluation?

**Correct Answer: D. Poor judgment and difficulties with safety issues.**

**Incorrect Answers:**

A. Negative, self-deprecating comments and depression.

B. Slow responses and cautious behavior.

C. Hesitancy and fearfulness.

**Rationale:**

A patient with a right CVA will often demonstrate impulsive behaviors that manifest poor judgment and disregard for safety. Negative, self-deprecating comments and depression can be evident when a person incurs a disability but these behaviors are not necessarily indicative of a right CVA. Slow responses, and hesitancy and fearfulness and cautious behavior are indicative of a left CVA. The person's behaviors can appear slow because of the hesitancy caused by perceptual or motor planning problems.

**Type of Reasoning: Inferential**

This question requires one to draw conclusions based on the information presented, which is an inferential reasoning skill. Questions that ask about what to expect from a diagnosis are essentially asking one to infer information, even though one cannot be 100% sure. For this situation, the most likely symptom of this patient would be poor judgment and decreased safety. If answered incorrectly, review the typical presentations of right versus left CVA.

510

## B139 C6

A young adult with a 10-year history of serious and persistent mental illness is being discharged home in two days. The client collaborates with the care coordination team to plan discharge with the client's primary family members. The team consists of a psychiatrist, a registered nurse, a social worker, an occupational therapist, and an OTA. The team conducts a pre-discharge family meeting to provide family members with information to assist them in supporting the client's recovery. What is the most relevant information for the occupational therapist and OTA to provide to the client's primary family members in this meeting?

**Correct Answer: A. Family role activity suggestions and potential adaptations.**

**Incorrect Answers:**

B. The therapeutic effects and potential side effects of medications.

C. Advocacy strategies and consumer/family resources.

D. Family dynamics information and family support groups.

**Rationale:**

The occupational therapist and OTA are the members on the identified care coordination team who are most qualified to provide information about role activities and potential activity adaptations. The ability of a client to engage in meaningful activities in the home and resume relevant role activities can facilitate positive family functioning and support recovery. The other choices are all relevant foci for discharge planning but the other members of the team can provide this information.

**Type of Reasoning: Inferential**

One must determine the most relevant information for occupational therapy practitioners to provide to the family of a person with serious and persistent mental illness prior to discharge home. This requires inferential reasoning skill, where one draws conclusions based on information presented. In this situation, the most relevant information to provide is family role activity suggestions and potential adaptations. If answered incorrectly, review discharge planning guidelines and the functional impact of serious and persistent mental illness. The integration of this knowledge is required for a correct answer.

## B140 C1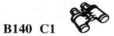

A six year-old child receiving OT services refuses to work on any project except an airplane model that requires multiple steps for completion. The OTA and the occupational therapist have determined that the child would be unable to complete the model. Which should the OTA do during the next intervention session?

**Correct Answer: C. Break the project down into accomplishable segments and instruct the child to complete one segment at a time.**

**Incorrect Answers:**

A. Allow the child to work on the model and provide maximum assistance as the child completes the project.

B. Explore with the child why completing the model is all the child wants to do and provide alternative project choices.

D. Explain to the child several reasons why the selected model is not the best choice for the child and provide alternative project choices.

**Rationale:**

The child is in the concrete operational phase of cognitive development according to Piaget. It is best to give specific information with clear guidelines at this age. Allowing someone to do a project or activity that he/she cannot accomplish is inappropriate. The OTA can use his/her activity analysis skills to break the model down into achievable steps which allow the child to successfully engage in the activity of interest. The exploration of motivation and the rational explanation of a decision require higher cognitive abilities that are consistent with Piaget's formal operational period, from age 11 through the teen years.

**Type of Reasoning: Inductive**

Clinical knowledge and judgment are the most important skills needed for answering this question, which is an inductive reasoning skill. An understanding of the cognitive development of a six year-old is important in choosing the best solution. In this case, breaking the project down into segments the child can complete and telling the child to complete one segment at a time is the best action. Review cognitive development guidelines, especially the concrete operational phase if answered incorrectly.

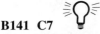

**B141  C7**

A seven year old child with spina bifida at the C-7 level receives home-based occupational therapy services. Which ability is most relevant for the OTA to focus on during intervention?

**Correct Answer: A. Dressing the lower body.**

**Incorrect Answers:**

B.  Dressing the upper body.

C.  Brushing teeth.

D.  Playing table top games.

**Rationale:**

An individual with a spinal cord lesion at C-7 has difficulty dressing the lower extremities. At seven, a child is typically independent in dressing; therefore, an intervention to increase the ability to dress the lower body is age appropriate. An individual with a C-7 lesion is independent in upper extremity dressing, personal grooming, and table top activities; thus, no intervention is warranted.

**Type of Reasoning: Inferential**

One must determine the most relevant intervention approach for a child, given the diagnosis provided. This requires inferential reasoning skill, where one must draw conclusions based on the information presented. In this situation, dressing the lower body is the most relevant intervention. If answered incorrectly, review levels of spinal cord injury and their corresponding functional abilities. Understanding how these capabilities would impact on the ADL for children with cervical spina bifida is required to correctly answer this question.

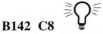

**B142  C8**

Following an exacerbation of post-polio syndrome, a client is referred to occupational therapy for a wheelchair evaluation to enable independent mobility. The client wears bilateral hip-knee-ankle-foot orthoses (HKAFOs) to provide support during independent transfers and brief standing periods throughout the workday. The client's insurance is Medicare. What is the best seat width measurement for the OTA to recommend for the client's wheelchair prescription?

**Correct Answer: D. Two inches wider than the point across the individual's hips or thighs while wearing orthoses.**

**Incorrect Answers:**

A.  Two inches wider than the widest point across the individual's hips or thighs.

B.  Four inches wider than the widest point across the individual's hips or thighs while wearing orthoses.

C.  A standard adult seat width to ensure Medicare reimbursement.

**Rationale:**

Two inches wider than the individual's widest measurement with the orthoses on will allow for ease of movement in and out of the chair. If the width of the orthoses is not included in the seat measurement the chair will be too tight. A standard width adult chair would not meet this individual's needs. Four inches added to the measurement while wearing orthoses would significantly increase the width of the chair. This can complicate mobility in hallways, office spaces and through doorways. Medicare does reimburse for wheelchairs that are prescribed based upon an individual's measurements.

**Type of Reasoning: Inferential**

One must have knowledge HKAFOs and wheelchair prescription guidelines in order to arrive at a correct conclusion. This is an inferential reasoning skill where knowledge of clinical guidelines and judgment based on facts are utilized to reach conclusions. In this situation, the OTA should recommend a seat width two inches wider than the point across the person's hips or thighs while wearing the orthoses. If answered incorrectly, review wheelchair prescription guidelines and use of HKAFOs.

512

**B143 C5**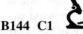

An OTA provides home care services to a neonate with significant developmental delays. Two hours before the next scheduled home visit, the child's parent informs the OTA that one of three older children has developed the chickenpox. While the other children do not show signs of chickenpox, the parent expresses concern that they are contagious. Which is the OTA's best response to this situation?

**Correct Answer: B. Complete the scheduled session using airborne precautions.**

**Incorrect Answers:**

A. Cancel the scheduled session and reschedule after two weeks have passed.

C. Complete the scheduled session using standard precautions.

D. Complete the scheduled session using droplet precautions.

**Rationale:**

There is no need to cancel the scheduled session. Standard precautions are used in all clinical situations. Chickenpox is a disease transmitted by airborne droplet nuclei that remain suspended in the air; therefore, airborne precautions are warranted. Wearing respiratory protection (i.e., a mask) provides sufficient protection. Droplet precautions are used with individuals known or suspected to be infected with serious illness microorganisms transmitted by large particle droplets that can be generated by the person during talking, sneezing, coughing (e.g., rubella, mumps, pertussis, influenza).

**Type of Reasoning: Evaluative**

One must weigh the possible courses of action and then make a value judgment about the best course to take. This requires evaluative reasoning skill, which often utilizes guiding principles of action in order to arrive at a correct conclusion. For this case, because there is the presence of an airborne virus, the OTA should complete the session using airborne precautions. Review transmission-based precautions for airborne viruses if answered incorrectly.

**B144 C1**

A toddler attends an early intervention program as a result of developmental delay. Over the past two weeks, the toddler has successfully completed the activities the OTA has provided in order to develop a palmar grasp. Which action should the OTA take next in response to the child's progress?

**Correct Answer: C. Provide activities to develop a radial palmar grasp.**

**Incorrect Answers:**

A. Continue providing the child with the activities to refine palmar grasp.

B. Review the initial evaluation with the occupational therapist to determine new goals.

D. Provide activities to develop an ulnar palmar grasp.

**Rationale:**

The child has exhibited mastery of a palmar grasp. The next developmental level of grasp after a palmar grasp is a radial palmar grasp. Ulnar palmar grasp is the developmental precursor to palmar grasp. If the initial evaluation determined there was a need to work on the development of grasp, intervention can proceed to the next level without re-evaluation or the establishment of new goals.

**Type of Reasoning: Deductive**

One must recall the developmental guidelines for children in development of grasp patterns. This is factual knowledge, which is a deductive reasoning skill. In this case, after development of a palmar grasp, the next level is radial palmar grasp. If answered incorrectly, review development of grasp patterns in children.

**B145  C2**

An OTA constructs a splint for a 12 year-old child who fractured the radius and ulna. The child becomes angry and pushes the OTA as the OTA attempts to mold the splint onto the child's arm. What should the OTA initially do in response to the child's behavior?

**Correct Answer: D. Remind the child of acceptable behaviors within a clinical setting.**

**Incorrect Answers:**

A.  Ignore the behavior and continue with the splint construction.

B.  End the session and document the child's behavior.

C.  End the session and notify the parents of the child's behavior.

**Rationale:**

The most appropriate initial response is for the OTA to help the child regain control so that he/she can receive needed services. Providing information to the child on the appropriate behavioral limits of a clinical setting enables the OTA to establish a professional relationship with the child. The child is of sufficient age to understand limit setting. Ending the session is premature because this does not provide the child with the opportunity to modify his/her behavior and be fitted for the needed splint. Ignoring the behavior would be inappropriate. The child's anger and loss of control must be handled in a direct, non-threatening manner.

**Type of Reasoning: Evaluative**

One must weigh the possible courses of action and then make a value judgment about the best course to take. This requires evaluative reasoning skill, which often utilizes guiding principles of action in order to arrive at a correct conclusion. For this case, the OTA should remind the child of acceptable behaviors within the clinical setting. Review behavioral intervention guidelines and establishing a professional relationship with children if answered incorrectly.

**B146  C6**

An older adult who is recovering from a cerebral vascular accident attends occupational therapy two times per day. The intervention environment is highly structured and not over-stimulating, yet the client's mood often changes abruptly. Within one session, the client will laugh and then become tearful with no apparent precipitant. What should the OTA document these behaviors as potential signs of in the client's daily progress note?

**Correct Answer: D. Emotional lability.**

**Incorrect Answers:**

A.  Early Alzheimer's disease.

B.  Anhedonia.

C.  A response to auditory hallucinations.

**Rationale:**

Emotional lability describes abrupt changes in mood without external precipitants. It is often observed in persons recovering from CVAs. Anhedonia is the inability to experience pleasure. There is no information in the case that would substantiate a conclusion that the individual is developing Alzheimer's disease or is responding to the internal stimulation of hallucinations.

**Type of Reasoning: Analytical**

This question provides symptoms and the test taker must determine the likely cause for them. This is an analytical reasoning skill, as questions of this nature often ask one to analyze a group of symptoms in order to determine a diagnosis. In this situation the symptoms indicate emotional lability, which should be reviewed if answered incorrectly.

**B147  C3**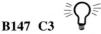

An older adult with rheumatoid arthritis is provided with a functional hand splint to help prevent deformity. The OTA also advises the individual about actions that can be taken to help prevent deformity. Which of the following is most important for the OTA to advise the individual to do?

**Correct Answer: B. Maintain active range of motion.**

**Incorrect Answers:**

A.  Avoid fatigue.

C.  Increase muscle strength.

D.  Do passive range of motion exercises.

**Rationale:**

The maintenance of active range of motion is a primary anti-deformity technique. Passive range of motion and resistive exercise to increase strength are contraindicated for individuals with RA. Avoiding fatigue is helpful from an energy conservation perspective but it does not prevent joint deformity.

**Type of Reasoning: Inferential**

One must link the individual's diagnosis to the recommendations presented in order to determine which recommendation is best to prevent deformity. This requires inferential reasoning, where one must draw conclusions about the likely course of action for a diagnosis. In this case the most appropriate recommendation is to maintain active range of motion. Review deformity prevention activities for persons with rheumatoid arthritis if answered incorrectly.

**B148  C8**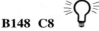

A school-based OTA consults with a teacher regarding a non-speaking student who uses a wheelchair and an augmentative communication device. The teacher reports that the student is making many errors on the communication device but that no difficulties had been observed when the student used the device in the past. Which is the most effective initial action for the OTA to take in response to the teacher's report?

**Correct Answer: C. Evaluate the position of the student in the wheelchair and the device on the wheelchair.**

**Incorrect Answers:**

A.  Advise the teacher to contact the student's parents and recommend that they bring the child to a physician for an examination.

B.  Reassess the student's motor and communication abilities.

D.  Reposition the communication device.

**Rationale:**

Even minor changes in a person's positioning can impact on his/her access to an assistive device; therefore, the OTA's initial action must be to evaluate the position of the student and the device. Based upon the results of this assessment, the OTA may provide recommendations for positioning the student and/or for placement of the device. Referring the student's parents to contact a physician for a physical examination, reassessing the student's motor and communication abilities, and repositioning the communication device are not steps indicated at this time.

**Type of Reasoning: Inferential**

One must determine the most likely cause for the communication difficulty, given the diagnosis and limitations of the student. This requires inferential reasoning skill, where one must draw conclusions based on the information presented. In this situation, the OTA should evaluate the position of the student in the wheelchair and the device on the wheelchair, as improper positioning can affect use of an augmentative communication device. If answered incorrectly, review positioning of augmentative devices on wheelchairs.

**B149  C2**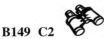

Several residents of a skilled nursing facility report that they are bored with their individual daily range of motion exercise programs. The OTA collaborates with the physical therapist to design a group to attain the goals of the individual exercise programs. Which would be most beneficial for the OTA to recommend incorporating into the proposed group?

**Correct Answer: A. Several exercise videos with diverse exercise styles and music.**

**Incorrect Answers:**

B.  The residents performing gentle range of motion on each other.

C.  Exercises in rhythm to a marching band video.

D.  The provision of coffee and cake after the group.

**Rationale:**

Adding variety can stimulate interest and socialization. Group members can select videos that are of personal interest. Clients should not do hands-on treatment with each other. A marching band video may be at a tempo that is too vigorous for some residents. Providing coffee and cake does not address the need to increase interest in performing daily ROM exercises.

**Type of Reasoning: Inductive**

One must utilize clinical knowledge and judgment to determine the exercise approach that best addresses the resident's concerns. In this case, providing several exercise videos with diverse styles and music is best. If answered incorrectly, review exercise programming for older adults in skilled nursing facilities

**B150  C6**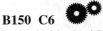

An individual with obsessive-compulsive personality disorder participates in a vocational program. The client asks the OTA to speak to the supervisor of the transitional employment program (TEP). The client is concerned that compulsive behaviors are interfering with job performance and may result in the loss of a new TEP placement. Which is the OTA's best response to these expressed concerns?

**Correct Answer: D. Schedule an appointment with the client and the TEP supervisor.**

**Incorrect Answers:**

A.  Instruct the client to speak directly to the TEP supervisor about the right to receive reasonable accommodations.

B.  Schedule a re-evaluation of the client's work behaviors and skills.

C.  Assure the client that it is natural to have initial difficulties at a new job.

**Rationale:**

Meeting with the individual and the TEP supervisor will enable the OTA to provide support for the client's concerns. The OTA can also facilitate a dialogue about the specific difficulties the client is experiencing from both the employee and employer perspective. This will help the OTA analyze the situation and can provide a basis for making recommendations for accommodations, if needed. Instructing the client to speak directly to the work supervisor ignores the client's request for the OTA's input. In addition, knowing one's rights for reasonable accommodations as provided by the Americans with Disabilities Act (ADA) does not equate to knowing what accommodations will help with work performance. A complete evaluation of the essential functions of the job and the person's skills and abilities must be completed prior to determining the nature of accommodations. Re-evaluating the client's work behaviors and skills does not address the client's stated concerns. In addition, TEP placements are typically made after an extensive evaluation process. This information would be readily available for the OTA to review, if needed. While it is natural to have initial difficulties and concerns when one begins a new job, reassuring the client of this reality does not address the client's request for the OTA's support.

**Type of Reasoning: Evaluative**

This question requires professional judgment based on guiding principles, which is an evaluative reasoning skill. For this situation, the OTA should schedule an appointment with the supervisor and client in order to analyze the situation and make any needed recommendations. Review transitional employment guidelines and fostering success in individuals if answered incorrectly.

516

**B151  C4**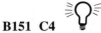

An OTA working in a school system conducts a series of educational workshops for parents of children with attention deficit and sensory processing disorders. The series focuses on principles of sensory integration (SI). Which of the following is most beneficial for the OTA to recommend the parents provide in the home environment?

**Correct Answer: C. A balance between structure and freedom so the child can direct his/her own actions.**

**Incorrect Answers:**

A.  A wide range of sensory stimuli including auditory, visual, and tactile, to increase awareness and responsivity.

B.  Minimal auditory, visual, and tactile sensory stimuli to decrease distractibility and responsivity.

D.  Clear directions and structured limits to organize behavior and promote adaptive responses.

**Rationale:**

A key principle of SI theory is to structure the environment to match the child's capabilities. This "just right" environment enables the child to direct his/her own activity participation which can then facilitate skill development. Sensory processing disorders may present along a continuum of under-responsivity (hyposensitivity) to over-responsivity (hypersensitivity) of multisensory processing and sensory seeking. Environments and activities must be tailored to the specific child. The design of an environment to increase awareness or to decrease distractibility is more consistent with a compensatory remediation approach. Providing structure and limits is more consistent with a behavioral approach.

**Type of Reasoning: Inferential**

One must have knowledge of attention deficit and sensory processing disorders and sensory integration guidelines in order to arrive at a correct conclusion. This is an inferential reasoning skill where knowledge of clinical guidelines and judgment based on facts are utilized to reach conclusions. If answered incorrectly, review sensory integration treatment guidelines for children with attention deficit and sensory processing disorders.

**B152  C8**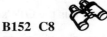

The family of a two year-old in a spica cast asks the OTA to modify the child's car seat. The child cannot fit safely in the car seat due to the cast. Which action is best for the OTA take in response to this request?

**Correct Answer: B. Recommend the family purchase a car seat designed for a child with a spica cast.**

**Incorrect Answers:**

A.  Pad the area between the car seat and the child's back with a pillow to accommodate for the lack of hip flexion.

C.  Cut down the sides of the car seat to allow the cast to hang out of the sides of the car seat.

D.  Tell the family to use the current car seat and tighten up the straps to hold in the child.

**Rationale:**

The child needs a car seat adapted for a child in a spica cast that has been crash tested. A variety of specialized car seats are available. OTAs and other pediatric care providers can become trained in fitting specialized car seats. Padding the area between the child and the car seat and cutting the car seat would invalidate the warranty and is unsafe. The current car seat is not safe and cannot be made safer by tightening the strap.

**Type of Reasoning: Inductive**

The test taker must determine the safest course of action in this scenario, which requires clinical judgment, an inductive reasoning skill. Being able to predict what may happen as a result of such actions, the test taker should conclude that purchasing a car seat made for a child with a spica cast is the best and safest choice. If answered incorrectly, review pediatric adaptive car seats.

## B153 C3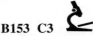

An OTA conducts a standardized sensory evaluation of an individual recovering from a left cerebral vascular accident. The individual has right hemiplegia and expressive aphasia. During the evaluation of stereognosis, which should the OTA have the client use to identify responses to the testing stimuli?

**Correct Answer: B. A set of identical objects.**

**Incorrect Answers:**

A. Pictures of the objects.
C. Cards with "1" and "2" printed on them.
D. Cards with "yes" and "no" printed on them.

**Rationale:**

Stereognosis is the ability to identify objects through touch and cognition. Having an identical set of objects from which the individual can select an object that matches the test stimulus will enable a person with expressive aphasia to participate in the evaluation. The person can point to the object to indicate his/her response Cards with "one" and "two" printed on them would be relevant assists for the evaluation of two point discrimination. Cards with "yes" and "no" printed on them would be relevant assists for the evaluation of light touch. Presenting the person with pictures to indicate a response requires the ability to generalize the object to its symbolic representation. This ability may be compromised in an individual with a CVA. It is more accurate to have exact matches of the objects used during the evaluation for this will not require the interpretation of pictures.

**Type of Reasoning: Deductive**

This question requires recall of testing guidelines based on factual knowledge. This is a deductive reasoning skill, where recall of facts is essential to arriving at a correct conclusion. In this scenario, the only appropriate method for identifying the response to a stimulus in stereognosis testing is to use a set of identical objects. Review guidelines for stereognosis testing for patients with expressive aphasia if answered incorrectly.

## B154 C6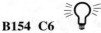

A woman with chronic depression and her spouse attend a discharge meeting with the OTA following the wife's six-week hospitalization for a major depressive episode. They state that they have few activities in common and spend little time together. The wife retired two months ago and her spouse continues to work full time. Which of the following should the OTA encourage this couple to do first to address this concern?

**Correct Answer: C. Explore activities enjoyed together and alone.**

**Incorrect Answers:**

A. Immediately participate in one activity together.
B. Become involved in their own individualized activities during the day.
D. Delay planning activities until the depression is totally resolved.

**Rationale:**

Assistance with an exploration of activities is a priority given the wife's recent hospitalization for depression. Her life has changed significantly with the loss of her worker role due to retirement and the resultant change in the amount of time spent alone. It will be important for her to explore activities enjoyed alone so that her retirement and time separated from her husband will be enjoyable and meaningful. Exploring activities that the couple enjoy together will assist both in the maintenance of their relationship and in the establishment of a new activities pattern. Immediate participation in one activity together is premature for there has been no determination of shared interests. While involvement in their own individualized activities during the day may be helpful, this also must be done after their involvement in treatment planning and activity selection. A delay in planning activities until the depression is totally resolved is contraindicated. The wife has chronic depression and needs treatment now.

**Type of Reasoning: Inferential**

One must infer or draw conclusions about a likely course of action, given the information presented. This is an inferential reasoning skill, where knowledge of a therapeutic approach is essential to choosing a correct solution. In this case, the OTA should begin with exploration of activities that the individual and her spouse have enjoyed together and alone. Review meaningful activities and activity exploration for individuals with depression if answered incorrectly.

518

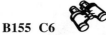

**B155  C6**

An individual attends a community day treatment program to assist in recovery from major depression. The client has fair eye contact and responds verbally to interactions initiated by others. Cognition is intact. Which group level is best for the OTA to recommend this client attend?

**Correct Answer: A. Project.**

**Incorrect Answers:**

B.  Parallel.

C.  Cooperative.

D.  Mature.

**Rationale:**

A project group utilizes short term activities that require the participation of two or more people. Tasks are shared and the focus is on interaction rather than task completion. This level is appropriate for someone who is socially responsive to others with intact cognition. A parallel group does not require any interaction for task completion. This group is too low-level for this individual because it would not provide the opportunity to use and build existing social skills. Cooperative and mature groups require members to be self-expressive and meet socio-emotional roles. These groups are too high-level for the individual at this point.

**Type of Reasoning: Inductive**

One must utilize clinical knowledge and judgment to determine the group level that most appropriately facilitates interaction with this individual. This requires inductive reasoning skill. In this case, a project group is most appropriate to facilitate sharing and interaction. If answered incorrectly, review types of groups, especially project level groups

**B156  C8**

An adolescent student with Duchenne muscular dystrophy and depression is being evaluated for a power wheelchair. Which is the most important area to be considered during the occupational therapy evaluation of the student to determine the student's readiness for the wheelchair?

**Correct Answer: C. Cognitive skills.**

**Incorrect Answers:**

A.  Level of interest.

B.  Fine motor skills.

D.  Postural control.

**Rationale:**

Cognitive skills include alertness, spatial operations, judgment, decision-making and problem solving, which can be affected by depression. Since these abilities are needed for the safe operation of a power wheelchair, it is essential that the OTA assess the student's cognitive level. The student's level of interest can help engage him in mobility training but it is not the most important area to assess. Fine motor skills and postural control are likely absent due to the progression of Duchenne muscular dystrophy. Wheelchair adaptations can compensate for decreased fine motor skills and poor postural control.

**Type of Reasoning: Inferential**

One must determine the critical skills needing to be assessed prior to providing a power wheelchair. This requires inferential reasoning, where one must infer or draw conclusions based on the information provided. In this situation, the student should be assessed for cognitive skills as this is the most important element in determining the safe and appropriate use of the device. If answered incorrectly, review power wheelchair prescription guidelines.

**B157 C2**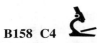

An OTA conducts a caregiver education workshop on positioning techniques for family caregivers. At the conclusion of the class, the caregivers will be expected to utilize the skills taught. Which is the most effective method for the OTA to use when teaching these techniques?

**Correct Answer: C. OTA demonstration of techniques followed by a lab with caregivers practicing positioning on each other.**

**Incorrect Answers:**

A. OTA demonstration of general techniques followed by individualized discussion with each caregiver.

B. An oral multimedia presentation including PowerPoint slides and handouts of positioning techniques for diverse disorders.

D. A question and answer session to address the specific individual positioning concerns of the caregivers.

**Rationale:**

A variety of teaching methods including demonstration, practice, and discussion has the best chance of reinforcing learning in a diverse group. Using only oral teaching methods will not likely enable the participants to develop the needed positioning skills. Psychomotor skills are best learned by practice, not lecture or question and answer. Feedback should include both knowledge of performance and knowledge of results.

**Type of Reasoning:  Inferential**

One must infer to draw a conclusion about the best approach for educating a group of individuals. Because the group may have differing needs and abilities in learning information, one must provide a variety of approaches to delivering the information. Inferential reasoning requires one to use knowledge of therapeutic approaches to determine which approach will result in the most effective outcome. For this case, demonstration of the techniques by the OTA and the caregivers practicing the techniques on each other is most effective. Review principles of teaching and caregiver education if answered incorrectly.

**B158  C4**

An OTA working on a sub-acute rehabilitation unit implements intervention with an older adult who recently incurred a cerebral vascular accident. The evaluation completed by the occupational therapist states that the individual is exhibiting signs of a flexor synergy in the right upper extremity. Which motor pattern will the OTA most likely observe during the initial intervention session?

**Correct Answer: B. Scapular adduction and elevation, shoulder abduction and external rotation, elbow flexion and forearm supination.**

**Incorrect Answers:**

A.  Scapular abduction and depression, shoulder adduction and internal rotation, elbow flexion and forearm supination.

C.  Scapular adduction and elevation, shoulder adduction and external rotation, elbow flexion and forearm pronation.

D.  Scapular abduction and elevation, shoulder abduction and internal rotation, elbow flexion and forearm supination.

**Rationale:**

The correct answer describes the components of typical flexor synergy pattern. The others have movement patterns that deviate from this traditional description.

**Type of Reasoning: Deductive**

One must recall the typical flexor synergy pattern in the upper extremity in order to arrive at a correct conclusion. This requires deductive reasoning skill, where factual knowledge is essential to choosing the correct solution. The typical pattern is scapular adduction and elevation, shoulder abduction and external rotation, elbow flexion and forearm supination. If answered incorrectly, review flexor synergy patterns of the upper extremity.

520

### B159 C2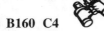

An individual with borderline personality disorder is admitted to the hospital following a suicide attempt. After attending an OT orientation group, the patient tells the OTA, "You are the only therapist who has ever been really helpful." The patient asks to meet with the OTA privately on a regular basis instead of the assigned primary individual therapist. Which action is best for the OTA to take in response to the patient's request?

**Correct Answer: A. Refer the patient to the assigned primary individual therapist.**

**Incorrect Answers:**

B.  Agree to meet with the patient since a positive therapeutic connection has been expressed.

C.  Tell the patient that an OTA provides only occupation-based group treatment.

D.  Explain that this type of manipulative behavior is not acceptable.

**Rationale:**

The patient must be referred to the primary individual therapist assigned to his/her case. Although the patient has responded favorably to the initial OT group session, this does not preclude the patient's need for individual therapy. On inpatient psychiatric units, OT practitioners often serve as primary individual therapists in addition to their group therapist role. However, the assignment of caseloads is not (and cannot be) based upon patients' requests. Labeling the individual's behavior as manipulative is judgmental and can be considered antagonistic.

**Type of Reasoning: Evaluative**

This question requires professional judgment based on guiding principles, which is an evaluative reasoning skill. For this situation, the OTA should refer the person to the primary individual therapist for individual therapy. If answered incorrectly, review individual versus group therapy guidelines for inpatient psychiatric settings.

### B160 C4

An adult is hospitalized in the recovery phase of Guillain-Barré syndrome. The patient complains of tingling, aching and weakness in both hands, causing difficulty in grasping grooming supplies. The patient requests relief from the hand symptoms. Which action should the OTA take to address the patient's concerns?

**Correct Answer: D. Educate the patient about sensory deficits and related adaptive ADL strategies.**

**Incorrect Answers:**

A.  Provide soft tissue massage to both hands prior to grooming activities.

B.  Apply hot packs to both hands and complete stretching exercises prior to grooming activities.

C.  Refer the client to a neurologist for follow-up of possible condition regression.

**Rationale:**

Guillain-Barré (GBS) is characterized by ascending motor weakness in the limbs, usually beginning in the hands and feet. Paresthesias and pain are also a common occurrence. The best approach for this patient is to educate the patient about the sensory deficits that are common to the condition and provide adaptive strategies for ADL so the patient is successful. Soft tissue massage will not remedy the aching in the hands as the inflammation of the peripheral nerves must decrease for this to resolve. Hot packs are contraindicated in this situation due to the potential for burns from altered sensation. Referral to a neurologist is not needed as the symptoms are typical of the syndrome.

**Type of Reasoning: Inductive**

This question requires the test taker to understand the nature of course of Guillain-Barré syndrome in order to determine the best approach to address the patient's concerns. In this case, because the patient's symptoms will require time to improve, the OTA should educate the patient about the sensory deficits and adaptive ADL strategies. If answered incorrectly, review information on the recovery phase of Guillain-Barré syndrome, especially sensory deficits of the hands.

**B161  C4**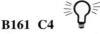

A person with a traumatic brain injury is assessed to be at the level of 2 on the Glasgow Coma Scale. Which should the OTA use to initiate intervention with this person?

**Correct Answer:  B. Sensory stimulation.**

**Incorrect Answers:**

A.  Demonstrated directions.

C.  Verbal cues.

D.  Hand-over-hand assistance.

**Rationale:**

A level of 2 on the Glasgow Coma Scale is just one level above a completely non-responsive coma.  As a result, a person at this level has severe deficits. The person can open his/her eyes in response to pain and make incomprehensible sounds; therefore, intervention begins at the sensory stimulation level.  The other choices are at levels that are too high for this individual.

**Type of Reasoning: Inferential**

One must determine the most likely intervention approach for a person, given the diagnosis provided and level of functioning. This requires inferential reasoning skill, where one must draw conclusions based on the information presented. In this situation, the OTA should begin with sensory stimulation, given the level of 2 on the Glasgow Coma Scale (GCS). If answered incorrectly, review intervention activities for individuals with TBI, especially a level of 2 on the GCS.

**B162  C1**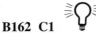

An OTA collaborates with an occupational therapist to design intervention activities for an 18 month-old toddler with multiple developmental disabilities. The child has been assessed as delayed by 6-8 months in all developmental parameters. Which intervention approach is most effective for developing the toddler's play skills?

**Correct Answer:  B. The use of toys that are visually and auditorily stimulating.**

**Incorrect Answers:**

A.  The use of toys that encourage creative play.

C.  Participation in a small parallel play group.

D.  Engagement in activities that use sensorimotor skills prerequisite to play.

**Rationale:**

Providing toys that are visually and auditorily stimulating will help engage the child in the intervention process. As the child explores the sensory properties and characteristics of these toys, he/she will engage in activities that will facilitate developmentally appropriate play. Through this process, the child will develop sensorimotor and cognitive skills. Many toys that provide visual and auditory stimulation also provide opportunities to explore relationships between actions and objects (e.g., striking a colorful keyboard to produce music). The exploration of relationships between actions and consequences is typical of the cognitive development of a 9-12 month-old, which is this child's developmental age. Creative play occurs developmentally at 4-7 years, so this option is not developmentally appropriate for this child. Placing a toddler with the developmental age of a 10-12 month-old into a parallel play group is not age appropriate. Engaging the child in activities that use sensorimotor skills prerequisite to play would not achieve the stated aim of developing play skills. It is more effective to directly use play activities during intervention to develop play skills.

**Type of Reasoning: Inferential**

One must infer or draw conclusions about a likely course of action, given the information presented. This is an inferential reasoning skill, where knowledge of a therapeutic approach is essential in choosing a correct solution. In this case, the OTA would likely initiate intervention with toys that are visually and auditorily stimulating, given the child's diagnosis and delays. If answered incorrectly, review intervention approaches for small children with developmental disabilities.

**B163  C3**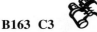

An individual with complex regional pain syndrome (CRPS), Type I presents with severe pain and pitting edema in the right hand. The individual has a secondary diagnosis of degenerative joint disease (DJD). Which should the OTA initially recommend to the person to address these concerns?

**Correct Answer: C. Elevation of the affected hand above the heart.**

**Incorrect Answers:**

A. Passive range of motion of wrist and fingers.

B. Retrograde massage from distal to proximal.

D. Retrograde massage from proximal to distal.

**Rationale:**

Elevation of the affected hand above the heart will promote venous and lymphatic drainage and decrease the hydrostatic pressure in the blood vessels. Retrograde massage is performed in a centripetal direction. It is not the initial treatment when severe pain is present. Passive range of motion is not advisable for persons with DJD.

**Type of Reasoning: Inductive**

This question requires one to determine the best recommendation for addressing the patient's symptoms. This requires inductive reasoning skill, where clinical judgment is paramount to arriving at a correct conclusion. For this situation, the OTA should initially recommend elevation of the affected hand above the heart. If answered incorrectly, review treatment guidelines for patients with CRPS Type I and pitting edema.

**B164  C5**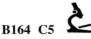

An OTA has scheduled a discharge planning session with an individual recovering from hip replacement surgery. In preparation for this session, the OTA reviews the nursing reports and learns that the person has mycobacterium tuberculosis which is currently in the dormant phase. Which type of precautions should the OTA use when entering the patient's room?

**Correct Answer: A. Standard.**

**Incorrect Answers:**

B. Airborne.

C. Droplet.

D. Contact.

**Rationale:**

Standard precautions are observed in all clinical situations. The additional use of airborne precautions is required when working with persons known or suspected to be infected with a serious illness transmitted by airborne nuclei that remain suspended in the air and can be dispersed widely by air currents within a room. When in the active phase, mycobacterium tuberculosis (TB), measles, and chickenpox are transmitted in this manner. Airborne precautions include the use of a respiratory isolation room and the wearing of respiratory protection (i.e., a mask) when entering the room. Airborne precautions are not needed when TB is dormant as is the case in this scenario. Droplet precautions are used for persons known or suspected to be infected with serious illness microorganisms transmitted by large particle droplets that can be generated by the individual during talking, sneezing, coughing (e.g., rubella, mumps, pertussis, influenza). Contact precautions are used for persons known or suspected to be infected or colonized with serious illness transmitted by direct contact (hand or skin to skin contact) or contact with items in the patient's environment.

**Type of Reasoning: Deductive**

One must recall the guidelines for standard and transmission-based precautions. This is factual knowledge, which is a deductive reasoning skill. Because the mycobacterium tuberculosis is dormant, one should recall that this is no longer an airborne illness and only standard precautions need to be observed. If answered incorrectly, review standard precautions and transmission-based precautions, especially guidelines for working with individuals with active vs. dormant tuberculosis.

### B165  C4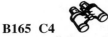

A Sensory Profile completed by a caregiver indicates that a 6 year-old child has modulation impairments and sensation seeking patterns. The OTA observes the child frequently wandering, bumping objects in the room, and fidgeting. The child has low muscle tone. Which is the best intervention approach for the OTA to provide to improve this child's deficits?

**Correct Answer: D. Sensory experiences that focus on proprioceptive, tactile, and vestibular input in the clinic and a sensory diet program while at home and school.**

**Incorrect Answers:**

A. A written sensory diet to the family and teachers which includes strategies to increase sensory input into the child's daily routine.

B. An obstacle course that focuses on proprioceptive and tactile input while crawling on hands and knees and encouraging high physical activity at home.

C. Sensory experiences to the child that include proprioceptive activities that focus on body awareness and grading control during play activities.

**Rationale:**

The use of skilled clinical observation is important with children. Because they create sensation for themselves, their behavior tells us what sensory input they need. Children who rock and fidget require vestibular input to help them attend and learn. Children with proprioceptive problems often rely on visual and/or verbal cues to know how to move their bodies and they often appear clumsy, bumping into objects in their environments. Children with low muscle tone frequently have difficulty registering proprioceptive input and require more intense input into their muscles and joints. More intense tactile, proprioceptive, and vestibular input will help this child pay attention and stay with an activity for a longer period of time before moving on to another activity and help improve body awareness and kinesthetic sense. It is also important to provide caregivers with a written sensory diet to implement on a daily basis in the child's home and school environments for carryover.

**Type of Reasoning: Inductive**

This question requires one to draw upon knowledge of effective therapy processes in order to determine the best approach for this child. This requires inductive reasoning skill. In this situation, the OTA should include sensory experiences that encompass proprioceptive, tactile, and vestibular input in the clinic and a sensory diet at home and school. If answered incorrectly, review sensory integration and sensory modulation guidelines, especially the Sensory Profile.

### B166  C8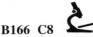

A religious congregation obtained private funding to build a ramp so that members with disabilities can attend services. The entrance to the congregation's building has six steps with a rise of 7 inches each. Which is best for the OTA consultant to recommend for construction of this ramp?

**Correct Answer: C. 32 feet long with a 4'x4' landing at the ramp's mid-point.**

**Incorrect Answers:**

A. 32 feet long.

B. 48 feet long.

D. 48 feet long with a 4'x4' landing at the ramp's mid-point.

**Rationale:**

A ramp should provide one foot of slope for every foot of rise. Six steps that have a rise of 7 inches results in a total rise of 32 inches. A 32 foot ramp may be too long for some individuals to independently access. Therefore, a landing at the ramp's mid-point would be best to allow the opportunity to safely take a rest break.

**Type of Reasoning: Deductive**

One must recall the guidelines for ramp construction in order to choose a correct solution. This is factual knowledge, which is a deductive reasoning skill. For this scenario, construction of the ramp should be 32 feet long with a 4' x 4' landing at the ramp mid-point. If answered incorrectly, review ramp construction guidelines of the International Code Council's accessibility standards.

## B167  C4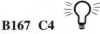

An OTA instructs the direct care staff of a rehabilitation unit on proper positioning techniques for a patient following the occurrence of a left CVA. In which of the following positions should the OTA recommend the patient's right affected arm be placed when the patient is sleeping in side-lying on the unaffected side?

**Correct Answer: B. Protracted with arm forward on a pillow and the elbow extended or slightly flexed.**

**Incorrect Answers:**

A.  In 90 degrees of humeral abduction and 15 degrees of internal rotation.

C.  On the person's side, adducted and internally rotated.

D.  In 90 degrees of abduction of the humerus with neutral rotation.

**Rationale:**

The best position of the upper extremities for sleeping or bed rest is to place the affected arm on a pillow in a comfortable position. Excess abduction can cause the joint capsule to loosen and reduce the stability of the humeral head in the glenoid fossa. It is important to avoid traction of the affected arm to ensure adequate positioning of the humerus with the scapula and to prevent subluxation. Correct positioning means putting the involved arm in slight abduction. Ninety degrees of abduction is excessive.

**Type of Reasoning: Inferential**

One must infer or draw conclusions about the optimal positioning of the affected upper extremity in side-lying. One must understand the reasons for the positioning of the extremity in order to prevent further problems from developing, which requires inferential reasoning skill. In this situation, positioning the extremity on a pillow in slight abduction is best.

## B168  C4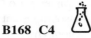

A client recovering from a traumatic brain injury reports frequently losing place when reading. Upon evaluation, the client exhibits difficulty with the letter cancellation task. When reviewing the evaluation results with the occupational therapist, which visual ability should the OTA report as deficient?

**Correct Answer: A. Scanning.**

**Incorrect Answers:**

B.  Imagery.

C.  Cognition.

D.  Memory.

**Rationale:**

The behaviors described relate to the ability to scan. Visual imagery is the process of making a mental picture of information so that it can be remembered. Visual cognition is the ability to mentally manipulate visual information and integrate it with other sensory information. Visual memory is the retrieval and recall of information that has been stored and encoded.

**Type of Reasoning: Analytical**

This question provides symptoms of a deficit and the test taker must determine what these symptoms indicate. This requires analytical reasoning skill, where one must consider all of the pieces of information provided and draw conclusions about what that means as a whole. In this situation, the symptoms indicate deficits in visual scanning ability. If answered incorrectly, review the definitions of visual perceptual skills and the symptoms of visual perceptual deficits.

**B169  C2**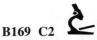

An OTA provides home-based services to a child with developmental delays. The child picks up and puts away toys when reminded by the parents and mimics the parents when they dry dishes and fold clothes. The family has identified a goal of including the child in home management activities. Which activity should the OTA introduce next during intervention?

**Correct Answer: A. Wiping tabletops.**

**Incorrect Answers:**

B.  Sorting laundry.
C.  Making a bed.
D.  Taking out trash.

**Rationale:**

Picking up and putting away toys when reminded and copying the parents when they do domestic chores are home management task skills that are typical of two year-old children. When working with a child with a developmental delay, the OTA would use a developmental frame of reference. According to the typical developmental sequence of home management tasks, wiping spills an ability of three year old children. Therefore, the next activity the OTA should work on with the child is wiping tabletops since this is consistent with normal development. The other options are too high a level at this point for this child. Sorting laundry is 4 year-old skill, making a bed and taking out trash are 5 year-old skills.

**Type of Reasoning: Deductive**

One must recall the developmental sequence of home management tasks and the developmental frame of reference in order to arrive at a correct conclusion. This is factual recall of information, which necessitates deductive reasoning skill. For this situation, the OTA should introduce wiping tabletops as the next developmental activity. If answered incorrectly, refer to Chapter 5 and developmental sequence of home management tasks, as well as the developmental frame of reference. The integration of the knowledge is pivotal to answering the question correctly.

**B170  C3**

A patient incurred a traumatic upper extremity amputation. During pre-prosthetic treatment, the OTA molds the contours of the residual limb to shrink and shape it in preparation for a prosthesis. Which method is most effective for the OTA to use?

**Correct Answer: A. Wrapping.**

**Incorrect Answers:**

B.  Percussion.
C.  Intermittent compression therapy.
D.  Massage.

**Rationale:**

Wrapping by applying an elastic bandage to the residual limb in a figure-of-eight pattern will reduce the volume of the residual limb and shape it for a prosthesis. Intermittent compression therapy is used for edema but not residual limbs. Percussion and massage are used to desensitize a residual limb.

**Type of Reasoning: Analytical**

This question provides a description of an intervention method and the test taker must determine the likely definition of the described method. This is an analytical reasoning skill, as questions of this nature often ask one to analyze a descriptor to determine the specific method being defined. In this situation the intervention method is that of residual limb wrapping, which should be reviewed if answered incorrectly.

526

## B171  C3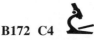

A patient with fibromyalgia is receiving occupational therapy to reduce pain and promote flexibility during ADL tasks. The patient expresses the intent to discontinue treatment based on information obtained during an online search which questioned the value of therapy for fibromyalgia. Which of the following actions should the OTA do first in response to the patient's statements?

**Correct Answer: D. Inform the patient that online information can be inaccurate and provide literature about the benefits of therapy for fibromyalgia.**

**Incorrect Answers:**

A. Confront the inaccuracy of these statements and provide current evidence-based research about the benefits of therapy for persons with fibromyalgia.

B. Reassure the patient that the physician has ordered therapy; therefore, it will be beneficial.

C. Respect the patient's wishes and discontinue occupational therapy, offering to provide therapy in the future if symptoms exacerbate.

**Rationale:**

It is common for patients to seek out more information about their condition. The internet can be informative and resourceful. It can also be inaccurate, incomplete, and misleading. OTAs are responsible for making sure patients have accurate information about their conditions in order to make informed decisions. In this case, the OTA should inform the patient of the inaccurate information and provide accurate information about exercise related to his/her condition. It is not as beneficial to directly confront the inaccuracies of this information with the latest research. This stance can be overwhelming and lead to the person feeling belittled. Reminding the patient of the physician's orders does not respect the patient's feelings or address his/her concerns. Discontinuing treatment overlooks the need to provide accurate information first to ensure the patient is making an informed decision.

**Type of Reasoning: Evaluative**

This situation requires one to consider the AOTA Code of Ethics guidelines of beneficence, nonmaleficence (do no harm) and autonomy (the right to refuse). This necessitates evaluative reasoning skill, where the test taker must determine a proper course of action that respects the rights of the patient, while doing no harm. In this situation, the OTA should inform the patient of the inaccurate information and provide accurate information about the benefits of exercise. If answered incorrectly, review the AOTA Code of Ethics, especially beneficence, nonmaleficence, and autonomy.

## B172  C4

An OTA is providing intervention for an individual recovering from a CVA who has residual body neglect. The OTA is using a deficit-specific approach to intervention. Which type of activities is best for the OTA to use with this client?

**Correct Answer: D. Bilateral using both upper extremities.**

**Incorrect Answers:**

A. Unilateral using the affected upper extremity.

B. Unilateral using the non-affected upper extremity.

C. Tasks that require right/left discrimination.

**Rationale:**

A basic principle of intervention for body neglect, according to a deficit-specific approach, is to provide bilateral activities. During these activities, the OTA can guide the affected extremity through the activity, if needed. Providing unilateral activities does not work on the identified deficits. The provision of tasks that require discrimination of right/left is indicated for spatial relations dysfunction.

**Type of Reasoning: Deductive**

One must recall the guidelines for use of a deficit-specific approach for body neglect. This is factual knowledge, which is a deductive reasoning skill. In this situation, the most appropriate activities for the OTA to use under this approach are bilateral with use of both upper extremities. If answered incorrectly, review deficit-specific approach to treatment of CVA.

**B173 C1**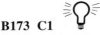

An OTA is treating an eight month old child with mild developmental delay. The child exhibits normal cognitive development. The child has developed adequate static sitting balance but has poor dynamic sitting balance. The OTA implements intervention by positioning the child and having the child find a toy that is covered with a cloth. Which positioning and toy placement are most beneficial for the OTA to use with this child?

**Correct Answer: A. Sit the child between the OTA's extended legs and alternate placing the covered toy to the child's right and left side.**

**Incorrect Answers:**
B.  Sit the child in a child seat and alternate placing the covered toy to the child's right and left side.
C.  Lay the child in a prone position and place the covered toy in front of the child.
D.  Lay the child in on the right side and place the covered toy to the left of the child.

**Rationale:**
Having the child sit between the OTA's extended legs can enable the OTA to easily provide postural support to the child as needed. Placing the covered toy to the right and then left of the seated child will facilitate the child's sideward protective extension response. Sideward protective extension in sitting is a functional, protective reaction that typically occurs at 7 months and persists in normal development. Sideward protective extension is a key component to the development of dynamic sitting balance as it protects the child from a fall. This reaction also supports the body for unilateral use of the opposite arm. Sitting the child in a child seat would provide too much support and would not provide the child with the 'just-right' challenge to develop dynamic sitting. Laying the child in a prone position and placing the covered toy in front of the child would help facilitate a prone on elbows position. If the child has begun to sit, this position would have already been mastered so this intervention is not needed. Laying the child in on the right side and placing the covered toy to the left of the child would facilitate rolling. If the child has begun to sit, rolling would have already been mastered so this intervention is not needed.

**Type of Reasoning: Inferential**
One must recall the developmental milestones of infants and infer the best choice for positioning in order to choose the correct solution. For this child, who just achieved static sitting balance, positioning that provides postural support during dynamic sitting activity with facilitation of the protective extensive response is most beneficial because this skill is essential for dynamic sitting. If answered incorrectly, review the motor developmental milestones of infants.

**B174 C6**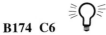

An OTA implements a sensorimotor group for six individuals with chronic schizophrenia. What is the most beneficial activity for the OTA to include in the group?

**Correct Answer: D. Parachute games.**

**Incorrect Answers:**
A.  A discussion of the importance of exercise.
B.  Relaxation activities.
C.  Tai Chi.

**Rationale:**
A sensorimotor group utilizes active, gross motor movements. Parachute games facilitate such gross motor mobility. Discussion and relaxation activities can be relevant activities but they do not meet the criteria of a sensorimotor group. Tai Chi is a slow, gross motor movement.

**Type of Reasoning: Inferential**
In order to arrive at a correct conclusion, one must consider the sensorimotor needs and diagnosis of the group members, and the characteristics of the provided activities. This requires inferential reasoning skill, where one must draw conclusions based on evidence presented as to which activity would be the best. In this situation, a parachute game is the only activity which meets the needs of the clients. Review sensorimotor group activities for individuals with chronic schizophrenia if answered incorrectly.

## B175 C2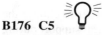

When performing a chart audit for an on-site accreditation visit, an OTA realizes that a date of service was documented wrong. The OTA had provided this service under the direct supervision of an occupational therapist. Which actions are best for the OTA to take?

**Correct Answer: C. Put a single line through the incorrect date, write the correct date of service, and then initial and date the correction.**

**Incorrect Answers:**

A. Use white out to remove the incorrect date, write the correct date of service, and then initial and date the correction.

B. Write the correct date over the incorrect date and then write the supervising occupational therapist's initials.

D. Meet with the supervising occupational therapist to discuss the need to correct this documentation.

**Rationale:**

Medical charts are legal documents that cannot be altered without accountability. Therefore, the error found must be acknowledged with the date of correction and the initials of the person making the correction. According to established guidelines for documentation, charting errors should be corrected by drawing a single line through the error and initialing and dating the chart. The permanent removal of an error by using white-out is not acceptable nor is it acceptable to place another practitioner's initials on documentation. There is no need for the OTA to meet with the OT supervisor to discuss this situation. The OTA can make the needed correction according to established documentation standards.

**Type of Reasoning: Evaluative**

This question requires one to evaluate the merits of the four possible solutions in order to determine which response is consistent with documentation standards of practice. Evaluative reasoning skills are utilized whenever one must make a judgment about a best course of action. For this type of situation, drawing a single line through the incorrect information with initials and then making and dating the correction is consistent with established guidelines for OT documentation, which should be reviewed if answered incorrectly.

## B176 C5

An individual with a body mass index (BMI) of 35 is joining a community-based wellness program conducted by an occupational therapist and an OTA. When formulating an individualized wellness plan, which condition should the occupational therapist and OTA take into consideration as an increased risk for this person?

**Correct Answer: B. Hyperthermia during exertion.**

**Incorrect Answers:**

A. Hypothermia during exertion.

C. Rapid weight loss during the initial weeks.

D. Increased anxiety and depression.

**Rationale:**

A patient with a body mass index of 35 is considered obese and is at increased risk for hyperthermia during exertion. Weight loss will occur after the person actively engages in a wellness program that includes lifestyle redesign, a nutritional diet, and exercise over an extended period of time, not just in the initial weeks. An individualized wellness program should decrease anxiety and depression, not increase them.

**Type of Reasoning: Inferential**

This question requires one to infer a patient's risk factors based on the diagnosis provided. This is an inferential reasoning skill, as one must determine what may be true of a patient, although one cannot be 100% certain. In this case, the patient is likely to have hyperthermia during exertion. If answered incorrectly, review risk factors for patients with obesity.

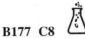

## B177  C8

A patient is recovering from a right CVA resulting in severe left hemiplegia and visuospatial deficits. The person's left lower extremity has pitting edema. Which wheelchair would be best for the OTA to recommend for this patient?

**Correct Answer: D. A hemiplegic chair with an elevating leg rest on the left.**

**Incorrect Answers:**

A. A powered wheelchair with a joystick control and dual elevating leg rests.

B. A lightweight active duty wheelchair with dual elevating leg rests.

C. A one-arm drive chair with an elevating leg rest on the left.

**Rationale:**

A hemiplegic chair has a low seat height ($17^1/2$ inches as compared to the standard seat height of $19^1/2$ inches) and is the best choice for this patient. The patient can propel it using both the unaffected hand and leg. An elevating leg rest for the left side is needed to address the edema in the patient's left lower extremity. There is no need for an elevating leg rest for the right lower extremity. A one-arm drive wheelchair has both drive mechanisms located on one wheel. A person can propel this type of wheelchair by using one hand. A one-arm drive wheelchair is contraindicated for patients with cognitive or perceptual deficits (as in this case) as they can be confusing to learn to propel accurately. The electric wheelchair with joystick would also be difficult for a person with visuospatial deficits. In addition, an electric wheelchair is significantly more expensive, less transportable, requires increased maintenance, and would be difficult to justify for reimbursement.

**Type of Reasoning: Analytical**

A number of important symptoms are described in this exam item and the test taker must analyze all of the symptoms (not just some) in order to make the best choice in wheelchair prescription. When balancing the edema issues, hemiplegia, and visuospatial deficits, one must conclude that a hemi chair with elevating leg rest provides the safest, most effective means of mobility and addresses all the deficits mentioned. If answered incorrectly, review wheelchair prescription guidelines.

## B178  C1

A client has a 3-year history of multiple sclerosis. One of the client's disabling symptoms is a persistent and severe diplopia, which leaves the client frequently nauseated and unable to complete desired activities. Which adaptive strategy is most effective for the OTA to recommend the client use during BADL and IADL?

**Correct Answer: D. Wear an eye patch on one eye.**

**Incorrect Answers:**

A. Wear magnifying glasses.

B. Wear prism glasses.

C. Close both eyes and initiate movements without visual guidance.

**Rationale:**

Double vision (diplopia) can be managed by patching one eye. Patients are typically on an eye-patching schedule that alternates the eye that is patched. Loss of depth perception can be expected with eye patching but is not as disabling as diplopia. The other options do not correct diplopia.

**Type of Reasoning:  Inferential**

The test taker must infer or draw conclusions about how the four possible treatment options will be the best remedy for diplopia. This requires knowledge of the condition of diplopia and how eye patching is the most effective choice for remedying the condition, which is an inferential reasoning skill. For this case, the OTA should recommend that the client to wear an eye patch. Review information about treatment of diplopia if answered incorrectly.

**B179  C6**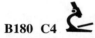

An older adult is admitted to a skilled nursing facility following a fall that resulted in a fractured hip with open reduction, internal fixation. The resident lived alone in a second floor apartment and was unable to return home. The resident is extremely agitated over being in a nursing facility. During the first OT session, the resident angrily yells, "Leave me alone, I just want to get out of here!" Which is the OTA's best initial response?

**Correct Answer: C. Calmly and supportively acknowledge the resident's feelings.**

**Incorrect Answers:**

A. Explain the benefits of active engagement in occupational therapy.

B. Console the person by stating that it is likely this nursing facility placement is only temporary.

D. Advise the OT supervisor that a psychiatric evaluation should be requested to assess the resident's mental status.

**Rationale:**

This resident has just incurred an injury that has resulted in the loss of his/her home. It is natural for the resident to be angry and upset over the unanticipated placement in an institution. The OTA should not be surprised by this outburst and should respond in a calm and supportive manner to acknowledge the resident's feelings. This is an effective use of interactive reasoning and can effectively assist with building rapport. While it is important to explain the benefits of active engagement in occupational therapy, the resident's ability to adequately process this information will be diminished by his/her distraught state. Therefore, calmly supporting the person is the best initial response. Once rapport has been attained the OTA can more effectively explain the OT process to the resident. Consoling the resident by stating that the nursing home placement is only temporary is not truthful since the OTA cannot know what the residential outcome will be for this person. Advising the OT supervisor that psychiatric evaluation should be requested is not appropriate. There is no information provided in the scenario to indicate a need for a mental status evaluation.

**Type of Reasoning:  Evaluative**

In this type of question, one must assess the value of the four possible choices. In this scenario, the test taker should be able to determine that an agitated newly admitted resident will require a calm and supportive approach to reduce agitation and build rapport. This type of question requires one to weigh the strength of statements, which is an evaluative reasoning skill. If answered incorrectly, review guidelines for building rapport, especially in individuals with agitation.

**B180  C4**

An OTA is implementing intervention with a child with developmental delay characterized by hypotonicity. According to the Rood approach, which is the first stability pattern that the OTA should facilitate during intervention?

**Correct Answer: B. Neck cocontraction.**

**Incorrect Answers:**

A. Roll over.

C. Quadruped.

D. Prone on elbows.

**Rationale:**

Neck cocontraction requires simultaneous activation or contraction of the neck flexors and extensors. It is essential for head control. Roll over is an early mobility pattern and occurs when the arm and leg on the same side of the body flex as the trunk rotates. It is utilized to elicit lateral trunk responses. The positions of prone on elbows and quadruped are stability patterns that develop after neck cocontraction. The prone on elbows position provides trunk and proximal limb stability. The quadruped position develops limb and trunk cocontraction.

**Type of Reasoning: Deductive**

This question requires recall of guidelines and principles, which is factual knowledge. Deductive reasoning skills are utilized whenever one must recall facts to solve clinical problems. In this situation, the OTA should facilitate neck cocontraction in this child, as this is the first stability pattern in the Rood approach. Review Rood treatment approach, especially stability patterns in children if answered incorrectly.

## B181  C2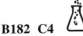

An OTA conducts an after-school transition skills group with adolescents with a diversity of disabilities. One of the student's behavior is very different than in prior groups (e.g., difficulty focusing when typically serving as the group initiator, making statements that are irrelevant to the topic at hand). The OTA smells a strong alcohol scent on the student's breath. Which action should the OTA take in response to this situation?

**Correct Answer: D. Call for a school aide to escort the student to the school's on-site health care facility.**

**Incorrect Answers:**

A. Directly ask the student if the student has been drinking.

B. Initiate a group discussion about the effects of substance abuse on occupational performance.

C. Proceed with the group and report suspicions of alcohol use at the next transition planning team meeting.

**Rationale:**

The OTA must ensure the student's safety. The medical staff of the school's on-site health care facility can evaluate the student to determine the cause of the student's atypical behavior and alcohol-smelling breath. These symptoms can be the result of alcohol use or an indication of ketoacidosis. In either case, it is best for the student to receive a medical evaluation and the corresponding care. The other options do not address the student's need for a medical evaluation and they can be disruptive to the group process for the other group participants.

**Type of Reasoning:  Evaluative**

This judgment question requires one to determine what will not only address the situation at hand, but protect the student from future harm. The test taker must choose the answer that addresses the situation immediately and with the professionals who hold ultimate responsibility for the patient. Evaluation questions are challenging in that one must evaluate the merits of each statement and conclude what will result in the best possible outcome. Review first aid procedures and symptoms of ketoacidosis if answered incorrectly.

## B182  C4

A patient who incurred a right CVA asks for a bottle of water to drink. The OTA gives the patient a bottle of water but the patient is unable to open it. The OTA provides instruction on opening the bottle but the patient remains unable to complete the task. After the intervention session, the OTA observes the patient independently open the bottle and drink from it. Which deficit is most accurate for the OTA to report to the occupational therapist as needing further evaluation?

**Correct Answer: B. Ideomotor apraxia.**

**Incorrect Answers:**

A. Anosognosia.

C. Unilateral neglect.

D. Somatagnosia

**Rationale:**

With ideomotor apraxia, a patient cannot perform a task upon direction but can do the task when on his/her own. Anosognosia is a more severe form of neglect that is demonstrated by a lack of awareness and denial of the severity of one's paralysis. Unilateral neglect is demonstrated by a failure to respond to or report unilateral stimulus presented to the body side contralateral to the lesion. Somatoagnosia is a body scheme disorder that results in diminished awareness of body structure and a failure to recognize body parts as one's own.

**Type of Reasoning: Analytical**

One must have a firm understanding of the difference between the cognitive-perceptual deficits of apraxia, neglect, and agnosia in order to arrive at the correct conclusion. Doing so requires one to assess the differences between these deficits and determine the likely reason for this deficit, which is an analytical reasoning skill. Review the definitions of these terms and other perceptual deficits associated with CVA if answered incorrectly.

532

## B183  C8

An OTA is working with a non-ambulatory elementary school-aged child who demonstrates moderate to severe extensor spasticity and limited head control. Which is the most beneficial positioning device for the OTA to recommend for this child to use in the classroom?

**Correct Answer: B. A wheelchair with a back wedge and head supports.**

**Incorrect Answers:**

A. A wheelchair with an adductor pommel.

C. A supine stander with an abduction wedge.

D. A prone stander with an abduction wedge.

**Rationale:**

A wheelchair wedge and head supports will position the child's trunk and head in slight flexion. This will help decrease the child's extensor tone and is the most beneficial positioning recommendation for this child. An abduction pommel or wedge controls scissoring of the legs which often occurs with increased extensor tone. However, these positioning devices do not provide the head or upper truck support that is needed for effective functioning in the school environment.  In addition, supine and prone standers would not facilitate the child's ability to integrate into the classroom setting since most elementary school tasks are done at a desktop.

**Type of Reasoning:  Analytical**

The test taker must determine which of the four possible positioning devices is most effective in addressing the child's issues. This requires knowledge of wheelchair seating and positioning and properties of spasticity in children. For this case, the OTA should recommend a wheelchair with a back wedge and head supports. If answered incorrectly, review information on seating and positioning for children with spasticity.

## B184  C2

An OTA provides bed-side BADL training to a patient recovering from multiple injuries incurred during a motor vehicle accident. The patient's children arrive for a visit and ask the OTA to let them look at their parent's chart while they wait outside the room for the session to conclude. Which response is best for the COTA to make in response to this request?

**Correct Answer: A. Tell the family members that they must have the permission of their parent before they can look at the chart.**

**Incorrect Answers:**

B. Give the family members the chart and let them read it.

C. Tell the family members they cannot see the chart because they could misinterpret the information.

D. Tell the family members to go ask the supervising occupational therapist for permission to look at the chart.

**Rationale:**

According to the Health Insurance and Portability Accountability Act (HIPAA), the OTA must obtain the person's permission prior to sharing any information about the person's status with family members or significant others.

HIPAA does allow providers to use their clinical judgment to determine whether to discuss the person's case with others if the person cannot give permission or objects. Documentation for this decision is essential (e.g., person is at risk of harming self due to lack of judgment; consultation with a specialist is essential to ensure quality of care). All information used or disclosed about a person's status must be limited to the minimum needed for the immediate purpose. There is no need for the OTA to advise the family members to speak to the occupational therapist. The OTA can directly inform the family of the HIPAA guidelines.

**Type of reasoning: Evaluative**

One must weigh the courses of action presented and determine which approach will result in the most effective outcome and follows federal guidelines for protecting patient privacy. This is an evaluative reasoning skill. For this situation, having knowledge of HIPAA guidelines, the OTA should tell the family members that they must have the permission of their parent before they can look at the chart. Review HIPAA guidelines for protecting patient privacy if answered incorrectly.

**B185  C6**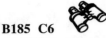

An OTA conducts a task-oriented activity group for adolescents recently diagnosed with anorexia nervosa. Which is the best activity for the OTA to include in the initial session of this group?

**Correct Answer: D. Composing lyrics and melody for a group song.**

**Incorrect Answers:**

A.  Making cards to send to veterans in a local hospital.

B.  Baking cookies for the residents in a homeless shelter.

C.  Performing low impact aerobic exercises.

**Rationale:**

A task-oriented group utilizes a psychodynamic approach to increase participants' understanding of their needs, values, ideas, feelings, and behaviors. Activities are selected and designed to facilitate self-expression and the exploration of feelings, thoughts, and behaviors. Composing a song is a self-expressive activity that allows each member to contribute his/her thoughts and feelings. It is an activity that can be stopped to discuss behaviors, feelings, and issues that arise during the group. The other activity choices do not provide this self-expression opportunity. In addition, baking and exercising are not the best initial activities for a person with eating disorders.

**Type of Reasoning: Inductive**

Clinical knowledge and judgment are the most important skills needed for answering this question, which requires inductive reasoning skill. Knowledge of the diagnosis and most appropriate activities for a task-oriented group are essential to arriving at a correct conclusion. In this case, the most appropriate initial activity is composing lyric and melody for a group song. If answered incorrectly review task-oriented activities for adolescents with anorexia nervosa.

**B186  C3**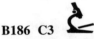

A patient has extensive full-thickness burns to the dorsum of the right hand and forearm and is being fitted with a splint to support the wrists and hands in anti-deformity position. In which positions should the OTA construct this splint?

**Correct Answer: A. 35 degrees of wrist extension, 70 degrees of MCP flexion, IPs in extension, and thumb in abduction.**

**Incorrect Answers:**

B.  Neutral wrist position with 90 degrees of MCP flexion and 30 degrees of IP and thumb flexion.

C.  30 degrees of wrist flexion with MCP and IP extension and thumb opposition.

D.  Neutral wrist position with MCP and IP extension and thumb in abduction and opposition.

**Rationale:**

The anti-deformity splinting position for the wrist and hand includes 30 – 45 degrees of wrist extension, 70 degrees of MCP flexion, IPs in extension and thumb in abduction. The other positions do not meet these criteria.

**Type of Reasoning: Deductive**

This question requires one to recall the protocol for anti-deformity position splinting after burns, which is a deductive reasoning skill. Deductive reasoning skills are often utilized when one must recall facts to solve problems. For this case, the splint should be constructed in 35 degrees of wrist extension, 70 degrees of MCP flexion, IPs in extension, and thumb in abduction. Refer to splinting guidelines for burns if answered incorrectly.

**B187 C2**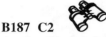

A school-based OTA is teaching orientation and mobility skills to an adolescent with a degenerative visual disorder. Which is the most effective motivational technique for the OTA to use with this student?

**Correct Answer: C. Treat the student as an adult and incorporate the student's orientation and mobility goals into intervention sessions.**

**Incorrect Answers:**

A. Provide concrete structure and frequent feedback to ensure accurate orientation and safe functional mobility.

B. Keep sessions short to allow time for emotional adjustment to orientation and mobility challenges.

D. Limit anxiety by practicing the techniques in a quiet and self-contained environment; e.g., an empty classroom.

**Rationale:**

Adolescents prefer to be treated as adults. The most important (and most effective) motivational technique is to incorporate the student's goals into the intervention sessions. Too much structure will limit the student's trial and error learning which is vital to learning and retaining orientation and functional mobility skills. The length of intervention sessions should be determined by the student's established goals, the methods identified to attain these goals, and the student's progress towards goal attainment. Throughout the orientation and mobility training sessions, the OTA can incorporate the therapeutic use of self to help the student emotionally adjust to the challenges of the situation and effectively deal with any anxiety he/she may be experiencing. Using a quiet self-contained environment can be a helpful intervention approach when first introducing orientation and mobility techniques but it is not a motivational strategy.

**Type of Reasoning: Inductive**

This question requires one to utilize clinical judgment to reach a sound conclusion, which is an inductive reasoning skill. For this question, the test taker must consider the age of the individual in order to determine the best motivational techniques. In this case, treating the patient as an adult and incorporating the patient's goals into the plan of care is best.

**B188 C4**

A 6 year-old is diagnosed with Duchenne's muscular dystrophy. The family establishes a goal of maintaining the child's leisure and social participation. Which is the best activity for the OTA to recommend the family pursue with this child?

**Correct Answer: D. Recreational swimming.**

**Incorrect Answers:**

A. Electronic sports (e.g., Wii bowling).

B. Adapted little league baseball.

C. Wheelchair basketball.

**Rationale:**

Recreational swimming is a social and leisure activity that the child can participate in with family members and friends. It can also be helpful in maintaining the child's functional level as long as possible. Even when the child's Duchenne's progresses, swimming will often remain an activity that can be successfully pursued. The eye-hand coordination to play electronic sports games will likely be too difficult for the child with Duchenne's. Baseball and basketball also have mobility and coordination requirements that would be difficult for this child. In addition, at 6 years of age, wheelchair use due to Duchenne's is not usual.

**Type of Reasoning: Inferential**

In this question, one must make a link between the diagnosis, the age of the child, and the appropriate interventions. Here, swimming is appropriate because the child is ambulatory and it encourages the maintenance of function for as long as possible. Questions such as these require one to draw conclusions based on evidence presented, which is an inferential skill. If answered incorrectly, review leisure activities for children with muscular dystrophy.

**B189  C8**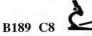

An OTA completes an ergonomic examination of a computer programmer and the programmer's workstation. Which is the best recommendation for the OTA to make for to ensure the programmer uses ideal wrist and elbow positioning?

**Correct Answer: B. Use a keyboard rest to maintain a neutral wrist position.**

**Incorrect Answers:**

A. Elevate the keyboard to increase wrist flexion.
C. Lower the keyboard to increase wrist extension.
D. Add armrests to support elbows in 90 degrees of flexion.

**Rationale:**

Work involving increased wrist deviation from a neutral posture in either flexion/extension or radial/ulnar deviation has been associated with increased reports of carpal tunnel syndrome and other wrist and hand problems. Therefore, using a keyboard rest to maintain a neutral wrist position is the best recommendation for the OTA to make to ensure the programmer uses ideal wrist and elbow positioning.

**Type of Reasoning:  Deductive**

This question requires one to recall the proper ergonomic guidelines for workstation function. This is factual information, which is a deductive reasoning skill. In this scenario, it is important to prevent wrist and elbow dysfunction by facilitating neutral wrist positioning when using a keyboard. Review ergonomic workstation evaluation guidelines if answered incorrectly.

**B190  C6**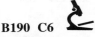

An OTA uses behavior modification techniques to help shape the behavioral responses of students with behavioral disorders. Which action is most consistent with this intervention approach?

**Correct Answer: A. Provide frequent positive reinforcement for all desired behaviors.**

**Incorrect Answers:**

B. Reprimand the students every time an undesirable behavior occurs.
C. Allow each student enough time for self-correction of the behavior.
D. Encourage the teaching staff to tell the students which behaviors are correct and which are not.

**Rationale:**

Behavioral modification is best achieved through use of positive reinforcements for all desired behaviors. Negative behaviors should be ignored. Self-correction is not a form of behavior modification.

**Type of Reasoning:  Deductive**

For this question the test taker utilizes knowledge and recall of behavioral modification techniques to choose the correct answer. This necessitates the factual recall of guidelines, which is a deductive reasoning skill. For this scenario, the OTA should provide frequent positive reinforcement for all desired behaviors, which is aligned with behavioral modification guidelines. Review behavioral modification guidelines if answered incorrectly.

536

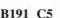

## B191 C5

An OTA works with an acute care rehabilitation patient with diabetes and a below-knee (BK) amputation to learn how to effectively perform home management tasks while wearing a BK prosthesis. When taking laundry from a front-loading washer and placing it into a top-loading dryer, the patient reports feeling weak, dizzy, and somewhat nauseous. The OTA notices that the patient is sweating profusely and is unsteady when standing. Which is the best immediate course of action for the OTA to take in response to the patient's complaints and these observations?

**Correct Answer: B. Administer orange juice for developing hypoglycemia.**

**Incorrect Answers:**

A.  Return the person to the unit of care due to an insulin reaction.

C.  Call a nurse to administer an insulin injection for developing hyperglycemia.

D.  Have the patient sit down until the orthostatic hypotension resolves.

**Rationale:**

Hypoglycemia, abnormally low blood glucose, results from too much insulin (insulin reaction). It requires accurate assessment of symptoms and prompt intervention. Having the patient sit down and ingest an oral sugar (e.g., orange juice) is the best immediate action for the OTA to take. Once the patient is stabilized, the physician should be notified. Profuse sweating and nausea do not usually accompany orthostatic hypotension.

**Type of Reasoning: Inductive**

The test taker must determine first what the cause is for the patient's symptoms and then what is the appropriate course of action. Questions such as these utilize one's clinical judgment and diagnostic thinking, which is an inductive reasoning skill. One should recognize that these symptoms are indicative of hypoglycemia and require immediate administration of sugar to relieve symptoms. Review first aid guidelines for hypoglycemia if answered incorrectly.

## B192 C1

An elderly person has lost significant functional vision over the last four years and complains of blurred vision and difficulty reading. The patient frequently mistakes images directly in front, especially in bright light. When walking across a room, the patient is able to locate items in the environment using peripheral vision when items are located to both sides. Based on these findings, which visual deficit should the OTA report the client is exhibiting?

**Correct Answer: D. Cataracts.**

**Incorrect Answers:**

A.  Glaucoma.

B.  Presbyopia

C.  Hemianopsia.

**Rationale:**

Cataracts are a clouding of the lens which results in a gradual loss of vision. Central vision is lost first, then peripheral. There are increased problems with glare and a general darkening of vision with loss of acuity and distortion. Glaucoma produces the reverse symptoms: loss of peripheral vision is first (tunnel vision), then central, progressing to total blindness. Presbyopia is a visual loss in middle and older ages that is characterized by an inability to focus properly and blurred images. Hemianopsia is field defect in both eyes that often occurs following CVA.

**Type of Reasoning: Analytical**

In this question, symptoms are presented and one must make a determination of the most likely diagnosis. These types of questions require analysis of the meaning of information presented, which is an analytical reasoning skill. For this situation, the symptoms are indicative of cataracts. Refer to information on visual deficits associated with aging if answered incorrectly.

**B193 C5**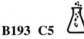

An older adult is referred to occupational therapy for ADL training. During a dressing session, the OTA notices a persistent area of redness over the sacrum that is still evident after the patient has been upright for 30 minutes. Which of the following does this observation indicate?

**Correct Answer: A. A stage I pressure ulcer.**

**Incorrect Answers:**

B.  A stage II pressure ulcer.

C.  A stage III pressure ulcer.

D.  A stage IV pressure ulcer.

**Rationale:**

A stage I pressure ulcer is characterized by a defined area of persistent redness (as in this example). Additional changes include alterations in skin temperature (warmth or coolness), tissue consistency, and sensation (pain, itching). A stage II ulcer involves redness, edema, blistering and hardening (induration) of tissue. The skin is open and inflammation extends to the fat layer with superficial necrosis in advanced Stage II lesions. Stages I and II are considered partial thickness ulcers. A stage III pressure ulcer is a full thickness skin lesion extending down to the muscle; the ulcer margin is thickened. A stage IV pressure ulcer extends down to the bone and includes bone destruction.

**Type of Reasoning: Analytical**

This question provides a description of a condition and the test taker must determine what the symptoms indicate. This is an analytical reasoning skill. For this case, the symptoms described indicate a stage I pressure ulcer. Review pressure ulcer stages, especially stage I, if answered incorrectly.

**B194 C8**

A young adult with a T9-10 spinal cord injury wishes to engage in sports activities. Which wheelchair features are best for the OTA to recommend to this client?

**Correct Answer: C. An ultra-light rigid frame with a low back.**

**Incorrect Answers:**

A.  A heavy-duty foldable frame with a high back.

B.  An ultra-light foldable frame with a high back.

D.  A heavy-duty rigid frame with a low back.

**Rationale:**

Sports competition wheelchairs are usually made with rigid construction and very strong lightweight materials. A folding wheelchair does not provide the stability needed for competition sports. A low seat back enhances the user's upper body/arm movements. A higher seat back is indicated for patients with decreased trunk control (not a factor in this example). At T9-10 this patient has partial innervation of the abdominals (innervated T6-12) and full innervation of the upper extremities.

**Type of Reasoning: Inductive**

One must utilize diagnostic reasoning and clinical judgment to determine the best type of wheelchair for a patient with T10 paraplegia who wishes to participate in sports. This requires inductive reasoning skill. For this case, the OTA should recommend an ultra-light rigid frame with a low back. Review wheelchair prescription guidelines if answered incorrectly.

**B195  C3**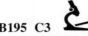

An OTA has established service competency in completing biomechanical evaluations. The OTA evaluates a person who complains of persistent wrist pain after painting a house three weeks ago. The patient demonstrates signs and symptoms consistent with de Quervain's tenosynovitis. Which assessment measure should the OTA use to confirm the diagnosis?

**Correct Answer: A. Finkelstein's test.**

**Incorrect Answers:**

B.  Phalen's test.

C.  Froment's sign.

D.  Craig's test.

**Rationale:**

Finkelstein's test is specific for reproducing the pain associated with de Quervain's tenosynovitis of the abductor pollicis longus and extensor pollicis brevis. Froment's sign is used to identify ulnar nerve dysfunction. Phalen's test identifies median nerve compression in the carpal tunnel. Craig's test is used by physical therapists to identify an abnormal femoral antetorsion angle.

**Type of Reasoning: Deductive**

This question requires factual recall of knowledge of provocative tests for de Quervain's tenosynovitis. In this case, the appropriate test is Finkelstein's test, which reproduces the pain of the APL and EPB tendons associated with de Quervain's. Refer to provocative testing of the hand or wrist and de Quervain's tenosynovitis if answered incorrectly.

**B196  C1**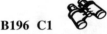

An older adult with persistent balance difficulty and a history of recent falls (two in the last 3 months) receives home care OT services. During the initial session, which client factors are most important for the OTA to consider?

**Correct Answer: D. Sensory functions and sensory organization of balance.**

**Incorrect Answers:**

A.  Spinal musculoskeletal changes secondary to degenerative joint disease.

B.  Cardiovascular endurance and level of dyspnea during IADL.

C.  Mental functions of attention and orientation during functional mobility.

**Rationale:**

A critical component of balance control is sensory input from somatosensory, visual, and vestibular receptors and overall sensory organization of inputs. With age, these systems undergo changes that can compromise the person's balance and safety. Therefore, these are the most important client factors for the OTA to consider during intervention. There is no information in the scenario to indicate that the person has a cognitive deficit, degenerative joint disease, or a cardiopulmonary disorder.

**Type of Reasoning: Inductive**

This case scenario requires the test taker to combine knowledge of the somatosensory system and possible reasons for falls in order to arrive at the correct conclusion. A key facet of this question is in the terms "initial session" and "most important." These words should cause the test taker to focus on what should come first in a sequence of intervention events and what is most important for the patient. This requires the use of clinical judgment, which is an inductive reasoning skill. For this case, sensory functions and sensory organization of balance are most important. Review intervention approaches for balance deficits in older adults if answered incorrectly.

**B197  C4**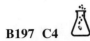

An OTA provides OT services in a patient's room. The patient has left hemiplegia and is able to recognize the OTA after the OTA talks with the patient for awhile. The patient is unable to recognize the faces of family members when they enter the room to visit. The family members become upset by this behavior. Which deficit should the OTA explain to the family members as the most likely reason for the patient's behavior?

**Correct Answer: C. Visual agnosia.**

**Incorrect Answers:**

A.  Ideational apraxia.

B.  Anosognosia.

D.  Somatognosia.

**Rationale:**

All of the choices are indicative of perceptual dysfunction. This patient is most likely experiencing visual agnosia, which is an inability to recognize familiar objects despite normal function of the eyes and optic tracts. Once the family members talk with the patient, he/she will likely be able to recognize them by their voices. Ideational apraxia is the inability to perform a purposeful motor act, either automatically or upon command. Anosognosia is the frank denial, neglect, or lack of awareness of the presence or severity of one's paralysis. Somatognosia is an impairment in body scheme.

**Type of Reasoning:  Analytical**

In this question, one must recall the meaning of the four choices provided and apply them to the patient's symptoms described above. This requires analytical reasoning, which often requires one to determine the meaning of symptoms or deficits. For this situation, the symptoms are indicative of visual agnosia, which should be reviewed if answered incorrectly.

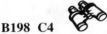

**B198  C4**

An OTA works with an individual recovering from traumatic brain injury who demonstrates behaviors consistent with Level VII of the Rancho Level of Cognitive Functioning Scale. The client is a resident in a transitional living program. Which is the most important focus for the OTA to include in the client's intervention plan?

**Correct Answer: B. The development of strategies to accurately and safely complete IADL with minimal assistance.**

**Incorrect Answers:**

A.  The provision of a high degree of environmental structure to decrease confusion and ensure safety.

C.  The development of adaptive techniques to accurately and safely complete BADL with moderate assistance.

D.  The provision of maximum assistance to accurately and safely complete IADL.

**Rationale:**

A person at Level VII of the Rancho Level of Cognitive Functioning Scale is able to appropriately complete highly familiar tasks such as BADL with minimal assistance. At this level, the person can learn to use strategies to accurately and safely complete IADL with minimal assistance.

**Type of Reasoning:  Inductive**

While this question does require one to recall the Rancho Level of Cognitive Functioning Scale and the guidelines for treatment provided within these levels, one must utilize inductive reasoning skill to determine the most important focus for intervention within the individual's current abilities and limitations. This necessitates clinical judgment, which is an inductive reasoning skill. For this case, the OTA should focus on the development of strategies to accurately and safely complete IADL with minimal assistance. Refer to the Rancho Level of Cognitive Functioning Scale if answered incorrectly.

### B199  C2

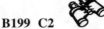

A two month-old infant with bilateral hip dislocations is being discharged home from an acute pediatric facility. The occupational therapist and OTA have developed a home program for the parents of this first-born child. Which is most important for the occupational therapist and OTA to assess before instructing the parents in the details of this home program?

**Correct Answer: D. The parents' degree of anxiety.**

**Incorrect Answers:**

A. The child's insurance reimbursement plan.
B. The parents' level of formal education.
C. The family's home environment.

**Rationale:**

Prior to providing the parents with detail about the home program, the occupational therapist and OTA should assess the parents' level of anxiety since excess anxiety could impact upon their comprehension and retention of the instructions given. This is an appropriate use of interactive reasoning and can help build rapport with the parents. This can contribute to increased compliance with the prescribed home program. While the other factors may also be considered, they do not represent immediate priorities for hospital-based instruction.

**Type of Reasoning:  Inductive**

This question requires one to utilize clinical judgment in order to determine the most important item to assess before instructing the parents in a home exercise program. This requires inductive reasoning skill. In this case, it is most important to determine the parents' degree of anxiety and attention. Review home program development guidelines in pediatric settings if answered incorrectly.

### B200  C8

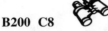

An individual incurred a back injury while working as a stock person for a large warehouse distribution company. The individual's level of productivity is just below the warehouse minimum standards. The individual complains of pain when lifting the heaviest of boxes. The individual frequently becomes angry and verbally abusive in response to directions or feedback. What is the most important initial focus for this client's work hardening program?

**Correct Answer: B. Developing the client's affective work behavior skills.**

**Incorrect Answers:**

A. Increasing the client's productivity to meet minimum standards.
C. Increasing the client's productivity to exceed minimum standards.
D. Developing the client's strength and ergonomic lifting abilities.

**Rationale:**

Affective work behavior skills include social responsiveness, attitude toward the job, and relationships with supervisors and co-workers. The individual is exhibiting significant deficits in these areas by becoming agitated and verbally abusive. These behaviors put the client at risk for not being able to maintain employment upon return to work. Increasing work productivity and developing ergonomic lifting abilities and strength can be addressed during the course of the work hardening program. The individual's inappropriate work behavior skills must be immediately addressed for the individual to be able to benefit from this program.

**Type of Reasoning: Inductive**

This question requires one to determine the best approach for improving function for a patient in a work hardening setting. This requires inductive reasoning skill, where clinical judgment is paramount to arriving at a correct conclusion. For this situation, given the individual's behaviors, the OTA should develop affective work behavior skills. If answered incorrectly, review treatment guidelines for individuals in work hardening settings, especially work behavior skills.

**Notes**

**Notes**

**Notes**

**Notes**

**Notes**

**Notes**

**Notes**

**Notes**

**Notes**

**Notes**